DATE DUE			

THE SEARCH WITHIN

THE SEARCH WITHIN

THE INNER EXPERIENCES OF
A PSYCHOANALYST

Theodor Reik

Introduction by Murray Sherman, Ph.D.

JASON ARONSON, NEW YORK

150.19
R27s
104435
april 1978

LIBRARY OF CONGRESS CATALOGING IN PUBLICATION DATA
Reik, Theodor, 1888-1969.
    The search within.
    Reprint of the 1956 ed. published by Farrar, Straus and
Cudahy, New York: with new introd.
    1. Reik, Theodor, 1888-1969. 2. Psychoanalysis.
I. Title.
BF173.R423   1974   150'.19'50924   74-997
ISBN 0-87668-138-0

Manufactured in the United States of America

Contents

Theodor Reik:
The Man

Theodor Reik was the "human" psychoanalyst par excellence. More than any other analytic writer he put himself into the forefront of his writing. Reik consistently made an explicit point of writing in the first person singular, and made even more of a point of inserting his own shortcomings and pecadillos into what he said. But he was also explicit in saying that he was only presenting small "fragments" from his life and that in writing about oneself one must often sacrifice literal truth and disguise facts for the sake of a larger reality. Reik said, "We must remember Goethe's phrase that a fact in our life is important not when it is true, but when it is meaningful."

Reik lived several lives, as do most of us. He was one man to the literate public, another within the psychoanalytic community, and still another in his personal life. Moreover, Reik had several different personal lives—i.e., the one he wrote about, the one his wife and children saw, and the one that could be termed his own inner, or secret, life. As Reik also recalled, Goethe said, "The course of my life remained mostly a secret even for my friends."

Reik addressed himself to the essence of psychoanalysis —the unconscious, or the secret life of mankind. He had an uncanny talent for uncovering thoughts and feelings that lay deep in forgotten years. This was Reik's genius and he illustrated it over and over again in what he wrote. It is not too much to say that Reik devoted his entire life to a search for the unconscious both in others and in himself. He believed that psychology began with "the search within," and a large part of what he discovered stemmed from explorations of his own psyche. The title of this volume could therefore stand as a symbol of Reik's major devotion to psychoanalysis.

Still, one may ask about the limits of self-discovery. With even the strongest of talents, how close can one approach the core of one's own being? It is a mercy that we see ourselves but faintly as in a shimmering pool; the closer we come to inner truth, the more the sun shines directly in our eyes. We must fight fiercely and even blindly for crumbs of self-knowledge.

Theodor Reik wrote about psychoanalysis and he wrote about himself. He explored his consciousness in order to reach the unconscious; he devoted a lifetime to this paradoxical task. On one hand, there was much of an apparently simple nature that Reik did not recognize in himself or, in fact, in others. Yet, he was able to uncover vast territories of mind that were hitherto unknown. This is the true paradox of psychoanalysis. It holds forth profound discoveries in the guise of banal facts and necessary illusions. Freud often said that it had been his ironic destiny to make scientific discoveries out of simple matters that nursemaids had known since the dawn of time.

I first met Reik at a professional seminar in psychoanalysis which went on for many years. The seminar was an informal one and was sponsored by Dr. Ruth Berkeley and attended largely by students and graduates of the National Psychological Association for Psychoanalysis. It was my pleasant task to drive Reik to and from these and other meetings, and thus I got to know him in a rather more personal way. But Reik was inordinately difficult to approach in any personal way, despite the fact that there was a quality of immediate and penetrating intimacy to his being.

It is not an exaggeration to say that I learned almost all I know about the unconscious from Theodor Reik, both from his books and from being with him. But Reik the man remained largely a mystery and it was partly for this reason that I decided to write a biography of him. Reik was entirely cooperative in that he granted me a number of interviews and also engaged the cooperation of his sister Margaret and his three grown children.

Reik's books have yielded a certain amount of autobiographical information, much of which is contained in this volume of *The Search Within*. My own relationship with him and the interviews with his children provided another order of information and a vastly different point of view. I also met with a woman who had an intimate friendship with Reik from 1947 until he died in 1969.

The picture Nora gave of Reik was almost completely different from any other. The coalescence of these different lives into a biography remains to be done, but here I shall present fragments from the separate lives of Theodor Reik.

The emphasis will be upon the different and usually contradictory impressions he made in different places. Reik's readers have one view of him, his colleagues another, his students still another. In his family life and love relationships an almost totally different Reik emerges, and there is little evident overlap in these separate lives of Theodor Reik. This fact is not unusual in itself but as a pioneer contributor in psychoanalysis Reik has brought us a particular message about the unconscious. In these days of anti-intellectualism and mindlessness, the concept of the unconscious reaffirms man as a creature who responds on several different levels of consciousness—a person in depth. Man's consciousness has always been taken for granted, but Freud's discovery of the unconscious has added a totally new dimension to man's being. If Reik's life can provide clues to his genius for divining the unconscious, it will amply repay our attention and study.

I have had certain misgivings in deciding what facts and what images to commit to paper. This job was made easier when I was asked to speak about Reik at one of a series of professional meetings devoted to the lives and contributions of famous psychoanalysts. Reik was the first analyst selected for presentation.* His son Arthur and his daughter Miriam were asked to speak about their father and I also spoke. Much to my surprise (although a surprise is unconsciously prepared in advance, according to Reik), both Arthur Reik and Miriam Reik spoke very openly about the contradictory pictures and impressions and reactions they had to their father. They contrasted the bitterness and alienation within their own families to the genial and witty man who appeared in Reik's books but not in their lives with him.

In order to illustrate Reik's inconsistencies and seeming contradictions, I shall quote a particular episode recounted by him in *Curiosities of the Self* (1965). This gives a rather typical picture of

---

*Sponsored by the New York Center for Psychoanalytic Training and held January 28, 1972.

Reik's family life as he himself wrote about it. Then, since Miriam Reik herself also spoke of this same episode, I shall quote from the tape recording of her presentation and then compare and discuss the two versions.

Reik writes:

In general my mood in those weeks following my seventy-sixth birthday was one of discouragement and depression. It was the spring of my discontent. I tried to escape that mood by taking a walk, and then and there I decided to visit my younger daughter Miriam who lived not far away. She offered me coffee, but I refused and began to talk. I told her that I had been feeling depressed and was often thinking how I had wronged some people and hurt their feelings, and I perhaps felt poignant remorse—now when it was much much too late to do anything about it. And then I began to talk about Miriam's mother. I had often been cruelly inconsiderate to her and often short and impulsively abrupt, perhaps even offensive. It was a kind of shameful confession poured out, but without humility.

I told Miriam that I must have made her mother suffer. (Did I suffer too? I don't know.) I confessed to Miriam that I had not often visited her mother in the nursing home where she spent her last years, that I had neglected Maria more and more; yes, that there were many days when I did not even think of her. I worked and enjoyed life; I slept with other women—I had almost forgotten that I had an incurably ill wife in a nursing home not very far from where I lived. When the thought of her occurred, I sometimes felt ashamed, but I nevertheless did not visit her. I sometimes fooled myself into believing that perhaps she did not even want to see me. But I knew, of course, that this was not true—at least during the first months at that nursing home on West End Avenue.

All this I told Miriam. It was a moment, or rather an hour, of truth—"all my sins remembered," as with Hamlet. It was not only a confession, but also a self-accusation; but, strangely enough, told and formulated without emotion, as if I spoke of the omissions and mistakes of a stranger, yes, like a prosecutor speaking of the deeds of a defendant.

I knew all the while I was speaking that Miriam had been aware of all my omissions and mistakes for years, since she visited her mother in that nursing home as often as possible. She must have often wondered about the strange behavior of her father and must have accused him of neglecting her mother. Now she sat opposite me, listening, and not saying a word.

Toward evening I said, "I must go now." I kissed my daughter; she accompanied me to the door, waiting while I rang the bell for the elevator. When the elevator arrived at the floor, Miriam said, "One must forgive oneself too."

Walking home, I wondered about this daughter of mine. From where had she got this wisdom? My depression receded by and by, as I walked through the streets in the calm of the evening. It was like coming out of a tunnel. I repeated to myself, "One must forgive oneself too." (pp. 53–54)

I now cite the verbatim transcript taken from the tape recording of Miriam Reik's address:

. . . [My father's] common sense, which many people have remarked on, his humanity, his wisdom, his warmth, and so on, which I am very used to hearing about in meetings and other people's impressions, were absolutely missing when it came to his expressing himself rather than expressing his observations about mankind.

I thought I would give you just one more example of a time in which he did try to say something a little bit more personal. It's an incident which he retells in one of his last books, *Curiosities of the Self*, and it refers to an experience he had with me. I will tell you the story as it is in the book and then come back to it in another way. In the book he says that on the occasion of his seventy-sixth birthday he was depressed, had thoughts about death in connection with thoughts he also had about his two marriages. Both my brother's mother and my mother were long dead. In this depressed mood, this mood of self-recrimination about the wrongs he had done to them, he decided to take a walk and found himself walking in my direction and came to visit me.

And in the book he says that he came on a surprise visit and sat down for an hour with me—I wonder why he chose an hour (laughter from audience)—but he sat down for an hour with me and poured out all his confessions, his sins, of how he had mistreated his wives, of how terrible he was, and so on. And that he poured this all out in a bloodless, unemotional, affectless fashion. He then got up to leave and as he left I said to him, "One must forgive oneself." And with that he went off and slowly his depression lifted, which he very generously attributed to my remark. I forget in what connection he brings up this incident in the book.

It's a very nice incident, I think, and I'm happy to have been of some therapeutic help to him in that moment and alas it's not true (laughter). There are two mistakes in the story, one an error of omission and one a cunning addition. So let me retell the story as it actually happened and I will draw a point from it.

He did, as a matter of fact, show up at my apartment that day on his seventy-sixth birthday, which was a great surprise to me. He already had some difficulty at that point in moving around—his age—and he was not accustomed to just dropping in. He did show up and I distinctly remember him standing at the door with a beret jauntily pulled over one side of his head, and he was clutching in his hand a paper bag which he held in front of him, and he looked altogether like a little boy who had been sent to the grocery and was bringing back something he bought. And as he came in, he thrust this paper bag at me and said, "Here, your mother used to love peaches." So this was the error of omission. He doesn't write about the peaches, and it's significant because my father had not mentioned my mother for many years and before that had only asked about her rather vaguely. She was long dead as I said. So I was astonished: Not only did he recall her, but he did so with a very concrete detail of her likes and dislikes. It was a recollection that must have gone back to much balmier times in their relationship. So this was the error of omission; you'll see how it works out in a moment.

The error of addition concerns the fact that when he came into the apartment he sat down and he didn't say a word. He sat for an hour but he didn't say one blessed word. He was completely depressed and gloomy and unresponsive. I tried to chat with him and asked him how he was, what not, told him what was going on with me. He was absolutely unresponsive and then he abruptly got up to leave. And it was perfectly clear to me, without being an analyst, that he had come to me for something. He was unaccustomed to dropping in and since he was clearly depressed, he was looking for me to do something and I was at a complete loss and very desperate because I would have liked to have helped him but he wouldn't say a word. So I assumed that it was somehow connected with these peaches, which, as a matter of fact, it turned out to be. But as he was leaving, in desperation to say something nice I did indeed say that he also had to forgive himself. Where I got the thought I don't know. And he broke out in smiles and he trotted off. And I never knew that the whole incident had any significance for him at all until it appeared in the book in this highly distorted form, in which he says that he had made this huge confession, of which he had not said one word. The whole confession was wrapped up in that bag of peaches, and my remark was a sheer stroke of luck.

But what emerges from this is that anybody reading *Curiosities of the Self* and seeing where he says he made this confession would think that everything I said earlier in this talk was wrong, that he did indeed speak about himself freely. But he didn't. This was an addition he made for purposes of the book. And it leaves me to conclude that the most private things he said, that he had to say, the most personal things that he confessed, were confessed in fact in only the most public places, which [are] his books. If it weren't for his books, I would know very little about him. So those of you who have read his books know just about as much as I do. Now, I have a feeling, I can't substantiate it any way . . . that the only place where he felt free, the place he could overcome that particular block in communication, was in his books, where he probably felt he had control over what he said. There he could strike out what he didn't want to say, he could arrange material, and there was no danger of his emotions becoming too strong. . . .

The main inconsistency, of course, is the "confession," which Reik describes minutely in his book but which Miriam Reik says never occurred at all. This seeming inconsistency is resolved as soon as we recognize that the confession occurred just as Reik wrote about it but that it transpired only in his thoughts; he was unable to speak openly to the daughter he loved but could not approach. Reik was waiting for Miriam to share the peaches with him in some way that would have resembled the sharing he recalled with his wife Maria. Unconsciously, Miriam must have known this but she could not speak the words until her father was safely on his way out of the apartment. At that point Miriam brought up the peaches (although she does not say how), and her remark, "One must forgive oneself too," took on particular significance in this connection. It was this oral connotation of the forgiveness that helped Reik over his depression.

There are a number of other significant comparisons between the two versions but I can mention only a few here. When Reik states in his own version that "[Miriam] sat opposite me, listening and not saying a word," he was projecting his own silence, that actually did occur, in terms of an identification with Miriam. There were many identifications and counteridentifications between the two, which are expressed in the rivalries and antagonisms described by Miriam.

Miriam's own resentments come forth in the various belittling phrases she uses to describe her father, but her basic identification with Reik is shown by the candor and search for truth that her remarks indicate. With this extent of iden ical yearning between them, it was no wonder that they could speak but little. The father-daughter bond was much more intimate than words could express. Still, Reik had this same problem with many other people and with much the same basis. He was able to establish an unconscious identification based upon a bond of secret understanding of the unspoken lives of many persons he met or for whom he wrote.

I mentioned that I used to drive Reik to our seminar meetings. Here members presented cases from their practices, and Reik illuminated the therapeutic interaction by his inimitable insights into the unconscious, which were especially striking in his interpretations of neurotic symptoms and of dreams. After these discussions a sumptuous repast was served in which Reik participated avidly. But much the same kind of silence existed between Reik and the seminar members as Miriam described above. Reik would inquire about how practice was going and engage in small talk, and the conversation was rarely more personal than just this. Very strangely, the only times Reik asked me about my practice was when it was going poorly, never when it was going well, and I often felt compelled to say things were going well when in fact they were not. In this superficial sense there was also a somewhat strained atmosphere at the seminar. But we all loved Reik quite intimately. We recognized that he had devoted his entire life and his own love to psychoanalysis and that he was giving us the opportunity to take away a small share of his genius for delving into the unconscious. We somewhat resembled Reik's family, none of whom doubted that their father loved them deeply despite the constant tension he caused.

In my drives with Theodor Reik, to and from the meetings, the sense of strain somehow disappeared. He was relaxed and so was I. The situation recalled my relationship with my mother, with whom I generally felt antagonistic and at odds except when we were riding together in a car. I can remember any number of times from the ages of six to ten when the family was at a picnic and I would be nagging my mother for something she was unable to supply, and then we would enter the car for the ride home, and I would lay my head in her lap and she would hold it tenderly and I would relax and sleep. In my memory, this never happened except in a car.

With Reik I was able to exchange jokes, anecdotes, and small bits of gossip or incidents taken from reading or from practice. He, in turn, would share his thinking about a book which he was writing, inquire about tidbits of gossip, and also speak from time to time about incidents from his own family life. There was one strange encounter between us that I still ponder in some puzzlement.

One evening as we were driving home, Reik, who was an inveterate smoker, offered me a cigarette. I was not a smoker but he made me an offer I could not refuse. Reik took the cigarette, placed it directly at my lips, and said, "Here, Murray, have a smoke." And before I knew exactly what was happening, he had lit the cigarette and I was smoking. This incident continued to occur for perhaps several years and it took place whether we were alone in the car or others were with us. Since as far as I know, I was the only person whom Reik engaged in this cigarette ritual, we were all quite amazed. These remained the only occasions when I smoked but finally, after a long time, I refused the cigarette. Reik then turned to me in genuine amazement and exclaimed, "Ach, Murray, so you've given up smoking. How did you do it?"

The cigarette was Reik's way of getting through to me. It may have been somewhat similar to the peaches with Miriam. He had a number of other ways, most of them verbal rather than behavioral, but they were all surprising and effective in conveying Reik's intimacy to one's core of being. This was Reik's way of reaching into the unconscious and it was an important part of what made him a psychoanalyst. He did not plan his words or behavior but rather used remarkable intuition (a word he objected to) in responding with instant appropriateness to the exact psychological moment.

One of Reik's idiosyncracies was his proneness to give direct advice when it was least expected and when it seemed almost inappropriate. When confronted by students with ordinary human dilemmas, Reik would respond with aphorisms or homilies, and one might not know how serious he was. He was completely serious. One topic which preoccupied Reik for many years was the battle of the sexes. He devoted much writing to "The Emotional Differences of the Sexes" (*Of Love and Lust,* Part IV) and also wrote *Sex in Man and Woman: Its Emotional Variations* (1960).

Perhaps Reik's most quoted insight in this area was, " . . . men are afraid that they will not be men enough and women are afraid that they might be considered only women."* He also said that men had three roles available to them: as fathers, as husbands, and as workers in their careers, and it was enough if they were successful in two of these.

In looking for insights such as these, students would often ask Reik how to deal with "impossible" wives or difficult marriages.

Of Love and Lust, p. 423.

More directly, he would be asked how to deal with a wife who was sexually frustrating. At times, Reik would quote Freud's advice about being "abstinent under protest," but more frequently he would simply say that we should "get a mistress." At such times he would smile and say that if all the wives who said they would kill themselves if they discovered their husbands were unfaithful did so, the streets would be littered with corpses.

Today Reik would be called a chauvinist and he would cheerfully agree. At the time, some of us were still able to be shocked by Reik's directness; others took his advice. As Reik notes in his own writing, he consistently managed throughout both marriages to find other attachments. Some of these were casual, others were intimate and enduring. His relationship with Nora was close from almost the very beginning.

The picture that Nora painted of Reik, in my talks with her, was one of fulfilling romance and almost constant harmony. The only conflict stemmed from Reik's constant fear that Nora would leave him. All the acrimony and bitterness that characterized both of Reik's marriages were totally lacking in his life with Nora. And correspondingly, all the intimacy and expressiveness that were denied his family emerged when he was with Nora.

One could, of course, question this picture as one that was romanticized and glossed over but, among other evidence, there is a college composition which Nora's daughter wrote about Reik as the man she knew from his visits with her mother. She titled the composition "Tayo," which was her spelling of her mother's address to Theo. The composition follows:

. . . He first came into our lives when I was six or seven years old. I used to watch him striding up the street toward our house—a tall, very impressive old man with a military carriage, and hatless in all weather.

He has a striking face with unusually piercing eyes. I would say that he looks very much like Bruno Walter—assuming that Bruno Walter were always badly in need of a haircut.

Also, Tayo's impressiveness is very much in spite of his clothes, for he looks always as if he had picked up odds and ends of trousers and jackets from a missionary barrel, put them on, and over them thrown the same ancient trench coat that he has worn for years. He is oblivious to clothes and has a suspicious attitude toward men who are fussy about them.

He is delightful with children. We three . . . were all enchanted by him, especially since our parents were separated and we saw very little of our father.

We were all rather solemn children except when we were with Tayo, who used to delight in involving us in ridiculous arguments. He insisted that clocks go to clock school to learn how to tick. The arguments over this went on for weeks. Once, when my little brother was taking his nap, Tayo went out into the garden and hung large gumdrops on the dogwood trees. When he woke up to find the trees in bloom, he was enraptured.

Tayo brought us many records of his favorite Viennese songs, and would sit singing along with the records in a cracked but sweet voice. The old songs made him cry. We were all embarrassed when this happened. We were not used to a person so free-flowing in his emotional reactions as Tayo is.

He is invariably kind and understanding to everyone. Once my mother, dressed to go to the opera, suddenly decided that she would not go. Her dress was old, her hair looked awful, and she too was old and awful. Turning to Tayo, she cried, ". . . and don't give me any of your *gemütlichkeit!*"

Tayo looked very sad and spoke very quietly, as he always does when he feels something deeply. I was about ten years old then, and I remember feeling sad too; and envious when he took my mother's hand and said, "To me you will always be beautiful, even if dressed in newspapers!"

I have many other recollections of Tayo, some of them quite recent. Last year I asked him what he would do in a certain situation if he were a schoolteacher. He answered, "To all the girls who wear long hair and full skirts and never talk, I would give 'A.' To girls who wear short hair and pants (Bermudas) and always talk, I would give failures."

Perhaps it is time to say who Tayo is. He is the famous psychoanalyst, Dr. Theodor Reik. I know that he is a famous man; a great psychoanalyst and writer, a complex intellectual, and a cultured man-of-the-world. I know it, but I can't really feel it. To me, he is our Tayo, a lovable old man, humming Viennese songs off-key, wandering through our house leaving a trail of books, papers, neckties, ballpoint pens, and cigarette ashes, hanging gumdrops on the dogwood trees, and saying quietly to my sad, nervous mother, "To me you will always be beautiful, even if dressed in newspapers!"

If we put these different pictures of Theodor Reik together, we find that the autobiography he presents in *The Search Within* is a combination of all of them. He simply neglects to separate his parts as husband, father, lover, teacher, psychoanalyst.

When Reik wrote of his sentimental affection for his wife, these were feelings that emerged when he was with Nora, although he felt affection for Maria that he could not express directly to her. Neither could Reik verbalize his profound affection for his own children, although he continually gave evidence of his love for them. Nevertheless, his deep affection for his children came forth far more directly with Nora's children than with his own. This was the deep tragedy in Reik's life, and of course it affected all who were personally involved with him.

The only place where Reik was able to combine the contradictory parts was in his role as psychoanalyst. Here he met some patients as the warm, understanding father, others as the intimate lover, and still others as the cold, detached mother. It may have been Reik's capacity for combining these extremes of character that gave him his genius for divining the unconscious. For within his secret self these extremes and contradictions were resolved. Reik never regarded himself as a distant, unapproachable father because in his own inner thoughts he was communicating with those around him even if the words remained unspoken. Within his own inner life he was in touch with deep feelings about himself, and to an exceedingly unusual degree Reik did live within his own being. His fantasies were intense, self-sustaining, and sometimes self-deceptive. Reik was able to see into the very depths of other people but this capacity also included being oblivious to much that was on the surface of others and also of himself.

Reik's need to live his life inwardly rather than openly was another key to his being in touch with unconscious phenomena. In his inner self the contradictory pictures faded into fantasied self-images, and later these images reemerged as startling insights which he described in his writing. This may well be another root of the unconscious in each of us.

Since Theodor Reik spent most of his life exploring and confronting the forces of the unconscious, we can learn much from his views of himself and others, especially as we compare these with the pictures other people had of him. Now we turn to Reik's life and his insights into the unconscious.

MURRAY H. SHERMAN

New York City

Author's Note: A Portrait Comes to Life

I T IS just two o'clock in the morning. I am still sitting at my
desk struggling with the book that has occupied me for many
years. I am discouraged and tired. My eyes are burning. I should
like to bundle up the pile of manuscript and notes, stuff it into a
file and be done with it. Then my eyes chance upon the portrait
that hangs above my desk. The light falls on the head, and for a
moment it seems as though Freud were alive again. I see him
again at his desk, see him stand up, come forward and extend his
hand to me with that bold, characteristic gesture. I see him shuf-
fling the manuscripts on the desk aside, opening a box of cigars,
and holding it out to me.

I have stood before this portrait, paced up and down the room,
and now I have returned to it again, strangely moved. I remember the day the Viennese etcher Max Pollak first exhibited it at
Hugo Heller's galleries. That must have been in 1913. A dimly
lighted room. In the foreground, on the desk, antique bronzes
and figurines, dug up out of the ruins of centuries, phantoms of
the past. They stand out starkly against the picture's white border. Freud's head, bent forward slightly, outlined distinctly.
The eyebrows lifted as though in deep attention. Ridges on the
high forehead and two deep furrows running down from the
mouth to the short white beard. The eyes gaze into the beholder
and yet see beyond him. How often have I looked into those eyes.
They have an expression of hardy quest, as though their gaze had
wholly merged into their object; and yet they valued that object
only for the knowledge it gave. One hand holds the pen loosely,
as though the sudden vision of a long-sought answer has interrupted the writing. The other hand lies slack on the paper. The
light from the window at the side of the room highlights but one
side of the forehead. The face is in shadow, with only the eyes
gleaming steelily. . . . There suddenly come to my mind some

words of his. It was during a walk, and I had asked him how he felt when he first captured the psychic perceptions contained in *Totem and Taboo*. I probably spoke rather floridly, saying something about an overwhelming joy, for he answered, "I felt nothing like that; simply an extraordinary clarity." . . . He was an unusually keen observer with a deep respect for the data of the senses, but he had the gift for intuitive perception, for unconscious observation which belongs to an obscurer realm. Rembrandt has been greater than any artist for strictness and exactitude of faithful observation of what he has seen, yet the French have called him a *"visionnaire."* It was darkness that disclosed to him the wonders of light. Of Freud too we may say what the art critic Eugène Fromentin wrote of Rembrandt: *"C'est avec de la nuit, qu'il a fait le jour."*

How often since that first momentous visit I sat with him at this desk. (I remember that important occasion in 1912 when I announced to him that now that I had my Ph.D. I intended to study medicine. He advised me strongly against it, saying, "I have other things in mind for you, larger plans." He insisted that I go on with my psychoanalytic research work.)

For a moment the figure in the etching seemed to be alive, seemed to step out of the past into the present. For the space of a few quickened heartbeats I thought: He is alive.

I know, now that the impression has passed, that I am called again to fulfill the demands of the day.

For me the demand of the day is to continue my work, to write those books which I have so long borne within me, to complete the researches I have begun. That moment when Freud's picture seemed to come to life now assumes more than momentary meaning. His memory has given me new heart, has set before me his example, his unerring and tireless striving.

"The demand of the day"—that is one of Goethe's favored expressions. My glance wanders from the picture of Freud to the bust of old Goethe that stands on the bookcase. One day in April of the year 1825 the seven-year-old Walther von Goethe came with an album in his hand to the famous poet who was his grandfather. Many ladies and gentlemen of the Weimar Court had already inscribed mottoes in the little book. Among them, for example, Frau Hofmarschall von Spiegel had written down one of the melancholy sentences of Jean Paul: "Man has two and a half minutes; one for smiling, one for sighing and a half for living for in the middle of this minute he dies." The seventy-six-year-old poet thoughtfully reading the line felt some reluctance against the false emotional allure of the dictum. Abandoning himself to the inner protest against the sentimental wisdom, he took up his pen and, while Jean Paul's sententious apportionment of human life still echoed within him, he wrote in his already somewhat shaky hand, with its free, generous flow:

> Sixty of them in each hour,
> A thousand in a single day.
> Child, may you soon discover
> All you can do along the way.

PART ONE

From Thirty Years with Freud

From Thirty Years with Freud

I

I HAVE set down here memories garnered through the thirty years of my closeness to Freud, years during which his work and his personality were an invaluable inspiration to me. The memories and impressions recorded here are largely of personal matters. They dwell on Freud chiefly as man and scientist, and not on the substance of his scientific work. My own life work and my books may testify to what profound effect Freud's scientific work has had upon me. I have no ambition to write a biography of Freud. I wish simply to set down certain impressions of the days when he lived and wrought good. Often, when I am musing over certain ideas, I surprise myself thinking that I shall write to him about them. I wonder what he will think about them—I find myself considering how to phrase the problem, and I hear myself murmuring the salutation under my breath, "Dear Herr Professor . . ." And then I remember that he is no longer here. When I now read presentations of Freud's personality in books and articles, I am often reminded of a little story I heard as a boy in Vienna. The father of a peasant had died and the son, an Austrian Peter Simpleton, wished to possess a picture of the dear deceased man. The boy wandered to Vienna, found a well-known painter and described to the artist what the father looked like, giving full details of the shape of the face, the colors of hair and eyes and so on. The painter promised to deliver the picture. When the naïve boy returned to the studio after a few weeks he broke into sobs before the finished portrait and cried, "Poor Father, how much you have changed in such a short time!" Reading many books and magazine articles of those last years that pretend to give a correct picture of Freud's personality amazes us who have known him: how much the man has changed in such a short time!

3

Certainly I do not wish to vaunt an intimacy that did not exist. In his books and in conversation Freud often named me as one of his friends. But I myself have never ventured to claim that I was one. One is not "intimate" with a genius, however familiarly he may speak to one as a friend. In conversation with me Freud was never circumspect or aloof; he was always friendly and personal—more so than ever in the last years. But there was always a barrier. My late friend, Dr. Hanns Sachs, admitted that he had the same feeling. In the beautiful eulogy he wrote after Freud's death he closes with the words: "He was, so to speak, made out of better stuff than ordinary people." In this, however, I was at odds with my friend. It would be truer to say that Freud was made of the selfsame stuff as all of us. But he molded and shaped and worked this paltry material with unceasing labor and self-education, strove until he formed himself into some greater figure, of a stature unique in our age.

Let us avoid making a legend of him. He himself would not have wished it. On the occasion of his seventieth birthday, his disciples were preparing a birthday celebration in Vienna. Then came the sudden death of Dr. Karl Abraham, whom Freud perhaps considered his most talented follower. Freud had heard of our preparations and asked us to abandon them. "One does not celebrate a wedding with a corpse in the house," he said. He requested me to speak the funeral address for Abraham at the meeting of the Vienna Psychoanalytic Society. Freud himself was present, of course, but because of his illness he refrained from speaking. After I had given the address he pressed my hand silently, but on the way home he commended me for mentioning not only the virtues of our friend, but his faults also. "That is just the way I would have done it, Reik," he said. "The proverb, 'De mortuis nil nisi bonum,' is, I think, nothing but a relic of our primitive fear of the dead. We psychoanalysts must throw such conventions overboard. Trust the others to remain hypocrites even before the coffin."

No, let us have no legends woven around Freud. His human weaknesses, or his human qualities, manifested themselves in little traits left over from his earlier development. They were never conspicuous. He was capable of much love, but he was also a good hater. He tried to suppress his desires to avenge injustices he had received; but often they broke forth in a word, a gesture or an intonation. In old age, despite his self-control, more than one bitter word broke through the bars. "Men are a wolf pack," he could say at such times, "just a wolf pack. They hunt down those who would do good for them." Such remarks startled us. But at such times he always spoke without strong emotion. These remarks sounded quite matter-of-course, like a final, calm judgment. Once—and only once—I saw him terribly angry. But the only sign of this anger was a sudden pallor and the way his teeth bit into his cigar. He could utter curses and vituperation as well as any one of us, but he preferred not to. Once, when I was railing against a certain professor of psychiatry for his shabby conduct, Freud merely smiled. He nodded in agreement when I used an expression that implied the man came from no human ancestry; but he restrained his own anger. I once asked him how he had endured the hostility of a whole world for so many years without becoming enraged or embittered. He answered, "I preferred to let time decide in my favor." And he added, "Besides, it would have pleased my enemies if I had shown that I was hurt."

He was not insensitive to neglect or slights. It hurt him that he had not yet received official recognition in Vienna itself, at a time when the whole world already honored him. But he would never air his feelings except in a casual joke. Once a Vienna tax collector challenged his income tax statement and pointed out that Freud's fame was spread far beyond the borders of Austria. Freud wrote in reply, "But it does not begin until the border."

He was not vindictive, but he did not forget injuries. For many years he kept away from the Viennese Medical Society, the members of which had once jeered at him when he lectured before them on the psychic genesis of hysteria. He once asked me to look up something in a magazine. I found that the volume containing this magazine could be obtained only from the Medical Society, and since I needed a letter of recommendation in order to use their library I asked him for one. He promised to write it for me, but forgot, which was very unusual with him. I reminded him, but he forgot again. Finally he confessed, "I couldn't bring myself to do it. My resistance was too strong."

He once said to me that character was determined essentially by the prevalence of one drive over others. In his personality, the particular impulse which would incline a man toward being a healer was not nearly so strongly developed as his impulse to knowledge. He had nothing of the *furor therapeuticus* that so many doctors manifest. He repeatedly said to us that three tasks were "impossible"—to govern, to educate, and to heal. By this he implied that these actions are wholly in the ideal domain. As a matter of fact, he was not over-happy about becoming a physician. But the desire to contribute some vital addition to mankind's volume of knowledge awakened early in him; this desire was already clearly defined when he was still in high school.

His capacity for self-control was extraordinary. He once said that we are indebted for our cultural achievements to great personalities with powerful impulses who had the gift of curbing them and turning them to serve higher ends. In his excellent essay on the "Moses" of Michelangelo he has shown us an example —or rather an ideal—of such an instinct-ridden genius who tamed his raging emotions.

He invariably expressed impatience or irritation by twisting these emotions into a wry joke. It must have been in one such moment of annoyance with us followers, with our rivalries and petty quarrels, that he cried, "Oh, if all of them had but a single backside!" With this parody of Nero's cruel sentiment he diverted his own anger.

Experience bears out that there is a kind of functional relationship between literary and oratorical gifts. Master stylists are seldom good speakers; ability to express oneself in the one form seems to hamper expression in the other. Freud was a masterful stylist. His prose, with its lucid, tranquil, richly associative flow, merits comparison with that of the great writers. Freud revised the well-known maxim to: *"Style est l'histoire de l'homme."* By that maxim he did not mean merely that literary influences fashioned the style of the individual, but that the development and experiences of an individual do their part in molding his style.

Certainly, he was not a powerful orator; and, in fact, he disliked speaking. He always had to overcome a certain resistance before delivering a lecture. His speaking manner had nothing of the demagogic about it, nothing of the impulsive or the emotionally winning. In its sobriety and lucidity, its slow, logical development, and its anticipations of objections, it had none of the qualities which sway the masses. On the other hand, it possessed all the qualities which convince unprejudiced, sympathetic, thoughtful listeners. There was something curiously compelling about the very uncoercive manner of his speech. His lectures at congresses and scientific meetings could not be called lectures in the rigid academic sense. They were, rather, free accounts of his experiences and researches. Their manner was conversational instead of formal. He once wrote to me that when he lectured he chose one sympathetic person from among his audience and imagined that he was addressing this person alone. If this person was absent from among his listeners, he would not feel at ease until he had found someone to understudy, so to speak. This attitude explains the direct-address form of his lectures and the manner in which he anticipated objections, formulating the doubts and questions of his audience as though he could read their minds. This direct approach is carried over into his *General Introduction to Psychoanalysis* where it can be easily detected.

He always spoke extemporaneously. He prepared for a lecture simply by taking a long walk during which he reflected on his subject. He never liked us, his assistants and disciples, to read our lectures from manuscript. He believed that the reading distracted the attention of the listener and handicapped his identifying himself with the lecturer. He thought this capacity for identification would be encouraged if the lecturer spoke freely, developing the train of his ideas as they came to him at the moment. This would be true even though he had often reviewed these ideas in his mind, for in speaking he would be re-creating them. This kind of lecturing was particularly easy for Freud because of his astonishing memory, a memory which in his earlier years was almost photographic.

Sometimes he would begin his lecture with an assertion that seemed patently improbable, and then he would so support this assertion by the citing of a number of cases that no attentive and just listener could disagree with him. I remember once that he made just such a statement, which sounded starkly unbelievable, and then went on to admonish his listeners not to reject it prematurely as paradoxical or impossible. "Do you remember," he said, "how in Shakespeare's play, when the ghost of the king cries, 'Swear!' from within the earth, Horatio cries out, 'O day and night, but this is wondrous strange!' But Hamlet replies, 'And therefore as a stranger give it welcome.' So I too shall ask you first to give welcome to the things that here rise so strangely from the tomb of the past."

He lectured in a measured, firm, and pleasant voice, although in later years he was often forced by his illness to break off suddenly to clear his throat. His language was unadorned. He rarely used adjectives, preferring understatement. The rich current of thought flowed along without any marked rise and fall of his voice. I never heard him become sentimental or emotional. He had so strong a desire for clarity that he could not help making everything clear to his listeners, and where he could not, he would frankly point out the obscurities of the problem. In order to make his points clear and concrete he was fond of adducing analogies from everyday life. In a lecture given in 1915, where he was discussing the place of masturbation in childhood and in the life of the adult, he first waived all moral evaluations of this sexual activity and insisted on considering the problem only from the standpoint of purpose. He drew the following analogy: "Bow and arrow were once, in prehistoric times, man's only weapon, or at any rate his best weapon. But what would you say if a French soldier of today went into battle with bow and arrow instead of a rifle?"

In the discussions which followed lectures of the Psychoanalytic Society he usually was the last to speak. He rarely failed to find a friendly word for the analyst who had lectured, but he also freely offered criticism which was always *suaviter in modo, fortiter in re*. I remember a lecture by a young colleague which, instead of being an examination of the problem, presented merely pretentious plans for the treatment of scientific questions. During the lecture Freud, who sat next to me, slipped me a sheet of paper on which he had written: "Does reading menus fill your stomach?"

In the midst of a serious discussion he would often surprise us with a humorous remark. In a lecture before the Vienna Psychoanalytic Society the New York analyst, Dr. Feigenbaum, once showed that even the speaking of intentional nonsense, which often happens in card playing, for example, can by analytic study be shown to convey unconscious rhyme and reason. Freud remarked that though it is no easy task for men to produce deliberately absolute nonsense, still everyone knows that the books of German scholars are full of effortless and unconscious nonsense.

After a lecture he gave (sometime in 1910) on the problem of sex, there was raised in the course of the discussion the question of a practical solution for the sexual dilemma of young students. For, on the one hand, psychoanalysis had shown that sexual abstinence was one of the most important factors in the formation of neurosis. On the other hand, the economic circumstances of most students made it impossible for them to marry early. Morality forbade the seduction of young girls, the danger of infection made sexual intercourse with prostitutes inadvisable, and so on. Freud's advice to the young students was, "Be abstinent, but under protest." He felt that it was imperative to keep alive the inner protest against a social order which prevented mature young men from fulfilling a normal instinctual need. He drew parallels between this attitude and that of the French Encyclopedists of the eighteenth century who, though submissive outwardly to the power of the Church which ruled their age, dedicated themselves to tireless protest against its overwhelming and unbearable force. Like Anatole France whose writings he loved, Freud did not believe in sudden and violent revolutions. (He cherished the lofty wisdom of France's writings as well as the subtlety and wit of his art. I remember Freud laughing aloud when I, in a discussion of feminine feelings, reminded him of a remark in a novel of Anatole France. In *Monsieur Bergeret à Paris* a young man attempts to seduce a lady. Anatole France, the connoisseur of women, concludes his description as follows: "He came to her again, took her in his arms, and covered her with caresses. Within a short time her clothes were so disarranged that —aside from any other considerations—shame alone compelled her to disrobe.") Freud put more faith in the steadily mounting, continuous force of patient resistance to bring about ultimately changes in the social order. He believed, also, that psychoanalysis, by making men more straightforward and upright, was one of these reforming forces. He often reiterated that in regard to money and to sex men are hypocrites. In both these realms they refuse to confess their true needs.

He was convinced that an individual's sexual behavior provided the prototype of his attitude toward other aspects of life. Once, while we were discussing a case of neurosis, he related an example he had met with outside his practice. This example was memorable because it involved two famous contemporaries. The mathematician and physicist, Christian Doppler, of the University of Vienna, had early done remarkable scientific work; it was he who made the discovery now known throughout the world as Doppler's principle. Later his scientific creativeness ran dry, or ran aground. His work became trivial; much of the time he busied himself working out riddles and was unable to publish anything of scientific significance. Freud traced this striking development to the fact that, though Doppler's marriage was extremely unhappy, for "moral" reasons he could not attain the inner freedom to seek a divorce. The emotional conflict arose out of Doppler's acquaintance with a young girl toward whom he was strongly attracted; but he had decided to resign himself and continue his life at the side of an unloved wife.

Freud contrasted this attitude with that of Doppler's contemporary, Robert Koch. Koch, who was at first a young health officer in a small German city, had won considerable fame with the publication of his first scientific papers. He had made a good middle-class marriage with a woman whom he respected but did not love. Later he met a girl whom he truly loved and Koch resolved to have a frank and friendly discussion with his wife. He requested divorce, and she finally consented. He married the girl, who proved to be a courageous and understanding companion through life. Happy and fulfilled in marriage, he pursued a scientific career that grew steadily in importance. He made great discoveries in regard to tuberculosis, sleeping sickness, and malaria, and contributed to medicine those theories and methods which will forever be associated with his name. Freud respected Koch's behavior in the emotional crisis of his first marriage as a

sign of greater strength of character. More than that, he felt that
it sprang from a higher morality than Doppler's, a morality
whose values were honesty and courage.

I was constantly amazed anew at the extent of Freud's reading
and the diversity of his knowledge. He read in almost every
branch of science. He followed with great interest the progress
of medical and biologic research, and read widely in archeology
and history, keeping up with current developments in all these
fields. Until almost the last he was a tireless reader. It was a thing
of wonder to me how a man whose days were crammed with so
many hours of exhausting analytic work, and whose nights were
largely devoted to writing, could find the time for such extensive
reading. Nor was this reading in the field of science alone. He
loved biography and the best work of contemporary writers like
Romain Rolland, Arthur Schnitzler, Franz Werfel, and Stefan
Zweig.

I remember once talking with him about a drama of Stefan
Zweig's, *Jeremiah*, which had just appeared. I expressed the
opinion that a drama making use of related material, *Der Junge
David* by Richard Beer-Hofmann, was far superior to Zweig's
work. Compared to Beer-Hofmann's work, I said, the Zweig
drama was very feeble. Freud was surprised at this criticism. He
told me that such an attitude was altogether strange to him, for
he never drew comparisons in matters of aesthetic pleasure. (As
a matter of fact, I believe that this is an attitude he adopted later
in life.)

For analogies in his scientific work he usually called upon
physics, for that science deals with the interplay of forces; but
he also drew comparisons with chemistry and biology, and with
archeology, which was particularly interesting to him. Let me recall a comparison he used when we were discussing the function
of trauma in the structure of the neuroses. Freud mentioned the
theories of Charles Lyell and George Cuvier, the great geologists.
He disagreed with Cuvier's theory of cataclysms, which held that
changes in the surface of the earth are wrought by great catas-
trophies. He inclined to Lyell's theory that such changes are
produced by constant forces working imperceptibly over periods
of thousands of years. I remember another time he drew an

analogy fom geology. We were discussing how in psychoanalysis only the psychic reality holds sway, while the material reality is altogether minor—so that, for example, it does not matter whether a patient really dreamed a dream or only imagined it. From this we went on to discuss the psychic significance of the lie, particularly the lie in children. Freud pointed out that children's lies are frequently composed for an imaginary gratification of desire. From this point of view it is psychologically unimportant whether we are dealing with lie or truth, since the boundary between them—in analysis, though not in life—is vague and shifting. He added, "Imagine that the human eye could behold at one glance all the changes that have taken place over eons in the surface of the earth. To such a vision the boundaries between hill and valley, water and land, would become vague and strangely immaterial."

Until ripe old age Freud was receptive to all new ideas and original thoughts in psychoanalysis. He met them without prejudice, even when he did not agree; but he required a long time to feel at home in new views. Although he always evinced a lively and open-minded interest in all intellectual changes, he left it to the younger generation to extend psychoanalysis beyond the specific limitations that he had set himself.

He impressed upon us that it was almost always a bad omen when a neurotic patient accepted with enthusiasm the results of analysis. The best attitude toward analysis or any other new and radical scientific views was, he maintained, a friendly skepticism. Consider, he would say, the way housewives tell a good oven from a bad one. The bad ones are those that heat up right away, but also cool rapidly. The good ones, however, grow warm slowly and hesitantly, but hold their heat for a long time.

This was his own attitude toward innovations in psychoanalysis; in his later years he usually avoided expressing an opinion on newly published analytic works. He needed a long time for a well-considered verdict. He was tolerant enough to appreciate others' efforts in analysis along paths that did not interest him, although he himself would never venture out upon such paths. After a lecture by one of our colleagues on broad problems of character neurosis, he remarked that he had limited himself to

narrower aspects of the subject, but that the new generation
would wish to explore more remote regions. "I myself have always sailed upon inland lakes. But good for them who are striking out into the open sea."

Whence comes the view so prevalent in America that Freud was
dogmatic? Throughout thirty years I never noticed a single trait
of narrow-mindedness or dogmatism in him. In this book I have
included a letter of his (his reply to my criticism of his Dostoyevsky essay) which testifies that he was critical of his own work and
freely admitted weaknesses where they existed. He was intolerant
only toward false tolerance. He insisted that psychoanalysis, as a
science, should adhere to its own methods, and he tried to keep it
free of the methods of other sciences.

I often had long talks with Freud about the qualifications and
education of the analyst. We were agreed that a medical education is inadequate for the profession of analyst. In the course of
the conversation, Freud pointed out that poets (Shakespeare,
Goethe, Dostoyevsky) and philosophers (Plato, Schopenhauer,
Nietzsche) had come closer to the fundamental truths of psychoanalysis than had the physicians. He once informed me that the
natural scientist and philosopher, Paracelsus (1493-1541), had advanced a theory of neurotic therapy which was akin to that of
psychoanalysis. This scientist, who had been persecuted as a
quack, had recommended a strengthening of the ego as a counter-
poise to the instinctual forces which are morbidly expressed in
neurosis. "Just what he himself understood by it, I don't know,"
Freud added, "but there is no doubt as to its correctness."

On the question of the education of the analyst Freud differed
with me. He found my views too exacting and had more respect
than I for the value of instruction. He admitted, however, that
the personal inclinations and talent of the individual were more
important than is generally conceded. In a conversation on
Dostoyevsky he smilingly granted my assertion that this poet had
more psychological talent than the whole International Psychoanalytic Society; but he felt that Dostoyevsky was a phenomenal
case. I replied that all instruction and control analysis was in vain
if it were offered to individuals who had no innate gift and did
not possess that "psychic sensitivity" he had once spoken of. He

nodded to this, but insisted that the talent of understanding unconscious processes was more widespread than I would have it,
and that analysis augmented and developed this talent. We finally agreed that the ideal would be for those who were born
psychologists to learn the analytic method and be able to practice
it. We have said we have to seek out such "born psychologists" not
only in the circle of psychiatrists and neurologists. In my opinion
they will be as few and far between there as anywhere else.

Freud occasionally was pessimistic about the future of psychoanalysis. I am told he once said that analysis would suffer a
lingering death after his own death. Such a moody remark was
certainly only the reflection of momentary bad humor. In later
years he was always confident and optimistic. He knew that the
science he had created would not disappear. He knew also that
that science would undergo modifications and corrections, would
be supplemented and considered from new angles. But what
Freud mined from the profoundest depths and abysses of the
psyche will endure, and his work will continue with ever more
fruitful influence upon the life of individuals and of nations.
Above all, his method of research will endure; that method which
accords such critical attention to apparent trivialities, the method
whose objects are the inconspicuous, the hidden, and the veiled.

Here is not the place to discuss the development of his
thoughts. Greek mythology tells the story of the Augean stable,
wherein three thousand oxen were kept, which remained un-
cleaned for thirty years. The misconceptions and distortions, the
falsifications and misrepresentations to which psychoanalysis was
subjected in its popularization threaten to transform the magnificent house that Freud built into a stable similar to that of King
Augeas. It too was not cleaned for thirty years and was, alas,
frequented by more than three thousand oxen during this time.
To clean it is a task compared with which Hercules had an easy
job.

A small circle of those who were Freud's followers will teach the
new generation. He knew that after a short period of lying fal-
low and of being overrun by confusion, disturbance, and ob-
scurantism, psychoanalysis would come into its own in the lives of
civilized peoples. In his last book he saw a great vision of the fate

of Moses and his mission, a fate that may well be his own. Does he not prophesy the great work of his little circle? He recounts the tale of the Levites, who stood fast in all perils, defying all the forces that opposed them to save the intellectual heritage of a genius for the millenniums to come. Is this not an outline of the task of his little group of followers? Freud's death does not mean the beginning of the end of psychoanalysis, as his foes aver, but rather the end of the beginning.

The deepest and final memory Freud left with us is the memory of his utter sincerity. He dared to pursue to the end thoughts which some few had encountered, but at which most men had turned and run—thoughts on sex and the sexes, on life, love, and death, and on the powerful instincts that live beneath the pitiable artifices we invent to conceal them from ourselves and others. He faced the psychic processes in himself and others without fear and favor. He was more courageous than his time. And these qualities—talent, utter honesty, and the ability to consummate his thoughts—seem to me the qualities with which are endowed those rare human beings whom we call geniuses.

II

NEARLY FORTY-FIVE years had passed since, with pounding heart, I first ascended the steps of Number 19 Berggasse and stood face to face with Freud. At the time I was a student of psychology at the University of Vienna. About a half year previously our fine old professor, Friedrich Jodl, had for the first and last time mentioned Sigmund Freud's name in his lectures. Research into the psyche at the time was completely under the aegis of experimental psychology. When we thought of psychic processes, we thought of them in terms of laboratory work, tests, experiments with stimuli and blood pressure.

Professor Jodl had been lecturing to us for weeks on Wundt's laws of association. At the close of his lecture he mentioned offhandedly, with a keen ironic smile, that there was one instructor in our city who asserted that there was a type of forgetting that did not follow Wundt's laws, but the laws of a psychic process he called repression. We students also smiled ironically, for like our professor we were confident of our knowledge of the human soul.

Some time later a book by this instructor fell into my hands. It bore the title, *The Interpretation of Dreams*. I began to read, but soon laid the book aside. It seemed altogether preposterous —was I not a student of Wundtian psychology? But a few days later I took it up again—I had left it lying on my desk next to Ziehen's textbook of psychology—and this time I read on and on, fascinated, to the last line. In the following weeks with growing wonder I read everything this author had published. Here was the psychology that had been sought so long, a science of the psychic underworld. Here was what I had looked for when I first took up the study of psychology in spite of all the warnings of practical people. Here was something derived not from psychology textbooks but from the premonitions and visions of Goethe, Shakespeare, Dostoyevsky, Schopenhauer, and Nietzsche.

Some months later I stood for the first time in the room where Freud worked, stood by his desk, surrounded by Egyptian and Etruscan figurines, excavated trophies of a long-dead world.

In the following years scarcely a week passed that I did not see him. The lectures in the old psychiatry clinic in the Lazarettgasse, the discussions of the Vienna Psychoanalytic Society and, later on, the Wednesday evenings at his home (for he was then already ill and received only his closest co-workers on these occasions— "From time to time I like to see the young ones," he said, quoting Goethe)—these are unforgotten and unforgettable times.

One who was not close to Freud cannot conceive of the stature of the man, for he himself was greater than his work, that work which embodies the profoundest insights into the psychic life of man that have yet been attained. Many, throughout the whole wide world, know how kindly, helpful, and loyal he was. I can still see his smile as he appeared unexpectedly one day in our apartment in Berlin, after toiling up four flights of stairs. It was in 1915, I had just married and was poor as only a Doctor of Philosophy can be. Freud brought the news that the Psychoanalytic Society had decided to award me the prize for the best scientific work in the field of applied psychoanalysis. It was like a fairy tale, and the most miraculous feature of it was Freud's smile. Clearly, it made him happy to hand me the sum of money, which was not large but to me in my circumstances at the time seemed like a fortune.

Shortly before Hitler's invasion of our Austria I saw him for the last time. This was after an interval which I spent in Holland. I still, at fifty, felt as I rang the bell the joyful expectation that had surcharged me as a boy of twenty.

I found him greatly changed, his skin withered and his eyes deep-sunken. His hands, as he opened a cigar case, seemed no more than skin and bones. But his eyes, his curious and penetrating eyes, were as lively and kindly as always. In conversation he showed all his old eager interest. Every sentence he spoke was characteristically his. We talked of the problems of our science, and it seemed to me that the wisdom of old age in this man had revealed to him mysteries whose existence I had not even suspected. After a long discussion of psychoanalytic problems, our conversation turned to questions of the day. Freud realized how precarious was the situation of Austria, and he was very doubtful that she could maintain herself. He felt no fear for himself, but he foresaw a dark future.

Only a few of his remarks shall be recorded here. He knew that psychoanalysis might well suffer seeming defeat for a long time. But then its effect would be profounder than ever. He was not surprised by the brutality and blind cruelty of the Nazi regime. It seemed as though he had anticipated it and was armed to meet it. What surprised him, however, was the intellectual attitude of the majority of Germans, whom he had thought more intelligent and capable of better judgment. While we were speaking of race prejudice, he said smilingly, "Look how impoverished the poet's imagination really is. Shakespeare, in *A Midsummer Night's Dream*, has a woman fall in love with a donkey. The audience wonders at that. And now, think of it, that a nation of sixty-five millions have . . ." He completed the sentence with a wave of his hand.

We spoke of the Jews and their destiny. (At the time he was still working on the manuscript of the Moses book.) He was not downcast. "Our enemies wish to destroy us. But they will only succeed in dispersing us through the world." Averse to nationalistic prejudices, he loved his people and he did not believe that this persecution would break their will to live. When I commented on the tragedy of Jewish destiny, he replied with a smile, "The ways of the Lord are dark, but seldom pleasant."

While on this subject, I should like to record Freud's reply when a London weekly requested him to express his opinion, to be published in a symposium, on the Nazi persecution of the Jews. Freud refused, citing a French proverb:

> *Le bruit est pour le fat,*
> *Le plainte est pour le sot;*
> *L'honnête homme trompé*
> *S'en va et ne dit mot.*

He did not show much surprise at the outbreak of hatred for the Jews. When he learned that in Berlin his books, together with those of Heine, Schnitzler, Wassermann, and so many others, had been solemnly consigned to perdition and burned, he said calmly, "At least I burn in the best of company."

A journalist reported in the New York *Times* Freud's comment on his own fate at this time. " 'They told me,' he said, 'that psychoanalysis is alien to their *Weltanschauung,* and I suppose it is.' He said this with no emotion and little interest, as though he were talking about the affairs of some complete stranger."

It is well known that he was not indifferent to the fate of his own people. He hailed the reconstruction going on in Palestine and wrote to the Jewish organization, Keren Hajazoth, on June 20, 1925: "It is a sign of our invincible will to live which for two thousand years has survived the worst persecutions. Our youth will carry on the fight."

If I here describe some more personal moments of this last conversation, I do so to show how charmingly and spiritedly the octogenarian expressed himself. I want to give some hint of the graciousness of his mind and the modesty and kindliness of his character. We were speaking of my latest book. He praised it in words that I still cherish in my memory. He freely criticized some of my ironic judgments of the ideas of certain colleagues. Later on I explained, "I don't care much what my colleagues think of my books. For me your opinion is the vital one. Only what you say to me is important." "You are very wrong, Reik," he answered. "You must regard your colleagues' opinions of your work. I am no longer important, I am already an outsider—I no longer belong . . . You know," he added after a short pause, "your position is so unreasonable. You remind me of the hero of a fairy tale I once read—where was it?

"A barber in the Orient, let us say Bagdad, often heard his customers talking of a beautiful princess in a faraway land who was held captive by a wicked wizard. The brave man who would free the princess was promised both her hand and a great kingdom. Many knights and princes had set out upon the adventure, but none had succeeded in reaching her. Before the castle in which the beautiful lady was imprisoned there lay a vast, gloomy wood. Whoever crossed this wood would be attacked by lions and torn to pieces. The few who succeeded in escaping these lions were later met by two terrible giants who beat them down with cudgels. Some few had escaped even this danger and after years of travail had reached the castle. As they rushed up the stairway, the wizard's magic caused it to collapse. It was said that one brave prince had nevertheless managed to ascend into the castle, but in the great hall where the princess was enthroned a fierce fire raged which destroyed him.

"The adventurous barber was so deeply impressed by these tales of the beautiful princess that by and by he sold his shop and set out to liberate her. He had singular good fortune; he escaped the wild beasts, overcame the giants, and survived many other adventures, until at last he reached the castle. He strode over the stairway, although it toppled beneath him, and plunged intrepidly through the roaring flames that were threatening to consume the hall. At the end of the great hall he could dimly see the princess. But as he rushed across the room and drew near the figure, he saw a gray old woman supporting herself on a cane as she sat, her face full of wrinkles and warts, her hair drawn back in sparse, snow-white strands. The brave barber had forgotten that the princess had been waiting sixty years for her deliverer . . . No, my dear Reik, you are wrong in setting such store on me and my opinion. You must listen to what the colleagues say about your work."

That was Sigmund Freud's way.

III

THE MEMORIES that form the major part of this chapter emerged during the last years on different occasions and sometimes by most surprising detours. Some were immediately recognized, others acknowledged only after some time. A few were obviously continuations of conscious thoughts as, for instance, those stimulated by reading the biography of Freud by Ernest Jones. The period Jones describes antedated my acquaintanceship with Freud, whom I first met in 1910, but the reading of the book renewed impressions I had received in later years. These reminiscences varied in character: sometimes they were clear recollections of things he had said. The perception frequently was accompanied by the visual image of Freud sitting at his desk across from me, or giving a lecture in the psychiatric clinic in the Lazarettgasse, or walking beside me afterward on the way home. On rare occasions I even remembered the precise place where he had spoken this or that sentence, as if the locality itself had some significance. Now and then his voice was recalled, its timbre, the intonations and inflections, the modulation of a sentence, even the clearing of his throat. Along with this auditory memory there came to mind how in later years he coughed, took out his handkerchief, and thoughtfully looked at the sputum for a moment. (Gestures are very rarely remembered, but Freud did not use many gestures.) Associations easily to be guessed lead from here to the time when I heard Freud mention cancer: he spoke of the eagerness of young psychoanalysts to help their patients, to free them as quickly as possible from their neurotic, often painful symptoms. He declared that suffering is a biological necessity and pointed out that some physical illnesses—for instance, cancer—are so dangerous because the signal of suffering is absent in their first phases.

Many of these recollections occurred to me during psychoanalytic sessions with patients, either while listening as they communicated certain experiences or while I was giving an analytic interpretation myself. Sometimes such a memory occurred when I was giving a lecture or a seminar, trying to get some idea across to the young people who study psychoanalysis. Whenever such reminiscences emerged, I told my students what Freud had said on this or that occasion. In analytic sessions, from out of somewhere a sentence from the lips of Freud summarizing an emotional attitude or explaining a dynamic unconscious process would occur to me, as if to help me to understand the actual situation. In other cases a memory occurred to me after I had said something explaining the secret meaning of a dream or formulating a psychological insight in a poignant sentence. I then suddenly became aware that it was my voice that spoke, but that he had said this same thing in a conversation.

I often remembered on such a detour an apt simile he had used or a surprising insight, and the *mot juste* he had found was sometimes pronounced by me as if it had been my own, only to be recognized as Freud's expression later on. In those early years we followers of Freud were often criticized because we identified ourselves with our master. We did, of course, but one is tempted to ask: What else should we do with him? Moreover, the process of identification is psychologically by no means as simple as the critics imagined; it has its unconscious motivations and aims and naturally has also its hostile aspect. At the end of the emotional process it is almost meaningless to decide what belongs to the object of identification and what to the transformed ego. The Talmud reports that Moses, after his descent from Sinai, was so filled with the spirit of God that he said, "I am giving you the Law." Students of a Hassidic rabbi once asked him to interpret this passage which seemed blasphemous to them. He answered with a fine parable: A merchant wished to undertake a journey. He hired a clerk to replace him in the interval and let him work at the counter. He himself made a practice of remaining in the adjoining room. From here he might often hear the apprentice saying to a customer, "The master cannot give it to you at that price." The merchant thought the time was not yet ripe to leave the shop. The second year he heard the apprentice saying, "We cannot give it to you at that price." Still the merchant thought it would be wiser not to leave. At last, in the third year, he heard the clerk in the next room declaring, "I can't give it to you at that price." He felt then he could safely go on his journey.

Even everyday impressions sometimes bring back memories of Freud to me, as for instance the paper on which I am at the moment writing. I prefer very large sheets to those of smaller size. Freud also used such large sheets, and when I once asked him about this habit he declared, "When I have to restrict myself in so many directions in life, I want to have space and freedom at least when I am writing." The image of his large slanting handwriting, with its left to right ascending character, comes to mind together with a remark he once made about graphology. He told me once about a letter he had received from an unknown Russian lady who suffered from a serious emotional disturbance and had wandered for a long time from one psychiatrist to another. She had spent many months in treatment with Dr. P. Sollier in Paris and asked Freud whether he would take her as patient. She warned him in her (French) letter that she would be unable to speak of certain matters. After I had read this passage, he turned my attention to the patient's handwriting. "What do you think of it?" he asked. It was a strange way of writing, regular in its character, but conspicuous because each letter seemed to be bent to the left—as if the handwriting as a whole were leaning backward. "There is no doubt," said Freud, "that men also express their character through their writing. What a pity it is that its understanding is so ambiguous and its interpretation so uncertain! Graphology is not yet a scientific exploration."

The conversation about that letter brings to mind that Freud liked to use comparisons, similes and analogies when he sought vividly to illustrate what he meant. For example, this patient had expressed her eagerness to undergo analytic treatment provided she could keep certain things to herself. Freud spoke of the impossibility of such reservations in psychoanalysis and of areas set apart and withheld for certain reasons. "Let us assume that the police can enter any quarter of Vienna except certain streets or sections. Do you think that the security of Vienna would be very strong in such a case?" He was amused when I told him about a patient from New England who declared during the initial interview, "A gentleman does not speak of his mother or his religion."

Here are a few instances noted at random, which show Freud's liking for metaphor: About a patient who intermittently fought against a masochistic perversion, only to succumb to it when it seemed as if he had already conquered it: "He acts like a wanderer who returns home and who already sees the lights of his house from a distance, only to stumble into the last tavern on the highway." About the same patient who, after having been separated from his domineering wife, began a sexual affair with a very masculine woman: "He has broken the whip that lashed him to obtain a cat-o'-nine-tails for himself."

In speaking of the fact that, unavoidably, psychoanalysis often affects patients who seem to have adjusted themselves to intense inhibitions and symptoms so that they begin to feel anxious and emotionally insecure when old conflicts are explored in their analytic sessions: "Yes, psychoanalysis stirs them up. *Pour faire une omelette, il faut casser des oeufs* (To make an omelette, you have to break eggs)." Another comparison, used when, during a walk, we discussed the increasing difficulties one meets when exploring the repressed motivations and origins of neurotic disturbances: "When you dig into this sandbank as those children over there do, the work is at first easy, but when one gets deeper into the ground it becomes stony and often seems as if the spade cannot penetrate." A similar comparison was used when he spoke of digging a shaft into the depths, or making a mine with regard to analytic exploration. Once he spoke of the future of psychoanalysis and said that the analysts and the researchers of endocrinology and allied sciences are being compared to groups of workers who build a tunnel from opposite sides and will meet in the middle of it. He often used comparisons from archeology and from research into early phases of mankind; for instance, when he called early infancy the prehistory of the individual. He liked to take his comparisons from everyday life. When I once spoke of a patient who in a violent scene threatened to leave her husband, Freud said, "Dishes are never eaten as hot as they were cooked." Discussing the part unconscious resistances have in reaching certain insights, he said, "It takes hardly more than a day and a night to reach Verdun from Berlin by train. But the German army needed many months to make the journey. There were the French divisions that considerably slowed the march."

I sometimes heard Freud quote from literature in his conversation. Here are two examples: I spoke of a patient who had definite walking difficulties of a psychosomatic kind. I mentioned to Freud that some doctors had suspected that these difficulties in walking were initial symptoms of multiple sclerosis. When I then related that the man often had short phases in which there was not the slightest trace of his walking symptoms, Freud remarked, *"Die war's nicht, der's geschah."* ("That was not it, if that happened.") The line is from a poem by the old Austrian poet Friedrich Halm (1806-1871) about love. The line asks: "And tell me how does love die?" And the answer is: "It was not love if that happened." In such poetic language Freud rejected the diagnosis of multiple sclerosis.

On another occasion I told him that I could not interpret an element in the dream of a patient in which apples played a significant part. Instead of answering, Freud quoted from the Walpurgis Night scene in which Faust dances with a young witch and says:

> Once came a lovely dream to me
> I saw there an apple tree,
> Two lovely apples on it shone;
> They charmed me so I climbed thereon.

The beauty answers:

> The little apples men entice
> Since they were in Paradise.

> I feel myself with pleasure glow
> That such within my garden grow.

These lines—quoted, of course, in German—provided the inter-pretation that had eluded me.

In a discussion about the psychopathology of criminals Freud emphasized the differences between neurotic and criminal per-sonalities. He said that as long as there were no individual ana-lytic case explorations of delinquents, analogies with the attitude of neurotic patients had only a very restricted value, since certain traits, conspicuous in criminals, appeared in the emotional life of neurotics sporadically isolated "as veins in the ore."

He once said that men who are terrified at the idea of the possibility of incest with their mothers will be only weakly potent or impotent because they "shy from this potentiality as a horse does from his own shadow." He added that a little of one's mother is to be found in any woman.

He was far from considering psychoanalysis as a help or cure in all cases of emotional conflicts and often felt that analytic treatment was not indicated. In a case known to me in which a husband had deserted his wife, who in her unhappiness asked Freud for analytic help, he said, "That is a calamity like another ("*C'est un malheur comme un autre*") and one has to deal with it as with others. Psychoanalysis cannot help, perhaps resignation is the right answer."

For a long time Freud mistrusted all attempts at short cuts in analytic treatment and occasionally made sarcastic remarks about some analytic innovations. We once visited the newly furnished consultation room of one of our colleagues. Freud, pointing to the very broad couch, said smilingly to me, "That is rather for group analysis."

I remember that one of the first patients he referred to me was a young man with serious nervous complaints. The patient had told me in the first interview that he had violin lessons with a well-known virtuoso. At one of the next analytic sessions he brought his violin case with him and put it on my desk where my manuscripts were. When I told Freud about it, he blamed me because I had charged the patient too low a fee. Freud interpreted the placing of the violin case as symptomatic action in which the patient had expressed his unconscious contempt toward me, to whom he paid so much less than to his music master. When I told Freud later about certain features of this case, he expressed the opinion that the strange behavior of my patient was perhaps to be traced to some unknown traumatic events of his childhood which he unconsciously remembered. Much later this conjecture was confirmed: the uncle in whose house the boy had been brought up told me a secret which had been kept back from all members of the family. The mother of the patient had become insane and had treated the boy very badly. The patient had no conscious knowledge that his mother had died in an asylum.

I have often wondered about Freud's attitude to women. He certainly did not share the American concept of equality of the sexes, and was of the opinion that the man should take the lead in married life. He spoke of America as a matriarchy in which women have the real rule. He was old-fashioned in his gallantry toward women and showed in his conversation a deep insight into their emotional life. Sometimes I heard him joke about them. In a variation of a colloquial sentence Viennese women used when they were shopping he said, "A wife is expensive, but you have her a long time." Another time he said jokingly that a woman who feels restless consults a physician or goes shopping.

He once compared the analytic process, in certain masochistic cases in which the patient has unconsciously subjected himself to a severe punishment for his thought-crimes, to a legal procedure in which the analyst takes the case to the court of appeals, pleads that the verdict of the superego was too severe, and recommends a milder judgment. He also compared the process of analysis with the task of the re-education of the individual who vacillates between the demands of his drives and those of the society incorporated within his superego. In enlarging upon this conflict in one of his lectures, he gave vivid instances of those opposite tendencies that have their battleground within the soul of neurotic patients. Occasionally in informal discussion he spoke like a conversationalist rather than an academic teacher, presenting ingenious comparisons of such conflicts with situations which seemingly were very distant. The conversationalist was then transformed into a raconteur. The metaphor and the simile were re-placed by a story in which both understatement and wit played a part.

I recall a lecture in which he spoke of the clash between the justified demands of society for renunciation of certain satisfactions and the power of biologically determined instinctual drives. He compared that conflict with a story about the town of Schilda. The citizens of that town, in old German folklore, were known as rather silly in their pretense of deep wisdom, and many foolish actions are reported of them. They once bought a horse for work on the municipal plot. After some time the mayor and the town council decided that the horse was too expensive because it ate too much hay and oats, and they cut down its daily ration. The horse continued to work, and the citizens, still unsatisfied with the saving reached, determined to retrench its food ration still more. The horse was apparently still workable, whereupon they cut the feed ration even more. Then they set to wondering whether the horse might not work without any hay or oats. The experiment was performed and the horse died the next day. Thus, remarked Freud, it is certainly necessary to restrict demands of our sexual and aggressive drives in the interest of society, but human nature does not allow this renunciation to transgress certain limits. A variable measure of instinctual gratification is necessary, if man is to remain emotionally healthy.

Freud considered it necessary that the patient to whom the first analytical interpretations were given be psychologically prepared for them. He felt that the psychoanalyst should introduce his interpretation by remarks that would serve to give the patient an elementary insight into the contrast and conflict between the organized and conscious ego and the repressed. "It would be as obviously nonsensical to tell an unprepared patient that he once had incestuous desires for his mother as to tell the man on the street that he sees things standing on their heads."

In the discussion of a case presentation in which an analyst had told a patient some very unpleasant things in a seemingly brutal manner, Freud remarked that such a technique ought to be called aggressive rather than active. Enlarging on the manner in which first interpretations in analysis should be communicated to the patient, he told us the following story: The Shah of Persia once had an anxious dream and summoned the dream-interpreter, to whom he told the content of his dream. The magician said, "Alas, O King, all your relations will die and after them you will die!" The Shah got angry and ordered the dream-interpreter decapitated. He then summoned a second interpreter and told him the dream. "Hail, O King," said this man, "you will survive all your relatives!" The Shah ordered that a hundred gold coins be given to the second dream-interpreter.

Often a bit of practical wisdom or common sense was expressed by Freud by comparisons. Once when someone wanted to give up a job without any hope of getting another or better one, Freud said, "You do not throw out dirty water unless you know you can get some clean." In one of the cases discussed at the meeting of the Vienna Psychoanalytic Society the patient had long and detailed conversations with a friend about her analysis. Freud told the young analyst that he should energetically discourage such discussions. "Much valuable material will be lost to the analytic treatment if you allow the patient to continue that. When you want a river to have a powerful waterfall, you do not dig channels to take water away from it."

I remember Freud speaking of an American physician who came to Vienna to undergo psychoanalytic treatment, but considered his analysis as a kind of byproduct and gave priority to studies of other disciplines. Freud said that, for the time being, analysis should have priority for that physician, adding, "Analysis, in such a case, is like the God of the Old Testament and does not allow that there are other gods."

About a young physician who boasted in a letter that he had sacrificed all other interests to the study of psychoanalysis, Freud said, "That is not a merit: to choose analysis is part of one's destiny."

He warned us not to discuss the positive transfer provided it did not take those forms which interfered with the progress of the therapeutic procedure—that is, unless it showed itself as resistance. "Don't forget that those positive feelings are the wind that moves our mills."

Once during the first World War the ambiguous role the Poles played was discussed. Freud was amused when someone said, "The Poles sell their country, but they do not deliver it." Freud laughingly commented, "The result is that the Poles are truly patriots!"

I remember that he read an article of a colleague and called its style "tasteless as matzos." When he criticized someone, which was rare, he was always direct. I remember when Hermann von Kayserling, the writer of the *Diary of a Philosopher* and the leader of the School of Wisdom in Darmstadt, visited him and began to talk about psychoanalysis in a rather superficial manner, Freud said, "You do not understand that, Count."

In his critical remarks about books and articles he unerringly put his finger on the weak spot, not only in regard to their content, but also their presentation. Sensitive to every shade of stylistic peculiarity, he reached conclusions from the manner of writing as to the personality of the writer, even to certain hidden qualities as well as shortcomings. He felt, for instance, that a certain author whose excellent intelligence he admired spoke or wrote down to his readers. I remember he occasionally quoted a witty remark of Karl Kraus, the well-known satirical Viennese writer, adding that Kraus was a highly intellectual person who was very aggressive and malicious.

I know he had a low opinion of the American mentality of the 1920's and said it was very superficial and satisfied with labels and slogans. He characterized it once as having the character of adolescence and showing "an unthinking optimism and an empty activity." He was not in the least impressed with the Freud craze which at the time was in vogue in this country, and always pointed out that the enthusiasm of American intellectuals for psychoanalysis was only possible because they did not really understand the new science. He told me that, with a few exceptions, psychoanalysis in this country had not made any remarkable scientific contributions to depth-psychology.

In emphasized contrast to the attitude of the American Psychoanalytic Association, he was, until his death, of the opinion that psychoanalysis is not a medical science but belongs to psychology. At one of the Wednesday evenings when we, a selected group of his students, met at his home, I remarked in a discussion that the future of psychoanalysis would be in the study of history, anthropology and the social sciences, and that the analytic therapy of neurotic and psychotic disturbances would be obsolete in the year 2000. To the astonishment of almost all present—some are still alive—Freud entirely agreed with me. He said, "There is no doubt that the main task of therapy of the neuroses will be dealt with by means which new discoveries in the area of inner secretions will provide. I hear the steps of endocrinology behind us and it will catch up with us and overtake us. But even then psychoanalysis will be very useful. Endocrinology will then be a giant who is blind and does not know where to go, and psychoanalysis will be the dwarf who leads him to the right places."

While he showed himself always warm and was interested in my private life, he was reserved and reticent about himself. Only after his seventieth birthday did he begin to speak freely about himself and his private life, and told me some interesting memories. My impression is that he was really shy and overcame it by a kind of emphasized spontaneity.

When I first made his acquaintance he was interested to hear that I was working on a book on Flaubert's *The Temptation of St. Anthony.* He knew the work very well and admired its writer. Shortly after my book was published in 1912—it was the first psychoanalytic doctor's thesis in Europe—he suggested, during a walk, that I should write a psychoanalytic monograph on Emile Zola. He knew an astonishing amount about Zola's married life and about his two illegitimate children, and about Zola's compulsive way of working which produced the most thorough study of the theme with which his novels dealt. Freud told me then about some very interesting features of Zola's compulsions. I have always regretted that I made no notes on that conversation. Only much later did I realize that my resistance against writing the monograph had its main source in my unconscious reluctance to accept Freud's suggestion, an infantile hesitancy to receive a gift from a father-representative. Strangely enough, it was Freud again who helped me much later to arrive at this insight. He once spoke in another context of typical characteristics of the defiant attitude of an adolescent son toward his father: "That unconscious reluctance goes so far that the son does not want to owe anything to his father, not even his life. Do you remember the typical theme in fairy tales and folklore of a young man saving a king or duke from highwaymen who want to kill him? You easily recognize in such veiled shape the unconscious defiance of the son who wishes to give back to his father the life he owes him."

Whenever, later on—especially after my arrival in America in 1938—I became discouraged, I would bolster myself by remembering that Freud often and freely said to me and others that he had high expectations in regard to my future research work. Looking back now, when the end of work is in sight, I find myself ashamed at how little I could fulfill those expectations. Yet I know I have done the best that as poor a man as Hamlet was able to. Such a retrospective glance renews the awareness of what a stroke of luck it was that I met Freud when I was in my early twenties, and that I could work with him so long. It was a great time because it was a time lived with a man who was great.

IV

IN THE PREFACE to the Hebrew edition of *Totem and Taboo*, written in 1930, Freud states that he does not understand the sacred language, that he is as alienated from the religion of his forefathers as he is from any other and that he cannot share nationalistic ideals—yet he feels that his personality is Jewish and he does not wish it to be different. Asked, "What is still Jewish in you since you have renounced all those features common with your people?" he would answer, "Still very much, perhaps the main thing." He added, however, that while he could not, at the time, put that essential character into clear words, he thought that it certainly would become accessible to scientific insight later on.

The great psychologist never attempted to explore those vague, yet definite emotional and mental traits that are so difficult to grasp, but a few sentences, spoken in answer to a speech at his seventieth birthday celebration at the B'nai B'rith in Vienna, circumscribe those characteristics. On this occasion, too, Freud confessed to being an infidel Jew and rejected a feeling of national superiority as disastrous and unjustifiable. But he added, ". . . there remains enough that made the attraction of Judaism and of the Jews irresistible, many mighty emotional forces, the more powerful, the less able to be caught in words, as well as the clear awareness of an inner identity, the secret of the same inner construction." He gratefully acknowledged that he owed to his Jewishness the two qualities that became indispensable on his difficult road. As a Jew he felt free from many prejudices which restricted other people in the use of their intellect, and as a Jew he was prepared to go into opposition and to renounce a conformity with the "compact majority." Posterity has recognized that it was this intellectual freedom from convention and this independence of thought that enabled him to write those eleven volumes that "shook the world." It was that readiness to remain in splendid isolation and to stand alone against an army of antagonists which made it possible to carry his research forward, unperturbed and unafraid—a Jewish knight in the shining armor of the integrity and courage of his deep-rooted convictions.

In the excellent book *The Life and Work of Sigmund Freud* by Ernest Jones, the significance of the Jewish element in Freud's personality is not fully considered. Only two short paragraphs of the volume are dedicated to that essential part of the great explorer's background. Jones, who belonged for forty years to the small circle of Freud's co-workers, is not only a scholar and skillful writer, but also an honest man. As the only foreigner of that intimate circle, he could remain more objective than the others. The same fact prevented him, who lived outside the culture pattern in which Freud was born and bred, from properly understanding the Jewish element in Freud's personality. A biography is not an inquiry in depth, and that shortcoming does not diminish the value of Jones's work which emphasizes that Freud "felt Jewish to the core and it evidently meant a great deal to him." "A Gentile," says Jones, speaking for himself, "would have said that Freud had few overt Jewish characteristics, a fondness for relating Jewish jokes and anecdotes being the most prominent one."

It seems that the great man had inherited his sense of humor, his skepticism and the high evaluation of Jewish wit from his father, the wool merchant Jakob Freud, who had the habit of pointing a moral by quoting a Jewish proverb or anecdote. Jakob Freud was admired by his son who became a raconteur of those Jewish stories long before he became interested in the psychoanalytic exploration of wit and its relation to the unconscious. Already in 1897 Freud writes to his friend, the Berlin physician Wilhelm Fliess, that he has begun to collect "profound Jewish stories." It is not without significance that this communication follows a comparison which alludes to one of those anecdotes: he reminds the friend that they share a wide area of research ("you the biological and I the psychological") like the two *schnorrers,* one of whom gets the province of Posen.

The correspondence with Wilhelm Fliess* presents an excellent picture of Freud as a younger man who turned his interest, at first hesitatingly, later determinedly, to the new field of psychopathology. In those intimate letters in which Freud freely speaks of his personal and professional life as well as of his recent research, Jewish jokes are again and again quoted or alluded to. In 1897 he expresses the hope that he will arrive at the basic insights into the psychology of the neurosis, if his constitution can stand it. Here is an allusion to the well-known anecdote in which a destitute Jew sneaks into the express train to Karlsbad (the Czechoslovakian health resort) without a ticket, is caught, thrown out at each station and each time more and more brutally treated. At one of his stations of suffering an acquaintance sees him and asks where he is journeying to. The answer is: "To Karlsbad, if my constitution can bear it." Allusions to the same joke also occurred to Freud later when he interpreted one of his dreams.

A few other instances: Freud reports in a letter that he had been mistaken in one of his earlier theoretical assumptions about

* Freud, "Aus den Anfangen der Psychoanalyse," *Brief an Wilhelm Fliess* (London: Imago Publishing Co., 1950).

the etiology of hysteria and he ought really be dissatisfied and depressed. His hopes of fame, of riches and independence, of
security for his family and himself were frustrated since that
concept about hysteria had proved erroneous: "Now I have to be
again quiet and modest and have to worry and to save. There
the little anecdote from my collection occurs to me: 'Rebecca,
take the dress off; you are no *kalle* (bride) any more.'" A year
later he sends the friend a part of his self-analysis, the first in
the history of science, and remarks that it is entirely directed by
the unconscious in accordance with the principle of Itzig, the
inexperienced horseman, who is asked, "Where do you go?" and
answers, "How should I know? Ask the horse!"

Students of Freud's style in which the personality and its history are reflected could have discovered that the same joke still
influenced the shaping of a comparison twenty-three years later.
In Freud's book *The Ego and the Id,* published in 1921, the relation of the ego, which represents reason and common sense, to the
id, from which our drives emerge, is compared with that of the
rider to the horse which he tries to bridle. The simile is extended: "As the rider who does not want to be separated from his
horse frequently can't help leading it where it wants to go, thus
the ego usually fulfills the will of the id as if it were its own."

While Freud was writing his *Interpretation of Dreams* he
considered it impossible to disguise his own dreams, but he was
unwilling to renounce his most important discovery on account
of such discretion. In this dilemma, he reported to Fliess, he behaved like the rabbi who was asked by a couple for advice about
what they should do. They have a rooster and a hen, wish to have
roasted chicken for the holiday dinner and cannot make up their
mind which of the two animals they should kill. "If we kill the
rooster, the hen will feel hurt, and if we kill the hen, the rooster
will be grieved. What should we do?" The rabbi decides: "Kill the
rooster!" "But then the hen will be grieved!" "Yes, that's true,
then kill the hen." "But, rabbi, then the feelings of the rooster
will be hurt!" "Well, let him feel hurt."

When Freud sent the first sheets of the finished book to the
printer in 1899, he was dissatisfied with his own work and remembered the joke in which Uncle Jonas is congratulated by his

nephew, who has heard that he is engaged to be married. "And what is your bride like, Uncle?" "That's a matter of taste. *I* don't fancy her."

The monumental book on the interpretation of dreams was published in 1900. Five years later Freud's *Wit and Its Relation to the Unconscious* appeared. In this work, whose psychological profoundness has not yet been fully appreciated, he takes much of the material for his analytic exploration from the source of Jewish jokes. We find here stories about *schadchen* and *schnorrers,* rabbis and unlearned people, poor and rich Jews; cynical,. sophistical and skeptical jokes. It is obvious to any reader that the writer loves those Jewish anecdotes, familiar to him since his boyhood. Here are examples of subtle and coarse, pessimistic and hopeful Jewish wit, of genuine Jewish humor and of wit whose essence is generally human and of which only the accessories are Jewish.

In sharp contrast to so many previous attempts at evaluating and interpreting the character of Jewish humor, Freud's point of view is pervasively psychological. In penetrating the façade of those precious stories, in demonstrating their technics and in revealing their means and methods, he shows their emotional meaning. In their psychoanalytic interpretation he arrives at the recesses of the heart that beats in them. Cautiously removing layer after layer, he demonstrates their secret tendencies, their social and individual skepticism, their knowledge of the quintessence of life and the profundity of their views. In the combination of an incomparable psychological perceptiveness and of independence of thinking, this explorer looks at the Jewish wit from an elevated point of view, aware of its national and religious as well as of its social premises, yet seeing in it expressions of all humanity and humanness. He comments on the self-irony of Jewish humor: "I do not know whether one often finds a people that makes so unreservedly merry over its own shortcomings." He contrasts stories invented by Jews and directed against Jewish social and religious manners and mannerisms with jokes made by anti-Semites making fun of the same foibles and failures. Those jokes, made by Gentiles who ridicule the Jews, "are nearly all brutal buffooneries in which the wit is spoiled by the fact that the

Jew appears as a comic figure to a stranger." The Jewish jokes which originate with Jews know and acknowledge the weaknesses of their people, "but they know their merits as well as their short-comings." In a conversation, Freud agreed with me that the self-ironical and sometimes even self-degrading character of Jewish humor was psychologically made possible only under the premise of an unconscious or preconscious awareness of the high value and worth of one's people, of a concealed national pride. Only a person who stands on an elevated place can jump down. Only a proud man can stoop to ridiculing himself.

In my thirty years of friendship with Freud I heard him, of course, frequently tell a Jewish anecdote or quote a witticism, but it was never for its own end, never for mere amusement. In most cases the comical story was used as illustration to a point he had made, a comparison of a certain situation or behavior pattern or as an instance of the human experiences we all share. It was as if he brought the joke forward as an example of how wisdom is expressed in wit and—much more rarely—wit in wisdom. Most of the instances I remember were quoted in connection with subjects we had just discussed in our conversation which concerned private matters or professional problems as well as scientific questions. Some of those witty stories compared actual situations of that time with various aspects of the troubled life of the Jews. The need to make something very clear let him call up some funny Jewish anecdote from the treasures of his almost photographically faithful memory. On rare occasions such illustrative or comparative purpose was replaced by some whimsical or satirical trend in which he made fun of the stupidity or hypocrisy of some antagonist.

It is regrettable that the psychological inquiry into the secret meaning and significance of Jewish wit as revealed in Freud's classical book has not been continued in psychoanalytic litera-ture. Very few psychologists have recognized the ramifications of Freud's exploration of this kind of humor. While he was still alive, I published several articles on Jewish humor in which I resumed his research and tried to discover new characteristics of Jewish wit. In a conversation with me, Freud acknowledged that I had succeeded in pointing out two features he had not emphasized. "We laugh at those stories, but Jewish wit is not merry in its character. It is a kind of humor that leaves sadness in its wake. One of those profound proverbs proclaims: 'Suffering makes one laugh too.' Another characteristic feature of a Jewish joke is its emotional intimacy, a special atmosphere in which it is born and bred."

Here are a few instances which show occasions on which Freud remembered a Jewish story and the special manner in which he used it. I discussed with him once the case of a patient whom he had referred to me for psychoanalytic treatment. The young man suffered from a compulsion neurosis, especially from syphilophobia, a fear of being infected by spirochete, and had developed a complicated system of measures to protect him from the danger of venereal infection in everyday life. He refused, for instance, to sit down on a chair where a person had sat who could have been acquainted with another whom he suspected of having syphilis. The patient found out that on a certain occasion his parents had taken a man who was the uncle of such a suspected person to the theater in their automobile. The patient refused to use his parents' car any more. Pointing out the possibility of infection by touch, he insisted that they buy him a car of his own. In discussing the secondary gains of the neurosis, the different advantages the patient gains from his illness after it is established, Freud told a Jewish anecdote: A man in an insane asylum rejects the food there and insists on having kosher dishes. His passionate demand is fulfilled and he is served food prepared according to the Jewish law. On the next Saturday the patient is seen comfortably smoking a cigar. His physician indignantly points out to him that a religious man who observes the dietary laws should not smoke on Saturday. The patient replies, "Then what am I *meschugge* (nuts) for?" Since Freud told me that story I have often quoted it to patients, illustrating that they get various secondary compensations in the form of attention, love and even financial support from others from whom they expect help as a result of their neurosis.

I still remember the occasion on which Freud told a story about Moses, because it was the first time he mentioned the theme of the Egyptian nationality of the leader, the theme he many years later dealt with in his book on Moses and monotheism. We discussed the typical forms of the myths of the birth of the hero which Otto Rank described and analyzed later on in his well-known book. Freud told me that the feature which recurs frequently in those myths—namely, that the hero is drawn out from a lake or a river—is a symbolical expression of the delivery process of the infant. He interpreted the situation as an archaic presentation of the embryo's position in the mother's womb, surrounded by amniotic fluid, and pointed to the stories in which the stork pulls babies out of the water. Returning to the origin of Moses, he quoted the following story: The boy Itzig is asked in grammar school, "Who was Moses?" and answers, "Moses was the son of an Egyptian princess." "That's not true," says the teacher. "Moses was the son of a Hebrew mother. The Egyptian princess found the baby in a casket." But Itzig answers, "Says she!"

It was during the Psychoanalytic Congress at Munich in 1913 (my God, is it really forty years ago?) that Freud told me another Jewish story, this time stimulated by the scientific conflict with C. G. Jung which came into the open at the sessions of the congress. It had become quite clear that Jung and his school were in full regression from the essential findings of psychoanalysis, and that they were reinterpreting and misinterpreting the discoveries of Freud which they had acknowledged before, in the sense of a new "higher" concept. They wished to be recognized as psychoanalysts although they had replaced the concept of the libido, of the energy of the sexual drives, by a vague, general idea of the force of life, had put a general conflict between it and inertness in the place of the struggle of the ego and of the drives which psychoanalysis made responsible for the neurosis and so on. Freud spoke with me of Jung's disavowal of the importance and significance of sexuality for the etiology of the neurosis. He had mentioned before the fact of Jung's theological history to which he attributed a decisive role in the new concept denying the forces of sex. It was perhaps this factor, as well

as Jung's previous leanings toward anti-Semitic views, which
brought a Jewish story to Freud's mind: A rabbi and a parson
decide to found a new common religion. The new faith is to be
established on the basis that the two priests will agree on certain
compromises and concessions. The parson begins with the demand: "Instead of Saturday, Sunday has to be observed." The
rabbi agrees. "In place of Hebrew, Latin has to be the language
of the service." "Good," says the rabbi. The parson enumerates
other concessions concerning rituals and religious observances.
The rabbi concedes them too. At the end it is his turn, and the
pastor asks, "And what are your conditions?" "I have only one,"
replies the rabbi. "Jesus Christus has to be radically removed."
The meaning is clear: all those changes the pastor suggests concern only external things, are not essential for the differences
between Judaism and Christianity. But if Jesus Christus is "radically" out, what remains then but Judaism? Freud, by thus comparing the attitude of the rabbi with that of Jung, wanted to convey that Jung, in removing the decisive role of sexuality from the
concept of psychoanalysis, brings the new science back to the
views of old psychiatry.

Here is another instance of a discussion of scientific problems
at which the memory of a Jewish joke occurred to Freud when
he tried to find a simile for a certain attitude. The joke emerged
as an afterthought by way of an illustration to an idea, but was,
as always, poignant and pungent. We were speaking of a group
of neurotic cases in whose symptomatology manifestations of
instinctual drives are blended with expressions of unconscious
guilt feelings. Freud pointed out that such an *entente cordiale*
between the demands of the drives and the powers of conscience
can often be discovered in the psychology of masochistic and
obsessive characters. He told me of a case in which a grossly selfish tendency, which was conscious, was put into the foreground
disguising an intense unconscious need for atonement and punishment. "Do you remember the anecdote of Jacob at the synagogue on Yom Kippur?" Freud asked. The premise of that story
is based on the fact that seats for the service on the High Holidays
have to be paid for, and poor Jews often cannot afford the price.
Jacob pleads with the sexton at the door of the synagogue to let

him enter because he has to convey an important business message to Mr. Eisenstein who is attending the service. But the sexton
is adamant in his refusal, saying, "I know you, you *gonnif*
(scoundrel)! You only want to get in to *daven* (to say your
prayers)!"

On another occasion Freud introduced a new point of view
into the interpretation of Jewish humor, a point of view which
was not considered in his book on wit. I told him a comical story
I had heard at that time in Vienna. In the middle of the night the
superintendent of the house of the Spanish ambassador in Vienna
is awakened by the repeated ringing of the bell of the palace.
He finally opens the door and finds two well-groomed, dignified
gentlemen who say again and again one sentence: *"Wir syn zwa
Spanische Granden"* ("We are two Spanish grandees"). The
Viennese is astonished to hear them repeat those words pronounced in unmistakably genuine Yiddish, but understands,
finally, that the two men ask him urgently to waken the ambassador, to whom they bring an important message from Spain.
The ambassador, at last brought to the scene, greets the two men
with great respect: they are really two Spanish noblemen of
highest rank who have brought a diplomatic message from the
king. The Viennese superintendent hears them converse with the
ambassador in pure Castillian, and learns that the two men who
cannot speak German had run into a Polish Jew on the express
train from Madrid to Vienna. They made him understand who
they were, that they would arrive at night in Vienna and asked
him what they should say in order to get their message to the
ambassador.

Freud not only liked the little story, but thought it worthy of
an analytic interpretation at which he arrived by bringing the two
Spanish grandees in intimate connection with the Polish Jew
whom they encountered. He told me that the concealed meaning
of the anecdote becomes transparent when one assumes that the
two Spanish noblemen could have been Jewish. That means that
one would have to look at the situation of the story from the point
of history. There was a long phase in the history of the Spanish
and Portuguese Jews during which they really became noblemen,
served the kings of Spain in high functions, were diplomats and

statesmen and so on. The Maranos, baptized Jews and descendants of Jews, played a very important role at the Spanish court. Seen in such a historical light, the secret meaning of the story becomes revealed: there is a subterranean tie between the two Spanish noblemen and the Polish Jew, a tie represented by tradition and origin, the same which connects the Ashkenazim and the Sephardim. It is not accidental that the two Spanish grandees were confused with Jews by the Viennese superintendent who is taken aback by what they tell him.

In his analytic investigations Freud often follows the development of Jewish wit back from mirth to misery, from the fanciful to the fateful. He shows us the unbroken spirit, the pride and dignity of his people because also from the ridiculous to the sublime it is but one step.

V

THE FOLLOWING three critical essays deal with Freud's writing in the 1927-1930 period. I have selected those on which Freud commented in letters or conversation. These essays were originally lectures given during those years in the Vienna and Berlin Psychoanalytic Associations.

I shall not attempt a précis of Freud's essay, *The Future of an Illusion,* but rather an interpretation of the main themes. I hardly think it valuable to restate Freud's ideas here. I shall more or less play the accompaniment to his melody.

When we carefully study Freud's essay, we shall become aware of three main divisions. The first concerns itself with present cultural conditions, the second discusses religion, and the third offers a picture of a future culture. We feel that the first division was originally intended to be the outstanding one; that Freud meant to develop it further. One passage seems to confirm this supposition.

The composition of the whole, proceeding from broad problems of civilization to a single cultural question, is admirable. Artfully, and yet with utter naturalness, everything inexorably centers around those problems which are most dear to the author. There is the eloquent overture, expressing the wish that we may get some inkling of the remote destiny of our culture. Then follows a passage dealing with the general cultural situation, mainly from the psychological point of view; the consideration of the conditions which engender culture; the description of the psychological requirements of civilization—the renunciations, prohibitions, lacks, and compensations. Finally, Freud indicates what is the most significant element for the psychic inventory of a culture: its religious ideas. If we prefer to imagine this work as a symphony, this introduction represents the first movement. Here Freud sets forth a comprehensive psychological picture of the present state of culture. Sterling clarity and wisdom inform this picture, which for us serves the purpose of a cross section, disclosing all the strata formations of a culture. *Totem and Taboo* gave us an analytical account of the dark origins of our institutions. Here the institutions themselves are characterized.

The future may judge this introduction, this all-embracing, serene portrayal of our culture, to be the most important essay Freud ever wrote. But not for the sake of its discussion of religious problems, for these will be problems no longer. Critics, fettered as always to the present, may embroil themselves with Freud's attitude toward religious questions. But we can afford to take the longer view. Unmoved by opposition from analysts and non-analysts, we will continue to insist that this rich and profound introduction rather than the discussion of religion is the most valuable section of Freud's book.

Let us compare this book with the one preceding it. Wherein lies the special value of this study about lay analysis? What part of its content will be considered its most significant one after twenty or fifty years? Perhaps the penetrating discussion of the problem and the elucidation of Freud's point of view? Not at all. Its significance will lie rather in this fact, that the essence of analysis is here represented with an impressive clarity never before reached. The whole realm has been looked at closely by eyes that have not overlooked anything.

The main section of the new book treats first the singular nature of religious ideas. It contains nothing with which we are not familiar from other writings of Freud. Even the role of infantile helplessness in the genesis of religion is not new, for Freud had discussed it previously in "Leonardo da Vinci."

What follows is a dialogue, handled with the same conversational grace and sharpness that we have come to know from personal association with Freud. An opponent is introduced who follows the author's thought processes and extends or contradicts them. This opponent and gainsayer is no stranger to us; he played the same part in Freud's earlier essays. He was not always personified, but he was always present. In all his works Freud anticipated objections, replied beforehand to arguments. This alternate examination and self-assertion was a sign of his strict self-criticism.

Let us consider the opponent for a moment. As always, the interlocutor is a cultured intellectual with the highest moral sentiments, accessible to reason, and not intolerant of strong emotions. Still, our impression is that this time Freud has treated his opponent somewhat cavalierly. The opponent might have raised more cogent objections and questions. Freud might have chosen a sounder opponent—say, from among the real opponents of his ideas. I could, for example, conceive as a really competent opponent one of those subtle Catholic priests with whom it is a delight to debate. These are men full of life's wisdom and gifted with a remarkable intellectual sensitivity. They have been pupils of the stern logic that derives from Thomas Aquinas.

At one point in Freud's debate there is no longer any basic cleavage between the two opponents. Suddenly Freud writes that their disagreement is not irreconcilable; it will vanish with time. He could never have forced such a conclusion in a dispute with a priest trained in the dogma. Here the end would have been unrelenting disagreement. But perhaps Freud deliberately wished to present a cultured, worldly scholar as the type of his opponent. We must not anticipate his intentions.

But even accepting this type of opponent, the discussion still should have taken a different turn. The attitude of an intellectual of our times toward the religious question is insincere, and it cannot be made straightforward through discussion. The cultured class of mankind, or more strictly, the intellectual upper class, evince the same shamefacedness and evasiveness toward their religious needs that they do toward their sexual and economic needs. Indeed, in the religious realm these needs are often more equivocal, harder to name for what they are. The pious man and the freethinker are frequently not so far apart as they seem. They have their insincerity in common. The religious man believes and does not reflect too much on his faith. The freethinker does not reflect too much on his lack of faith because he does not reflect very much about anything. We might sum up this strange attitude toward religion by saying that most educated people do not believe in God, but they fear him. Although science has proclaimed that God is dead, he lives on underground. And this is where scientific analysis must begin its work. The corpse must be exhumed and we must determine whether it is really dead. There is little doubt that official disbelief can live very comfortably alongside of unofficial belief.

This unconscious insincerity regarding religion would naturally alter the course of the conversation. The opponent would probably accede to most of Freud's arguments and demonstrations, declare that he was himself an atheist, and yet cling unconsciously to the faith he had denied. It would be especially hard to reason with him just because he apparently shares our views. Similarly, many obsessional neurotics will accept fully all the results of analysis, but will nevertheless cling to their illness.

Freud assures us that he himself considers his book quite harmless. He warns, however, of the fierce reactions it will call forth and of the discrediting effect it will have upon psychoanalysis. Since the appearance of *The Future of an Illusion* I have heard all kinds of objections to it, and none of them has been from the religious point of view. I am prepared to refute them all, but I shall spare the religious objection, for these contradict themselves. The first assertion is that religion is unimportant today and that Freud exaggerates its importance for the human soul. I do not believe this. I think the importance of religion in the psyche has not yet been sufficiently appreciated or investigated by psychoanalysis. Freud is still arguing in the spirit of the eighteenth century, these objectors claim; his reasoning continues the direct tradition of the Enlightenment. It is all so old-fashioned. Note that here, for once, psychoanalysis is attacked for lacking originality. *O quae mutatio rerum!*

Freud has, of course, emphatically indicated that views similar to his have been the common property of many great men. Nevertheless, that objection is all at sea. What a difference there is between Voltaire's passionate *"Écrasez l'infame!"* the trenchant, rationalist phrases of the French Encyclopedists, and the quiet, objective argumentation of Freud. And where, in the literature of the Enlightenment, do we find a study of the psychologic source of religious ideas? Where do we find an analytic explanation of them and an appreciation of the human meaning behind them?

Like the former objection, also the second is voiced by people who are apparently completely in agreement with Freud's religious views. They accept Freud's presentation, but immediately they point to the metaphysical value of religion. They claim that it contains transcendental truths in symbolic form; that it expresses the Absolute.

This argument brings back through the window what has already been thrown out the front door; for what here appears as a transcendental absolute is nothing but disguised, emasculated, and intellectualized religion, in its true form an object of shame. Moreover, it is easy and convenient to make statements about the transcendental because they need no proof and by their very nature admit of none. These objectors know everything about the transcendental that has ever been known; that is, nothing at all.

The last objection grants the logic of Freud's reasoning but challenges his right to extend to the collective psyche conclusions that have been derived from individual analysis. Now, psychoanalysts have often discussed this methodological question. What precautions are necessary in translating the results of individual research to the realm of folk psychology? What limitations must be imposed on such translation and what heuristic justification does it nevertheless have? We certainly do not wish to overlook methodology. But it is gradually becoming clear that up to the present methodology has always been the best scientific excuse for doing no scientific work at all. Nowadays it is possible to devote oneself to restful vacancy of mind without danger of reproach; for it is easy to impress the philosophic layman with the declaration that one is busy with considerations of methodology. It has become a pretext against all unequivocal statements. Methodology is the most convenient haven for intellectual sterility.

I have expounded these objections because they represent the position toward religious problems of many cultured persons. What is common to all of them is the sidetracking of the main question. Moreover, we see that these objections all correspond to typical defense reactions that we meet in analysis. The first, which holds that religion is unimportant, is the exact counterpart of the minimizing defense mechanism, the reduction to triviality. The second, which insinuates metaphysics to the fore, corresponds to dual conviction in obsessional neurosis. The third objection, which emphasizes the methodologic point of view, represents the forepleasure stage of intellectual activity. This is a sort of Hamlet compulsion which inhibits all real scientific work by continuous delay of action. But all these objections show the common feature of the first: acceptance of Freud's reasoning. None of those who raised these objections took issue from the standpoint of the believer; but every one of them unconsciously was a believer.

To my mind, then, the enemy acts, not so much by frank resistance to Freud's essay, but otherwise; paradoxically, by that very preliminary intellectual acceptance which is his façade, a fortress behind which resistance can develop. A concession is made so that it will not be necessary to draw the logical conclusions. This implies that the book will not alter the mental indolence and inner insincerity which dominate our society.

Since we are in the midst of considering religious problems, it will not be inappropriate if I remind you of the miracle of St. Anthony's fish sermon. It is recounted in the Book of Saints, and we also have it in the simple, lovely verse of our great collection of German folk poetry, *Des Knaben Wunderhorn*. The saint finds the church empty and goes to the fishes to preach to them. The carp come swimming up, and the pike, the cod, the crab. The tortoise,

> . . . as a rule
> A slow-enough fool,
> Rose from the depths in a hurry
> To hear the saint's story.
> Each and every word
> Delighted the cod.
> Fish great and fish wee,
> Of high and low degree,
> Turned their heads to the east
> Like reasoning beasts.

And then the close, so powerfully and bitterly expressed in Mahler's F Major chords:

> The sermon now ends;
> Each on his way wends—
> The pike remain thievish,
> The eels much love lavish,
> Upside-down walks the crab,
> Carp eats all he can grab—
> The sermon was nice
> No one thinks of it twice.
> Each goes on as he begun
> And my story is done.

There is another point we must raise. Freud emphasizes that psychoanalysis as a method of research is impartial and that the defenders of religion may also use it to determine the affective significance of religion. Certainly we will all agree to this. But analysis depends upon who practices it; and the situation is considerably changed when we are attempting to analyze the content of truth in religion. When a priest practices analysis, he does not cease to be a spiritual shepherd, and gradually the original aims are displaced, the ideational base shifts and contradictory tasks arise. When this happens, psychoanalysis pays the piper. Undeniably, many priests have shown a broad under-standing of analysis. But along with this is an inflexible, though cleverly concealed desire to put it to work in the service of the only Holy and Apostolic Church. For the first we thank them; for the second we say, no thank you. Everyone who has followed the literature knows that the Church is preparing to take over psychoanalysis. But it cannot be denied that the Church is one of the strongest repressive forces in our society. When it utilizes analysis, it places it in the service of repression. In our practice we have often noted how an obsessional neurotic not only cleverly weaves newly acquired knowledge into his system, but often uses it to enlarge his obsessional patter. This is precisely what happens to analysis in the service of religion.

It it all very well to be tolerant toward the religious view, but we must guard against extending our tolerance also to analytic aberrations. One of our Berlin colleagues recently wrote that analysis, like religion, has the same basic belief in goodness; both demonstrate how powerful and triumphant the good is in us all. Certainly we cannot object to this, providing we stipulate that analysis can also demonstrate precisely the opposite. One might believe in a world order in which the good is unmercifully pun-ished and evil is its own reward. If our distinguished colleague clearly sees the hand of God guiding human destiny, we shall not venture to question him. But we may add mildly that the direc-tion in which that *digitus paternae dextrae* points is extremely dubious.

At another point in Freud's discussion we should like to expand on his remarks. He points out that religion also may give license to sin freely once more after repentance. The brood-ing Russians have concluded from this that it is necessary to sin in order to partake of divine grace. But this is the attitude not only of certain Russian types. Long ago, in the beginnings of Christianity, there were many gnostic sects, such as the Cainites, the Carpocratians and others, whose contempt for the flesh went so far that they determined to gratify all its lusts in order to destroy it. Many a girl was burned on a medieval stake because she had been accused by a priest of valuing her hymen too highly, thereby prizing a thing which was of no value with respect to her eternal salvation. The Holy Mother Church often emphasized that asceticism was sinful. Only wanton pride inspired one to free oneself from the eternal curse of the flesh which God, in His inscrutable counsel, had made man's fate since the days of Adam. The Church here enjoins sinning. *Extra ecclesiam non est salus.*

Freud's passages on the future of religion and its slow, fateful dissolution are so clear and impressive that we need only draw the reader's attention to certain portions. There are sentences here which in their courageous directness, their monumental weight, and diamond-hard clarity, are reminiscent of the opening of the Beethoven C Minor Symphony. Thus destiny knocks at the door of a culture.

We turn now to the last section of Freud's book. Here he considers what the future will be like after religion disappears as a significant element in our cultural complex. The ideal of psychology, the supremacy of the intellect, will then take hold; education for reality will begin. The man of the future will confront with resignation the limitations of his own nature and will renounce all illusions.

Here, together with the opponent, we recognize the logic and importance of Freud's ideas; but our skepticism prevails. We feel inclined to counter not with a harsh "no," but with the gentle *"Je doute"* of Renan. While we cannot but agree with Freud that religion is doomed, that it has run its course, we cannot help doubting the suggestion that men are capable of living without illusions. Education for reality is certainly a consummation most devoutly to be wished; but the most striking attribute of reality is its unpleasantness. We secretly feel that reality is something others should accept. The illusion of religion will vanish, but another will take its place. The supremacy of the intellect which Freud foresees would never be more than superficial; basically men would still be guided by their instinctual desires. We do not deny the possibility that men will some day be ruled by science. But they will still be men, which is to say, frail, inconstant, more or less unreasonable beings who are the slaves of their instincts and who will never cease to strive after ephemeral pleasure. And men will continue to pray, "Lord, give us this day our daily illusion."

Experience must have convinced Freud that science has not made the scientists any better; that they are neither more patient nor happier nor even wiser. Science is by no means identifiable with the scientists. Freud himself once wrote the following lines which indicate that this view was not entirely strange to him. "If another form of mass education replaces religion, as socialism seems at present to be doing, the same intolerance against outsiders will persist. And if the scientific viewpoint ever gains a similar hold over the masses, the result will be no different." The rule of reason was instituted once before to the accompaniment of "Ça ira," and in its honor several thousand heads fell under the guillotine. The supreme intellect will at best be established as a puppet king for the powerful government of the instincts. I am afraid that the rule of reason will never prevent anyone from being utterly unreasonable. Freud overestimates both the extent and the strength of human intelligence. It is, in essentials, hardly different from the animal's intelligence; and in many instances even this comparison seems a low form of flattery.

Freud points out that the supremacy of the intellect is only possible if mankind undergoes a profound change. He emphasizes the fact that the human psyche has certainly undergone a development since earliest times and is no longer what it was at the beginning of our history. He counts among these changes the introjection or "internalization" of the outward compulsion, the creation of the superego. No one denies this development, but development does not necessarily mean progress. What appears as progress subjectively is succeeded by retrogression, by reactions which annul all that has been attained and which distort its shape. The course of human history may be compared with a gigantic pendulum which swings back and forth as senselessly and unpurposefully as the life of the individual. The skeptic will even venture to question whether the strengthening of the superego is indeed such a valuable achievement of civilization. Perhaps this very internalization of outward compulsion has given birth to ego impulses which either gradually smother the ego or break forth in a destructive explosion. At any rate, we see that in neurosis the demands of the superego restrain the individual from the work of civilization as effectively as the demands of the ego. Indeed, these demands not infrequently coincide. The main question is one of proportion. The oversevere superego is just as cruel as external compulsion. It has ruined just as many lives and prompted just as many murders. The differences are not as fundamental as appears at first glance. We must remember that metamorphosis of the instinctual impulses from outer to inner compulsion does not imply any decrease in intensity. In fact, the process of repression itself strengthens these impulses. Further, in an organism which has been refined and differentiated by cultural evolution, stimuli of lesser intensity bring about the same effects which in a cruder, more resistant organism must result from extremely powerful stimuli. God has provided that the elephant can bear loads which would break the back of a horse. A blow which to a primitive man would have been like the prick of a needle would overwhelm a modern civilized man like a hammer blow. Perhaps man would actually be better off if God had not granted him the right of reason.

In discussing the possibilities of cultural evolution Freud points to woman's intellectual limitations, which result, perhaps, from sexual prohibitions. But the peculiarity of feminine mental processes does not imply inferiority. Analysis tells us, of course, that sexual censorship exercises a significant influence upon the thought functions. However, that is not conclusive proof that it alone is responsible for the special character of feminine intelligence. Perhaps here, too, peculiarities of the psychophysical structure, anatomical differences which prevent their using their intelligence in the by no means always reasonable manner of men, account for the fact that women do not think as men do. Certainly, they have their feet more firmly on the ground and are far more submissive to reality than men. We would not have much trouble finding both religious men and unbelievers who agree with the opinion of St. Jerome: *"Tota mulier in utero."*

We suspect, however, that the supremacy of the intellect must fall because of the fundamentally unchangeable nature of man and the power resistance this will offer to any attempts of the intellect at aggrandizement. Freud has shown us clearly that religion makes many claims which it cannot prove. Nevertheless, in all justice we must admit that there are exceptions to this. Religion tells us, "Blessed are the poor in spirit." And this assertion is by no means hollow. Many believers splendidly demonstrate the truth of the maxim. We need only summon to mind the many pious men and saints who were especially beloved of God. But life itself also testifies to the truth of this precept. I shall never forget the happy, indeed rapturous expression of a poor idiot at a psychiatric clinic, and the reflection of it, alas so faint, upon the face of the physician who was treating him. Nay, I do not believe that, for the sake of intelligence, men will renounce stupidity. Like "liberty, equality and fraternity," unreason is a sacred, inalienable human right. The history of all countries, and especially of our beloved Austrian fatherland, proves that men know how to defend this principle, if necessary with sword in hand.

Freud believes that the voice of the intellect, faint though it may be, will eventually make itself heard. And he believes this will be a great event. He also foresees that the great god Logos will not be all-powerful. But unlike his opponent in the dialogue, he does not feel that this is sufficient reason for despairing of the future of mankind and renouncing all interest in the world and in life. Here we may venture to interject that renunciation does not follow from a less optimistic conception of the future, for our interest in life and in the world is stirred mainly by other than intellectual factors. It is fed by powerful instinctual aspirations. Even though we believe that after us comes the deluge, we may still retain intense interest in this life—perhaps even more intense because of that belief.

We feel inclined to say that in the first part of this essay Freud has imparted knowledge. In the latter part he has made a confession of faith. We shall not withhold our great admiration for this brilliantly delineated picture of the future; but it seems to us less compelling than the foregoing. Moreover, it is admittedly more dependent on subjective factors than the rest. It is not outside the bounds of possibility that this picture of Freud's will become reality; but it is certainly striking that his view of the future in the main seems to conform to our wishes. Whereas the main section of Freud's essay shows the future of an illusion, we may say with little exaggeration that this last section presents the illusion of a future.

We might presume to sketch another picture of the future, without abandoning analytic principles. Human civilization is essentially constructed like an obsessional neurosis; it begins with reaction formations against the suppressed instinctual currents. The longer a civilization lasts, the more successful are these restrained impulses in gaining the upper hand; the scales tip steadily in their favor. We can study this process in the decline of Greco-Roman civilization. On the one hand, the Logos as represented by Socrates and the doctrine of Sophrosyne in Greece and by Marcus Aurelius and by the Stoics in Rome, was literally the highest principle. On the other hand, the instinctual forces which had been so long dammed up began to overflow the walls which reason had already undermined—and wrought the destruction of this civilization. Other peoples of unassailed vitality, less spoiled by civilization, following their instincts with untroubled confidence, not yet exhausted by the struggle with the forces of repression, were then able to deal this civilization the death blow. Then the cycle begins again, for all that is here brought forth anew "deserves in the end nonentity." There is nothing to oppose this assumption that our civilization faces the same destiny; that the culture of our little peninsula of Asia will also collapse within a measurable space of time and that more vital and primitive peoples will bring about its end. It is one possibility among many others, and no more unlikely than the others. It is well to remember, of course, that Freud also has presented his picture of the future not as a prophecy but as a suggestion worthy of consideration. He emphatically warns us against taking these reflections for more than just that.

The future is closed to us; we labor on our corner of civilization like those weavers who never see the tapestry they are weaving. We do our work because we have no choice and—we will not deny it—because it gratifies us. The ultimate wisdom remains, "Cultivons notre jardin."

Mankind, in the course of its historical development, has suffered three great disillusionments and humiliations. Let us compare the positions which the representatives of these three disillusionments have had toward religion. Copernicus, who proved that our planet had small claim to be considered the center of the cosmos, closes his book with an impassioned hymn to God, the creator of the heavens and the earth. Darwin, who forced man to surrender his title of the "crown of creation," still clung to religious belief as a sort of reservation against his theory of evolution. Freud shows religion as an illusion which should be eliminated from our concept of culture.

The devout and cautious Copernicus did not dare to publish his work. But during those same years a liberty-loving man, Florian Geyer, became the leader of a movement which demanded freedom from the compulsion of the Church and justice and equality for all men; a movement which abjured all the consolations of heaven and stood stoutly for the principle that our kingdom is of this world. His plain, straightforward, uncomplicated mind had not yet grasped that profound necessity which, in the words of Anatole France, decrees that "the law in its majestic equality forbids both rich and poor to sleep under bridges and to steal bread." Because of his outrageous ideas he was hunted and cut down like a mad dog by the henchmen of the throne and Church. Within these four hundred years there has been no real change; despite all appearances we still live in an era of intellectual coercion. But through those four hundred years the words I have seen engraved on the sword of Florian Geyer still glow with fire, and these words might well stand as motto for Freud's essay, "*Nulla crux, nulla corona.*"

The foregoing critical discussion was first delivered at one of our Wednesday meetings in Freud's home in December, 1927. He was in complete agreement with me about my condemnation of methodological evasions and said, "Those critics who limit their studies to methodological investigations remind me of people who are always polishing their glasses instead of putting them on and seeing with them."

However, Freud rejected my pessimistic outlook. Although he admitted that his more favorable prophecy did not apply to the immediate future, he said that "in the long run" he had faith in the critical and intellectual capabilities of man. He thought these would not fail to fulfill themselves. In the discussion he also conceded that there were useful illusions which advanced civilization; he granted that in the past religion had been valuable as a force for education and progress; but he believed that now it had become a brake upon the progress of civilization and must be cast aside. After the meeting he said smilingly to me, "You are not at all the skeptic you think you are. I would call you a positivist, because you are so thoroughly convinced that man will not progress."

VI

Now I am going to discuss Freud's interpretation of *A Religious Experience* and generalize on the psychological significance of his little essay.

It must be emphasized that the material on which his interpretation is based is extremely scanty. It consists of a brief epistolary communication. The facts are as follows: One day Freud, in the course of an interview, expressed his indifference to the life after death. Shortly afterward an American physician wrote to him recounting a religious experience which he hoped would have some telling effect upon the skeptic. The physician told of how, when he was yet a student, he had been profoundly moved at the sight of the corpse of an old woman with a serene lovely face; and how this event had determined his religious views. When he saw this corpse on the dissection table the thought had suddenly flashed through him: No, there is no God. If there were a God he would never have allowed such a sweet-faced, dear old woman to lie dishonored in the dissection room. This was not the first time he had doubted the teachings of Christianity; but on this afternoon he resolved he would never enter a church again. An inner voice had admonished him to think well before he denied God.

And his mind had replied to this inner voice: If I can be shown with certainty that Christian doctrine is true and that the Bible is the Word of God, I will accept it.

In the course of the next few days God instructed his soul that the Bible is God's Word, that all the teachings about Jesus Christ are true and that Jesus is our sole hope. "After this clear revelation I accepted the Bible as the Word of God and Jesus Christ as my Saviour. Since then God has revealed himself to me by many indisputable signs." The young physician then expresses the hope that God will reveal the truth to Freud's soul also.

Freud, in attempting to interpret the story on the basis of this scant psychological evidence, takes the situation in the dissection room as his clue. The corpse of the old woman reminded the young physician of his dearly loved mother. The mother-longing of the Oedipus complex is aroused, and is accompanied by revolt against the father. The unconscious desire for the destruction of the father found its way to consciousness in the form of doubt of God's existence. This is possible because of the associative and affective connection of the two concepts: God—father. The mother-longing could be translated to the reason as justifiable rage at the abuse of the maternal object, especially since the child's mind believes that the father abuses the mother in sexual intercourse.

This new impulse, then, is no more than another guise of old emotions which have been transferred to the religious realm. And this impulse suffers the same fate as the old emotions. It subsides under the tremendous pressure of inhibition. The psychic conflict ends in complete submission to the will of the Father-God. The young physician becomes and remains a believer.

This remarkable interpretation has been met with the criticism that the paucity of material disallows such far-reaching conclusions concerning the emotional processes of the young physician. I think, however, that in spite of this handicap Freud has successfully and lucidly established the connection between the impression at the sight of the corpse and the subsequent religious conversion. We must admit that the insufficiency of the material obviated an investigation into the details of the psychic process. For psychological analysis it would certainly have been preferable if we had possessed more exact and exhaustive information about the mysterious conversion. However, it may be in the nature of things that the conversion remain mysterious. Dogma maintains that conversion is a process which is psychically and psychologically all but incomprehensible, since, for the most part, it is a manifestation of God's Grace. St. Augustine has impressively described how, at death, Grace inclines the soul of the sinner toward the Faith (if this be his destiny), and how divine virtue takes possession of the human will *"indeclinabiliter et insuperabiliter"* so that it is transformed into a new will.

The physician's letter was written a long time after the experience; nevertheless, in this case the analysis was unable to take into account either the later changes induced by memory or the psychic stratification, both of which would be necessary for a thoroughgoing analytic investigation.

Let us try to explore some of the lesser elements which Freud's more general analysis passed by.

Whence comes the profound impression made by the naked corpse of the woman? Freud's answer is that the sight of the naked old woman reawakened the mother fixation. The memory of the mother, therefore, stirs up mingled feelings of tenderness and sensuality. When we consider that the corpse is lying on a dissection table, we see good reason for diagnosing that there is also present a strong sadistic component of the sexuality of the young man. This sadistic element, transformed into intellectual aggressiveness, later proceeds to question the divinity. When, at the sight of the corpse, there flashed through his mind the thought that there is no God, not only was the mother-longing completed by the revolt against the father, but there was also a transference of the sadistic impulse back to the original object of childhood.

In other words, the sight of the dead woman, who here unconsciously appears as a mother-surrogate, did more than revive longing for the mother. It also stirred the negative Oedipus complex and permitted the counter-impulses, intensified by reaction, to press to the surface of the psyche. Only after that sadistic reaction does the mother once more appear to the physician as the "sweet-faced, dear old woman." Not until then is the old Oedipus reaction allowed to appear in its original intensity and form: as revolt against the father. It is by no means immaterial that it was a dead woman, a naked corpse which prompted the old emotions. The sight of the corpse, by reawakening the unconscious sadistic impulses, also caused the revival of the whole emotional constellation of the child. As soon as the one instinctual goal had been attained by the revolt against the Father-God, this regression could take place.

It is noteworthy that the religious conversion of the physician proceeded from a sight experience. The analyst is well acquainted with the intimate connection between the peeping impulse and desire for knowledge, the investigatory impulse. The child frequently experiences the frustration of the earliest forms of this impulse when he is punished for improper desires to look at what he is not supposed to see. Thus the little boy is scolded for his sexual curiosity about the body of his mother or his nurse. There is a regression to this early experience in the situation at the dissection table. Along with the unconscious memory of the mother, the old rage against the father is also aroused. The father always represented interference and prohibition to the child's sexuality.

It is significant that in the processes the physician describes, the sexual strivings appear to focus in the eye, while the forbidding and repressing forces take the ear for organ. The profound impression the sight of the woman's corpse made upon the young doctor was succeeded by doubts which manifested themselves in the form of an inner dialogue. A warning voice speaks within him and his mind replies to it. It is not hard to understand what aspects of the development of the child are here repeated. The inner voice is a manifestation of the superego, of the father of childhood who has been absorbed into the ego. It is he who warns against the release of the impulses and the defiance to God. Here, then, the uprising of obscure impulses is put down by the memory of the father's voice and of the voices of his representatives whom the child revered and dreaded: the teacher and the priest. There is a curious reaction to this prohibition. The ego ("my spirit") responds: If I can be shown with certainty that Christian doctrine is true and that the Bible is the Word of God, I will accept it. Such demand for proof is an old story for theology. Again and again characters in the Bible and in the other holy books plead for some proof of religious truths which will be accessible to their senses. They want signs and miracles, and signs and miracles are always vouchsafed them.

The counterpart of this religious phenomenon is to be found in obsessional neurosis. Often enough, in the treatment of obsessional neurotics, we meet with those characteristic dependent clauses which are presumed to establish the strange connection between such an omen and an expected or dreaded event. Psychologically, there is no great difference between the religious pattern of the American physician and the obsessional idea that seizes upon a neurotic patient as he walks down the street: "If the streetcar passes that lamppost before the automobile does, my father's operation will be successful." Cause and effect notions of this kind derive their affective value from the belief in the omnipotence of thought. Such ideas are always arising out of the inexhaustible reservoir of the unconscious. Yet in this case we may also assume that preconscious memories of the tradition of Christianity were responsible. At any rate, the profound, lingering influence of Christian doctrine is indicated by the fact that three times in close succession the Bible is spoken of as the "Word of God." ("If I can be shown with certainty that . . . the Bible is the Word of God"; "In the course of the next few days God instructed my soul that the Bible was God's Word . . ."; "After this clear revelation I accepted the Bible as the Word of God . . .") This inconspicuous, though for the analyst pointed, repetition serves as an unconscious confession. It leads us to believe that the reactionary tendencies may be traced back to the religious doctrines which were dinned into the ears of the child.

We can now reconstruct what went on in the psyche of the physician during those anguished days when God revealed to him that the Bible was His Word. By reaction, the religious doctrines of childhood have been lent increased effectiveness in the unconscious memory. This effectiveness is based originally on familiar phrases heard so often about the parental household and carrying with them powerful affective overtones. This is particularly interesting in this connection because it is these very religious doctrines which contribute, at a certain age, to over-coming the infantile Oedipus complex, thus paving the way for the child's entrance into the social order. Freud remarks that the conflict in the young physician seems to have manifested itself as a hallucinatory psychosis. We might add that this auricular hallucination of the young doctor's was a regression to religious phrases with an aura of strong emotion. The conversion took place through unconscious, affective cathexis of childhood impres-sions, especially those pertaining to childhood doctrines and symbolism.

The poet, wishing to present such an experience in dramatic form, quite justly reproduces in objective action the process which appears here as subjective. Though he can rely for symbols only on sense impressions, he will nevertheless manage to convince us that his character has been experiencing profoundly affective childhood impressions. The young doctor's mysterious conver-sion, with its undercurrent childhood religious impressions, may remind many readers of the Easter Eve scene in Goethe's *Faust*. Here the sound of the Easter bells in the church and the singing of the Easter choral, "Christ Is Risen," makes the doubt-ridden and despairing Faust remember the days of his childhood:

> This sound, habitual to my dearest youth,
> Now summons me again into this life.

It is these childhood impressions that make the sound of the bells and the choral song powerful, soothing, heavenly tones. In both situations the *"holde Nachricht,"* the "sweet message," is reinforced by the overtones of the childhood feelings it once aroused.

Though the release of the impulses has been accomplished and the unconscious memories reawakened, our young physician is once more seized with the old yearning. The religious teachings, the childhood fables which had gone to oblivion, become real to him again and he believes as fervently as he once had. The mother-longing is here isolated from the longing for the loving and protecting father.

This, then, is the inevitable result of the conflict; love alone cannot resolve it. Freud's conception of the emotional process may be schematically outlined in this way: Sight of the naked body of the dead woman—(unconscious) reawakening of the mother-longing; revolt (wish for the death of the father)—(conscious) doubt of the existence of God; revulsion against this and conversion by reaction. This outline requires a psychoanalytical supplement: the wish for the father's death (in the displacement: doubt of God) unconsciously provokes the release of intense effects in the young man, which essentially are nothing less than fear for his own life (fear of castration). These effects could not reach the consciousness; but they evidence themselves first in the emergence and later in the triumph of the admonishing inner voice. If we may translate unconscious processes into the language of consciousness, this is, roughly, the train of thought: If I revolt against the father and kill him (the Father-God), I shall be punished just as this woman was, who now lies on the dissection table. Our analytic experience gives us ample justification for these deductions that fill in the gaps in the emotional process. For analysis has indicated that fear is a reigning factor in the psyche.

Once the death wish has emerged (i.e., the doubt of the existence of God), the prevailing attitude is now no longer determined by ambivalence, but also by the alternation of defiance and unconscious anxiety. This vacillation between hatred and affection, defiance and anxiety, lasts for days. The denouement is a crisis in which the hate impulses, intensified by fear, attempt to force themselves into the consciousness in all their primitive might. And, involved as they are with the Oedipus complex, they threaten to drag this complex to the surface. At the height of this crisis the aggressive and hostile impulses are then thrown back upon themselves under the influence of the unconscious fear of castration. This is a re-enactment in a telescoped form of what took place when the Oedipus complex was first suppressed. Submission to God and the religious tradition are therefore conditioned by the re-emergence of the fear of castration.

The overpowering homosexual tendency of the young physician, in its highly sublimated, religious form, now makes him a proselytizer; he strives to unite his brothers ("brother physician" in the letter to Freud), to unite all mankind in love for the father. The "saviour tendency" is a well-known peculiarity among certain educated classes of the American people. How much stronger must this tendency become when the individual in question commands such profound and mysteriously won knowledge of the Absolute. But it cannot be completely concealed that even this all-embracing love is essentially nothing but a reaction to extreme rebellious impulses. Its explosive quality, its eagerness to convert, derives from those repressed aggressive impulses. Just so an unconscious desire betrays its intensity by the severity of the inhibition. The very violence is diverted to the service of the opposing factors. We can now understand the development in the unconscious of the young doctor's conversion as a regressive process. Thereby we have cleared up much of the mystery. Now we can also propound a better evaluation of the emotional situation which prevailed when the letter was written:

> The wild desires no longer win us,
> The deeds of passion cease to chain;
> The love of Man revives within us,
> The love of God revives again.

His religious faith, which has been gained at the cost of so much conflict and which is retained despite all the arguments of reason, is therefore the counterpart of the extreme rebellious tendencies from which it was wrested. The fathers of the Church would doubtless describe the psychic experiences preceding his eventual enlightenment as one of those salutary ordeals which so frequently precede the *conversio*.

Once more there wells up from the hidden sources of the psyche a wave of rebellion and anger, finally to be engulfed in the undertow. The young man's revolt against a cruel and tyrannical God yields under the pressure of psychic reaction. *"Die Träne quillt, der Himmel hat ihn wieder.*" ("The tears burst forth, and Heaven has regained him.")

So much for the psychological analysis of this case. Wherein lies the more general scientific significance of Freud's essay, the broader implications of this individual case? I believe that these four pages of Freud's essay analyzing this religious experience are a great advance toward a deeper general understanding of the conversion process. Modern religious science has collected a wealth of material on the psychology of conversion. These works treat of some of the points we must consider here.* William James finds the unconscious—which he conceives in the old, static fashion—of considerable significance in conversion. More recent literature on the psychology of religion deals with psychoanalytic findings as well. Nevertheless, the fundamental psychic processes of conversion were not clarified. However, we can understand them if we, disregarding the features peculiar to the case Freud has discussed, reflect upon the essential result of his analysis. It is well to proceed from cases just such as this, which are characterized by a sudden, mysterious illumination. When we arrive at an understanding of what motivates such *"conversione fulminea"* (so de Sanctis terms these cases, in contrast to the examples of *"conversione progressiva"*),** we shall also approach an understanding of the psychic processes in slower, more gradual conversions.

Analytic psychology now presents the remarkable conclusion that the most important prerequisite for conversion is the unconscious emergence of powerful hostile and aggressive impulses directed against the father; that these undergo displacement and are expressed as doubts of God. The essential feature of the conversion process consists in the emotional reaction against this uprising in the unconscious of hate and revolt. The affection

* Cf. Joh. Herzog, *Der Beruf der Bekehrung*, 1903; W. James, *The Varieties of Religious Experience*, 1903; E. D. Starbuck, *The Psychology of Religion*, 1910. Further, the well-known more modern works of de Sanctis, Girgensohn, Oesterreich, etc.

** Sancte de Sanctis, *La Conversione Religiosa* (Bologna, 1904), p. 53.

which has been born out of reaction to the "bad" impulses will then express itself in utter submission to the love object and faith in the doctrines, commands, and prohibitions it represents. The close resemblance between the effects of love and the phenomena of religious conviction will undoubtedly seem strange to conscious psychology; but pastoral theology for several centuries has accepted it as a matter of course. The turning point of the psychic process is the appearance of the unconscious fear (fear of castration) which follows in the wake of the emerging hate impulses.

Freud's little essay has great significance because it clarifies this process. Within his discussion of the individual case there lies the solution to the enigmatic universal case. Conversion arises out of an eruption of the impulses which provoke unconscious hate tendencies toward the father. This in turn sets in motion a whole mechanism of reaction through fear and affection. All the various metamorphoses of conversion—and the literature on the subject shows how many these are—can be included under this psychological explanation. Whether the psychic process is instigated by any special event, as here, or whether it results from prolonged conflicts, the ecstatic state of the ego is the product of that unconscious reaction.

This essay of Freud's has also opened broader vistas for religious science. Conversion is so closely related to revelation that the two expressions are frequently used interchangeably. It would be more accurate to say that the core of many cases of conversion is a kind of mysterious revelation. We do not realize the scope of Freud's little essay until we extend the results to the field of cultural history. The conclusions of this analysis prove to be valid also for phenomena of the collective psyche. Every revelation arises out of revolt against the divinity, and evinces that powerful reaction which results from fear and affection. The tradition of the Revelation on Mt. Sinai, upon which Jewish and Christian religion is based, tells how the Israelite tribes revolted against their chief, how they were intimidated and ultimately subjected. Here we have a personal, intrapsychic event represented as an external, historical happening; as uprising followed by threats and punishments which compel the people to obey. The voice of

Jahveh becomes audible and pronounces the commandments, the "Thou shalt" and "Thou shalt not." Psychoanalysis has shown that these at heart are nothing but the suppression of unconscious incestuous and insurgent impulses. What appears as *"veritates a coelo delapsae"* are distinctly of earthly origin and earthly motivation. Freud's theory about the case of conversion is equally valid for the Revelation on Sinai.

For this reason I have hopes that the young psychoanalysts of religion, whom the official religious psychologists superciliously condemn, will come to even more revealing, and perhaps conclusive, discoveries. We are still a long way from a thorough psychological understanding of the arcane ways of religion; but analytic research has come closer to piercing the mysteries than all previous research.

VII

THE essay "Dostoyevsky and Patricide" served as preface to that great Dostoyevsky edition in which the sources, outlines, and fragments of *The Brothers Karamazov* are compiled and critically evaluated.* Unquestionably, this was the proper place for this study which offers such original and important insight into the life and creation of the great novelist.

In their preliminary remarks the editors express their gratitude to Freud for composing "specially for the occasion this deeply penetrating analysis of Dostoyevsky and his *Brothers Karamazov.*" Does this mean that the essay was merely an occasional piece? In more than one sense it was. Certainly, the occasion gave Freud the opportunity to put old reflections into an appropriate form. And it is equally certain that the occasion did not evoke these reflections. But while we welcome the stimulus that led him to embody his thoughts in writing, it would have been preferable had

* F. M. Dostoyevsky, *Die Urgestalt der Brüder Karamasoff*, Editors: René Fülöp-Miller und Friedrich Eckstein (München: R. Piper & Co., Verlag).

they not been composed "specially for the occasion." For in that case, there is little doubt that Freud would have added some very welcome material and would have gone far beyond the bounds set by a preface. And some of his remarks which now seem somewhat forced interpolations could have been developed within a broader framework.

Freud first pays tribute to the richness of Dostoyevsky's personality. He describes him as a poet, neurotic, moralist, and sinner. It is as though Freud had slipped open a fan to reveal the curious lettering and interesting pictures on the folds. Little space is devoted to Dostoyevsky the artist, and Freud intimates that psychoanalysis must lay down its arms before the problem of the writer. But, we may assume, only before the biological aspect of this problem, before the question of special innate gifts. For psychoanalysis has a great deal to contribute in questions of artistic creation. It can explain much about unconscious instinctual forces and mechanisms, as well as the obscure psychic predispositions which govern conception and form. Indeed, it has already done a great deal in this field. We have found that the processes of artistic creation are far less inscrutable than has been thought, although they are still mysterious enough.

Freud feels that Dostoyevsky is most vulnerable as moralist. When we consider him as a moral man, we must seriously object to his ideal that only one who has experienced the lowest depths of sinfulness can attain the highest morality. He who alternately sins and then, in repentance, makes lofty moral demands of himself, has in reality greatly simplified matters. For what is morality but renunciation? Dostoyevsky's own life, Freud continues, was torn between alternate outbreak of the impulses and repentance.

Our first impression of this judgment is that it is stern but just. On second thought it seems sterner than just. Yet why does Freud's discussion of the concept of morality strike us as dubious and inadequate? It is because his negative statement seems to have more truth than his attempted positive formulation. We freely grant that his is not the highest stage of morality who alternately sins and then sincerely repents. But while once upon a time renunciation was the sole criterion of morality, it is now but one of many. If it were the sole criterion, then the upright middle-class philistine, to whose shabby imagination submission is natural, and to whose blunt senses renunciation is easy, would be morally far greater than Dostoyevsky. If we pursued this sentiment we would arrive at the proverb: A good conscience is the best rule of health. This is all very well, but it merely explains why there are so many sluggards, so many contented and satiated men who have gained "wretched self-complacency," as Nietzsche put it, out of renunciation. Renunciation in itself is, after all, not so important. What we respect is renunciation that is the victory over powerful impulses. We cannot overlook the intensity of temptation in our concept of that compromise we customarily call morality. Where there is no sin there is no religion. Religion would not last for a day if the heart of man were relieved of guilt (and affiliated ideas like taboo, unclean, and their like).

Let us not succumb to shallow and conventional judgments; we must perceive that morality resides in the struggle with drives and not in the victory over them. In this sense the criminal who abandons himself to his vicious instincts can in many cases be considered more moral than the solid citizen who escapes his instincts by renouncing them. Satan, too, was an angel like the others and he remains a great theologian before God—and against God. The concept of renunciation seems obvious only in the most superficial sense. Its full meaning unfolds to us only when we understand the part played by the instinctual goal. For psychologically, renunciation is another method of gratification of the instincts, a method which sacrifices crude material pleasure for the privilege of enjoying that pleasure in fantasy. The instincts are again victorious, but in sublimated form, and the victory can be attained at small cost. The differences between this kind of gratification and others are only quantitative.

Freud believes that Dostoyevsky's kind of compromise with morality is a typically Russian trait. In reality it is a universal human trait. Only in the extremes between one emotional state and the other is this a national peculiarity, that is, a quality dependent upon the history and destiny of a people. Such a struggle between the demands of the instincts and the requirements of society will take a certain form and have such an outcome according to the period and the culture of the community. In the case of

Dostoyevsky, these two factors have left their unmistakable imprint on his compromise with morality which is in itself a compromise. Throughout his life the great artist unconsciously stood in the heavy shadow of that unfortunate error which nineteen hundred years ago separated mankind into saints and sinners. The dominance of this view in his psyche explains the hypertrophy of his conscience and the radical swings between sin and repentance. We children of another age, which appears as a progressed one to simpler spirits, are no longer capable of fully understanding the psychology of the Russian people of this period. No one who has not grown up in this cultural milieu and has not early undergone the profound influence of Christianity can project himself into the feelings of these people. Religious upbringing added a new, more refined form of gratification of the impulses to the old ways: the voluptuousness of giving oneself up for lost, of knowing that one was damned. It is very hard for us to comprehend emotionally the orgies of passion and suffering which were the psychological aftermath of this attitude.

It was such factors that prescribed the fate of Dostoyevsky's instincts. They also were responsible in part for his moral views. Dostoyevsky would never, for example, have admitted that a man, however moral he be, can experience inner temptation without that experience being a surrender to it. He would take an even sterner stand than Freud's, declaring that the very appearance of forbidden impulses is in itself immoral. He would insist upon the letter of the Saviour's parable: he who merely looks with desire upon his neighbor's wife is an adulterer. This urgent moral imperative leads us to a strange fatalism, for sinning in thought is inevitable. Therefore, the sinful act does not matter. In fact, the unconscious guilt feeling requires it. Whoever knows himself damned has no reason to shun any of the byways on the road to hell. Nor has the hangman who is leading a murderer to the gallows any reason to expect that the condemned man will be docile and make no trouble. Dostoyevsky's life shows that he harbored such temptations and fantasies always with a deep feeling of guilt, and with spells of violent abandon.

To Freud's moral ideal—the complete renunciation as soon as the temptation appears—Dostoyevsky would rejoin that it was certainly the purest and most beautiful, but that God in His inscrutable counsel had not designed this way for mortal man. Numerous saints of the Church are precedents, he would say, that above all he who attains virtue through sin and repentance is pleasing to God. In the light of human frailty, Freud's moral program would seem superhuman to Dostoyevsky. And how the pharisees would distort and make a mock of it, extolling their own renunciation to God, and putting by all suggestions that they have anything in common with sinners.

It is understandable that, with such psychic predispositions, Dostoyevsky resolved this inner conflict by bowing completely before all secular and ecclesiastical authority. We may regret this, but we cannot condemn it. Freud points out that Dostoyevsky failed "to become a teacher and liberator of mankind; instead he joined forces with humanity's jailers." Freud adds, "The cultural future of mankind will have little to thank him for."

Now it is perfectly true that Fyodor Michailovitch Dostoyevsky sought the shelter of the old jail that he was used to from childhood. In keeping with his time and his milieu, he was not eager to inspect the spick-and-span new ones. Loving the old illusion, he did not care to exchange it for a modern one with the fine-sounding name of freedom. He saw that progress was marching stoutly along on the wrong track, and he chose to remain outside of the procession. He shared the admirable prejudice about a more splendid future for mankind; but he felt that life without religion would be as empty and meaningless as is reality. He preferred to cherish the old illusion—and we cannot take him to task for this.

"The cultural future of mankind will have little to thank him for." Very true, for everything points to this, that the men of the future will look upon thinking as a kind of infectious disease which prevents the possibility of being happy. (Perhaps they will discover with some satisfaction that already many of the scientists of our time have acquired immunity to this serious malady.) But whatever may be our opinion about this future, it is clear that gratitude will not be one of its virtues. We know that the men of our time are mediocre, capricious, petty, mean, and wretched. We know that they were thus in earlier times; and we have no reason to think that in the future they will be generous, resolute, noble, helpful, and good. If they should turn out so, they would have to thank Dostoyevsky from the bottom of their hearts. Not, however, for the religious and political goals he sought. (The Russian soul will not be the redeemer of the human race any more than the German soul.) The future will have very little use for his Christian or national program. But then, neither do the ethics of Homer, the Bible or Shakespeare govern our lives any longer. Today Goethe's political views seem provincial and antiquated to us. The close of his *Faust,* in which the Catholic heaven opens, impresses us as a painful discord amid music of the spheres. Schiller's nationalistic and social ideas have meaning only for adolescents. For the apostolic life of the older Tolstoi, whom we revere as a poet and psychologist, we have only pity and an almost superior tolerance.

The political and religious opinions of great poets are simply not important. Reforming mankind is not their task on earth, nor do they hold the future of humanity in the hollow of their hands. Heavy industry and munitions works are much more influential. Any petty boss in a political party can advocate political and social programs. The ward heeler's smile is mightier than the pen. Every statesman and political leader of today who helps the insulted and injured win their rights has a juster claim to the title of ethical liberator than the writer whose art portrays their wretched fate for us.

But the poet can show us human beings who are mirrors of ourselves and to whom we are mirrors. And on this stage of the world he presents the drama of the human condition, its coldness and darkness and effort, the rise and decline of our fates. He extracts some meaning from the misery of man as well as from his absurd aspirations and desires. Who can do this but one blessed of God—a writer like Fyodor Michailovitch Dostoyevsky, whose political and religious ideas seem so abstruse, limited, and foolish to us? That future civilization which may owe nothing to Dostoyevsky should nevertheless honor him for his creation of characters whose terrible and calm genius shakes the utmost depths of our souls. He has offered the men of the future insights that are almost visionary. He has offered them wonderful and strange emotions which surely are beyond the power of social reformers or apostles to give. His religious and political beliefs have come to nothing—his God has been dethroned long ago. But the prayer that was breathed by his creative spirit will be mightier than all the prayers he addressed to the God of the Christians. That prayer, in the words of the hymn of Hrabanus Maurus, goes:

Veni, creator spiritus:
. . . Accende lumen sensibus.

Freud's critical attitude toward Dostoyevsky, for whom, certainly, he has no great love, becomes gentler and more objective as soon as he leaves off making evaluations and steps into his own field of depth-psychology. Here there is no more caution, no more feeble argument, and he masterfully opens the hidden way to the life of emotions. All philosophical differences cease to matter, all divisions of period and culture disappear, and a man stands naked before us, shipwrecked in a tempest, but stranded on Prospero's island, where his most secret thoughts are recognized. Where Freud thinks as a psychologist and not as a moralist, he no longer bothers his head about the Commandments. He sees the man alone, suffering at the insufficiency of human existence, his genius caught in the snares of his environment.

It was merely by chance that a great writer was the object of this analytic study. The advantage and desirability of such an object is that the man reveals himself as other men cannot. Those revelations are often oblique and obscure, sudden flashes which illuminate one corner of his being, leaving the greater part in even deeper shadow.

But Freud's analysis of Dostoyevsky's unconscious attachment to his father fell like a long shadow upon his impressionable ego and colored forever after the nature and effects of his malady. The father's mysterious influence ruled his life and work. It was this force that drove him into the abyss and exalted him to the heights. With a few short strokes Freud draws a picture of the history of a man's psyche, of the determinants of his illness and of the meaning of his symptoms. Freud has thrown more light upon Dostoyevsky's being than has any literary critic or biographer.

The crowning point in this analysis is the explanation of the writer's malady. Freud shows how a powerful instinctual desire may turn about and attack the desirer himself; how in an epileptic fit the "other self" enters the ego and how the death of this other is well-nigh an experience of the death of the ego itself.

From this point the analysis broadens and by subtle degrees Freud approaches the major problem, the essence of this personality. He provides the long-sought explanation of the daemonic elements in Dostoyevsky's life and work. He shows them to be the play of hidden emotional forces against opposing impulses. The daemon is not alien to the ego, but merely alienated. Daemonic impulses are not newcomers in the psyche; they are merely the reappearance of old, submerged drives. The inner relation between Dostoyevsky's fate and that of his characters becomes clearer. In both there is waged the same struggle between elemental drives and the powers of conscience, a perpetuation of the more ancient struggle between the still feeble ego and the outer world.

Freud has wonderful insight into how such conflicts were bound up with Dostoyevsky's religious and nationalistic views, however apart they may seem. He shows us how they figured in both the personality of the writer and of his characters, for these latter are personifications of the potentialities of the ego. They are the developed offshoots of the ego. When Freud links up Oedipus, Hamlet, and the Brothers Karamazov, drawing comparisons between them as various facets of the same latent content, he thereby contributes profoundly to our understanding of the basic drives which impel men's lives, whatever the times, the culture, the race or the person. The laws have been obscure, but they are becoming ever more accessible.

The last section of the study concerns itself with an extremely interesting interpretation of Dostoyevsky's passion for gambling. Freud's surprising, but persuasive theory is that this passion is derived from the masturbatory compulsion in the child. The unsuccessful efforts to overcome the habit and the resultant self-castigation find their parallel in the compulsion to gamble. This observation illuminates a complex and little-understood aspect of Dostoyevsky's life.

We may notice an abrupt transition between this section and the main theme. Perhaps our impression is that the author has turned arbitrarily to this new subject because it interests him and not because it has any special connection with the whole. And yet there is a very definite organic connection. What inspires the efforts to suppress masturbation is nothing else but fear of the father. This Freud intimates in a single word at the end of the section.

Unfortunately, Freud breaks off his analysis at this point. Had he continued, I believe he would have pointed out how the gambling passion later assumes a form whose motivation and mechanisms are akin to certain obsession symptoms. Gambling, which never had as its end money or gain, becomes a kind of question addressed to destiny. It is a form of oracle which the modern psyche readily accepts, although this latent meaning does not become conscious. Now, recalling that destiny is the ultimate father-surrogate, we see the significance in the unconscious of this questioning. Originally it sought to discover whether or not expectation of evil was justified. In other words, would the threatened punishment for the trespass be carried out or would the angered father forgive the son? Good or bad luck stands as symbol of the answer. Observing the rules of the game is the psychological equivalent of obedience to the compulsive neurotic symptoms. Uncertainty plays the same role in gambling as it does in the compulsion complex. Take, for example, a game like patience. Here we can see clearly the oracular meaning, which is obscured in other games where new players may enter late and where the prime purpose seems to be gain.

We have certain criticisms to make, even as we realize that this is the most valuable psychological work on Dostoyevsky we possess. Our first criticism is directed to the section just discussed. In this section Freud adduces the example of a story by Stefan Zweig. Which are the connecting links? The following: here the gambling compulsion of Dostoyevsky, there the same passion in one of the characters of Zweig's story. Stefan Zweig has devoted himself to a study of Dostoyevsky. We must confess that these are few and very loose connections. They serve as the barest possible reason for dragging in such an illustration, but there is certainly no reason for the lengthy summary of the Zweig story. It seems strange that Freud, usually so good at ordering his material economically, should devote four pages out of a twenty-six-page study of Dostoyevsky—nearly one-sixth, that is—to a parenthetical illustration. With all due respect to Zweig's literary merit, we cannot help feeling that this is an error in proportion. It is as though a medieval artist painting the Passion of Christ should place in the foreground of the picture the bishop of his native diocese.

There is another criticism, perhaps equally minor. In his introduction Freud separates Dostoyevsky's personality into four principal aspects: the poet, the neurotic, the moralist, and the sinner. Should he not have given recognition to another aspect, that of the great psychologist? (Perhaps Freud includes the psychologist with the writer, yet it would seem worthy of special mention.) Ours is a time when every mediocre psychotherapeutic practitioner thinks the soul is an open book to him—and every assistant at a neurologic clinic who has read Freud with happy carelessness and thorough misunderstanding believes he knows the human mind up and down. In such a time as this, we feel, it would be fitting that one of the greatest psychologists should salute the writer who was one of his great precursors, a salutation out of his own solitude to the other's solitude.

In this study the rapid, compressed style of Freud's last writings is evident, but here, in harmony with the subject, it is fluid and emotional in spite of its density. Many of his phrases are stamped forever in my memory because they were expressed in a language which was a rare union of succinctness and comprehensiveness, forcefulness and delicacy, directness and richness of association.

Our ultimate impression remains that this study of Freud's has an honored place in the scientific literature on Dostoyevsky—and more. For this penetration into the deepest levels of the psyche, this revelation of a man's unique, hidden qualities and of the qualities he shares with all men—such vision is something new in applied psychology, something which did not exist before psychoanalysis.

4/14/29

. . . I have read your critical review of my Dostoyevsky study with great pleasure. All your objections are worth considering, and certain of them, I admit, have hit the nail on the head. However, there are some points I can advance in my own defense that are, you understand, not quibblings over who is right and who wrong.

I think you have applied too high a standard to this trivial essay. It was written as a favor for someone and written reluctantly. I always write reluctantly nowadays. I know that you observed that this was so. Naturally, I am not saying this to justify hasty or distorted judgments, but merely to explain the careless architecture of the whole. It cannot be disputed that the parenthetical Zweig analysis disturbs the balance. If we look deeper, we can probably find what was the purpose for its addition. Had I been free to disregard the place where the essay was to appear, I would certainly have written: "We may diagnose that in the history of a neurosis characterized by so severe a guilt feeling, the struggle with masturbation plays a special part. This diagnosis is completely confirmed by Dostoyevsky's pathologic passion for gambling. For, as we see in a story by Zweig . . ." That is, the attention devoted to Zweig's story is not dictated by the relationship of Zweig to Dostoyevsky, but of masturbation to neurosis. Still, it did take an awkward turn.

I will hold to my belief in a scientifically objective social standard of ethics, and therefore I would not contest in the least the upright philistine's right to call his behavior good and moral, even though he has attained it at the cost of little self-conquest. At the same time I will grant your subjective, psychological view of ethics. Although I agree with your opinions on the world and present-day man, I cannot, as you know, share your pessimistic rejection of a better future.

Certainly I subsumed Dostoyevsky the psychologist under the poet. I might also have charged against him that his insight was so entirely restricted to the workings of the abnormal psyche. Consider his astounding helplessness before the phenomena of love; he really only understands either crude, instinctive desire or masochistic submission and love from pity. You are also quite right in your assumption that I do not really like Dostoyevsky, despite all my admiration for his power and nobility. That comes from the fact that my patience with pathological natures is completely exhausted in my daily work. In art and life I am intolerant toward them. That is a personal trait, not binding on others.

Where do you intend to publish your essay? I think very highly of it. Scientific research alone must work without prejudices. With all other thinking it is impossible to avoid choosing a point of view, and naturally there are many possible ones. . . .

Freud gave me permission in 1929 to publish this fine letter. It serves as an excellent refutation of the stupid allegations about Freud's dogmatism and his pessimistic view of life.

The remark on Dostoyevsky's limited understanding of love gives me a welcome opening for quoting another of Freud's comments on love. "Les Cahiers Contemporains" published in Paris in 1926 a little book called *Au delà de l'amour* which contained a questionnaire on the essence of love beyond the realm of sex. Freud wrote:

My Dear Sir:
It is quite impossible for me to fulfill your request. Really, you ask too much. Up to the present I have not yet found the courage to make any broad statements on the essence of love, and I think that our knowledge is not sufficient.

Very truly yours,
Freud

PART TWO

The Confessions of an Analyst

The Confessions of an Analyst

WE ARE all proud of certain experiences and qualities, and ashamed of others, but we sometimes meet people who seem to be proud of things we would not boast of and others who are ashamed of qualities and circumstances over which there is nothing to feel disgraced. Self-observation and comparison of ourselves with these persons tell us that the same experiences or qualities would not awaken similar feelings in us. We speak of false shame and false pride when we meet with such inappropriate feelings.

The new psychology has added some significant features to the pictures of false pride and false shame. Psychoanalytic experience shows that men or women do not always know what they are ashamed or proud of. Qualities or experiences which most people are proud to have are anxiously hidden by some as if they were disgraceful. Other qualities are conspicuously exhibited, although most people would be embarrassed to mention them. There is more in such concealment or demonstration than meets the eye of the average observer. The opposite feelings of pride and shame are not independent of each other. There is a secret tie between them, and in most cases we discover that displaced or distorted shame is connected with false pride. A careful analysis which penetrates to the origin of these puzzling feelings often discovers that they owe their intensity to a process of displacement which shifts the emotional accent from important issues to apparently insignificant details.

Here is an instance from personal experience of false shame. For many years I carefully hid a fact which other people might have mentioned with harmless pride, namely, that in my nineteenth year I had read every line Goethe had published. I went through the *Weimarer*, or *Sophien*, edition, 55 volumes of poetic works, 13 volumes of scientific papers, the diaries in 15 volumes, and the letters in 50 volumes. I also read the many collections of Goethe's conversations, as well as most books and papers on Goethe which the Vienna University Library then had, and that was a considerable number of books. It is not important that I read all these volumes, but why did I never mention the fact? Why did I keep it secret as if I were ashamed of it?

There were many opportunities later on, for instance in conversations with literary friends and writers, to drop a remark about my Goethe reading. I remember such an occasion which came rather late. It must have been about 1926 or 1927, more than twenty years after my Goethe obsession. One summer afternoon, Franz Werfel, Alma Maria, the widow of Gustav Mahler who had become Werfel's wife, a friend, and I sat in the library of the beautiful cottage which the composer had bought in Breitenstein on the Semmering near Vienna. Mrs. Werfel pointed to the many volumes containing Goethe's letters and told me that Mahler used to say, "I reserve this reading for the years of my old age." During the ensuing conversation on Goethe I felt the temptation to reveal that in my nineteenth year I had read all of Goethe in print, but the impulse disappeared immediately. There were other such occasions, but with the exception of my own analysis I never spoke of my compulsive reading of Goethe when I was a youth. Why was I ashamed of it?

To understand my secrecy, I must revive an important part of my young years, and awaken painful memories of grief and repentance. I do not agree with those writers who assert that such resurrection of the past is not difficult. To change the tenses is easy only on paper, but not in emotional experience. To recall feelings and impulses one is ashamed of, to admit emotions to others which one has not even admitted to oneself, is by no means an easy task. Our memories are conveniently derelict in such matters and we are only too apt to forget not only events, but also feelings and tendencies we did not like in ourselves. The dialogue which Nietzsche once imagined should be varied in this sense: "Thus I felt and thought," says my memory. "This I could not have felt and thought," says my pride. And my memory gives in. Such compliance of our memories with regard to unpleasant recollections is unavoidable. When one endeavors with all moral courage and sincerity to reconstruct what has been suppressed and repressed, one should be satisfied with incomplete results and not expect to attain the impossible and complete reconstruction of the past.

As for my compulsive Goethe study, more than forty years ago, my memory is somewhat bolstered by reference to a concrete event of those days. The emotional experiences out of which my strange labor emerged are vividly recalled in reading a paper about them I wrote a few years later. In this paper I tried in retrospect to understand my odd behavior by means of the newly learned method of self-analysis. The paper lies on my desk now, as I write. It is entitled, "On the Effect of Unconscious Death-Wishes" ("*Ueber die Wirkungen unbewusster Todeswünsche*"). I wrote it in 1913, seven years after the experiences out of which my Goethe study emerged. This article was published anonymously in 1914 in Volume II of the *Internationale Zeitschrift für Aerztliche Psychoanalyse* edited by Sigmund Freud. A short footnote contains the following sentences: "Most of the following analysis is made on a person whose mental good health I have no reason to doubt: on myself. It would be petty, if we analysts would refrain from the analysis of our own fantasies after our master and some of his students have published interpretations of their own dreams. The personal sacrifice appears small compared with the profit·which could accrue to research out of such reports. It is to be hoped that the intellectual interest of the reader in these complex problems will lead him to forget that the person analyzed is the analyst himself."

The spirit of these sentences would be more commendable if the author had signed his name to his paper. I can partly excuse him, since in his analytic report some persons were mentioned who were then still alive. Reasons of discretion made it necessary to remain anonymous, but I suspect that discretion appeared to him then as the better part of valor. The young man however has become an old man in the meantime, and he thinks it is never too late for moral courage and for overcoming the fright we feel in facing up to our own thoughts. He still believes in what he wrote then, more than forty years ago, as his creed for psychological explorers. In the following paragraphs I shall follow that fragmentary analysis of 1913 as it was then published, supplementing it only as it concerns my Goethe study, which is, of course, not mentioned in the paper. Here are the events and experiences which preceded it, the soil from which this strange plant grew.

My father died of arteriosclerosis on June 16, 1906. I was eighteen years old. This blow hit me a few days before the final examinations that open the doors of the university to the students. In those days this final examination did not signify merely the completion of high school. In keeping with its name (*Maturitätsprüfung*) it marked the student's arrival at maturity, in addition to academic achievement.

(The subject in which I had been least successful during my high school years had been mathematics. When I returned to school, after my father's funeral, I often felt the glance of my mathematics instructor resting on me. I must have looked rather miserable because the old man, who resembled my father in figure and bearing, looked at me as though he felt sorry for me. On the day before the examination, he stopped me on the stairs of the school, said a few casual words, and slipped a little paper into my hand. On it were the questions he would ask me the next day. He said, shortly, "Adieu" and went downstairs. He died two days after the examination, of the same disease as my father. This episode was also woven into the pattern of my obsession-thoughts later on.)

The death of my father threw me into an emotional turmoil of the strangest kind. I did not understand then what had happened to me and in me. I was unable to grasp the meaning of the emotions and thoughts which beset me, and I searched in vain for a solution, groping about as does a blind man for the exit from a room.

The emotional conflict in me had its point of departure in the rejection of a thought which emerged on the evening of the day my father died. The beloved man sat breathing heavily and groaning in an easy chair. Two physicians were at his side and one of them ordered me to go to the pharmacy to get camphor for an injection. The pharmacy was about fifteen minutes distant, with no bus or tram available. I was well aware of the urgency of the order. I knew the injection should be lifesaving. I ran as if for my own life. I soon had to stop and catch my breath, and then I ran on again through the streets. Suddenly, the image of my father as already dead emerged in my mind. As I passed from running to quick walking, I excused myself because I was out of breath. But then it occurred to me how much depended on my speed and I ran the more quickly to make up for the lost seconds. I reached the pharmacy, and then I ran back. Near collapse, I stormed into our apartment. My father was dead. I still know that I was in a terrible panic as if stunned by a strong electric shock, and I threw myself before the body, in despair.

The next days were filled with grief and mourning. An increasing longing for the familiar face, for his voice and smile, for his kind words, tortured me. When I came home from school, I expected to see him in the living room and was again and again painfully reminded that he was not there. When I heard a funny remark or when I got a good grade, I thought, "I shall tell Father," and only after some minutes, in which I imagined he would enjoy it, did I become aware that he was dead. Then there emerged that doubt which had first occurred on the terrible evening. Could I have saved Father's life if I had run more quickly? The doubt soon changed into self-reproaches and guilt feeling. I asked myself often in those days whether I would trade my own life for his. I answered at first that I would, of course, gladly die, if he could live again. But this was internally rejected by the sophistical argument that my longing for him would not be appeased if I were to die.

The stake was then diminished in my thoughts and I said to myself that I would gladly sacrifice a few years of my life if I could have prolonged his. Inner sincerity forbade that I make myself believe that I was ready to bring about this sacrifice. At the end of such trains of thoughts and fantasies I had to admit to myself, with terror, that I was unwilling to sacrifice a single year of my life for him.

In the following weeks my guilt feeling increased when I caught myself laughing at a witty remark or enjoying a stimulating conversation. I thought it was wrong to forget even for a mom nt that my father had died so recently. The worst of all self-reproaches came soon afterward. To my consternation, a w ve of sexual excitement swept over me, against which I fought with all my might. I could not fall asleep because the power of th sexual drive tortured me, and though only a few days after my father's death, I searched for any opportunity to have sexual intercourse. When at last I found this opportunity, my self-reproaches became intolerable. They had the form: Now, when all my thoughts and feelings should be directed to the dear departed, I am indulging in sexual pleasure. The power of the sexual drive was, however, stronger than my will; each sexual act was followed by depression, self-reproach, and repentance. I remember that I shuddered then at myself. I did not consciously believe in immortality, or in a life in the beyond, yet I could not rid myself of the thought that my dead father knew all about me: that I had slowed my running in the hour of his dying and that I felt sexual excitement in these weeks of mourning.

I often had a kind of expectancy of impending calamity as if my father would punish me for my deeds. All this is too sharply expressed, too definitely stated. It really had the character of fleeting thoughts, of vague ideas that occurred to me again and again. But this is just the nature of incipient obsessions; it is in this typical form that obsessive thoughts first transgress the threshold of the conscious. Thus I feared or thought it possible that my father would let me become ill (and eventually die), and this obsession-idea made me especially afraid of venereal diseases. All these thoughts and fears were, of course, contradicted from within and rejected by reason; but what could reason do against the emotional powers which forced me to think and act as I did? I first realized how much method was in this madness; soon afterward, how much madness was in this method. When I began to study psychoanalysis a few years later, I recognized how many typical traits were in my attitude and that they had almost the clinical character of an obsessional neurosis. Obsessions and counter-obsessions fought each other in me, and I was for many weeks a victim of those strange thoughts, compulsions, and emotions.

Out of this situation emerged a compulsive way of working as the most conspicuous symptom. It was accompanied by the conscious wish to accomplish something extraordinary for my years. During my high-school years I had been rather easygoing concerning my studies. With the exception of a few subjects in which I was at the top I had been lazy and careless. My father had often been worried about me when I had bad grades in mathematics, physics, and chemistry. He expressed his anxiety that I would not amount to much, if I continued to take life so lightly.

The thought that I had caused him grief in this direction had, of course, occurred among my self-reproaches, but the decision to give myself entirely to study and work seemed to emerge independently from my remorse. I still remember that it suddenly occurred to me that I wanted to become famous—the connection of my ambition with the memory of my father emerged through a detour later on. I thought that I wanted to give honor to his name in making my own name well known.

I can recapture only rarely, and for a fleeting moment, a faint echo of the emotions I felt then. (Some years ago, a playwright in psychoanalysis described to me the first night of his first play. His parents had been poor immigrants and had lived poverty-stricken on the Lower East Side of New York, but they had made every sacrifice to give their children a good education. When the cheering first-nighters called the playwright to the stage, his glance fell at once on his parents. They cried. My patient said this moment was the greatest triumph of his life. Other successes followed, but nothing approached the satisfaction experienced in those few moments when he looked at the two old people while bowing to the applauding audience. While I listened to him, I had a vivid feeling of envy, and on this detour I recaptured the memory of an old emotion.) During the last illness of my father I had studied for that final examination with all my energy. I wanted to prove to him that I was capable of a great effort. I wanted to show him that I could achieve something. I had often studied secretly in the night because I wished to surprise him with the results of the examination. During the weeks after his death I had the bitter feeling that I had been too late. Destiny had not allowed me this chance to convince him that I could make a place for myself in the world of men.

I had a similar emotion when Freud died in 1939. In the political unrest of those years I had not published anything of value, and Freud had written in a letter dated January 4, 1935, "I hope that you will give us still very valuable accomplishments of the quality of your first studies." I had not told him that for several years I had been working on an extensive book investigating the psychology of masochism.* The book was almost finished when the news came that Freud had died in London. Again I had the feeling that a malicious destiny had, just a short time before its realization, thwarted my hope to show—this time to the admired man who had become a father-substitute—that I could achieve something of value.

After the death of my father I found myself compelled by an invisible power to study and work with all my energy. I could, of course, justify this sudden zeal by the fact that I was now a student at the university, but there was no doubt that I was propelled by a passionate ambition which had been alien to me until then. I must confess, somewhat shamefacedly, that ambition has remained a great force in my life and has decreased only in these last years which bring me near to the age at which my father died.

The situation in which I found myself was responsible for some of my new zeal. My mother, my sister, and I now had to live on the small income which the pension of an Austrian government official yields to the family after his death. I had to earn enough to support myself by giving lessons. It was necessary to finish my studies as soon as possible. While the lessons secured bread and butter, the work in psychology satisfied an early interest. I was soon able to support myself and become known as a successful student in scientific psychology.

If this new ambition was somewhat intelligible, another kind of decision appeared, as if it were dictated to me from within. It came as the surprise of my young life. I do not remember any

* *Masochism in Modern Man*, first published in 1941 (2nd. ed.; New York: Farrar, Straus and Co., 1949).

longer when and under what circumstances the mysterious impulse emerged. I only know that there was suddenly the inner command to read everything that Goethe had ever written.

The thought had all the characteristic features of an obsession-idea. It came, so to speak, from nowhere; that is to say, it emerged from unknown sources. It was as if an inner voice issued a command without revealing a motive. There were also no emotions connected with the thought, so it seemed. It was as sober as the promulgation of a law. There were, later on, many motivations and rationalizations, but I still know that the first version of the obsession-idea was simply the "order" to read all the collected writings of Goethe. The emergence of this thought would have been easier to explain if Goethe had then been my favorite poet. But if I had been asked whose poetry I loved most, I would have answered without the slightest hesitation, "Heinrich Heine's." I had also at this time become interested in the works of Dostoyevsky, Nietzsche, Hauptmann, and Schnitzler. In short, I was more interested in modern literature, which we students discussed with great animation, than in the classics. I had, of course, read many of the poetic works of Goethe during my high-school years, and I loved and admired them more than those of Schiller, whom the German literary critics then put side by side with the great Olympian. Like many of my student colleagues, I knew the first part of *Faust* and a considerable number of Goethe's poems by heart—a very modest achievement shared with so many people growing up in the German culture.

My decision was certainly not born out of the desire to read all that a poet had written. It must have contained a meaning unknown to me. I did not then search for the motivation for my thought; I submitted to it without the slightest protest. I remember that the thought appeared to me at first as a kind of whim or fancy, as an interesting project, and I tried to regard it at first as we do our good intentions. I tried to diminish the severity or strictness of the order. I had not the faintest inkling that the idea had the power of an obsession-thought. I did not know that the idea which I considered as a casual one had the importance of a solemn vow and had to be followed whatever the price and the sacrifice its realization demanded. It corresponds entirely to the character of an obsession when I describe the strange idea as fanciful and yet as important, vague, and definite at the same time. The thought revealed its true content and nature to me much later. What appeared at first as a whim or a caprice made itself the master or the tyrant whom I had to obey.

Many years later I understood what Goethe then had meant to me and why the mysterious order had been issued. Psychoanalysis had shown that for many cultured Germans and Austrians the figure of Goethe represents not only the "great man," but also the elevated father-figure for our unconscious thought. Freud traced the idea of the "great man" back to the father-image. He pointed out that the will power, the greatness of accomplishment, and the decisiveness of thought, and above all the self-sufficiency and independence of the great man are features of the father for the little boy. Also the divine unconcern, which can change even into inconsiderateness belongs to these traits. You must admire him, you can trust him, but you must also fear him. "Who else than the father of our childhood should be the great man?" (S. Freud, *Der Mann Moses und die monotheistische Religion*, 1939, p. 195.) Freud names Goethe besides Leonardo da Vinci and Beethoven as "great men."* It was thus the connection with the father-figure which, unrecognized, had propelled and compelled me to read all the writings of Goethe.

I have already indicated the compulsive character of my reading of Goethe in this my eighteenth year. The most significant features of the compulsion which unmasked themselves later on were: the exclusion of other reading, perfectionism, accuracy. Repeated

---

* It was strange to read much later in Freud's autobiography that it was Goethe whose influence made him decide to study medicine at the very age that I had the obsession-idea to read Goethe's collected writings. Freud reports that his father let him decide for himself what he wanted to study. "In those young years I felt no special interest in the position or the activity of a physician—by the way, not later on either. I was rather propelled by a kind of desire for knowledge which concerned human situations rather than objects of nature, and which had not yet recognized the value of observations for its gratification. The theories of Darwin, however, attracted me intensely, because they promised extraordinary progress in the understanding of the world. I know that a lecture on Goethe's beautiful paper 'On Nature' in a popular course, shortly before the final examination, brought the decision to matriculate in the school of medicine." (*"Selbstdarstellung,"* Gesammelte Schriften, XI, 120.)

reading was often demanded, out of fear that I might have omitted a word or a sentence.

As an example of these features I can mention that I conscientiously reread the first part of *Faust* and many poems which I knew by heart. I began then to recognize that the order or the vow had to be followed most literally. For instance, I could have read a considerable part of Goethe's works at home where we had an edition of his poetic works. This was forbidden. I had to read the Historical Critical Edition, which was published by order of the Grand Duchess Sophie of Weimar in the years 1887-1909 in 133 volumes, because only the reading of this complete and authentic edition fulfilled all the conditions of my vow or my obsession-idea. I had to read every word, even the most insignificant biographical note, all variants, and the smallest additions. I had to read all the letters and all ten volumes of Goethe's conversations, collected by Woldemar von Biedermann (1889-96). After having read all of Goethe's works, I had to expand my program. It was always possible that a biographer or a literary critic had quoted a remark or a line by Goethe not to be found in the complete edition. I therefore read all that I could find written about Goethe.

This reading had to be complete in the most literal sense: everything Goethe had written. I remember that a fellow-student once casually remarked that a certain bookstore in Vienna had two lines in Goethe's handwriting—the address on an envelope—in its window. I hastily said goodbye to him and ran through the streets to the bookstore, anxious to see the two lines of the address, and afraid a collector might have bought the envelope in the meantime.

I thus spent every free hour of my time, as much as lectures and tutoring permitted, at the university library. I was the first to arrive in the morning and the last to leave at closing time. It seemed that the inner order to which I was subjected demanded that I give all my free time to this reading. Social intercourse was restricted to a minimum, even the time for meals was shortened so that I could hasten back to the library. There was only work and no play. I remember that my attention sometimes lessened when I was tired or when my eyes began to pain. I had to read the sentence or paragraph twice in order to convince myself that I had really read it. Of course, I rationalized my compulsive activity. I tried to convince myself that only this kind of reading deserved the name of thorough study and that it was a test of my seriousness, of my capability to go to the end, to complete a task I had once begun. I was even secretly proud of the singleness of purpose which I considered a prerequisite for every achievement.

I forbade myself to read anything but Goethe, although I had wished so much to read the modern writers. This was how I reasoned with myself in order to justify the exclusion of other reading: One has to know and to appreciate the achievement of the greatest writer (besides Shakespeare) because only then can one measure and appreciate the writers of our time. Only comparing them with Goethe would enable me to think of their achievements in their real proportions. But I could not justify the necessity to read every line of Goethe, every bill written by him to a laundress, and every insignificant note to his servant. Since I kept my Goethe reading secret, nothing in my behavior revealed the strange compulsion which possessed me. My avoidance of social intercourse as far as possible could be easily interpreted as an expression of my mourning.

All that is reported here is, of course, an emotional situation which is recalled only in its main features, its psychological premises and its thought-content. It is very difficult for me to feel even any clear echo of the emotions which governed my life forty-six years ago. It is difficult to imagine now that I could not free myself from the enslavement of my compulsive reading. Whenever I now listen to the description of the strange compulsions of obsessive patients I think that the obsession I was subjected to when I was eighteen years old helps me to understand many of these puzzling traits.

There are two sides—really many more sides—to every story, and to this one as well. I guessed many things about my strange compulsion before my own analysis (1913), but only in my analysis did I recognize the true meaning of my Goethe reading. A childhood memory emerging in an analytical session helped me to understand another meaning which had remained unconscious. At a certain point of reliving my life in recollection, I remembered a little scene of my early boyhood years which I had entirely forgotten. When I was nine years old I kept a secret diary of what was happening in my young life. I wrote about my parents, my brothers and my sister, my teacher and my friends, but mostly about a little girl who lived in our apartment house and with whom I was "in love." One evening I had fallen asleep on the couch in our living room. An elderly couple, my sister's piano teacher and her husband, had come to see my parents and had played cards with my father. I woke up but pretended to be asleep because I heard the lady visitor mention my name. I caught a glimpse of my father holding my secret diary in his hand and reading a few paragraphs to the couple. The lady seemed to like my childish literary effort which described how I had encountered the object of my puppy-love on the stairs of our apartment house. The reactions of my parents were significant. My mother guessed who "she" was, and she guessed correctly! "It is Ella of the O. family who lives in the apartment below," she said. But my father said to his friend, "Well, perhaps he will become a writer or a poet." I was disturbed because my secret had been discovered, but I pretended to sleep on and I must have really fallen asleep again, because when my mother woke me the guests were gone.

What my father had said sometimes occurred to me again in the following days. It was a new idea and I am sure I had no clear notion what a writer was. The closest I could come to such an idea was conveyed by the life-size bust of Goethe which stood on a bookcase. It is significant that I bought a similar bust of Goethe in Berlin forty years later. It now stands on my bookcase. I knew the name of the man and I had heard him spoken of as a great poet by my father. I am almost certain that he was the only poet of whom I knew when I was nine years old. I must have connected the idea of becoming a great writer with his image. My compulsive Goethe reading originated, however, also in the unconscious tendency to know all about the great man of whom my father had spoken with much respect. His pride in me and his high aspirations for me had to be frustrated, but my belated obedience to his wishes found its expression in my compulsive Goethe study. If I could not become a great writer like Goethe, I could at least know all about him or—better still—I *had* to know all about him.

2

The famous Austrian literary critic Hermann Bahr defined Goethe philology as a profession like medicine or law.* It is difficult to convey the true meaning of Goethe philology to persons who did not live and breathe in the atmosphere of German literary scholarship before World War I. It is also doubtful whether so strange a plant as Goethe philology is to be found in any other pattern of culture. A Goethe philologist is a man who not only thinks but acts, breathes, and lives in the mental atmosphere of Goethe. His entire and only interest in the world is the worshiped poet, to such an extent that everything he does and everything that has happened to him is seen through Goethe's eyes. His own life and that of others is understandable only in terms of Goethe's sayings. All things and events of the past and the present are tested according to Goethe's view. Everything concerning the divine figure is of vital importance to him. The weather of the day on which a certain line in a poem was written or whether Goethe liked Teltower carrots is a question of life and death to him. The Tibetan Buddhists worship their Grand Lama to such an extent that even his excrement is held as sacred and is carefully preserved. In a similar sense everything Goethe did and said, were it the merest trifle, is looked at with considerable awe by the Goethe philologist who collects even the refuse of the great man's life and work.

I was indeed on the road toward becoming a Goethe philologist when I was eighteen years old. The psychological difference between those German scholars and myself was only that I did not worship their hero in the same way, though I too was possessed by him, as people in medieval times were considered possessed by the devil or by a demon.

* *Goethe Bild, Preussische Jahrbücher,* Vol. 185 (1921).

When I was eighteen, I had yielded to my obsession-idea but even when I was in bondage to my Goethe reading, I did not surrender without inner protest. Not all the parts of Goethe's huge published works interested me in the same degree. His life, perhaps his greatest work of art, had many phases which appeared unattractive to me. The statesman Goethe left me cold: I had no interest in his building of bridges and roads. His extensive geological and meteorological studies as well as his optical theories did not strike any chord in me. The physiognomical fragments failed to arouse my admiration and the anatomical discovery of the inter-maxillary bone left me indifferent. But also many parts of his poetry did not appeal to me. There were many verses in the second part of Faust which I did not understand. There were even parts of *Wilhelm Meister,* of *Werther,* of *Truth and Fiction,* which had no emotional effect upon me. I read and reread them. I could even admire their style, the choice of words, the construction of the sentences, the sequences and consequences of their thoughts, but the voice which spoke there did not speak to me. The wisdom and the profound penetration of Goethe's old age was only intellectually satisfying. What did I, a greenhorn, know about life? How could I appreciate that there, in a few lines, was the result of the emotional experience by incomparable perception, the fruit of the mental labor of a long life? So much was beyond me and I was easily bored with issues which I only "understood" without emotionally sharing the experience with the poet, the philosopher, and the scientist. When I read the same parts and passages in Goethe's writings many years later, they conveyed much that I had never seen in them before. They were entirely new to me as if I had never read them before. And yet I knew I had read every word of it when I was eighteen years old.

Between Goethe and the boy there was not only the difference in intellectual quality, that astronomical distance which separates the greatest genius from a mediocre mind. Not only the difference of age, maturity, background, and experience prevented my penetrating the depth of Goethe's thoughts. There was something in the character of the great man himself about which I felt uneasy. I often had an almost instinctive resistance to his way of thinking and feeling. Whenever I tried to understand his nature he often appeared to me as superhuman, sometimes inhuman, and very rarely human. Strangely enough, I loved and disliked him now more than I had before. For instance, I felt the passion in some poems as personal and as my own as if I had written them, and then there were passages in which I felt the detachment of a cold touch. There was an impenetrable wall around Goethe's personality, a remoteness, and an icy atmosphere.

Some traits of his character were merely disliked and others were condemned with the uncompromising decisiveness of an eighteen-year-old boy. There was his submission and servility to dukes and duchesses, to kings and empresses, his opportunism in certain situations, his coolness toward Kleist, Heine, and other young German poets. He seemed to favor mediocrity in poetry and music. Had he not been critical of Beethoven and Schubert whom he turned away, and had he not preferred insignificant, anemic, and academic composers? His rejection of the people's democratic demands, his aristocracy—or should I say upper-middle class "bourgeois" outlook?—contrasted with his storm and stress which knew neither measure nor modesty.

Those were not the only contradictory traits which disturbed me. The same man who had shaped the heartbreaking scenes of *Faust*, who had given incomparable expression to the misery of Gretchen, this same man, as a councilor of state, put his signature to the death verdict for an unwed mother who had killed her baby. Was he a God or was he a monster? He was indeed both; that made me shudder. Those terrible two words "I too," with which he introduced his approval of capital punishment, shocked me. There were other disturbing traits, both puzzling and terrifying, about the Olympian figure. There was passion along with cold egotism, an abundant imagination beside dry sobriety. There were so many contradictory and contrasting features that my vision was blurred.

Behind the figure of Faust's Gretchen and of many other of the feminine characters which Goethe created, there emerged the image of Friederike, seventeen years old, in all her loveliness and serene sweetness. When I reread *Truth and Fiction*, the romance of young Goethe with Friederike seemed the high light in the life of this college student. During my reading and daydreaming

I wondered about this young genius and I doubted again that he was human. If he loved Friederike—and his love for her seemed deeper and more tender than for all other women before and after—how could he desert her so coldly, so cruelly? I did not understand it and I did not understand him. I remember how spellbound I was when I read those pages in which Goethe calls up the memory of Sesenheim. I wished, of course, in the depth of my youthful feeling, to meet and love a girl as charming as Friederike. I knew I would not act as Goethe had in a similar situation.

I was forty years old—twenty-one years after my compulsive working through the Grossherzogin Sophie edition—when I read once again the story of the Sesenheim romance in *Truth and Fiction*. I saw it for the first time in its own light, illuminated from within. I read it with the eyes, the awareness, and the curiosity of a psychologist. For many years I had been a psychoanalyst, but it had never occurred to me that Goethe could be the subject of a psychoanalytical study, that the new method could be applied to the life and the work of the great poet. In my student years such an application would certainly have seemed to me presumptuous, even blasphemous. It was as if to think of "psychoanalyzing" God.

Such an avoidance even in thought was the more conspicuous since I had applied the analytical method in the psychological appreciation of the works of other writers. I had written two books which proved that crossing the bridge between the imagination of creative writing and analytical research brought valid and valuable results. My doctoral thesis, *Flaubert and His Temptation of Saint Antony*, published in 1912, was a contribution to the psychology of artistic creation. My admiration for the great gift of psychological observation of a contemporary Viennese writer was expressed in *Arthur Schnitzler as Psychologist* (1913). Quite a few shorter publications during the next ten years expressed my active interest in various psychological problems of writers and their works. Yet I had never looked at Goethe's life and work from an analytical point of view. It was, no doubt, a residue of my awe before this monumental figure, before one of the greatest minds of mankind.

Freud once pointed out in relation to Goethe how unjustified it would be to consider analytical research into the life story of a great man as an intrusion.* The biographer does not wish to degrade the hero but to bring him close to us. It is unavoidable that we will then learn of occasions in which the great man behaved no better than do ordinary mortals. His distance from us will then be diminished. Nevertheless, Freud insists that the endeavor of the biographers is legitimate. "The great man is only a continuation of the father and the teacher of our childhood, and our relation to these important persons was ambivalent, our admiration for them regularly concealing a component of hostile rebellion. This is psychological fate. It cannot be changed without violent suppression of truth. Our ambivalent feelings must be continued in our relationship to the great man whose life story we seek to investigate."

In the same address, delivered when Freud received the Goethe prize (1930), he admits that we analysts have not done so well in the case of this great man. That has its special reasons: Goethe was a poet, a fine confessor; but in spite of his abundant autobiographical writings, he was also a careful concealer of his real feelings. "The course of my life remained mostly a secret even for my friends," Goethe wrote in his *Campagne in Frankreich* (November, 1792). This sounds paradoxical in a poet who speaks as freely as did Goethe about his emotional experiences. But in speaking his mind and his heart he could conceal perhaps the most important things. He who reveals himself in some facts makes it easy for himself to conceal certain other personal matters which he may wish to keep secret.

Such deeper secrecy, which disguises itself under the mask of free expression and of confession, suggests why the abundant materials of Goethe's life history still do not lend themselves easily to analytical investigation. They are difficult to penetrate because the analyst must pursue the smallest unnoticed clues and indications, those little signs of which a person is not aware when he speaks about himself. Only attention and observation dealing with the inconspicuous, the most careful psychological evaluation of unconscious circumstantial evidence can find here valuable information. All other ways are blocked, all other methods of psy-

* *"Speech at the Frankfurt Goethe-House," Psychoanalytische Bewegung,* II, Heft 5.

chological investigation fail. The analyst can only hope that what is so carefully guarded will give itself away unconsciously.

There was another important reason why I never felt tempted to approach the life story of Goethe from the viewpoint of psychoanalytic psychology. He himself had often emphasized that he did not appreciate psychological analysis. In the same report in which he said his life remained a secret even to his best friends, he declared that he generally lived unconsciously, that is, without conscious self-analysis and self-observation. The reader should compare Goethe's attitude with the opinion of old Anatole France: "Far from knowing myself I always took trouble to ignore me. I consider the knowledge of oneself a source of worry, unrest and tortures. I came as little as possible to myself . . . As a small boy and as an adult, young and old I have always lived as far away from myself as possible . . . Ignore yourself: this is the first prescription of wisdom."*

Goethe spoke to Eckermann in April, 1829 about the claim to know oneself: "This is a strange demand which until now nobody has fulfilled and which in reality no one can realize. Man is with all his senses and drives directed toward the outer world and he has much trouble recognizing it as such and making it serve his purposes and needs. He knows about himself only when he enjoys himself or suffers. He learns thus merely through pains and pleasures what he must seek and what to avoid. After all, man is a dark being; he does not know whence he comes or whither he goes. He knows little of the world and less of himself. I do not know myself and God forbid I should."

To Chancellor Mueller in 1824 he spoke in the same vein: "I declare man can never know himself as an object. Others know me better than I do myself." These are strong words, especially to the ears and minds of a psychologist who expects psychological insights of the poet into himself. In his *"Sprueche in Prosa"*** Goethe asks: "How can one learn to know oneself? Never by self-observation, but by activity."

When I had read the Friederike story, at the age of eighteen, I was not concerned with understanding Goethe's behavior. I iden-

* Michel Corday, *Anatole France d'après ses confidences* (Paris, 1927), p. 58.
** *Gesammelte Werke*, LV, 224.

tified myself with another young man who loved and was loved by the gentlest and loveliest of girls, and I condemned this young man who deserted his sweetheart so casually. I called him a conscienceless egotist and disliked him. When, having passed my fortieth year, I reread the Friederike romance, I understood young Goethe much better. My approach to the experience was different. It was no longer sympathy or antipathy which accompanied my reading; a new interest competed with the esthetic pleasure: the curiosity of the psychologist.

When I read the story of the meeting of young Goethe with Friederike, how their romance started, developed, and ended, vague ideas about concealed motives of Goethe's attitude dawned upon me. They were not clear insights and at first did not have the character of psychological notions but were more in the nature of hunches. They were not definite enough to be formulated in words. They were preverbal, in that transitional phase from presentiment to recognition, fleeting impressions, embryos of thoughts. These first inklings became by and by more distinct, the impressions became condensed when I reread certain passages, compared them with the preceding story, and filled in the gaps with what I knew about Goethe's life from other sources.

These psychological hunches were at first without tangible substance and evidence. Unstable, they were difficult to grasp and threatened to elude me. When I decided to follow them, the task had more the character of reconnaissance than of recognition. I slowly became sure that there was a subterranean connection between certain actions. Something hidden strove to communicate itself in those pages of *Truth and Fiction,* but shied away from them at the same time. An unconscious process revealed itself by small signs, but another factor tried to conceal the clues. I was often thrown off the track after I had found it, but I pursued it to the end, to discover the unconscious facts behind the facts which Goethe's story reports. What had been a hunch originally, a dim preconception, had become an idea which could be examined, tested, and verified by scientific research. I published the study on Goethe and Friederike, which is the result of this psychoanalytic investigation, in 1929.

3

"All I have written and published are but fragments of a great confession." This sentence from *Truth and Fiction* includes, of course, the wonderful presentation of the idyl of Sesenheim written when Goethe had passed his sixty-second year. The magical power of his prose revives the story of love and sorrow of the twenty-one-year-old student. Weyland, a friend of Goethe's, wished to introduce him to the family of Pastor Brion who lived in Sesenheim, a friendly little village not far from Strassburg where Goethe studied. Goethe describes the old gentleman and his wife and speaks of their lively oldest daughter. When Friederike appears, "in truth, a star arose in this rustic heaven." Her lucid blue eyes and blond braids, her loveliness and grace, the serene clarity of her talk charmed the young poet. In walks and at festivals, in solitude and company, in conversations and letters, the two glided into the sweetest of enchantments. Goethe felt "boundlessly happy" and the leave-takings became more and more a painful prospect when he had to return to Strassburg from his many visits in Sesenheim. His letters contain some of the masterpieces of German poetry. It is as if his love for Friederike gave to his language a naturalness and plasticity hitherto unknown. But there were already premonitions of an early parting: "My passion increased as I recognized more and more the true worth of this splendid girl, and as the time drew near when I was to lose, perhaps forever, so much that was dear and good." At the time when the happiness of the two young people seemed flawless, Friederike fell ill. Then came the parting. He rode again as so often from Strassburg to Sesenheim to see Friederike once more. "Those were painful days, the memory of which has not remained with me. When, seated on my horse, I held out my hand to her, there were tears in her eyes, and I felt none too happy." It was not until much later that he wrote the letter of farewell. Friederike's reply "broke the heart. It was the same hand, the same tone, the same feeling which had been fostered for me and by me. Now for the first time, I felt the loss which she was suffering. I realized that there was no possibility, nothing I could do to soothe her grief. I saw her as though she were present, I constantly felt the lack, and what was worse, I could not forgive myself. . . ." He felt guilty: "I had wounded this purest heart to the quick, and the period of melancholy, repentance, combined with the absence of the quickening love to which I had become accustomed, was agonizing, nay, insupportable." Goethe began in the following years, when his feeling of guilt mounted, that poetic confession which reached its peak in *Faust,* where Friederike appears transfigured into Gretchen.

The description of the romance with Friederike does not explain what it was that caused Goethe to part from the beloved girl. None of the many biographers of the poet could detect any plausible motives for Goethe's deserting Friederike, who meant so much to him. Least of all those biographers who assumed that the young poet had seduced the girl. It is not doubtful any more that nothing of this kind happened. Yes, modern biography has made it clear that Goethe suffered from emotional impotence which he overcame only after having reached his fortieth year. The plays in which Goethe shaped the fate of the seduced and deserted girl, most touchingly that of Gretchen in *Faust,* present thus an emotional potentiality and not what really happened.

My psychoanalytic analysis of the young poet's motives took its point of departure from the discovery of an error in Goethe's autobiography. He introduces the description of the Sesenheim idyl by describing the profound impression Goldsmith's *The Vicar of Wakefield* had made upon him. In the figures of this novel, which his mentor and friend Herder read to him, Goethe found the fictional characters which came to life shortly afterward when he visited the family Brion in Sesenheim. The peaceful life of the rural clergyman and his family, the destiny of his lovable daughter Sophie who is seduced by the ruthless Burchell, prepared young Goethe for his meeting the family Brion. But we know that Goethe did not know Goldsmith's novel when he first visited Sesenheim. The parallel between Goethe and that seducer Burchell is more than conscious. Goethe emphasizes it and seems to indicate that it was why he felt so guilty when he deserted Friederike. The psychoanalytic penetration of this and other slips and distortions led to the conclusion that there must be another unconscious motivation for the long-lasting guilt feelings of the poet toward Friederike. A sideline leads to that secret: Goethe had a mysterious fear that a kiss of his would bring calamity and death to a girl. This superstitious fear tormented him when he kissed Friederike. His vivid imagination showed him the beloved girl already suffering from the effect of that curse. Torn between his desire for her and the fear that he could harm her, he experienced pangs of panic when Friederike became ill which seemed "to hasten the threatened calamity."

Afraid that she would die, he fled.

We see here the young poet as the victim not only of superstitions, but also of severe obsessional thoughts that he himself later on recognized as expressions of magical beliefs: "A kind of conceit supported this superstition; my lips—whether consecrated or accursed—seemed to me more important than they had been hitherto. . . ." The continued analysis of Goethe's biography brings further proof that his guilt feelings toward Friederike can be traced back to unconscious death wishes against the beloved girl. When he left her, he had a strange experience. Riding home, he saw himself in his fantasy riding on the same road, in a suit he had never worn. This "friendly vision" became reality when, eight years later, he visited Friederike again. Riding away from Friederike, the young man enjoyed the sight of the Alsatian landscape and felt relieved as if he had escaped a curse threatening calamity and death. I compared the mood described in that part of Goethe's autobiography with that of the fourth movement of the Pastoral Symphony to which Beethoven gave the title "Joyous and Grateful Feelings after the Storm."

Goethe remained the man in Friederike's life. She never spoke of him and remained single. She died in 1813, when she was sixty-one. Her grave at Sesenheim has the lines:

> A ray of poet's sun fell on her
> So rich, it gave her immortality.

4

When I reread the Goethe study sketched here, in 1938, ten years after it had been written, I was already in the United States and considering the translation of some of my books. I felt annoyed with myself while reading this one. My self-criticism concerned not only the things said in the book but also the manner in which they were said. It concerned the structure as well as several special parts of the study. I was impatient, for instance, with my frequent use of the editorial "we" in the scientific manner of German scholars. I would now prefer to say "I"—not in order to assert myself, but because I was tired of a modesty which I felt was almost indecent. There was, I found, a shifting from minor to major and back again in the book. The tempi were not kept. I found many other things to criticize.

Not only critical voices accompanied my reading; others of a different kind became audible, sometimes made themselves heard as counterpoints to the points made by self-criticism. I had suddenly come upon my own trail. I was surprised to come upon circumstantial evidence whose psychological significance could not be ignored. The clues were small and inconspicuous, but they could not be belittled. It was at first as if islands of an unknown landscape, long flooded, emerged from the sea. It was my past life returning and appearing suddenly in a new light. Most of the facts that I remembered had not been forgotten, but their significance, the connection between them and their psychological influence upon my life, had not been recognized. It was one of those "stillest hours" of which Nietzsche speaks when I faced facts now, certain experiences of my own, reflected in the study I had written. I had not known ten years earlier that I was speaking of myself when I tried to penetrate into the secret emotional life of a young man in love, dead almost two hundred years.

Psychoanalysis has claimed that we do not live, but that we are lived, that is, that the greatest part of what we experience is not of our conscious doing, but is "done" by unknown powers within ourselves. Psychoanalysis has asserted further that we realize only to a very small extent what we experience, or what is happening to us and in us. An experience is like an iceberg, its greatest part submerged, unknown to us while we live it. An event whose full psychological significance and bearing we were able to recognize would not deserve the name of experience. Its power would explode in a moment and it would be without deeper and lasting emotional effects. The stronger this conscious effect, the less enduring is the experience. What is strongest felt and expressed at the moment is doomed to perish soon. What is sensational is for the day. What is lasting needs a long time until it reaches the deeper levels of our emotional life. It takes many years before we recognize what our own experiences mean to us and what their psychological nature and repercussions, their effects and after-effects, really are. Nietzsche uses a beautiful metaphor: "Deep wells take a long time to realize what has fallen into their depth."

Strangely enough, even the psychological clues that emerged while I read my book at first appeared in the form of literary criticism. They occurred to me as I wondered about certain strange features of the material. There is a passage at the beginning of the book which I passed by in my first reading, but which re-echoed as if to recall something to mind. It occurs in a description of the scene in which Friederike appeared and young Goethe looked into her clear blue eyes. The features of Friederike, I read in my book, "become the prototype of a girl that calls up in every man's memory the charming and the most beloved figures of his youth." The image of Friederike as Goethe describes it in all its charming details was at once transformed into a familiar face: serious blue eyes looked into mine and the name Ella was in my mind. It was as if my own words had called up the dear figure, as a line spoken on the stage gives the cue for the appearance of the leading lady. Ella's image emerged suddenly out of nowhere and I saw her as I had seen her again, when I was a youth of nineteen. She appeared and stood alive before me, yet I did not think of her when I wrote the sentence about Friederike calling up in every man's memory the most loved figure of his youth.

I did not think of any particular girl; it was a general statement and the appropriate thing to write in this context. Perhaps I thought of her without being conscious of her, and her image in the background of my mind dictated the sentence. Perhaps the vision as I had met her first was only a re-vision. I wondered, dismissed the thought, and read on. And then I stopped again, astonished.

There is a chapter entitled "Joyous and Grateful Feelings after the Storm." It begins with the words: "About the same time that Goethe was sketching the plan for his autobiography, in Heiligenstadt, near Vienna, Beethoven was daydreaming the abundance of melodies into a symphony he later called *Sinfonia Pastorale*." I read that the Sixth Symphony might well stand as a counterpart of Goethe's description of the landscape and atmosphere of Sesenheim. "This is a hell of a transition!" I thought. The connecting links between this part of Goethe's biography and Beethoven's symphony certainly are few: it is true that both were conceived at about the same time. But what a leap from the parson's house in Alsace to the hills surrounding Heiligenstadt, from the Rhine to the Danube! The tunes of the Pastoral, as the musical counterpart of the idyl in Sesenheim! No doubt was possible any more. It was no accident. Such a connection in thought is unconsciously determined by associations of a very personal nature. "Involuntary" memories now crowded one another; image after image appeared before me as if the waves brought forth precious long-buried goods, from the depths of the sea to the shore. The excursion to Heiligenstadt; Ella and I walking from Klosterneuburg to the place where Beethoven conceived the tunes of the brook scene. Our first kiss. . . . No, it was no accident, I decided, when I read the title of another chapter, *"Freundliche Vision."* I swear I did not think when I wrote the chapter title that this was the title of the song by Richard Strauss. But now I seemed to hear Ella's warm voice singing:

Nicht im Schlafe hab' ich das geträumt

. . . the Strauss song . . . and I remembered.

And now I turned the leaves of my book again and read with new eyes. There was an abundance of personal, even of intimate things in it that I had had no inkling of. It was full of allusions to little events and sayings from the years of my courtship and marriage. There was an overflow of references to later experiences, even to Ella's ill-health, and I had not had the slightest notion of these hints. I had written a scientific study on a certain phase of Goethe's life, an objective psychological essay about an experience in the youth of a writer who lived two hundred years ago, and I had not known that I had written about my own experience, so similar to his. How many references to my own conflicts had invisibly crept into the objective report!

The astonishing thing about it was that the study of Goethe was objective and subjective at the same time, and that these personal references were so well concealed that they remained unknown not only to the reader but even to myself. And some of these references, especially in the chapter titles, were so conspicuous that they could scarcely be disregarded! It was as if those memories were put into the window and I had passed them by unobserved. There were not only the Beethoven symphony and the Strauss song, there was the chapter "Interlude." But *Interlude* is the title of a play by Arthur Schnitzler. Ella and I had seen a performance of it at the Vienna Burgtheater. There were other telltale titles calling up happy and tragic memories.

My attention turned slowly to psychological problems. What did it mean that I had become so interested in the Friederike story as a boy of nineteen, that I had lost this interest shortly afterward, and had regained it nineteen years later to such an extent that I wrote a study on the romance? Why had I not realized for so long that my own youthful experience had crept into the investigation of Goethe's period at Sesenheim? It was difficult to solve these two problems separately. They had to be dealt with together; it is easier to crack two nuts by working one against the other.

I also learned some unknown or unrecognized things about myself and about the most important aspects of my youth. I must write of it now and I hope to do so with the greatest objectivity of which I am capable. It is well known that such objectivity is highly limited by the nature of the subject and by one's own nature. Some of these interferences can be relaxed when the fragment of one's life that is to be presented is remote from one's ego, because of the passage of time and emotional developments of a decisive character. One's own experience then appears as if it belonged to another person, as if it belonged to another's life. The ego has changed to such an extent that it encounters its past self as that of a stranger. The example of Goethe himself who as a man of sixty years looked back at his romance with Friederike is itself one of the best examples of such an attitude. Yet Goethe, dictating to his secretary, sometimes had to control his tears.

The romantic experience I had at nineteen is told in the following chapters. It is viewed from a distance of forty-five years and is presented differently than if written after five or ten years. It is also likely that it is in its final shape because the ego loses its plasticity in old age. The picture of the past is not subject to great changes any more. The distance from my youthful experience is secured by other factors. The Vienna of my boyhood years does not exist any more. I said farewell to the place of my birth, twenty years ago. The home town was turned into a vision of hell when its citizens celebrated Hitler's entry into Vienna. *"Wien, Wien, nur du allein sollst die Stadt meiner Träume sein"?* The city of my dreams became the city of my nightmares. I have been living in the United States for many years now and consider America my own and my children's country. My first love, of whom the following pages tell, has rested for many years in the Vienna Central Cemetery. Almost all of the persons I shall refer to in these chapters are dead. I have married again. The external and inner circumstances of my life have changed since the time of which I shall write.

I have become a stranger to the young man who had these experiences and I believe I can tell the story as if it happened to another person. There is so little in common between the nineteen-year-old youth in Vienna who went forth into life and the old man approaching the end of the journey.

The experience of my youth has re-emerged again and again as if it wanted to be shaped and presented in the light of the insights I had gained. It was not only lack of moral courage and the discretion which, according to Freud, "one owes also to oneself" that made me postpone the writing of this psychological study. It was also the doubt that I would be capable of grasping any unconscious material, which is so elusive, reluctant, and recalcitrant against presentation. I feel, however, that I cannot afford to procrastinate any longer. An external date helped me to action: Goethe started his autobiography when he reached his sixtieth year. (I have passed sixty.) Did the old pattern of unconscious identification still persist?

It is certainly unnecessary to emphasize the decisive difference between the presentation of the romantic experience of Goethe, one of the greatest achievements of autobiographical writing, and my own. One of the greatest writers of all time has painted an incomparable picture of a youthful experience, the same experience which gave *Faust* to the world, and which became the subject of a poetic creation and magical reconstruction in the pages of *Truth and Fiction* dedicated to the Sesenheim time. This sketch will be a small contribution to psychological research using autobiographical material. The following chapters make my own experience the object of psychological investigation and analysis. The difference in objectives determines not only the divergence of style in presentation, but also the material to be presented. In Goethe's creative achievement persons and events are plastically placed before the eyes of the reader. The hidden emotions and thought-processes of the young man were only alluded to or presented in an indirect way, yet artistically in so much more powerful a manner than by direct discussion. The material events, the outside of an experience, have but a very small place in a psychological investigation. The emotional processes are the real subject of the exploration. Beauty and significance are the aim of the poet; understanding, the goal of the psychologist. What Goethe achieved in his magical description is not even within the reach of the psychologist. He is incapable of creating the atmosphere of fatefulness in his description. He cannot present his own experience in such a light that it becomes only an image of a general human situation. He has to be content with so much less and will be satisfied when he succeeds in finding and demonstrating a few of the hidden threads running through the texture of unconscious life.

Looking back at the experience of my youth, I could speak as the great poet does:

> Ye wavering forms draw near again as ever.
> When ye long since moved past my clouded eyes.
> To hold you fast, shall I this time endeavor.
> Still does my heart that strange illusion prize?
> Ye crowd on me? 'Tis well! You might assever
> While ye from mist and mark around me rise . . .

As to the poet, so memories bring back to me many familiar faces and

> . . . many dear, dear shades arise with you
> Like some old tale that Time but half erases
> First Love draws near to me and Friendship too . . .

And with those memories the present seems to withdraw and the past becomes alive again:

> . . . what I possess as if it were far from seeing
> And what has vanished, now comes into being.

II

1

WHEN the boy and the girl met, they were both children. My family then lived on the second floor of a modest apartment house in Vienna. We were of the lower middle class; my father was an employee of the railroad company, and the family often had difficulties making ends meet. Below us, on the first floor, in a larger apartment lived the family of the journalist, Mr. O. Mrs. O. was, it seemed, a kind, warmhearted, and simple-minded woman. She was of Jewish descent. Her husband was a social climber who was an anti-Semite. We could not decide whether this was because or in spite of his wife's Jewish origin. An elderly spinster aunt, the sister of Mrs. O., a tall, slim, severe-looking woman with a sour disposition, lived with the couple. The two daughters, Mary and Ella, attended the same grammar school as did my sister Margaret. Mary was two years older than Ella, who was a classmate of my sister's. We heard that the two girls were friendly, but were allowed to have only a selected few girls visit them. They were not allowed to play on the street and could walk in the park only if accompanied by their mother or their aunt. They had to keep much to themselves, as did the whole family. Their father, we were told, was a disciplinarian and had odd ideas about the education of girls. He considered it necessary that the two girls, children of nine and seven, always be escorted.

This father was much younger than my father, but was in contrast very dignified-looking. Also, in contrast to my father, he wore very elegant suits and behaved much as a man about town. We children often saw him on the street or met him on the stairway of the house. We wondered about the monocle he frequently pressed into his eye and through which he looked at us critically. All in all, his fashionable suits, his top hat, his cane with the golden knob which he would whirl around gave us the first idea of what a dandy was. My father and Mr. O. leaving the house about the same time often met and walked a few blocks together. They chatted in a friendly manner. I heard my father tell my mother that in his opinion Mr. O. was a snob and an upstart. Mr. O. called himself chief editor of the *Kurortezeitung* (a monthly for summer and health resorts); he seemed to be a wealthy man. He often spoke of his trips to Germany, France, and Italy, and he was really frequently away from home, sometimes for months on end. He seemed to be a great hunter and he showed several guns to my father who was not much interested but too polite to express his lack of enthusiasm. (Much later I heard my father quote a Jewish proverb whose melancholic wisdom remained in my memory: "What a blessing that not only the hunted but also the hunters get tired.")

Mr. O. often spoke of his friends to whose castles or hunting lodges he was invited. There were dukes and barons, Graf von

Kinsky and Fuerst Esterhazy and other members of the Austrian nobility. We children were deeply impressed. Mr. O. seemed to be on most intimate terms with all these high aristocrats. This friendship seemed to be reduced to rather superficial acquaintanceship later on, to something very far from familiarity. We realized, also much later, how right my father was when he thought that Mr. O. made people believe what he wished. He was chief editor of the *Kurortezeitung*, that was true enough, but he did not reveal that he was not only the only editor but also the only person who owned, edited, wrote, and sold this monthly magazine. The journal was mostly filled with articles secured by Chambers of Commerce and publicity agents for hotels, vacation spots, and health resorts. Its larger part was devoted to advertisements. Mr. O.'s far-distant trips had as their main purpose the securing of these advertisements and collecting the fees. I did not like the man, but of course, I had the respect of a boy of ten toward an adult. He interested me only as the father of the two girls, especially Ella.

We often heard the two sisters play the piano. Mary, who was two years older than her sister, was technically superior; but Ella's playing expressed more emotion. Ella also played the violin and sang with a warm and gentle voice many of the lieder by Schubert and Schumann, and later on, songs in French and English.

Both girls were tall and had very good posture. Both were blond, but Mary's hair was much lighter than Ella's. Mary was, without doubt, the prettier of the two. All her features were regular and her face was of a classical beauty. Ella's darker hair and her eyes of a deeper blue were, at first sight, overshadowed by her sister's doll-like prettiness, but you felt more strongly and more lastingly attracted when you looked at Ella. Mary was, it seemed, more lively and cheerful; her eyes sparkled and danced when she smiled. Ella was serious.

I fell in love with Ella when I was eight years old, but it was not love at first sight. I remember that I had seen her often enough on the street or had met her and her sister on the stairway without paying the slightest attention to her. Like other boys at this age, I was not interested in little girls and devoted myself more to football and was an active member of a gang, which had frequent feuds and fights with another gang in the alleys of a park called Augarten. A boy of eight years who seems to be interested in girls is looked upon as a sissy by other boys in Vienna as in New York. If I showed any pronounced attitude toward the two sisters at that time, it was cold contempt, the disinterested behavior of the superior male toward little girls.

One afternoon something strange happened. I was strolling home from school. I saw Mrs. O. and her younger daughter, Ella, who stood before the house talking with a girl friend. The two girls said goodbye to each other. At this moment I accidentally glanced at Ella's face and I looked at it as if I saw it for the first time. Her eyes were serious, but there was a smile around her lips that was of a loveliness and sweetness I had never before seen on a face. It was as if her features were suddenly illuminated from within. The contrast of the quiet and earnest eyes with this smile appeared to me of a unique beauty. It was at this moment that I fell in love with her. Much later I understood what I really wished in my boyhood daydreams. I wanted her to smile at me in the same way. All my childish and clumsy attempts to turn her attention to me had this goal. It was as if I silently implored her: Smile at me the way you did then at your friend!

Nothing in my behavior changed for some time. I played hide-and-seek with myself or I made a brave attempt to conquer my infatuation, but I know that I felt my heart beat faster whenever I saw her. It must have been a considerable time later when I had the courage to greet her in passing her on the stairs. I argued with myself whether she had nodded and it made me impatient to meet her again. From this time on I took my cap off to her and her sister as if it were merely the thing to do and not a most daring deed of a boy of eight.

People say that the years after puberty, the late teens and early twenties, are the times when romance blossoms. I believe that the romantic infatuations of those years are only like a second or even a third edition of an original work. The real character of romance is much clearer in childhood. When I think of those silly things I did to arouse the attention of my beloved, the foolishness of young men's passion seems almost to be wise.

I knew, for instance, approximately the time when the two girls went with their mother or aunt to shop or to take a walk. It could be accidental that I came down the street so that I met them and took my cap off to them. But having passed them, I turned into a side street and ran a few blocks ahead so that I met them once again and could greet them again. I thought I was artful in handling the situation; it dawned upon me only later that running into the same person twice or even three times within a quarter of an hour could rouse suspicion. I pretended, of course, that I strolled through the streets, but my casualness, my surprised glancing up when I saw the girls again, and my taking off my cap with a friendly smile—these were telltale giveaways. I am sure that I behaved so awkwardly at these chance encounters that it seemed pitiful.

Once—I was nine years old—I did a terrible thing. One winter afternoon I walked home from school as usual with my classmate and friend Otto. Suddenly and without the slightest provocation I threw him to the ground. We rolled in the snow, in a fight in which I was victorious on account of my surprise attack. The next day, my father got a very indignant letter from Otto's father, who demanded payment for his son's torn overcoat. I had behaved so crazily because I had seen a certain little girl at the first-floor window of our apartment house.

I was not aware then that my desperate attempts to arouse Ella's interest had the character of wooing. If I had known Goethe at the time, I could have said in his words, "When I love you, what does this concern you?" But my actions called my bluff. They were directed to the aim of awakening a friendly response, especially that smile. It never came. It is strange that I did not feel frustrated and disappointed in the six years that I so pursued the shyly beloved girl. Her sister Mary smiled in a friendly enough way at me and nodded vivaciously; but Ella's greeting was hardly perceptible. She looked at me and looked away immediately. Only once her eyes met mine and rested there for a few seconds. It was a glance whose significance I could not understand. It was the first and only time that I felt she looked attentively at me. I was puzzled by this look. What did it mean?

The same evening my father told my mother at the dinner

table that Mr. O. had bought a country house with many acres of garden and vineyard in Klosterneuburg, one hour from Vienna, and that the family was to move to this town in a few days. He added that Mr. O. had some silly idea that it was better for his daughters, approaching puberty, to live in the country where they would be protected from the many dangers which threatened girls growing up in Vienna. He planned to take them from public school and to let them be taught at home by private teachers. Ella was then ten years old.

During the six years of my first love I had never spoken a word to its object. Mrs. O. asked me several times about my progress in school and about the health of my mother. Once I even made some casual remarks to Mary, on the stairway, but I was tongue-tied toward Ella who stood silently beside her sister. Only much later did I realize how rude my behavior had then been.

I do not remember that the news that Ella and her family would move shortly or the fact that I would not see her any more produced any strong emotional reaction in me. The following months are only dimly remembered, but I know that I made a special nuisance of myself at home and in school and that my father often reproached me. It was rather a gloomy time, and I felt unhappy because I was a naughty boy and was often scolded. (But perhaps I was naughty because I felt unhappy?)

In the following years I did not think of Ella any more. Out of sight, out of mind. I followed the many interests of a boy of this age and later I had the usual troubles of puberty as did the other boys. I flirted, joked with, and kissed the girl friends of my sister. At home Mr. O. and his family were not mentioned any more. Ella's image, which had been so vivid before my mind for some years, had evaporated. There are things one must forget.

2

The period from the twelfth to the nineteenth year sees many and decisive changes in a boy's life. It is the phase in which he makes the transition from childhood to manhood.

I have already attempted to describe my reaction to the death of my father shortly after I had reached my eighteenth birthday, and my exclusive and compulsive preoccupation with Goethe's life and works. Whatever were the unrecognized thoughts underlying it, my Goethe compulsion lost its uncontested power over me by and by and I re-emerged from my solitude.

During my high school years I had a friend named David E. He was a year older than I, of a cheerful, easygoing temperament, popular with the boys as well as with the girls. He had become a young man about town just at the time when I became increasingly introverted; he was a realist while I was an idealist and a daydreamer. His versatility and smartness as well as his social poise contrasted with my shyness and slowness. He had decided to go into his father's furniture business. After we had passed our final examination we met but rarely.

Just at the time when I hesitatingly recovered the path to sociability I ran into him on the street and we took a walk together. Strolling along the avenue of trees in the Prater, we talked of our past school experiences and our plans for the future. He suddenly stopped and said: "Look, the other day two very pretty girls asked me how you are and what you are doing." He then told me that he had met Mary and Ella O. His sister, who had been a classmate of Mary's, was frequently invited to the country house of the O.'s. He then described to me the strange life the two girls had led. It seemed to him that their father was a fool who subjected his wife, his sister-in-law, and his daughters to his *idée fixe*. He did not allow them to speak to anyone but women. No man, old or young, was permitted to enter the house except the mailman, the gardener, and the grocer's boy. The two girls were strictly forbidden to speak to men. They could take a walk and occasionally shop in Vienna, but, of course, only if accompanied by their mother or aunt, who had given a solemn promise to keep every man at a distance from them. Calling him a son-of-a-gun, David asserted that Mr. O. seemed to have a very low opinion of women's virtue, that he wished the two girls to become old spinsters. To forbid two very attractive girls of nineteen and seventeen even to speak to young men was unheard of. The man was a dangerous lunatic, who really threatened to shoot any man who entered his sacred house. He should be put into the insane asylum at Gugging, near Klosterneuburg.

David then reported how he had met the two girls. His sister, who was sorry for Mary and Ella, had arranged the date. The country house in Klosterneuburg was in a side street. Near the church of the small town a narrow path led from the church hill upward along the large vineyard and garden of the O.'s. Near the top of the hill, a ten-minute walk and invisible from the windows, there stood a garden-house in which the girls spent many summer afternoons. There was a meadow, surrounded by fruit trees. Nearby, a small door in the fence of the garden was almost hidden by the boughs of trees hanging over it. The girls had opened this door which was to remain locked by order of Mr. O. David had visited the two girls and his own sister in this part of the garden and had spent an afternoon in their pleasant company some weeks previously. It was summer and it was good to be in cool, fresh country air as often as possible. He had frequently spent free afternoons in the beautiful garden in Klosterneuburg as the guest of the two girls. God forbid that Mr. O. should ever learn that a young man had entered his garden or had had a conversation with his daughters! With the discretion due such matters at the time, David made some remarks which gave me to understand that he was falling in love with Mary.

Returning from his vivid talk about the situation in Klosterneuburg to his initial remark, he told me that Ella had asked about me. The image of a little girl walking straight ahead and looking forward emerged and passed. I was suspicious of David who had liked to tease me in past years. Had his sister perhaps realized that I had been infatuated with Ella many years ago when I was a boy? In short, I did not believe David and told him to go climb a tree, preferably one of the apple trees in the garden in Klosterneuburg. But he insisted that he spoke the truth.

About a week later, to my astonishment, David appeared in the university library where, as he knew, I was to be found at certain hours still reading Goethe or about Goethe. He called me out and told me that he had been in Klosterneuburg again and that he had promised the two girls he would bring me to their garden. He added that they were both very curious about me and asked me whether the day after tomorrow, a Tuesday, was convenient for me. I had to trust him.

We took the train from the Franz-Josef Station and rode to Klosterneuburg-Kierling which had been familiar to me since my childhood. Arriving at the town, we took the bus which brought us to the church of the village Kierling. David led me to the path which went along the garden of the O.'s and we climbed up the hill and stood before the little door, half hidden by bushes, exactly as he had described it. And then we were inside the garden; there were the meadow, the big trees, the summerhouse, and the bench some steps away from it. And there was Mary, who greeted me. She was as I remembered her, only taller, a beautiful woman; there were the classical features and the light blond hair and the easygoing, cheerful manner.

We sat in the summerhouse and looked down on the church and the vineyards. It was early afternoon and all was quiet in the village. There was a spiral path, which led in curved lines from O.'s cottage upward to our spot.

"Where is Ella?" asked David. Mary pointed to the path which was roofed and covered on both sides by vines. "There she is," answered Mary. We caught sight of a figure in a blue dress which came nearer, and Ella suddenly stood before me. She was apparently a bit breathless from climbing the hill. I looked into her blue eyes which were deep as a mountain lake and then I heard her warm voice. "How do you do, Mr. Reik?"

I listened to this voice and felt as if the bell of the church down there in the village had begun to ring. There was at last the smile for which I had longed many years ago, that same contrast of the serious expression of the eyes with the smile around the lips which had fascinated me when the little girl had said goodbye to her friend.

I looked at her as if she were an apparition. Here was the girl I had known and yet a girl who was unknown to me. This feeling of the blending of strangeness and familiarity confused and startled me. The fusion of half-forgotten memories and of new impressions caused the sensation that I had experienced this situation before. Goethe must have had a similar feeling when he met Frau von Stein:

Speak! Why is it this destiny engages
Us in bonds that cannot broken be?
Surely once in unremembered ages
Thou wert sister or wert wife to me.*

The psychological difference was that I had really known this same girl when she was seven years old and that I saw her again as a woman with all the charms of sweet seventeen.

Ella wore a simple dress of light blue material. It followed the lines of the body. The wide skirt reached almost to the shoes, according to the fashion of the time. On her arm hung a straw hat with a wide brim. While David and Mary walked away, we sat on the bench and talked as if we had been old acquaintances. But were we not old acquaintances although we had never spoken to each other? Ella told me much about herself and her sister, how they had spent the years during which we had not seen each other. She had studied music and foreign languages, and was interested, it seemed, in literature. Just as now we spoke of my family and of hers. She told me that her father was frequently on his travels and that he always brought home nice gifts for both girls. College instructors tutored the sisters at their home. She asked about my studies and showed interest in my plans for the future. We exchanged memories of our childhood and of the people in the apartment house in which we both had lived. She told me that she had discovered Gerhart Hauptmann, whose *The Weavers* she loved, and I praised another writer whose plays and novels I had "discovered" in the meantime and whose name—Arthur Schnitzler—she had never heard. She was so natural and spontaneous, so sweet and friendly that I was overwhelmed. Where was the proud and haughy girl who had only once looked at me with a strange glance whose meaning puzzled me?

(Many years later Ella told me that my silly behavior as a boy had made an impression on her and that she had been aware that it was a kind of silent courtship. She had wished I would speak to her, but, of course, she could not speak to me first. Little girls

* Translation by Ludwig Lewisohn (*Goethe, The Story of a Man*, New York: Farrar, Straus and Company, 1949).

have their pride. Her indifference, she told me, had been pretense. She had often heard her mother and her aunt say a woman should never show a man that she cared for him, because he would lose respect for her. I understood later that she had for hours daydreamed about me, since the family moved to Klosterneuburg, and she showed me a snapshot of me as a boy of ten which she had secured from a girl friend. Ella had looked at it almost daily during these six years. She told me she had often whispered "Theodor" as if she could call me, and when David appeared, she hoped that her daydream would come true. On what meager diet can the illusion we call love live! An adolescent girl had spent years of her life daydreaming about a boy she had never spoken to and about whom she knew nothing but that he silently cared for her. And what a fool I had been! I had never suspected that I could be the object of her affection. Nothing in her behavior, not a single sign had shown that she paid attention to my clumsy admiration.)

It seemed she knew much about me and my family from the girl friends who had visited the sisters in those six years since they had moved to Klosterneuburg. We spoke of a hundred things and persons and we found we had many interests in common. David had to leave earlier than I. I stayed another hour chatting with the girls, who had brought sandwiches of ham and eggs from the house. But twilight descended upon the garden and I had to leave. Before saying goodbye, I asked Ella to sing one of the lieder which I had heard her sing in my boyhood. She nodded and extended her hand to me without speaking. Then she walked slowly down to the house with her sister along the vine-covered spiral path, and I followed her with my gaze until she was not visible any more. I left the garden and approached the house, as near as I could without being seen. And then I heard the first bars of the Schubert song. Ella accompanied herself on the piano. Her sweet and warm voice sang the well-known words, the familiar tune of the Schubert lied I had heard her sing in Vienna:

> *Du bist die Ruh*
> *Der Friede mild*
> *Die Sehnsucht du*

Und was sie stillt.
You are sweet peace and rest,
You are the haven blest,
You are that bliss of yearning
And all that cools its burning.

In this moment these simple verses conveyed to me the essence
not only of their gentlest creature but of all femininity—of what
is best in all women: that they are self-contained and that they
have the center of gravity in their own soul, in contrast to the
restlessness and destructiveness of men.

I had missed the bus to the station and I walked the two miles
apparently on the hard highway, in reality on clouds. The image
of Ella accompanied me. I saw her face and her eyes and her
smile before me. In my imagination I followed the lines of her
figure down the wide blue skirt. I compared this image to a blue-
bell in clumsy verses which ran through my mind. But again and
again the tune of the Schubert song emerged and I sang half
aloud, *"Du bist die Ruh."*

People who met the young man on the road and saw his silly
smile or heard him singing must have thought that he had
escaped from the asylum at Gugging nearby. But I did not care
about public opinion because I felt that I had discovered the
most precious secret in the world. I was sure that I was its only
possessor. Nobody could have convinced me to the contrary. I
was nineteen. No use to talk to me.

We were married seven years later, almost to the day.

3

During those seven years I would take the train from Vienna
to Klosterneuburg, the bus from the station to the village, and
I would walk up to that garden gate whenever Mr. O. was absent. (Much later I used to joke with my wife that I had served
seven years for her as Jacob had for Rachel, in the Holy Scripture.) Sometimes I could stay with Ella only half an hour or less,

but neither snow nor hail, neither cold nor heat could keep me away from Klosterneuburg. During those seven years I never set foot in the house of the O.'s and never spoke a word with my future father-in-law. Mary and Ella both implored me not to approach him. It would unavoidably mean the end of my visits, which had to remain a secret. After some months it became necessary to tell Mrs. O. about the clandestine visitor. She was terrified and so scared of her husband that she cried. She could be persuaded to keep the secret from Mr. O. only when Ella threatened to leave home and never to return. The aunt was, of course, not let into the secret. The people in the village must have wondered about the young man who, almost daily, in every weather, went up from the church square to a certain garden gate. They must also have seen him with the young girl through the gaps of the garden fence; but they did not give us away to Mr. O.—as though they respected our secret engagement.

As far as I remember, Ella and I made only two excursions together during those seven years. We were too afraid of being seen together by acquaintances of Mr. O., on the train or on the bus. It is strange but true that Mr. O. did not know about the clandestine visitor in his garden until Ella told him a few weeks before she came of age and left her home. (In Austria at this time people came of age at twenty-four years.) Mr. O. had a violent temper and was a bully toward wife and daughters, who were afraid of him. He would have perhaps made good his threat to shoot every man who trod upon his ground.

Our first excursion is as vivid in my memory as if it had happened yesterday. It was perhaps six weeks after my first visit to Klosterneuburg that we decided to make an excursion. We wanted to walk over the Kahlenberg, the well-known mountain, to Heiligenstadt, and return by a different road. We met at a certain place outside the village, where it was unlikely that we would encounter acquaintances of Mr. O. I still remember how lovely Ella was in a dirndl dress, walking toward me early that Sunday morning. The September sun was pleasant and we took our time. We walked slowly passing cottages and vineyards, chatting with the farm folk we encountered, often stopping to look at the view. We soon arrived at the wood and we began the ascent to the summit. Near the peak, we chose a spot among the pine trees, where we could rest comfortably and look down into the valley. Before us was the Vienna Wood, the vineyards around Nussdorf and Heiligenstadt, the small towns on the Danube, which looked like a silver ribbon, and there the city in which we both were born. Ella had modestly pulled her wide dirndl skirt over her ankles when she sat down. We were both silent. I smoked a cigarette and, as if under a spell, I looked at Ella's profile, following the beautiful curve from the hair to the throat. Her face was in repose, of the loveliness and serenity of a Botticelli madonna. I felt as if I had met the Holy Virgin on the Kahlenberg on a Sunday noon.

She seemed so remote, so out of reach, so far above me at this moment. In these last weeks we had become familiar enough; we had talked about so many things, but we had not spoken about our feelings toward each other. The girl had been friendly and natural, but would she not be as friendly with any other young man? I had so often wished to kiss her, but she seemed so cool, so self-sufficient and exquisite, that one did not dare touch her. I was shy and I was afraid she would be offended if I approached her. All around us was quiet; only the birds hopped from one bough to another. A gentle breeze made the grass and the meadow flowers bend with a rustling noise. It was as if nature held its breath in expectancy.

For a long time Ella looked quietly down into the valley without moving. It was as if she was far away in her thoughts. Slowly she turned her face to me and looked seriously into my eyes. At this moment I did not hesitate any more. What propelled me was stronger than my shyness. I took her into my arms and kissed her. It was only some seconds, but it seemed to me a small eternity until I felt that she lifted her face to me and that her lips responded to my kiss. I stammered words of love and endearment and did not want to let her go. I implored her to say something, to answer my passionate questions, but she only bent her head back and looked into my eyes, without speaking. And then came that slow smile, while the eyes remained serious, that smile known to me so well since I was a child, and she said in a low, but firm voice, "I have waited so long for this."

I was flabbergasted. I had never thought that she expected to be kissed by me. (What fools young men are in all these things! A young Parisian lady once taught me an unforgettable lesson: We were speaking about a friend of mine, who had no secrets from me. She took it for granted that he was in love with a certain girl. My friend had often talked to me about his emotions about different women. As a matter of fact, he had also spoken about that girl, but I had not received the impression that he felt especially attracted to her. I am sure that my friend himself would have denied it at the time. I therefore expressed my definite disbelief when the Parisian lady remarked that my friend was in love with the girl. My charming partner in conversation looked at me with a smile which expressed a mixture of pity and amusement, shrugged her shoulders, and said, *"Stupide comme un homme!"* A few weeks later, my friend had discovered to his great surprise that he was in love with that girl—a fact which had remained unknown to him, but not to the girl or to her friends. Women are ahead of us men not only in their sensitiveness about such feelings; they are also much more realistic about them than men, who are the true romantics. Not long ago an old lady said to me, "While a young man thinks over how to tell a girl that he worships her, she already considers how to furnish the drawing room.")

After the kiss my shyness had evaporated and I could speak freely about us and our future. The sun, the pine trees, the song of the birds, and all the sweet scents of summer were changed. The world was flooded with glory. Holding hands, we walked down the Kahlenberg and I felt boundlessly happy. We arrived at Heiligenstadt where we had lunch at a small restaurant. Later on, we passed a *Heurigen,* one of those inns where the wine of the year is served. Most of those places are in the open; people sit around small tables under trees, drinking the sweet wine which has grown on the surrounding hills and listening to the "Schrammel quartet." We too sat down and heard some of the familiar tunes played by the three violins accompanied by an accordion. When we walked along, we moved in the three-quarter measure of the tune following us.

The air was full of promise. The faces of men, women, and children coming our way seemed to be carefree and smiling. It was as if they all shared our happiness. We followed the Sunday crowd to a place where people danced to the playing of a small orchestra. It was a typical Austrian peasant dance, with its peculiar kind of merrymaking, not at all refined, but rustic and earthy, accompanied by jokes, laughter, and teasing. Sometimes a couple did more stamping than dancing and quite a few young men flung their girls into the air, to catch them again in their arms. We looked on; Ella said, "Isn't it exactly like a hundred years ago, when Beethoven composed the Pastoral here? There are the peasants; these are the same kind of dances as then."

I had not thought of Beethoven. This was indeed Heiligenstadt, where Beethoven composed his Sixth Symphony; the same place where he wrote his famous will, that somber, heartbreaking document of a suffering genius. "Let's hope that there will be no tempest as in the Sixth," I said, but the sky was cloudlessly blue and serene. As it was still early, we decided to walk on and we turned toward Grinzing. At a certain point Ella stood still and said, "But we must be near the Schreiberbach here." I had never heard of this brook.

"What is so remarkable about the Schreiberbach?" I asked.

"Don't you know?" She told me then that it was at the Schreiberbach, between Heiligenstadt and Grinzing, where Beethoven composed the brook scene. We asked one of the peasants we met where the Schreiberbach was. On the way there, Ella told me that Beethoven had heard in the bubbling murmur of that brook the lovely tune which the first violins play in the Pastoral. We found the brook. Ella told me (how much the girl knew about the great composer's life!) that later Beethoven had made an excursion to this very point with his loyal friend Schindler. He had pointed out this spot, and had added, "The birds composed with me," alluding to the joke of the bird song at the close of the movement. We returned to the Heiligenstadt station, where Ella took the train home and I another one to Vienna.

What had surprised me in rereading my objective study of Goethe was the sudden transition from *Truth and Fiction* to Beethoven's Sixth Symphony, the jump from Sesenheim near

Strassburg to Heiligenstadt near Vienna. What were the connecting links? Goethe wrote his autobiography about the time when Beethoven made his sketches for the Pastoral; the tunes of this symphony could well describe the rural idyl at Sesenheim. The movement after the storm expressed a mood similar to Goethe's, when he felt that he had escaped the doom of the curse. "Grateful Feelings after the Storm," the words that Beethoven had written in his score—the words which I had chosen as the title of that chapter—were appropriate to the picture of the young poet when the Alsatian landscape quieted and consoled him, after his leave-taking from Friederike. The threads between the Sesenheim story and the Pastoral were so slender that the connection between them appeared to be artificial. But the title, Beethoven's sentence, had emerged spontaneously and my thoughts had really led from Sesenheim to Heiligenstadt when I wrote that chapter. Now I realized that my own memories had unconsciously influenced my train of thought. The memory of our excursion to Heiligenstadt had determined the title of the chapter of my Goethe study "Joyous and Grateful Feelings after the Storm." This same memory made me introduce the Sixth Symphony into a psychological investigation of young Goethe's mood, as he rode away from Sesenheim. It cannot be accidental that the chapter described Goethe's situation after he left Friederike, while my unconscious thoughts had circled around the time when Ella and I first spoke of our love for each other. If we accept that our train of thought is unconsciously determined, then the contrast of the two situations must have its secret psychological significance. In that chapter the end of Goethe's romance is sketched; my memory of the excursion to Heiligenstadt marks the beginning of a romance.

But before we try to penetrate into this darker area, a tie between the two situations becomes clear, when one compares them. Goethe describes in the third part of *Truth and Fiction* how his journey through Alsace mitigated his sorrow and that he again found himself looking at the landscape. The sense for the beauty of nature had been sadly neglected in my education. My early interests were almost exclusively directed to human relations. Later, time and occasion to correct that deficiency were lacking.

I had been scarely aware of it until I met Ella. The excursion to Heiligenstadt is one of my earliest memories to recall that whatever little sense for beauty of nature I possess was awakened by her. She showed me the pretty or remarkable qualities of flowers and trees and the beauties of landscapes and views. I began to see shapes and colors in the country and found increasing pleasure in the observation of woods, rivers, and hills. I saw with her eyes. But was not my teacher the loveliest creation of living nature? When she made me see beauty in flowers and trees in the garden of Klosterneuburg, in the view from the Kahlenberg, it was as if the landscape surrounding us was only an extension of her own charm.

In contrast to Goethe, who received his best and most significant impressions through the eye, I was, as the French psychologists would say, a *"type auditif."* I was not just blind as a bat, but most of my impressions and memories were of an auditory character.

These psychological considerations lead me to comment on the differences between the presentation of the Sesenheim romance and my report. In Goethe's story the reader sees forms and colors of persons and things. It is as if what happened almost one hundred and eighty years ago, in Strassburg and Sesenheim, is resurrected, happens again before the reader's eye. It does not occur to me to compare my own poor presentation with Goethe's, in regard to artistic values. But it is noteworthy that most of the recollections presented here are connected with music. The transition from the story of the Sesenheim idyl to Beethoven's Sixth Symphony is only one of the significant examples.

In reading the first draft of these memories, I myself was surprised at how many of them are connected with music, with sounds and tunes. It is as if musical compositions are the pearls on which these recollections are engraved. This fact can be easily understood. The Vienna of my youth was the most musical city of the world. It was not only on account of the great tradition that the most prominent composers lived here and left their imprint on the cultural life of the city. A concert of the famous Vienna Philharmonic Orchestra, a first performance at the Opera (both directed by Gustav Mahler) were for weeks the subject of vivid discussion among the upper and middle classes of people. "Let me go where'er I will, I hear a sky-born music still"—Emerson's words could have described the atmosphere of Vienna at that time. There was scarcely a house out of which you did not hear song, piano, or violin. My own family, as well as the O.'s, were very interested in music. My mother and sister played the piano rather well and my older brother was an amateur violinist who won very favorable reviews after some public performances. I had been the only one in the family who did not play a musical instrument. But in my early twenties I could not hear enough music. Indeed my recollections of those years appear intimately connected with music; especially those memories which concern my romance with Ella, who was an excellent musician. When I listened to her playing a Mozart concerto on the piano or singing a Schubert lied, I felt as the Duke did in Shakespeare's play: "If music be the food of love, play on."

4

Most of the clues which proved that my own memories had sneaked into my objective study on Goethe are to be found in the titles I had given to the chapters. I had not searched for them; they simply occurred to me. For that reason, those personal experiences secretly found their way into the research. This very fact shows convincingly that we cannot keep secret thoughts to ourselves; they ooze out from us without our knowledge.

Later I understood why those hidden memory-traces gave themselves away in the chapter titles. The psychical mechanism of isolation was operating here. It is a defense mechanism which separates two spheres originally belonging together and isolates an idea from the emotions associated with it. Two areas of thought are thus prevented from having contact with each other. By putting an interval in time or place between the two areas of ideas, they remain apart. This isolation mechanism is operating in our daily lives. For instance, we try to exclude or eliminate emotional associations when we want to think objectively. To keep away personal thoughts from a scientific and objective task is necessary in the interest of logic. By this isolation the bridge between one sphere and the other is drawn; there is no longer any connection between them. I had written a psychoanalytic study on Goethe and nothing—or almost nothing—in its text showed that it had any connection with my experiences. But I had unconsciously given myself away in those telltale titles, which were set apart and had a place of their own. By this unconscious device of isolating, I had avoided recognizing that the two spheres of thought, the Sesenheim romance and my own, came in contact with each other. I had maintained the thought-avoidance so carefully that I myself had not recognized the subterranean connection until ten years later. The titles and the content of the chapters were thus separated, and their distance from each other helped to conceal the fact that there was a secret tie between the Goethe story and my own. What astonished me most was that these titles, which were so revealing, were at the same time so appropriate to the subject; were so well in keeping with the content of the chapters. They fitted so well that not the slightest suspicion could be aroused that they had another, personal meaning. In choosing them, I let hidden memories slip into my research. In isolating them, in setting them apart as titles, I had disconnected their emotional significance from the objective investigation. At the same time, the wording of the titles had made a significant contribution to the study.

Take, for instance, *"Freundliche Vision,"* the title I gave to the chapter describing the mysterious apparition Goethe had seen when he rode away from Friederike, the vision in which he had seen himself in a very elegant costume, riding back to her. Is the title not well suited to the content of that chapter? I knew, of course, when I wrote it that the *"Freundliche Vision"* is a song by Richard Strauss, a song I had heard several times. I chose it, or rather it occurred to me, because the words "Friendly Vision" gave the real, emotional content of the story; but I did not then think of how closely this title was connected with a personal experience. I had not forgotten this experience, but it had never occurred to me that it had its significance in this place. The disconnection thus amounted to a distortion, because it interrupted the electric current between the two emotional areas and made its existence unrecognizable not only to the reader but also to myself.

The Strauss song has its place in my recollections of the second excursion Ella and I made together. That was probably during the next summer (1908) and this time our destination was nearer to Klosterneuburg: the little town of Nussdorf, about two hours from Ella's house. We met near the Klosterneuburg station—it was again on a Sunday—and we again walked slowly on the highway. We had an early lunch of goulash and a glass of the famous Nussdorfer wine in a small restaurant on the roadside. The friendly innkeeper chatted with us in broad Viennese dialect (which we both spoke) for a little while and then left us alone. It was a small room, with a few tables nicely covered with white linen, ready to make the Sunday customers welcome. From the wall the picture of our old Kaiser Franz Josef looked benignly down on us. Against the other wall stood a piano. I asked Ella to play. She sat down and played a Mozart minuet. When I asked her to sing, she was undecided what she should choose. "Why not Schubert?" I asked. "The '*Heidenröslein*'?" She nodded and sought on the keys for the first bars. The next minute, I heard her gentle and expressive voice sing the well-known lied:

> *Sah ein Knab' ein Röslein stehn,*
> *Röslein auf der Heiden.* . . .

> Saw a boy a rosebud there
> Rosebud in the heather
> Tipped with dew and passing fair,
> Swift he ran to pluck it there
> In the golden weather.
> Rosebud pretty,
> Rosebud red,
> Rosebud in the heather.

> Said the boy "I'll pluck thee now,
> Rosebud in the heather!"
> Said the rose "I'll stab thee now,
> For my thorn is sharp, I trow.
> Bear it will I never."

Rosebud pretty,
Rosebud red,
Rosebud in the heather!

But the boy, he broke in scorn,
Tho she stabb'd him with her thorn
Yet she died that summer morn
In the golden weather.
Rosebud pretty,
Rosebud red,
Rosebud in the heather.

Ella's warm voice died away. We were both silent a moment, but then I spoke about the poem. I described to Ella how young Goethe had met the famous theologian and writer, Gottfried Herder, in Strassburg, and how the friendship with this older and matured man had amounted to a kind of mental revolution in the young genius. Herder had stated that poetry originates in the folk song and reflects the emotions and thoughts of the people. In contrast to most German contemporary critics, he despised the making of verses that imitated the smooth, gallant, and elegant French poetry. Poems, he said, should be born out of the true and deep feeling of the average man. Under his influence, young Goethe, who had until then made playful and frivolous verses in the French manner, began to compose those youthful poems which expressed his deepest emotions and experiences. Young Goethe began to collect old folk songs, while he wandered around in Alsace. The *"Heidenröslein"* was, no doubt, a poetic transformation of an old folk song to which Goethe had given a new shape. Herder published the *"Heidenröslein"* in 1773 for the first time in his magazine *Von deutscher Art und Kunst.* A stream of beautiful poems, masterpieces like "Welcome and Leave-taking," the "May Song," and others emerged, as if a floodgate had been opened. It was not only the influence of Herder that freed the young poet from the imitation of formalistic and conventional French poetry. He had fallen in love with Friederike, who was then seventeen years old.

I told Ella then and there the story of Sesenheim, and tried to give her a vivid picture of that romance, of its blissful beginning and its tragic end. I pointed out to her that Friederike was the primal image which lived in so many of Goethe's girl-figures, and which made him shape the loveliest of them all, Gretchen, in *Faust*. As far as I can remember, that was the only time I talked about Friederike to her. And did I talk! I must have given her a lecture like a professor of German literature. My compulsive Goethe reading had been done not so long ago. Where was there a boy of twenty who knew more about Goethe than I? No doubt, I wanted to impress my girl, to show off to her. I talked learnedly and, I am afraid, pedantically. I quoted chapter and verse and that literally, because I advised her which section of *Truth and Fiction* she should read and I recited Goethe's poems of the Sesenheim time which I knew, of course, by heart. I could give her the data when the young poet visited his sweetheart and when he left her.

I spoke about Goethe's experience with Friederike, without much psychological understanding, I am sure; like a young man who tells his sweetheart about the romance of another young man one hundred and eighty years before. I was a student of psychology, it is true, but I heard the name Sigmund Freud for the first time in a lecture of the following year.

"And what happened to Friederike afterward?" asked Ella.

I told her what I knew about it; that Friederike became a generally loved aunt and died as an old spinster, perhaps without having read the description of the Sesenheim romance in Goethe's autobiography. I also recited the beautiful lines on her tombstone. Ella listened without interrupting me. After I had told her about Friederike's destiny, she was silent and looked thoughtfully ahead. What did she think? It was as if she was far away in her thoughts.

What she said then—could it possibly have any connection with the story of Goethe and Friederike I had just told her? "Do you know any songs by Richard Strauss?" "No, but I do not like the man," I answered. I was a bit annoyed because I felt that she was not interested in my Goethe story or did not appreciate it. Why had she dropped the subject so suddenly and asked about something which was so remote from it?

As a matter of fact, at this time (1908) I had not yet heard any musical composition by Richard Strauss, and I really did not like him. I knew and loved only one of the contemporary composers, Gustav Mahler. A few months earlier, Mahler had yielded to the stupid intrigues of his enemies and had left Vienna, to go to New York. Like many young Viennese who realized that Mahler was a genius, I felt it as a cultural loss that the loved and admired man had left our city. Richard Strauss appeared to me as Mahler's victorious rival. The public of Vienna and of Germany preferred his operas and songs to Mahler's symphonies. He received all the appreciation and honor which, in my opinion, Mahler deserved. I had been a passionate "Mahlerite" and I had felt antagonistic to Strauss, because I had the impression that he was pushing forward and strove for cheap laurels.

Ella then told me that her father had made the acquaintance of Strauss in Dresden, and that the two men had become friends. She herself liked some of the songs by Strauss, for instance, "Freundliche Vision." The friendship of the composer with Mr. O. did not make me feel milder toward him. (The company he keeps!) And then we got into a real lover's quarrel and said a lot of silly things. I called Strauss a poseur and a "phony," a money-grasping man without conviction and integrity, and Ella repeated some of the stupid gossip she had heard about Mahler; that he was inhuman and tyrannical, and that he had many affairs with the singers of the Vienna Opera, whose director he had been. We argued about the merits and demerits of the works of both composers and their places in the music of our time. The funny thing was that Ella had never heard a composition by Mahler and I never one by Strauss. We suddenly realized how childish and silly our argument was, and began to laugh. We kissed and made up.

Ella then did the only thing which was reasonable in the situation. She went over to the piano and started to play. I still remember how the quietly floating tune of "Freundliche Vision" sounded and that she sang the words:

> Not in slumber did the dream arise,
> But in day's broad light I saw it all . . .

Our conversation, especially the argument into which we glided, often came back to me in later years. How did it start?

With my story of Goethe and Friederike. Later on, during the years of our marriage, we sometimes talked about Goethe. We saw *Faust* and *Tasso* together, and I read some poems to Ella; but, as far as I remember, Friederike and the Sesenheim time were never again mentioned.

Hearing the *"Heidenröslein"* had led to my talking about Goethe and Friederike, but why had I suggested this particular song? Schubert composed six hundred and three lieder—why just this one? He composed seventy-two Goethe poems, and among them are pearls like the *"Erlkönig," "Rastlose Liebe," "Wanderer's Nachtlied," "Der Fischer,"* the *"Mignon"* and the *"Suleika"* songs. Yes, he even composed a poem of Goethe's from the Sesenheim period—*"Willkommen und Abschied."* Why then did I wish to hear the *"Heidenröslein"*? I do not believe in accidents in a choice like this. Psychoanalysis has convinced me that there are undercurrent, unconscious thoughts which determine why our mind goes in one direction and not in the other. When Goethe wrote the poem, he had thought, of course, of Friederike. The plucking of the heath rose is a symbolic expression for the deflowering of a girl. Was not my unconscious mind directed to the same aim? Did I not choose the *"Heidenröslein"* because my train of thought ran along the same road? And then I had talked about the Sesenheim time, about the romance of the two young people, and of Goethe's leave-taking after he had fallen in love with the girl.

Without having an inkling of a notion that I thought this, I must have unconsciously hinted at such a possibility in my case. I myself must have unconsciously played with the idea of flight. There was, I am now sure, a subtle threat in my telling Ella the story of young Goethe and Friederike. It was as if I conveyed the possibility that I could leave her as Goethe left his sweetheart. Nothing was further from my conscious mind than such a possibility, but the logical—and more than this—the psychological sequence of our conversation does not allow any other interpretation. It was as if I had expressed in a hidden and subtle manner: You see, Goethe left Friederike because she did not yield to his desires, because she did not give herself to him. The fact that I wanted to hear the *"Heidenröslein"* and then told the story of

Goethe's romance—that Ella and I were about the same age as that other young couple and in a similar situation—only points to the psychological truth that the undercurrent of my talk contained this secret meaning.

Ella had silently listened to my story, but I felt somehow that her very silence expressed disapproval and condemnation of the subject of my tale. You sense such unspoken emotions in the atmosphere. It was not only disapproval of young Goethe's attitude but also of my own, because she must have unconsciously felt that his behavior betrayed a psychical potentiality in me. (But did I not—consciously, at least—disapprove of Goethe deserting his sweetheart?) She had then asked what had happened to Friederike afterward, and I had told her. Did she not unconsciously identify herself with Friederike, compare herself with Goethe's girl? She must have thought of us two, of our future and of what would happen to herself. It was a moment in which the unconscious of one person spoke to that of another, without words and beyond words. While she sat there quietly, her hands in her lap, looking ahead of her, she must have thought: What has destiny in store for me? Will I be another Friederike?

And then she had asked me whether I knew any songs by Richard Strauss, and I had felt annoyed as if she had paid no attention to what I had told her in words and without words. She had turned away from the subject and from me, it seemed then. But now when I look back at it, her thinking of the "Friendly Vision" did not mean a withdrawal from the problem, which we had not discussed but which we both secretly had in our mind. It was the continuation of our theme in another direction. She had pursued her train of thought, but it had led her to another station. She had turned away from the picture of Goethe's desertion and Friederike's loneliness in her thoughts, but not from us two. She had been led to another, happier image, to the "Welcome Vision":

Nicht im Schlafe hab ich es geseh'n . . .

to the dreamlike song, which calls up a friendly vision indeed of a young married couple walking arm in arm to a beautiful, cool cottage, in the summer. If I had been able then to look below the surface, to "listen with the third ear," I would have recognized that Ella, instead of envisioning a possible future like Friederike's, had turned to this other, more promising vision before her mind. She did not want to face the music, or rather she wanted to face another one, the tune called up by the Strauss song!

Not in slumber did the dream arise . . .

But I did not know that when I was twenty. What did I know then about the thoughts and the deep feelings of a young girl? I merely had the impression that she wished to drop the subject and had turned to a song by Richard Strauss, whom I did not like.

When I try now to reconstruct what perhaps went on in her mind, sensing rather than reasoning, when I now consider what was hidden in her reaction, as in a concealed answer to an unspoken question, I can perhaps guess what she may have been thinking. She rejected the unconscious suggestion hinted at in my speaking of the *"Heidenröslein"* and Friederike, the suggestion of intimate relationship, which the song indicated. Her thoughts must then have gone to her father, in whose eyes a love affair would have appeared as criminal. . . . She thought that her father was at the time on a journey and in Dresden. . . . He had sent her some songs by Strauss, whom he knew personally, from there. . . . "The Welcome Vision" is one of these songs. . . . The image which this song calls up is of a young couple, in their beautiful garden and their quiet house. Her thoughts, which had repelled the possibility of a future like Friederike's, were attracted by this other vision of future happiness.

I was young, unfeeling and cruel. I did not guess what went on behind her clear forehead. If youth but knew . . . I had unconsciously interpreted her silence and her question about Strauss as lack of interest and withdrawal of affection. At the same time, it amounted to a rejection of what was concealed in my talk. In reality it was as if I had said, "I want you to become my mistress or I shall leave you," and she had said, "No, I want to be married," because that was what the *"Freundliche Vision"* unconsciously meant.

In the argument about Strauss and Mahler, the concealed conflict between our views had been continued. In striking at Strauss, I had hiddenly attacked her father, had called him "phony" and "poseur." She had called Mahler tyrannical and sensual or even lecherous; she must have meant me, without knowing it. All my anger against Mr. O. must have broken forth in displaced aggression against the composer, who was his friend. She had unconsciously defended her father, when she protected Strauss, and had rejected my views which were so contrary to her father's. I had insisted that Mr. O., as well as Strauss, had to be brought down a peg; she had said that Mahler and I were conceited and intolerant. The quarrel about those two was only on the surface. In reality it concerned a much more important contrast, one which was more personal and more vital and had to do with the core of our relationship. It was a clash of wills behind the clash of opinions about two musicians. Not what we thought of them, but what we thought of each other had a concealed expression in this lover's quarrel. It was a communication between our unconscious thoughts.

I do not know how far the reconstruction attempted here is correct. If it did not hit the target, it at least struck near home. It was really ridiculous, I thought later on, our first quarrel. We had argued about Mahler and Strauss, of all things! But we had been reconciled and we had kissed each other. All's well that ends well.

5

But it did not end so well. It was still early afternoon when we left the inn at Nussdorf. We walked around in the little town and finally arrived at a public dance hall. Its door was open and we could see many couples dancing waltzes. I had danced at student balls during the last winter, but I had never danced with Ella. I asked her to go in to the hall with me, but she hesitated to enter the place, which was respectable enough. Was a trace of ill-humor or injured feeling left in her? I took her arm and led her into the wide hall.

Just when we entered, the orchestra began to play "Roses From the South," a favorite Strauss waltz. We danced well together and we enjoyed it. When the waltz came to an end, the people clapped their hands and forced the orchestra to strike up the next waltz immediately.

"Let's skip this one, darling," Ella asked. But I had my arm around her and the tune carried me away. Inconsiderately I insisted that we dance at least this last waltz. In the middle of it, I felt that Ella's hand, which lay lightly on my shoulder, had glided down. Panic-stricken, I looked at her face, which seemed suddenly changed. It appeared swollen, the lips almost blue. She fought to get her breath.

"I can't. I can't any more," she said. It took an effort to say these words. It seemed that she would fall to the ground the next minute. I carried her to a neighboring room, where she sank down on a couch. I was very frightened, watching her gasp for breath. The beloved eyes were closed, and she seemed unable to answer my worried questions. I wanted to call a physician, but she did not allow me to.

"Give me only a few minutes. I'll be all right," she said. Slowly she recovered her breath and looked as she had before the dance. She explained that she had sometimes had such attacks. They lasted only a few minutes and had no bad aftereffects. She seemed all right now. I insisted that she rest half an hour, and she smilingly complied. We sat there quietly and listened to the orchestra, which played familiar Viennese tunes. When I asked her how she felt, she seemed in a good mood, but I sensed some sad undertones in her gaiety. After some time, she wished to take the train home. I took her to the station and saw her off. Comfortably installed in her compartment, she spoke to me and blew me a furtive kiss, when the train began to move.

I had planned to stay much longer with Ella. There was time on my hands, so I decided to walk from Nussdorf to Vienna. Marching along, I thought of Ella but I was not worried any more about her. Her sudden illness was perhaps due to the heat in the dance hall or to the glass of wine, because she never drank alcohol. It occurred to me also that our argument had upset her and perhaps caused her attack. I felt guilty. Why had I hurt the beloved girl? I reviewed our conversation, which still preoccupied my thoughts. There was something in our argument which I could not fathom. . . . Why, we had talked about Goethe and Friederike—what was there to get upset about?

I had decided to follow the course of the river on my march to Vienna. "On the beautiful blue Danube," I murmured mechanically as I walked along and looked at the waves, which rolled along and looked rather grayish in the light of the approaching evening. And then suddenly verses of Goethe's "To the Moon" came to my mind. I was not Goethe-possessed or Goethe-crazy any more at the time, but our conversation of this afternoon had, of course, brought my thoughts back to him again. I was speaking the lines half aloud. To my own surprise, they were verses of a lost love, of looking back at a happy time of romance which had tragically ended. Walking along the Danube, I was reciting:

> Echoes murmur once again
> Of days bright and dour,
> Hold me between joy and pain
> In my lonely hour.
>
> Flow, beloved river, flow!
> Joy from me has gone,
> Old embraces perished so,
> Troth that was undone.
>
> Once I had the better part,
> Things that precious be,
> And that haunt the tortured heart
> Unforgettably.
>
> River, roll the dale along
> Without pause or ease,
> Answering unto my song
> With thy melodies . . .*

* Translated by Ludwig Lewisohn, *Goethe*, 1949.

Why was I depressed? It suddenly occurred to me that Mrs. O. had told me a few months ago that Ella had had rheumatic fever as a child, and that she had to be careful not to overexert herself. Dr. W., the family physician in Klosterneuburg, had assured Mrs. O. that Ella's heart functioned almost normally, as long as she was not subjected to great physical demands. I thought that Ella's indisposition was perhaps due to a heart ailment, but had not Mrs. O. told me that there was nothing seriously wrong with Ella's heart? Had Ella not recovered within a few minutes? Perhaps she had to be cautious and remain aware of overexertion and excitement. I argued with myself that I was unduly worried and that Ella was basically healthy. I decided to dismiss these unfounded scruples and to think of more pleasant things, for instance, of Ella's and my future together. I called up her lovable image. It was as if I had invited her to accompany me on my lonely walk.

When I came to the suburbs of Vienna, evening had already descended upon the city. The streets were full of the Sunday crowd, of people enjoying themselves. Young couples sat at tables, on which wind-protected candles stood in the open air, and listened to and sang with the three fiddlers and the accordion player. I still remember that I heard the people sing one of the Viennese hit songs of those days, and I remember the tune and the words in Viennese dialect:

> 's wird schöne Maderl'n geb'n
> Und mir wer'n nimmer leb'n.

> There will be beautiful girls galore
> And we shall not live any more.

A strange characteristic of the Viennese folk songs of that time —special features of their words and their tunes—differentiated them from the songs of other people. Mostly in waltz-measure, they were simple and tuneful. Their artistic value might be small, but they represent Vienna and the Viennese of that era so well that hearing them after many years still awakens nostalgia for the past. What characterizes them is a mixture of enjoyment of life and sentimentality. In the middle of a vivid expression of *joie de vivre,* even of an ecstatic feeling, the thought of death emerges. But the feeling of the fleetingness of life does not lead to gloom, but functions as a stimulus to enjoy life, which is so short. It is a vivid *"memento vivere"* (Goethe's expression). There is a permanent vacillation between the two moods and often enough a blending of them. The one does not exclude, but includes the other. The thought that death is near leads to all intensification or reinforcement of the pleasures of life, to a kind of orgiastic "I should worry" feeling. It is stranger still that this reminder of death results sometimes in a softening of anxiety and grief, in a kind of sorry humor or glad sadness.

This special mixture is typically Viennese and it is not restricted to the folk songs. You will hear it in the Viennese dances by Beethoven, in the middle of a movement of Mozart's or Schubert's symphonies, in the scherzi and adagios of Bruckner and Mahler and the waltzes of Johann Strauss. Once an acquaintance visited Schubert, whom he found composing. "Why do you always make such sad music, Mr. Schubert?" asked the visitor. "Do you know any merry one?" answered the composer.*

Yet unalloyed sadness is not to the taste of the Viennese. They needed a long time until they began to like the North German Brahms, because he appeared to them stodgy, heavy, and obtuse. I remember being told that one of Brahms's Viennese friends, the journalist Julius Bauer, used to tease him: "When Johannes is in a specially good mood, he composes a song, 'The grave is my greatest joy.' " That character of the Viennese people impregnated their daily lives and even pervaded politics. When near the end of World War I the united German and Austrian armies had suffered decisive defeats, the Viennese satirist Karl Kraus once characterized the different moods in the two capitals thus: "In Berlin the situation is considered serious but not desperate; in Vienna, desperate but not serious." This is exactly what so many Viennese folk songs express. Death looks over the shoulder of people on their most beautiful holiday, but the nearness of the end invigorates their enjoyment of life. This is the kind of folk

* Jessica says: "I am never merry when I hear sweet music." *Merchant of Venice* (Act V, scene 1).

song that was sung in Vienna, sad and glad at the same time. It is the same mood which found the words:

> There will be beautiful girls galore
> And we shall not live any more.

(The same mood emerges in the last movement of Mahler's *Song of the Earth.*) Walking along and pursued by the familiar melody, I suddenly felt very depressed. Life appeared empty, no future was promising and the end was near. Was it only this tune and these words which cast a gloomy spell upon me when I walked home through the streets in the evening? A feeling of the evanescence of life and of the nearness of death went with me. It was as if a shadow had fallen upon my young life. There was no escape from this feeling of impending calamity. Tomorrow was doomsday, so it seemed.

I tried to reason with myself, but I could not shake off my depression. Now, from a distance of more than forty years, I can well understand or, rather, I can now reconstruct what had caused my depression. During the afternoon an unconscious death wish against Ella must have emerged, was energetically rejected, and had been turned against myself. Perhaps the process would be better described this way: The slight annoyance I had felt in Nussdorf had, in its continuation into the realm of the unconscious, resulted in a murderous wish: You should die! Such impulses, surprisingly emerging from unconscious depths against persons near and dear to us, accompany our most tender and loving attitude toward these persons. Only people who do not want to penetrate into those dark recesses of the mind, or who play hide-and-seek with themselves, deny the existence of these subterranean tendencies or disavow their emotional significance.

No doubt, I was myself one of those people because I had not the slightest idea of what took place within me. I was only aware of a sudden feeling of gloom. The way to such an intense emotion is well known to psychoanalysts. The death wish against Ella had been repressed as it threatened to become conscious. In its place emerged the emotional reaction, dictated by my affection for her and my guilt feeling—death fear for myself. My own death would be the only atonement possible for the evil wish that had occurred to me. My melancholic mood and that astonishing feeling that death is close by had nothing to do with any danger threatening from without. Instead my mood reflected the danger from within. When Ella suddenly felt ill, there must have been a moment of panic, of intense superstitious fear that what I had thought could become a reality: that Ella would really die. In the thought of death for myself, fear of retaliation had hit back at me. The folk song I had heard had been the last link in a chain. It is noteworthy that the song's melancholic reminder (in three-quarter measure) that there will be beautiful girls and we shall be dead is a reversal of my thoughts. Had I not wished that Ella should die and I live on?

It is conspicuous that psychoanalysts, as far as I know, have not yet recognized that mental preoccupation with the problem of death is strongest in our youth. From puberty until the early forties, rather than later, these thoughts are prominent. It seems that fear of death then slowly decreases and, if the thought occurs, has another character: fear of dying. The two emotions have to be differentiated. The first, fear of death, seems almost a metaphysical anxiety. It is really a problem of an obsessional kind, namely, thought-preoccupation with the question of what death is and what it means. It is akin to other problems on which obsessional thinking is often concentrated, like that of immortality, of existence of the soul, of a beyond and of reincarnation. It is clear that this fear of death is connected with the thought of nonexistence, of the *néant,* with the menace of annihilation and nothingness. It is the same kind of mental preoccupation, of mysterious fear, doubts, and questions, that Hamlet puts into his famous monologue. It is not fear of dying which frightens him, but whether to be or not to be, what dreams may come in that sleep of death. "The dread of something after death" puzzles the young prince.

The fear of dying is psychologically very different from this metaphysical fear of death and of the end of individual existence. It has nothing to do with such problems as that of immortality of the soul, reincarnation, and so on, and is of a realistic character.

Man is afraid of suffering and suffocating, of the only real enemy he has on earth. In maturity, especially in old age, the fear of being dead is evaporated and only the fear of dying remains. Young people often risk their lives as if they were not afraid of dying, although the thought of not living fills them with terror. Old people, on the other hand, seem not to be worried about not existing; yes, they sometimes wish not to be any more, not to carry on a life which has become burdensome. What they are afraid of is the last struggle. Is it not paradoxical that youth, the time of life that is remotest from death, is so haunted by the one problem, while old age, in spite of its nearness to death, is almost free from it?

My answer to this question is founded on my psychoanalytic experience of more than forty years. It is, of course, not accidental that this question emerged in connection with the analysis of my own preoccupation with the theme of death, as described in this chapter. I believe that the prominence of thoughts about death, the brooding and speculation about death, is an unconscious re-action to secret aggressive and murderous thoughts and impulses. Such anguish occurs to young, temperamental people when their strong wishes and desires are frustrated. Aggressive impulses then emerge against parents and teachers, in short, persons of author-ity. Under the influence of guilt feeling, those unconscious tend-encies often revert against oneself and finally take the form of intense preoccupation with the abstract problem of death, which makes its highly personal origin unrecognizable. What emerge now are speculations, doubts, and meditations about death as such; only rarely, about one's own death. The intensity of this preoccupation with the death problem corresponds to the inten-sity of the drives of lust and power, sex and dominance which insist on immediate gratification. When the impulses and tend-encies toward sex and ego satisfaction become less urgent, as in old age, when their force becomes less imperative, then the fear of death as such, of death as punishment and atonement, the pre-occupation with the death problem decreases. It is not accidental that Hamlet's profound meditations on death emerge when he plans to kill the King, and that in connection with it even suicidal impulses occur to him. His thoughts on death, all his reflections and doubts about "the undiscover'd country from whose bourn no traveler returns," are generalized thoughts about his own death as atonement and punishment for murder in thoughts.

When that sudden sadness hit me, when gloom and despair without any apparent reason engulfed me, I was twenty years old. My desires were most urgent and my impatience when they were not satisfied was great, my love as strong as my hate, my rage as immediate as my tenderness. But also the severity of the inner demands on myself and my moral self-condemnation were not yet mitigated. I had become prey to the moral reaction that had set in after murderous impulses against my sweetheart had threatened to reach the threshold of conscious thinking.

That evening I slowly walked through the streets of the suburbs of Vienna. Having arrived at home, I ate dinner with mother and sister. I felt sad and tired from my long walk from Nussdorf to Vienna so I went to bed early. How I could sleep when I was twenty! Whatever disappointment, grief, or misery the day had brought me, I could quickly fall asleep. Looking back now, when sorrows about the present and anxiety about the future often keep me awake, I almost envy the young man who could so easily fall asleep. That day I had been deeply unhappy before going to bed. Some dark power seemed to reach out for me and clutch me; life had seemed hopeless and all lost, but I—what a blessing!—fell into a long, uninterrupted sleep.

The "pursuit of happiness" is a butterfly hunt. Butterflies can be caught, but they cannot be kept alive at home for a long time. Happiness is restricted to hours, if not to minutes. The feeling one has when one glides into a deep sleep marks one of those happiest moments. It does no credit to life when the upshot of it is that happiness in it can be attained only in forgetting it. In the end, love and friendship, fame and achievement lose their lure and a low voice in us speaks: "Sleep, what more do you want?"*

* The five stanzas of Goethe's "Night Song" end with these words.

6

Psychoanalysts of all countries agree that long engagements in which young couples decide not to have sex relations and isolate themselves are psychologically unhealthy. Kissing and embracing cause sexual excitement, and desires are roused which cannot be gratified. Such frustrated excitement is especially harmful when this state lasts many months. I am of the opinion that young people in such a situation should either avoid being alone together for a long time, or they should break through and have sexual intercourse.

Take our case. Here we were together almost daily, fair weather or foul, alone and unobserved. In winter, we were enclosed in the summerhouse, which was then boarded up, planked in like a chalet, and dark. We kissed and embraced each other, of course, but there was nothing of what is technically known today as "heavy petting." Ella did not want this and I respected her wishes. Her upbringing had filled her with strong sexual inhibitions, but there must have been intense fears and scruples in myself, also. And this went on for seven years! What a waste of energy, what a luxurious and, properly seen, silly effort and restraint! How much better would it have been for both of us if we had broken through! The harm caused by permanent, frustrated desire was so much more serious than the doubtful service to a conventional, moralistic code. (But you cannot be young and wise.) We both became nervous and fidgety. I had the impression that the situation was tougher and more difficult for me than for Ella; but who can say that his own view in such things is right?

In those years, I considered sexuality as a kind of enemy rather than as a powerful and strength-giving source of enjoyment. It was not a friendly power, but an evil demon against which one had to fight. It was the "thorn in the flesh." I was uncomfortable and I wanted, not sexual gratification, but to be free from this persistent stimulation. I wanted to be able to work, to study and to write, to think of worthwhile things, to achieve something. I fought this battle with myself for almost three years. I worked and studied like a slave, and I tried to divert my thought from the images which emerged again and again, but I could not get rid of them. Nowadays psychoanalysts speak much about the "sublimation" of this drive, but I do not believe that the crude sexual urge can be "sublimated." Sex has such a terrific singleness of purpose. Finally, I gave up the fight. I had a few brief intimacies with different girls, none of whom had more than a fleeting and purely physical appeal to me. I had, of course, met the same difficulties as other young men in similar situations. There was the risk of making a girl pregnant, the fear that she could become emotionally involved with me, and the fear of venereal disease. When I met a decent girl, and wanted to "make love" to her and nothing else, she wanted to be told that I loved her. But I was not able to pretend that I felt tenderness while I felt only sexual desire. My aim was so much more modest; but without being loved no "nice" girl would be ready to go to bed with me.

After a few interludes, some of which were successful nevertheless, I met Vilma. She was a woman of (she said) thirty-five years, and had become a widow two years before. She was thus twelve years older than I and she had a son who was exactly ten years younger than myself. (Psychoanalysts will not fail to point out here, that Vilma, mother of a boy and so much older than I, was a mother-representing figure and that she was the object of an unconscious incestuous desire. "Elementary, my dear Watson" or "my dear Dr. E." or "my dear Dr. K.," as the case might be!) It is significant that my memory has not retained the details of how and where we met. I still remember that, shortly afterward, I made a pass at her and was rejected. A few weeks later, on a visit to her apartment, I tried my luck again and was even more energetically rejected. After this, I sat there silently when, to my great astonishment, Vilma gently took the cigarette from my hand, sat suddenly on my lap, threw her arms around me, and kissed me on the mouth.

(Do we ever understand women? Vilma told me later that when she had rejected me, I had looked like a disappointed and sullen little boy, with defiant lips. She said that she had then urgently wished to kiss me on these lips! I am smiling, because it just occurs to me what a patient of mine, a young newly married man, told me the other day. He and his wife were dressing in the morning when the young woman, standing before the mirror and examining her appearance, asked him, "Do you love your elbow?" My patient, telling me about it in his analytic session, shouted, "Did you ever hear such a silly thing? Do I love my elbow! It is as fantastic as if you were asked whether they have fancy dress balls on Sirius. What is there to love or not to love about an elbow? I am sure that such a thought has never occurred to a man since the beginning of creation.")

That evening Vilma gave herself to me, and we had an affair off and on for the following three years. Vilma was rather tall and slim, had light blond hair, vivacious eyes, and long, slender hands. She was the "sweet little girl," as Schnitzler has painted her, fifteen years after her first adventure. I was not her first lover after she had married, as I found out, nor was I the last. She was not very intelligent but sly and shrewd. She had the cajolery of a cat and similar morals. She lived in a tiny apartment, kept very clean, in the slum section of Vienna; had a small pension left by her husband and earned a little money as a dressmaker. She said she did not want to marry again because she did not wish to sacrifice her independence. What attracted her to me was, I believe, that I was young and intelligent and perhaps that I was rather shy with women—at least until after the first kiss.

Vilma made no demands on me. She was always ready when I wanted her, but the trouble was, and she sensed it, that I did not want her but just a woman. On many evenings I left her after a lustful hour, determined not to come back; but a few evenings later I found myself again on the trolley car that led to her house. When I was there, all intentions to restrain my desires evaporated. The swishing of her skirts, the silken underwear, and the smoothness of her flesh, the touch of her breasts, did things to the young man for which he was sorry half an hour later. I rarely stayed more than an hour with her, sometimes less, but she seemed to be content with this. She was at first subtly, and later on less subtly, exciting.

When we were together, I knew, while she talked about a hundred inconsequential things, that she thought of sexual intercourse as much as I. She had her own way to lead up to it, either by caressing me while she sat on my lap, or by showing me her own increasing excitement. Much more experienced than I was, she made me believe that the sexual initiative was on my side. She preferred the lecherous aspects of sex and tried successfully to awaken the taste for it in me. I remember an occasion when I once rang the bell to her apartment and she told me, when she opened the door, that her mother, who had come to see her, was in the next room. I wanted to leave immediately, but she led me to the dark bathroom and, while she talked to her mother through the door, she half undressed herself. We had sexual intercourse there, she sitting on the table and I standing. This situation, she told me later, was the most exciting for her during our affair. She was not a lady and just this was then sexually stimulating. It seems to me that there is only one situation in which a woman can use four-letter, "dirty," and very vulgar words: a few minutes before the orgasm. The habits and manners are different in the new generation. Vilma was not careful with her language in this direction, also outside the one situation. I still wonder why it did not disturb or sober me more.

She was, in so many directions, the opposite of Ella; very sensual, where Ella was chaste; mature and motherly, while Ella was girlish in every fiber of her nature. Vilma gave herself freely, while you always felt a certain restraint in Ella. Vilma was down-to-earth in behavior and language, while Ella was refined and ladylike.

Here was, it seemed to me at first, a convenient way out of an emergency situation. If I could not have satisfaction with Ella, to whom my real desire went, I could get it from Vilma. Here was an easygoing relationship, without obligation on her or my side, and with the mutual understanding that a deeper emotional involvement or a permanent tie was excluded. I had never said to Vilma that I loved her. Once, in an outburst of brutal frankness, I had even said that I often disliked her, and that my need for her was a purely sexual one. After a few months, I told her about my love for Ella and our clandestine engagement, but she had already sensed something of this kind and said, "I always knew I would lose you in a short time. Let's make it beautiful as long as it lasts." She accepted the state of things, put up with my moods and inconsiderateness, and never complained. And inconsiderate and sometimes brutal I was, especially when she wanted affection from me! I had none to give her, but this was no reason to be unkind. Or was it?

Did I feel guilty because I could not be tender, and take it out on her? I often wondered about why I had to succumb at least twice a week to this dark, imperative urge, which immediately evaporated after a release was reached. Why did this body first appear to me as the goal of my desires and a few minutes later appear to be without charm, just a body like others? Then I saw sharply the creases on the neck, the crow's-feet around the eyes, the blots and blemishes on the skin. (With the sensitiveness and delicacy of feelings most women have, Vilma never showed herself nude after sexual intercourse.) I knew that I would not have the same reaction with Ella, and strangely enough I sometimes felt resentful against her, as if she were responsible for my disillusionment in Vilma.

The Jews in East Galicia have a strange proverb: "If you eat 'Khaser,' let it be fat." Khaser is a Hebrew word and means "pork." The proverb proclaims: If you violate the sacred law, choose a fine, fat piece of the forbidden meat and enjoy it. In other words: When you do something that is forbidden, don't be a fool; relish it, get all the pleasure out of it. I knew this bit of practical wisdom since my childhood, but I was stupid enough not to make it my own.

In having the lecherous affair with Vilma, I "sinned" (thus I felt then) but under protest against that which drove me to it. I did what was forbidden, but I withheld my consent to it. I sinned with a bad conscience, as if this made the forbidden deed less serious or less real. But I made it only more senseless. I do not see that such an attitude is especially promoting the salvation of the soul or serving the morals. On the contrary, it is psychologically harmful—to commit a forbidden deed and then feel too guilty about it, because this intense guilt feeling becomes an unconscious incentive for committing the deed again. My remorse about my unfaithfulness to Ella had not the effect of making me faithful. It only made me feel unhappy. I agree with Nietzsche, who once stated that feeling remorse about what one has done is as futile and stupid as when a dog bites into a stone.

My reason told me that I had reached, if not an ideal, at least a tolerable solution to the problem which so many young men have to face. It presented itself as a clear, clean-cut division. One woman for the soul, the other for the body. (Maupassant's *Une Vie,* which I read then, shows such a picture.) But things are not as simple as they often appear to our reason, to which we sometimes attribute a totalitarian power in our psychical household.

I know that I have to interrupt the presentation of my story at this point, to meet the moral indignation of my readers. "What," they will say, "here is a young man in love with and engaged to a lovely and sweet young girl, who deeply cares for him, and he has a back-street sexual affair? How could he make his romance agree with such a lecherous adventure? Was he not ashamed of leading a double life? He confesses to being in love with this girl, while he indulges in sexual intercourse with that other woman! Is such a division psychologically possible and, above all, is it excusable?" Let me first state that I told myself these very things and I condemned myself then with more severity than my readers are inclined to. As a matter of psychological fact, I am now looking back at the young man I was then with more leniency and I am judging him with more clemency than I did then. I understand him better now than he understood himself then, when he was confused in a tangle of emotions.

I can partly explain to myself what the emotional situation was, between Ella and Vilma, with the help of an analogy which was taken from the field of physics and which I transferred to the area of psychology: the analogy with interference. We all know this expression from the disturbances which annoy us, when our radio reception is impaired by electrical causes, undesirable signals, etc. Interference is, however, a phenomenon not only restricted to sounds. It is also in general the mutual influence of two waves or vibrations which produce certain characteristic phenomena. When two trains of waves meet (for instance, on the surface of the water), the result is under certain conditions an increased intensity; under others, a neutralization or superposition of the waves. The action of one wave can, for instance, be neutralized or weakened by that of the other, or it can be twice what it would be without the other. Such encounter of waves in all media (for instance, in the air, the water, the ether) results in different figures, which are known as interference patterns. Still photography and slow-motion pictures can now give us an excellent idea of what these various interference patterns look like.

The physical term "interference patterns" seems to me very appropriate for the description of processes in which two different waves of emotion meet. I would like to borrow the name from physics and introduce it into the field of psychoanalytic psychology, because it fits so many emotional phenomena. The visual character of the phenomenon and its plastic nature recommend the expression for presenting the various and changing pictures in emotional conflicts. The waves of different feelings for Ella and Vilma fought each other and formed some strange interference patterns.

It often happened that I left Vilma and, on the way home, felt an intense yearning for Ella; such a strong urge to hold her in my arms, as if the union with her would purify me and sweep away all sordidness of my relations with Vilma. But it happened, also, that when I was with Ella, I sometimes felt a sudden urge to be with Vilma, to be engulfed by her desire, to enjoy her surrender.

I tried to "isolate" the one relationship from the other, to drown the thought of the one girl when I was with the other. I did not succeed, because the image of the one often appeared when I wanted to concentrate—in my thoughts and emotions—on the other. I did not call it up. It was uncalled for in more than one sense, but it emerged against my will.

There was also an attempt to bridge the abyss between the two women, and to find something Ella-like in Vilma.* I tried to imagine it was not she, but the beloved girl whom I held in my arms. I forced my fantasy to call up this other image, to give the satisfaction a quality beyond the physical one, and to make it deeper and more personal. The reality was too strong and I failed. But the other effort, to find something Vilma-like in Ella,

* We know the two mechanisms of isolating and connecting two different emotional and intellectual spheres best from the study of neurotic symptoms.

was unsuccessful, because I could not bring Ella down from the pedestal on which I had put her. I had to admit to myself that there was a sharply drawn line of demarcation not only between these two figures, but also between the two emotional areas of tenderness and sexuality. A last desperate attempt, to take a cynical view, to persuade myself that there was not much difference between one woman and the other in the sexual situation (do you remember "Cover their face with the Stars and Stripes and it is the same"?) was short-lived and vain.

Once I had decided not to see Vilma any more. I did not see her for two weeks. She wrote me pleading letters in which she said that she did not understand my behavior, and asked why I did not come, since she had done nothing wrong. Later, she must have sensed what my conflict was, because she once wrote that I should not think that I was unfaithful to Ella when I visited her, and that I should .not torture myself with superfluous scruples but enjoy life, and that the affair with her would not interfere with my love for Ella. Stronger than her emotional appeal was her sex appeal. I returned to her, to break with her, and returned again until I went to Berlin in 1913. I got some friendly lines from her a few months later, congratulating me on my wedding. Then I never heard from her again.

Before her twenty-fourth birthday, the date when she came of age, Ella told her father about us, listened silently to his raging and storming, packed her things, and followed me to Berlin, where we married. After seven years of being together almost daily, she was a virgin and I was a damned fool.

III

1

How far we are from our own experiences! How remotely we live from this hidden self, which is the core of ourselves, and which thinks and feels and acts in a manner quite different

from how we consciously are thinking, feeling, and acting! My
romance with Ella started when I was nineteen years old. My
book on Goethe was written when I had passed forty. Not before
I had passed fifty, more than thirty years later, did it dawn upon
me that there must be a subterranean connection between
Goethe's romance in Sesenheim, near Strassburg, and mine in
Klosterneuburg, near Vienna.

I never consciously thought of it during the experience (although it must have been several times near the threshold of
conscious thoughts, for instance, when I spoke of Goethe and
Friederike to Ella, in Nussdorf, and when she sang *"Heidenröslein"*). I did not think of it while I wrote the study on Goethe.
I spoke, of course, about Goethe and especially about my compulsive Goethe reading, in my analysis, which was in 1913—seven
years after I met Ella—but I had not the slightest inkling of an
idea that there might be a secret connection between Sesenheim
and Klosterneuburg. When I discovered those clues in my own
book, more than twenty-five years after my analysis, the first
notion emerged that my own experience was connected with that
of young Goethe, by some invisible threads. But before this, I
had not a drop of insight into what happened then to me and
in me.

It would tickle my vanity, as a psychoanalyst, if I could truth-
fully say that I early became conscious of this side of my experience. Since I do not want any embellishment or any "interior dec-
orating" of the soul, I must shamefully record the facts. I am
quite prepared to accept the criticisms of "colleagues," who think
I was lacking in analytical cleverness. I can now take their barbs,
blows, and broadsides imperturbably. (My head is bloody, but
still unbowed.) I am full of admiration for a speed with which
one rapidly understands one's own experiences and those of
others, but I have a suspicion that what can be so swiftly and
easily fathomed must be shallow.

When at last it dawned upon me what had happened more
than thirty years ago in Klosterneuburg, it was as if a curtain
were slowly pulled up. Finding those clues in the Goethe study,
and remembering the events and the emotions, was but preparatory work. The real questions appeared later on. What did it

mean that those unconscious memories emerged while I was investigating an early love experience of a poet of one hundred and fifty years ago? And why had I become interested in this subject now? Why did my own memories reveal themselves in those telltale titles of an objective, scientific study? In accordance with psychoanalytic principles, this could not have been accidental. There must have been a connection, in my unconscious thoughts, between Goethe's experience and my own.

The next answer, of course, would be that one experience was comparable to the other. But this answer is clearly wrong. Goethe fell in love, was haunted by many superstitious fears, and left his sweetheart after a few months. I waited seven years, and I married my beloved girl—not to mention the overflow of the dissimilarities, which are so apparent. There are so many and such clear differences that they put some possible similarities into the shadow.

Something warns me that I am in danger of making a rash judgment, as if my view is too hasty. Let us first look at our ages. When Goethe first met Friederike, he was just twenty years old; she was nineteen. When I met Ella, I was nineteen and she seventeen. In both cases it is the age of romance. Goethe was a student of law; I was a student of psychology.

There are a few similarities in the external circumstances. The friend, Weyland, who knew the Brion family, asked Goethe to come with him to Sesenheim. As Goethe reports in the tenth book of *Truth and Fiction,* the girls had asked Weyland about Goethe. (These two men usually had their meals together in Strassburg.) Weyland and he rode together from Strassburg to Sesenheim. There is a similar situation: when David invited me to Klosterneuburg and we took the train there together. There is, furthermore, the contrast between city and country. Goethe was born in Frankfurt and had stayed in Leipzig and Strassburg—all three big cities. Scenery and life in the village of Sesenheim were quite different. I was born and lived in Vienna. When I was with Ella, in the garden of Klosterneuburg, life had another atmosphere and another rhythm. A few miles from Vienna—as Sesenheim was from Strassburg—there was a different world, nearer to nature and yet not too remote from the cultural life of the great city.

There were specific similarities in the local features. Goethe reports, for instance, there was a little wood on a hill near the garden of the Brions' and "there was a cleared place with benches, from each of which one had a pretty view of the landscape. Here was the village and the steeple of the church, here Drusenheim and behind it the wooded Rhine islands. . . ." The young man sat there on a bench called *"Friederikens Ruh"* (Friederike's rest). From the garden of the O.'s, you looked down into the village. There was the steeple of the church, here Klosterneuburg, and behind it the Vienna Wood. We sat down on a bench which, as Mary told me, was called "Ella's bench" and was reserved for her, because she liked to sit there. In the Brion family was an older sister, whom Goethe calls Olivia, but who was really Maria Salomea. Goethe describes her as well formed, vivacious, and rather violent in temper, while Friederike was quieter than her sister. But this was exactly the difference between the temperaments of Mary and Ella.

There were other similar, small circumstances. When Goethe first visited the family in Sesenheim, Friederike had not yet come home and everybody awaited her. When I first visited Klosterneuburg, David, Mary, and I sat in the summerhouse waiting for Ella. Goethe describes Friederike as he saw her for the first time—the long blond braids, the clear blue eyes, the national Alsatian costume, the round white skirt, the bodice, and the black taffeta apron—"Thus she stood on the frontier between a peasant and a city girl. The straw hat hung on her arm, and thus I had the pleasure to see and recognize her at the first glance in all her loveliness and gracefulness."

But Ella also was blond, with large blue eyes, and Goethe's description of Friederike's appearance fits Ella's splendidly. When I saw her the second time, she wore an Austrian dirndl dress, and later on she preferred those rustic dresses when in Klosterneuburg. Friederike played the piano and sang Alsatian and Swiss folk songs—again a similarity to Ella. These are only a few of them, and their comparison is restricted to the first meeting. Later on, others became apparent, as Friederike's tubercular disease and Ella's heart ailment, similarities in temperament of the two girls and also of their two lovers. It is perhaps sufficient to enumerate only those similarities which must have unconsciously made an impression upon me, when I first saw Ella. I emphasize again that I had never consciously thought of a comparison between the situations, views, or persons, at this time or later.

I recognized the real character of the subterranean connection between Goethe's experience and my own when I remembered the story thirty years later, especially when I looked back on the first visit to Klosterneuburg. I remembered, namely, what Goethe said about the time immediately preceding the visit to Sesenheim. What an idiot I had been not to think of this in the first place, as it is so much more important than any real or imagined similarity! The reading of *The Vicar of Wakefield* had made a strong impression upon the young poet. The Vicar and his wife, their older daughter, Olive, beautiful and rather extroverted; and the younger, Sophie, lovable and rather introverted, the parson's house in rural surroundings, and the vicissitudes of the family— all these things left vivid traces in his mind. Goethe himself, looking back in his sixtieth year, wrote:

"The work I mentioned had left a great impression, of which I myself was not aware. I felt in agreement with that ironic mental attitude of Goldsmith, which soars above things, above luck and unhappiness, good and evil, life and death, and thus arrives at the possession of a truly poetic world . . . In no case could I have expected to be transported very soon from this fiction world into a similar, real one."

What Goethe here alludes to is, of course, the excursion to Sesenheim. When he saw himself with the pastor, Brion, and his wife, with Olivia and Friederike, he became more and more aware of the resemblance of the Alsatian family to the Vicar's. "My astonishment, about seeing myself really in the Wakefield family, was beyond description." It seemed that here were doubles of those figures in the Goldsmith novel. The conversation at table seemed even to enlarge the appearance of the family circle and of its environment. "As the same profession and the same situation everywhere, wherever they appear, produce similar, if not the same effects, several issues were discussed, several things happened similar to what had already taken place in the Wake-field family."

But this impression was not only Goethe's. His friend, Wey-land, who had introduced him to the Brion family, had realized it before Goethe. When the two young men were alone in the guest room, Weyland prided himself on having surprised his friend with the resemblance of this family to the Primroses. "Really," said Weyland, "the story is quite the same. This family can very well be compared with that, and you in your disguise can take over the role of Mr. Burchell." Weyland alluded to the villain in Goldsmith's novel, the young man who seduces the Vicar's daughter.

Young Goethe is not only aware of all these similarities, but also of the unconscious potentiality in himself of playing a role in Friederike's life similar to Burchell's in Sophie's. He sensed in himself the psychical possibility of seducing and deserting Friederike. He gave the most wonderful plastic presentation of this potential destiny, later on, in the tragedy of Faust and Gretchen. No doubt it is possible that Goethe flirted with the idea of reliving the story of *The Vicar of Wakefield,* as the French writer Brion says, *"de vivre un roman de Goldsmith."* For the reader of *Truth and Fiction* who can read between the lines, it is clear how strong this temptation must have been in the fantasy of the young poet.

All this was, of course, very well known to me. It had even occupied my thoughts a short time ago. Yet such knowledge was, so to speak, on another level from my own experience, was separated from it by an impenetrable emotional wall of isolation. Otherwise, how was it possible that for more than three decades, I had remained unaware of it; that I had wanted to relive a romance of Goethe's? When David told me about Ella and Mary, their cottage and garden in Klosterneuburg, and we went together to the village, I must have unconsciously thought of Wey-land, Goethe, and Sesenheim. So many things there reminded me of the idyl in Alsace, and all was emotionally prepared for the romance, as in the case of Goethe. Without having the faintest notion of it, I must have identified myself with him, as he described himself at this visit at Sesenheim. I saw everything and everybody with his eyes, and compared Mary with Olivia, Ella with Friederike herself.

It was less than a year before that I had been absorbed in thoughts of Goethe's Sesenheim tale, and my compulsive study of his works and life had reminded me again and again of Friederike, in these last months. I had reread the story of the young poet who had fallen in love with the gentle girl, and had been greatly moved by it. I was then near Goethe's age. What young man would not have wished to love and be loved as he was and as he had described it? And then all seemed to fit, as if it were a repetition of the Sesenheim story. If it did not fit, I unconsciously adapted it to Goethe's tale. I must have unconsciously compared his disguise as a poor candidate of theology with the secrecy of my visits to Mrs. O.'s garden. I can remember a characteristic feature, which shows how near the thought of Goethe was to the threshold of the conscious surface and that it was, nevertheless, prevented by strong inner powers from breaking through to this level. I still remember that in my first letter to Ella I compared life in Vienna with that in Klosterneuburg, and I wrote that the great city appeared to me so empty. Compare this with a passage from the letter young Goethe wrote to Friederike, after he returned from Sesenheim to Strassburg. "You would not believe that the noise of the city would grate on my ears after your sweet country joys. Certainly, Ma'mselle, Strassburg never seemed so empty as now." (I said, of course, "Fräulein Ella," instead of "Ma'mselle"!) It is clear that I must have unconsciously thought of Goethe's letter.

There was, however, a decisive difference and it explains from a psychological point of view why the story of Sesenheim, so well known to me in all its features, remained so long isolated from my own experience; why the threads did not become transparent to me. I was in love with Goethe, but my admiration for him was accompanied by strong resistance. I was, so to speak, his most recalcitrant reverer. And among the things I minded and resented in Goethe then was his behavior toward Friederike. How could he, who loved her so dearly, desert her so cruelly? With my wish to find a girl as lovely and charming as Friederike must have emerged a decision that I would never leave such a precious sweetheart. I would marry her and stay with her until "death do us part." It became clear to me that I must have repressed any thought of deserting Ella. This very thought interrupted the connection between his story and my romance and isolated the one from the other.

I recognized, so late in life, what had taken place so early in it: that the unconscious wish to experience something like Goethe in Sesenheim was an important factor in the genesis of my love, and that a subterranean resistance against the behavior of the young genius had contributed to my course of actions and my train of thoughts. There must have been many times when the temptation to desert Ella emerged in my unconscious thoughts. But when those thoughts threatened to become conscious, I drowned them immediately. After that excursion to Nussdorf, there were, I am sure, doubts about Ella's heart ailment, fears about the influence of her illness on our future common life. But I was one and twenty. . . . And I was unconsciously not as sure of my destination, nor as aware of the deeper needs of my nature, as Goethe was of his at the same age.

Looking back at this phase of my life, I am astonished at how great the influence of literature, especially of the great poets—as Goethe—was then on the lives of us young men. They not only prepared us for our experiences; they helped to shape them and to give them a certain development. We young men were not at all aware of this substructure of the house we then lived in.

I wonder whether literature will have a similar influence on the life of future generations. Fiction and poetry seem to decrease in their social function and certainly in their pattern-giving value for romance, which is as great an achievement of imagination as poetry. Will it not degenerate, if it is not nourished by appropriate food? But one need not be worried about the future generations. Even if poets should become extinct and all great writing were to disappear, other means would give food for romantic emotions, and would help to promote the birth of love. Future generations will perhaps . . . But here let me tell about my grandchild Loretta when she was three years old. The little girl was left alone in the room and played with her dolls, while the radio was turned on and a crooner sang. Suddenly, she came running into the kitchen to her mother, pointed to the radio, and said quite excitedly, "He says he loves me so!"

2

When I now look back at the years of my own romance at Kloster-neuburg, which is here compared with Goethe's stay in Sesen-heim, it seems there were an abundance of obsessional fears, doubts, and ideas such as Goethe felt. But the picture which presents itself to memory is neither distinct nor fixed. It is elusive and kaleidoscopic. While I know that I had then many obsessional thoughts, quite similar in character to those I later analyzed in Goethe, none of them becomes clear enough to be focused.

In this emergency of a psychologist facing wide gaps in his recollections, memory, which has failed me, gets an unexpected welcome support. In the paper, "On the Effects of Unconscious Death Wishes," written in 1913 and anonymously published in 1914, I tried to analyze some of those obsessional fears and doubts, those oracles and superstitious beliefs. This article speaks of certain obsessional thoughts, which occurred to the writer lately, and reports some events which happened only the other day. In other words, the compulsive and obsessive doubts and fears were almost present ones; were looked at and observed when they were new and fresh in my memory.

Reading this paper, I am meeting an unknown young man of twenty-four years. Was I this, really? No doubt, here is the unknown piece of a half-forgotten self, in cold print; its identity with myself now cannot be denied. But it seems, at first, as if this was a report about the thoughts of a stranger. In reality, it is only an I from which I became estranged. Yet, I remember the young man, his moods and his crises, very well, as I read this analytic paper in which he tried to give an account of some strange emotional phenomena of his own. Not only the authenticity of the self-observation and the identity of the observer are ascertained. It is also clear that these obsessional thoughts and fears are those which preoccupied my mind at the time. They are the special obsessions for which I was hunting in my memory.

Here is the report which I shall translate, omitting many points. "The girl whom I want to marry became seriously ill and I visited her in N. I had planned to return on a certain train from N. to Vienna. I departed, almost too late, on my way to the station, which is about half an hour distant from the cottage of Dora's parents." (Out of reasons of discretion, I had called the village N. instead of Klosterneuburg, and had given Ella the name of Dora, in this paper.) "During my march to the station, my thoughts were, as is understandable, occupied with the illness of Dora, which made me very worried. Suddenly, the following thought emerged: *If I do not walk now to my sister in K., Dora will die.* This thought became, by and by, so obsessive that I turned around when I was near the station N., in order to walk over to K. (three-quarters of an hour distant from N.) where my sister spent the summer weeks." (My sister, Margaret, spent the summer in the village of Klosterneuburg-Weidling.) I tried, in vain, to argue with myself and to convince myself that the thought was absurd. I was, nevertheless, afraid that the calamity would happen, if I did not follow the mysterious warning. In trying to find out what deeper motives should have propelled me to visit my sister, I remembered a note I had received from her a few days before. Having arrived at home, I reread it. This is its content:

Dear Theodor:

I forgot to tell you that we have to light Jahrzeit on June 28th. If you want it, I shall also light a candle for you; but come then on Friday, so that you are present at the lighting. If you do not come, I shall assume that you "light" for yourself. Please go to the synagogue, also.

Kisses,
Margaret

P.S. Would you not once go to the cemetery?

Let me first explain here that Jahrzeit is the name of a religious ceremony of the Jews, who light wax candles on the anniversary of the death of their nearest relatives. I had not been to a synagogue, and had not performed any religious ceremonies for many years now. I considered myself an infidel Jew, but I had not interfered with the religious beliefs of my sister Margaret. To please her, I had been present before at the ceremony of lighting the candles at the anniversaries of the deaths of our parents. Her letter had irked me, because I did not like to be told what I should do. Especially the postscript had given me reason to feel cross-tempered. My sister considered regular visits to the graves of our parents a duty. I sometimes had had arguments with her, in which I insisted on the view that true piety does not mean to visit the graves of our dear dead, but to live in a way which gives honor to their memory. I had said to her, "That our parents did not live in vain is shown through our existence. That they did not die in vain should be shown by our way of living."

I had been determined not to go to Margaret on this day, but my decision was now overthrown by my obsessional thought. It showed that I had attributed a real significance to the lighting of the candles on the anniversary of my father's death, against my conviction that the ceremony had symbolic meaning only. Following this train of thoughts, we arrive at a first correction of the text of my obsession-thought. In the shape in which the obsessional impulse first emerged, a connecting link is missing, which contains the most important fact and which can now be reconstructed and inserted into the train of thoughts. The complete text of my obsessive thought or fear is thus: *If I do not go to Weidling and if I do not honor the memory of my father, by "lighting," Ella will die.* This reconstruction of the original text appeared, of course, in the published paper. Why was it that this intermediate part—and, with it, the real reason of my visit to my sister—was left out?

That can be psychologically explained by the situation in which I found myself, and by the events just before the obsessional fear emerged. I have told how I could not see Ella at her house, even when her tyrannical father was not present. There was the aunt, who was the executor of his will and of his severe prohibitions, and even his wife, who had only reluctantly allowed us to meet in the garden. I could not see the beloved girl, who was now seriously ill. Her mother came into the garden to tell me news about Ella's illness. My exasperation at this abnormal situation and my fury against Mr. O. increased. At this visit in Klosterneuburg (Mr. O. was absent) I could not control myself any longer. I gave sharp expression to my indignation and to my rage, when I spoke to Mrs. O. My hostile attitude to Mr. O. was now intensified on account of Ella's illness, because I made him responsible for its aggravation. He should have called another physician, as the first symptoms of her illness appeared, not just Dr. W., the doctor from Klosterneuburg (whom I consciously appreciated), but the best specialist for heart diseases, Professor C., in Vienna. I accused Mr. O. in my thoughts; he spent plenty of money for his private pleasures on his journeys, but he was saving when the life of his daughter was at stake. How nonsensical and unjustified these accusations were can be realized from the fact that Mr. O. was on a trip and knew nothing of Ella's illness at this time. My excitement was increased by my fear that he was expected to return in the next few days; that I could then not even get any news about Ella's state of health, and that I would be tortured by uncertainty and worries.

I told Mrs. O. that if her husband were not half crazy I could visit Ella in his presence and could see with my own eyes how she was. It was inexcusably rude and I had offended the good woman. In this same conversation, she had reproached me for trying to estrange Ella from her father. She had added that such a way of acting was sinful. "Don't you know," she had said, "that the Bible says: 'Thou shalt love thy father and thy mother'?" "The Holy Scripture says nothing of this kind," I had replied, "because love cannot be ordered. It says only, 'Honor thy father and thy mother.' And even this you could only do when they deserve it."

All these thoughts must have echoed in me, on my way back from the O.'s cottage in Klosterneuburg to the station. They must have been the soil from which suddenly my obsessional thoughts sprang. From Ella's father, Mr. O., runs a subterranean thread to thoughts of my own father, who had died a few years ago, and to the commandment to honor one's father. On the way, my thoughts must have met with the remembrance of my sister's note, admonishing me to light the candles at the anniversary of Father's death, to honor his memory in a religious sense. And now, from the emotional underground of a religious belief I had thought I had overcome long ago, emerged the mysterious order to go to my sister and to light the candle in memory of Father. With this command was connected the menace that the person dearest to me would die if I did not fulfill my religious duty, or if I failed to honor his memory.

The student of human emotions, who is familiar with the psychoanalytic insights into unconscious processes, will here recognize that two inescapable conclusions are to be drawn from my obsessional thoughts. The first concerns the unconscious connection in my thoughts between Mr. O. and my own father.

In an earlier chapter, I pointed out that Mr. O. appeared to me in every way as the opposite of my father, when I was a small boy. He was elegant, yes, even a dandy; my father was neatly but poorly dressed and did not pay much attention to his appearance. He could, of course, not afford to be elegant. But I doubt if he would have dressed stylishly, if he had the means for it. He was poor and Mr. O. appeared, at least to us, wealthy and lived on a high standard, compared with that of our family. My father was an agnostic Jew, who scarcely kept any religious ritual, but had a deep feeling of emotionally belonging to the Jewish people. Mr. O. was, at least in his creed, a Catholic and an anti-Semite. He appeared to us children as cruel, not only because we became aware that he was a tyrant in his own family, but also because he went hunting—that he killed deer and hare. When accidentally the door to his apartment was opened and we children glanced into the hall, we saw big stuffed heads of deer, antelope, and bear on the wall, besides a whole collection of rifles and other arms. The impression that this made on us was a mixture of fear and admiration, a kind of distasteful respect. My father was gentle. Nothing could be less connected with his figure, in our thoughts or emotions, than cruelty or the idea that he would kill animals for pleasure.

In spite of these and many other features, which let Mr. O. appear as the opposite of my father, there was, in the production of my obsessive fear, a clearly discernible line of thoughts, which led from Mr. O. to my father. In that conversation with Mrs. O., did not the theme of honoring one's father appear? Was it not continued in my thoughts until it emerged in the form of a command, to light the candle for him? Here, toward Mr. O., I was full of hatred. I declined to honor a father who, in my view, did not deserve the name. There, toward my father, the urge to honor his memory had emerged, not only as a duty, but as an order. Toward the one, I had very conscious murderous thoughts and evil wishes; toward the other, my own father, I had affectionate and respectful feelings. According to all experiences we analysts make in our practice, we are led to a conclusion. I must have split the image of the original father-figure unconsciously into two parts, in such a way that all tender feelings were turned to my own father, while all hostile tendencies were directed against Mr. O. But both of these contradictory feelings and impulses were once, in childhood, directed to my father and formed the main emotional trends of an attitude which psychoanalysis calls ambivalence. In a typical manner, that what was once united in a single emotional attitude, toward one person who was loved and hated at the same time, appeared now divided and was allotted to two figures, who formed a contrast in my thoughts. The same distortion, by division, operates, for instance, in the fairy tale of "Hänsel and Gretel," in which the good mother is contrasted with the witch, who wants to kill the children. It is the same mechanism of splitting, which allows the great writers and poets to shape figures like Antonio and Shylock, Prospero and Caliban, King Henry and Falstaff—contrasting figures to whom they attribute emotions that contradict each other in the poet himself. When Goethe felt that

> . . . two souls contend
> In me and both souls strive for masterdom,
> Which from the other shall the sceptre rend

he personified the one striving in the figure of Faust, the other in Mephisto, the one in Tasso, the other in Antonio. To my knowledge, no analyst nor any Shakespeare commentator has yet pointed out that King Henry IV and Sir John present the two aspects of one figure. That the two persons are, so to speak, personifications of emotional potentialities of each other, becomes psychologically transparent, in reading the delightful scene (Part I, scene 4), in which Falstaff playfully acts the part of the King and speaks about Falstaff. The charm of the scene is even heightened, when later on the prince takes over the role of his father judging himself and Sir John: a forecast of his own future.

The evil wishes against Mr. O. form a great part of the underground out of which the obsessive thoughts emerged. When you consider its text, you will realize that there is a conflict implied between the duty to my father and my love for Ella. This conflict appears in the obsessional fear already as an emotional measure of protection. I have to light the memory-candle. Otherwise, Ella will die. Traced back to the original form, the connection between the two parts must mean: If I do not go to Weidling to do honor to my father, he will take revenge on me by letting my sweetheart die. Such expectations of impending calamity are typical emotions of obsessive neurotics. These fears emerge as emotional reactions against unconscious aggressive and rebellious wishes. I shall be punished for them, either by dying myself or by the death of persons very dear to me. Otherwise put, I am afraid, because I have unconsciously wished death to my father, and he could wreak his vengeance for it by letting my beloved girl die. This must be the real origin of the unconscious obsessive thought. In the later form, we already meet with a measure of protection against this magical threat. I must do him (or his memory) honor. I must show him affection and respect. Then he will be reconciled with me and will not deprive me of my love. The obsessional thought or the magical threat emerges in the shape so characteristic of this way of morbid thinking, in the form of an if-sentence, which announces a certain action or the performance of a certain duty and threatens calamity, perdition, or death, if the order or prohibition is not obeyed. *If I do not go to Weidling and if I do not light the candle, Ella will die.* The religious ceremony has thus the character of an atonement, of a petition of pardon for my unconscious death wishes against my father.

Is it not astonishing that the memory of my father is connected, in my thoughts, with Ella's illness, although my father could not yet know anything of my relationship with her? The unconscious supposition is, of course, the superstitious belief that my dead father knows all about my bad wishes against him, and also about my desire to atone for them. I remind the reader of a previous chapter in which my obsessive fear is described, that my dead father would punish me for my sexual indulgence, by venereal disease and death.

But the situation out of which the original obsessive thought sprang had nothing to do with my father, but with Ella's father, Mr. O. His wife had reminded me, in that conversation, of the duty to honor one's father. My thoughts had really taken their point of departure from my lack of respect, my dislike for, and my death wishes against Mr. O., and had led to honor to be given to my own father, only later on. The "day-remnant," the actual intermediate thought, was of the letter from my sister, admonishing me to light the candle in my father's memory. We have thus to reconstruct a primal form of the obsessional fear, which remained entirely unconscious and which does not concern my father but Ella's father. This unconscious text of the fear could be formulated thus: *If I do not honor Mr. O., Ella will die.* We meet here again with traces of a secret or unconscious identification of Mr. O. and my father, two persons who are not only sharply different, in my conscious thoughts and feelings, but appear also as opposites—the one hated, the other loved. We were thus led to assume that both feelings were originally present toward the one father-figure, from which Mr. O. was later split off as my prospective father-in-law. The hostile and aggressive feelings against my father originated in the prehistoric years of my childhood, and were later on displaced to this father-substitute.*

* The analysts will recognize that the case of obsessional thinking presented here confirms the analogy which Freud has shown between compulsive actions and religious ceremonial (*Gesammelte Schriften*, Vol. X). As I already pointed out in that paper published in 1914, this is striking, because the content of the obsessional thought is just a religious ceremony, and allows tracing back to the same psychical mechanisms of defense or protection. Lighting the candle has the unconscious meaning of a sacrifice to my father and should prevent him from punishing me for my unconscious death wishes against him. It is significant that this very ceremony confirms the result of my wish: Father

Nobody who knows the complicated nature and the overde-termination of psychical processes will be astonished at the fact that, in the analysis of my obsessional thought, other emotions also appeared responsible for the formation of its text. It was already mentioned that one of the main reasons for my hatred of Mr. O. was his violent anti-Semitism, which had taken the most absurd forms in the last years. (Remember, that was the time a certain young man, called Hitler, grew up in Vienna.)

3

I myself am astonished that I recognized the psychological meaning of my obsessional thinking so early, as a young man of twenty-five years, before I had been in analysis.

The anonymous writer of that self-analytical report gives an-other instance of an obsessional idea which emerged in these days of worry for Ella. Returning home one evening, I had the thought: *If I chat with Miss Daisy tonight, Ella will die.* Daisy is the daughter of my landlady, who had the friendly habit of com-ing into my room on some evenings to chat with me, which I, consciously at least, considered as an unwelcome interruption of my work. Immediately after the obsessive thought occurred to me, I had the impulse to lock the door of my room: in a literal sense, a measure of protection. Self-analysis, in this case, did not take its point of departure from this thought, but from the preceding feeling of jealousy, which had tortured me. This impulse was not only entirely unjustified, considering Ella's affection for me and her character, which I now knew for several years. It was the more absurd, since I knew that Ella just now was in bed, seriously ill, being taken care of by her parents.

Self-analysis and analysis of others has since made me realize that one of the unconscious roots of jealousy is the inner per-ception of one's own erotic temptation. This unconscious aware-

is dead. This compulsive action is psychologically analogous to the origin of sacrifice in all religion. Freud remarks that the significance of the sacrifice is "that it gives satisfaction to the father, for the insult inflicted on him, in the very action which continues the memory of the terrible deed" (*Totem and Tabu*).

ness of one's own sexual attraction is then projected to the love object, in a mechanism of rejection. It is as if I had refused to acknowledge that I was attracted to Daisy. It can be expressed in a formula: *No, I do not feel attracted to another girl, but she, Ella, is attracted to another man.*

Analysis of the obsessive connection I had made in my thoughts between my conversations with Daisy and Ella's condition leads to the original text of my idea. One arrives at it, when one fills in the gaps which made the unconscious meaning of the thought unrecognizable: *If I chat with Daisy tonight and feel attracted to her, Ella will die.* That means, of course, that I had unconsciously felt attracted to Daisy, who consciously did not appeal to me. The fear, the meaning of which is distorted by ellipsis and omission of intermediate thoughts, is: *If I become unfaithful with Daisy, Ella will die.* The unconscious death wish, which can easily be guessed beneath the obsessional thought, is directed against Ella, because the loyalty I owed her prevented me from responding to the advances that Daisy had made toward me. Unconsciously I wanted Ella removed, in order to have sex relations with Daisy. A memory, emerging then, helped me to reconstruct the missing links in the text of my obsessional thoughts.

Some time ago, Ella had told me about a dream of hers in which she caught me being intimate with another woman, and cried to me, "I can't stand this. I am going to drown myself in the Danube." My thought must have referred to the memory of this dream. Reconstructed, its text means: *If I chat tonight with Daisy and feel attracted to her* (so that I would like to become unfaithful to Ella) *Ella will be so grieved about it that she will commit suicide.* This thought occurred to me in a form distorted by omissions, so that it appeared as absurd or senseless. The emotion connected with it was, of course, fear that Ella could die. The impulse to lock my door should thus, in a magical sense, protect the life of the beloved girl. In reality, the measure of defense in barring the entrance has a secret meaning: To protect myself from my own drives, to defend myself against the sexual temptation.

This is, in general, the sense of obsessional measures of protection. They should secure the patients against the power of their own hostile and sexual wishes, which were felt to be incompatible with the demands of civilization and the moral claims of the individual, and are therefore rejected from within. Fear of retribution and punishment, threatening the life of the patient, or of persons dear to him, explains the intensity of the reaction against those unconscious impulses.

The anonymous report continues here, in analyzing another obsessional idea, which had its roots in the same emotional underground of jealousy. It is now difficult for me to recall this strong emotion of those days; but I was as jealous as the Moor of Venice. As with him, even the thought that my bride had deceived her own father for me was used as a reason for suspecting her, and worked upon me in those months as a slow but sure poison. After Ella's recovery, we paid a visit to my sister, who spent the summer nearby. We met there a few girls and boys. In a discussion which developed about a general question (I do not remember which one, and the report does not specify), the view I expressed was at variance with that of the company. My main antagonist was a young man who was very popular with the girls. In my antipathy toward him and forced by his good arguments, I led the expression of my opinion to extreme and even paradoxical consequences, so that all those present turned against me. Ella, also, rejected my attitude. It appeared to me that in her criticism of my opinion there was a certain sharp note and an inclination toward my antagonist. Upset, I dropped the subject of our discussion, with a wisecrack that was as cheap at is was farfetched.

When evening came, I accompanied Ella from my sister's back to Klosterneuburg. On the way, I tried to show her which (consciously unjustified) conclusions I had drawn in my exaggerated jealousy. The shortest way back from Klosterneuburg, where Ella lived, to Weidling, where my sister spent the summer, was a road over a hill, called "the black cross," because a marble monument was erected there, in the form of a cross. It had become dark by now. I felt a certain uneasiness, better known as fear, in walking on the path through the wood to the "black cross" because, at the time, there was some talk of a murder having been committed there. I thought that I would choose a more frequented detour through the city of Klosterneuburg. After I had said goodbye to Ella, I walked back to Klosterneuburg. When, on this way, I approached the spot where the ascent to the hill departed, a kind of obsessive command suddenly occurred to me: *You must walk the path across the "black cross."* I tried, in vain, to defend myself and to resist this mysterious order, appealing to my increasing anxiety. In the middle of the road, it became clear to me that this compulsive action presented a kind of trial or test, in the manner of medieval ordeals, in which God was supposed to determine the guilt or innocence of an accused person. The difference between ordeals and oracles was, in many cases (as in this one) often not very clear. The text of this obsessional ordeal, as it appeared now, was namely: *If Ella remains faithful to me, nothing will happen to me on this way. If she becomes unfaithful, I shall be attacked and killed.* I tried to overcome the reluctance against this second part of the alternative and against my anxiety, by telling myself that life without Ella's loyalty would be worthless to me anyhow.

The uncertain and displaceable character of the doubts operating in such thoughts will be made clear by the fact that the alternative was modified by me, after I had made half of the way. As no sign of an attack showed up, I imagined the following possibility, to determine the ordeal: *If I do not run into anyone of whom I feel afraid, Ella will remain faithful. In the opposite case, she will become unfaithful.* Accident decided that, near the end of the path, I should run into a man with whom I almost collided in the darkness. In a second, the alternative changed in my mind: *If he now gets rude, Ella will become unfaithful. If he does not make a fuss, Ella will remain loyal.* The man politely apologized and walked on. Strangely enough, the collision with him had the result of removing my anxiety for the rest of the dark road. Now a new doubt appeared. Did I feel afraid when I ran into him? Was the man suspicious of me? Might I conceive of the collision as a decision of the ordeal? It seems I could not acquiesce to the favorable turn given by destiny. The doubt in obsessional states is really the emotional area of infinite possibilities.

Self-analysis later on led me back to the discussion scene, which had been the origin of my present doubts. In the moment when Ella had turned against me and had approved of the view of my antagonist, I had felt a violent, fleeting impulse, which could have been translated in words like: *I hate her so that I could strangle her.* The intensity of this impulse is, of course, only explicable because I had conceived of Ella's words as an expression of her inclination to become unfaithful to me. My compulsive action, or rather the thought (I must walk the path over the "black cross") presents itself as a self-punishment for my murderous impulse. Because I wanted to kill Ella, I myself should be killed. Tooth for tooth, eye for eye, the oldest unwritten law of retaliation—of talion—operates here in the unconscious. Also, in the substitution of my obsessive thought, my own death is connected with a possible infidelity of Ella, as the death wish against her first emerged when I thought that she could turn her affection to somebody else. Many of such obsessive ordeals or oracles that appear in the thoughts of neurotic patients are emotional reaction-formations against aggressive wishes, and are originated in tendencies of self-punishment.

Not all unconscious oracles which were formed in my mind at the time were of such a somber character. That old article of mine mentions one which brings my mother back to my thoughts. In an early chapter of this book, I reported that she had correctly guessed the object of my puppy-love, at a time when no one could know of my secret and mute courtship. When, almost ten years later, I saw Ella again and told my mother about it, she seemed to be inclined to look upon my feelings as a passing infatuation of a nineteen-year-old boy. Later on, she realized that it was more serious, and began to be interested in Ella. My girl, accompanied by Mrs. O., paid a visit to my mother, who told me that she liked her well. It appeared to me full of significance that she kissed Ella cordially, when saying goodbye.

My mother was then already ill. After my father's death, she had lost most of her interests in life and did not leave the house. She lived only for her memories and caring for Margaret and myself. We saw her often in tears. She was mostly melancholic. When she became ill and the physician tried to give her encouragement, she answered him, "I am not afraid of death, Doctor. I am tired of life and would like to die." A few days before she passed away, she seemed to emerge from her melancholic mood and was inclined to speak to us.

Just before she fell into a coma, which lasted a few days, I had a conversation with her of which I frequently thought later on, as if it had been pregnant with many presentiments. It was a heart-to-heart talk, although much of it was spoken haltingly on both our parts. We spoke of my brother Otto, who, fifteen years older than myself, was destined to lead an embittered and joyless bachelor's life, which found its end when the Nazis killed him in Vienna. My mother said that he was often depressed, and she searched for reasons for his "nervousness." She said, "He will never make up his mind whether to marry a girl or not. Maybe he has already missed the bus." I asked, "Do you think I should marry early?" and she answered, "Yes, and you have already found the right girl." There were resemblances in the appearance and in character of Ella to my mother, and they had unconsciously determined the choice of my love object. Now, the approval of my mother had been added to my decision.

On the forenoon of the day of her death—she was in a coma—I sat near her bed and looked at her face, which seemed peaceful. The bell rang. It was Ella, with her mother. This visit appeared to me as a hint of destiny. My mother passed gently away, and to console me for the terrible loss, a successor was here, to whom I could give my tenderness. I was then twenty-two years old.

This is, it seems, the appropriate place to insert the letter Freud wrote me at the time:

Karlsbad, August 5, 1914

Dear Herr Doctor:

I cordially congratulate you on your wedding which has taken place in the middle of the turmoil of war. I certainly expect that you have found the right companion in Miss Ella. I hope that the neurotic phase of your life that has lost its meaning has now collapsed, and that your talent will freely work for the sake of our science and for yourself. You know that you can rely on me.

Cordially yours,
Freud

4

I had gone to Berlin to finish my analytic training, but the outbreak of the war made it necessary to return to Vienna. There our son Arthur was born, in 1915, and in the same year I was called to the army. I wish to insert here another of Freud's letters:

Vienna, May 25, 1915

Dear Herr Doctor:

Returned from my Whitsun trip, I shall not postpone any longer cordial congratulation to your dear wife on the happy occasion of the birth of your son. It is to be hoped that ahead of us lie better times than those in which we are aging.

I am very pleased also to see that at the same time your production in other fields has advanced remarkably. Your scientific achievements also deserve to experience better times.

I ask you to receive the enclosure as my contribution to the care of the dear confined one.

Cordially yours,
Freud

I had luck and could stay almost a year with my family while I attended officer's training courses in Vienna. All this time, and later also, on the front line in Montenegro and Italy, I continued my analytic research and wrote articles and books.

The year 1916 saw me as a young lieutenant in the Austrian army corps, which marched into Montenegro, the Balkan state on the southern frontier of Austria-Hungary. Our army had taken Cetinje, the capital of this country of the black mountains, and had occupied the greatest part of its interior. The Austrians are a belligerent people. Their history is full of wars. There are only few nations in Europe which can boast that they have not defeated the Austrian army. I do not want to speak of war, but of a personal experience in wartime.

We were then in Kolasin, a small town in the southern part of Montenegro, near the Albanian frontier. The resistance of the freedom-loving and brave mountain tribes had been broken only superficially. There were numerous ambushes and attacks upon small bodies of our troops, and behind every rock could be the enemy who knew how to shoot and to hit. A severe martial law, threatening the death penalty, had forbidden the natives to possess arms.

I once had to be present when an old man and his son, who had been held as hostages, were hanged in the marketplace. The old man walked with dignity to the gallows, and said a few words before the rope was put around his neck. I understood only the first word, *bredjen* (brothers), but I was told, later on, that he said he was glad to die for the freedom of his people. The grim spectacle made a strong impression on me, and I have been a decided opponent of the death penalty ever since. To this day, I cannot see that the government, any government, should be allowed to commit that lawful murder, misnamed capital punishment.

About a month later, I was ordered to function as defense attorney before the court of martial law. While the judge advocate and the prosecuting officers were lawyers in the Austrian army, the task of the defense attorney was, at the time, often assigned to officers whose civilian profession was not law. The defendant was a Montenegrin boy of seventeen or eighteen years who had been caught with a rifle in his hands by our soldiers. He had killed a man, apparently without any motive. The boy belonged to an Albanian tribe, to one of those half-civilized, black-haired people who have preserved primitive organization and law. In those mountains, the law of the clan is as alive today as in old times. In the frequent feuds between the clans, the revenge for murder is murder of a member of the hostile clan. The boy I had to plead for had been an avenger. A relative of his had been shot, and he had killed a man of the clan on which revenge had to be taken. I spoke with the boy through an interpreter. He could not understand how what he had done could be considered a crime. He had only obeyed the law of his tribe.

As his defense attorney, I tried to put all legal arguments at my disposal before the court. They were poor. I then attempted to make the deed of my client psychologically understandable. I pleaded before the officers who formed the court that the morals of these half-civilized mountaineers were different from ours, and that we had no right to judge others according to our ethical standard. I reminded the officers of the Holy Scripture. When, in ancient Israel, a member of one of the tribes was killed, it was not said, "The blood of one of us is shed," but "Our blood has been shed," because the common blood is the most important tie between the members of a clan.

While speaking, I felt under high emotional pressure. It was as if I were responsible for the boy's life, as if his fate depended on my pleading. I was never a good orator, but if I was ever eloquent, it was on this occasion. Dark motives identified me with this boy who had committed murder and thought himself justified in killing a man. No doubt, under the influence of these secret emotions, my pleading itself became emotional. I asked the court to consider that the reputation of our army, in this hostile country, would be helped if we did not obey the letter of the martial law, but tempered justice with mercy.

At this point, out of the deep well of forgetfulness, suddenly some verses occurred to me, verses which Goethe had once written into a copy of his drama *Iphigenia in Tauris*. I finished my passionate plea for the boy's life, asking my comrades that their verdict should be in the spirit of these words of Goethe:

> Go forth, and everywhere proclaim
> Whatever crime man does commit,
> Man's spirit does atone for it.

The officers were not unaffected by my plea. The judge advocate came over to me, shook my hand, and said, "You have spoken beautifully," but he added in a low voice, "You know that our hands are tied by orders." "Why then the farce of this court?" I replied, full of indignation.

While the court deliberated, I walked around and smoked, to steady my nerves. Behind the lines of our soldiers, who stood guard with fixed bayonets, the place was crowded with people: men, women, and children. I heard the buzzing of their voices, and I was aware that they talked about me. But their glances were not unfriendly. While I looked at these barren, bleak mountains around the town, I thought that we were surrounded by a determined enemy, hidden in these small houses and behind those rocks.

I asked myself, much later, why I had been so stirred up when I pleaded for the boy, why I had trembled and been aware of my inner tension, of heart beating, and of short breath. It became clear to me that my unconscious identification with the boy was founded on the fact that I, myself, had committed a thought-murder when I was about his age, that he represented an emotional potentiality of myself. He had done what I had only thought. If they took him to the gallows, I could say, "There, but for the grace of God, goes Theodor Reik."

I wondered why at the end of my speech those verses of Goethe's that I had forgotten suddenly emerged. They were certainly out of place in the sober, matter-of-fact atmosphere of a court of martial law. No doubt, I had pleaded for myself. The verses that had welled up in me were remembered from the time of my compulsive Goethe reading after my father's death when I was the same age as this boy. And Goethe's drama puts the murderer, Orestes, on the stage and shows how his terrible deed is atoned. And did not the old Goethe say there was no crime he thought himself incapable of committing?

I was called into the courtroom. The sentence was death by hanging. I went to my room and fell asleep. Later something propelled me to see the boy in jail. The verdict had been made known to him, and he had been visited by the Greek Orthodox priest. When I came into the prison, I found him sitting on the bench, his head sunk to his breast. I called him by name and put my hand gently on his black-haired head. He looked up, recognized me, and stammered only, *"Gospodine . . . Gospodine!"* ("Oh, sir!") And then he was on his knees before me, kissing my hand. They hung him two hours later.

Late that evening, when I returned from dinner at the mess hall, an old man in Montenegrin costume passed by me. He stumbled just when he was near me and I helped him up. He thanked me humbly, but in doing this he mentioned my name. I had never seen the man. It was strange that he knew me by name. At home, when I fumbled for matches in the pocket of my jacket,

I found a small package in brown paper, tied up with a thread; in it were twenty flashing gold coins. On the paper were a few words, written in cyrillic script, which I could not read. (An interpreter told me later on that the note said: "God bless you.")

What should I do with the coins? They were perhaps the life savings of those poor people. I was sure I could not find that man. He perhaps lived somewhere in the mountains, miles away. Should I give the money to my commander? That was certainly not the intention of the unknown giver. He wanted me to have it. But was it not treason to accept money from the enemy? I decided to keep the ducats. When I was on leave in Vienna much later, I sold them and used the proceeds to complement and improve the food for Ella and Arthur. "If this be treason, make the most of it."

I had, however, some serious conscientious scruples about another experience, which happened shortly afterward in Kolasin, that small town in the interior of the Cerna Gora (Black Mountains). . . .

Napoleon once played a kind of parlor game with a group of his generals and diplomats. Each of the persons present was to tell a story of some mean deeds he had done. When Talleyrand's turn came, the statesman started his tale with the words, "I have done only one mean thing in my life . . ." "But when will this end?" ("*Mais quand sera-t-il fini?*") asked the Emperor. Unlike Talleyrand, I believe I have done quite a few mean things or at least things I considered mean. The following tale presents one of them.

One evening a young, pretty woman approached me on the streets of Kolasin. She wore the braided and embroidered national garment of the Montenegrin women, but she seemed cleaner and more carefully dressed than the girls of the small town. I had not seen her before. "*Parlez-vous français, Monsieur le Docteur?*" she asked. I was, of course, astonished to hear a native of these wild mountains speak French. She told me then that she had been at college in Belgrade. She spoke better French than I and was, as was shown in our conversation, well educated. She was married to an officer who fought in the Serbian army against our troops. She had heard nothing from him for three years. He was, she said, perhaps dead for a long time. She asked me whether I would give her some bread. She was hungry. The Montenegrins were at this time half starved, and our army did little to help the poor people.

From then on, I often met Ivanka somewhere outside Kolasin —fraternizing with the natives was, of course, forbidden—and brought whatever food I could save for her. I tried to help her as well as I could—"*ça va sans dire.*" She lived with her in-laws in one of those miserable, one-window houses on a hill near Kolasin. Frequently now, I asked my orderly to saddle my horse and rode a few miles to a certain place in the mountains, not too far from the house of her in-laws, but also not too near to it. I brought her bread and other food in the saddlebag.

My horse was tied to one of the few trees and Ivanka and I sat on a rock and chatted. She told me about her home. She admitted frankly that last year she had been the mistress of an Austrian major who spoke Serbian. What should she have done? She did not want to starve. Once, she called herself a *coorva,* which is the Serbian word for whore. She seemed not only grateful for my help, but became obviously fond of me. We kissed, but something prevented me from going further until one evening she asked me whether I did not feel like "*faire amour*" with her. . . . She was natural, unashamed, and passionate. We then met regularly somewhere high in those mountains, where she knew every little path. "A loaf of bread, and thou"—the poet had not meant it this way. Ivanka sometimes sang one of those melancholy Serbian love songs. But her presence "beside me, singing in the wilderness" did not perform that miracle of transformation, that "Wilderness is Paradise Enow."

I did not feel guilty because I had a mistress. I was twenty-eight years old, many months away from home and sex-starved. But there were other things which made me feel very uncomfortable and awakened discomfort. She was the wife of another man, and sometimes I felt guilty toward the unknown husband. He was an enemy, but I did not hate the Serbians and Montenegrins. I was supposed to hate them, being an Austrian officer, but hate can be as little commanded as love. Often, in my imagination, I put myself in his place and I felt then a kind of hostility or resentment toward Ivanka. (I remembered a sentence of the Viennese writer Karl Kraus speaking of a man who imagined the jealous tortures of the husband he deceived so vividly that he felt he wanted to strangle his mistress.) Even the neurotic belief in magic retaliation from a punishing destiny occurred to me. Oftentimes, I thought it possible that Ella, in Vienna, would become unfaithful to me with an officer. Once, when I had a letter from her in which she wrote that our little son was sick, I was haunted for days by the fear that he would die as a punishment for my transgression. I really avoided Ivanka for a week, using some pretext. I tried, with some success, to overcome my obsessional and superstitious thoughts. Ivanka remained my mistress until I was transferred to the Italian front.

More than my adultery, the fact that I had used the emergency situation of a woman to get sexual gratification from her troubled me. I told myself that I was not her first lover and that she had offered herself to me, but this thought was cold comfort. If I had not taken her, I said to myself, she would have gone to another officer who would have made use of the opportunity. My God, why are the others not so conscientious! . . . *"A la guerre comme à la guerre . . ."* It bothered me, nevertheless. It had been a mean thing to do. But, I argued with myself, I saved her from starving. I could have saved her from starving without sleeping with her—this was the counter-argument. I got into a lot of ethical reflections and speculations. I pondered on the problem of whether a person is entitled to use another human being this way. I came to the conclusion that I was far from being a real Don Juan.

The doubt as to whether my behavior then had been mean sometimes occurred to me long after the first World War. I still know when it emerged in my thoughts the last time. That was perhaps twelve or thirteen years later, when we lived in Berlin. Someone had recommended to me a novel by the Berlin writer Georg Hermann, *The Night of Dr. Herzfeld.* I read a scene in a coffee house where a group of middle-aged bachelors and married men—writers, artists, and connoisseurs—regularly meet to banter and joke and discuss the state of the world. One evening, a woman in the uniform of the Salvation Army approaches the table of this group and holds the collection box out to them. She asks, "Please, for fallen girls!" One of the middle-aged men says casually, "I am giving directly."

I smiled, of course, when I read the witty remark, but then I thought of my first sexual intercourse. This was with a prostitute, and I was eighteen years old. Suddenly, the thought of Ivanka occurred to me. Yes, that had been mean and I felt ashamed of myself. (At the same time, the memory of her passionate sur- render emerged in after-enjoyment. How strange we human be- ings are!) But the thought bothered me not more than a few sec- onds and was quickly dismissed. I was now over forty, as those men in Hermann's novel, and I had become hard-boiled and a cynic. Or, at least, I thought of myself as a cynic.

5

Freud told me I could bring my bride to the psychoanalytic congress, in 1914, and we went together to this great meeting, where analysts from all countries assembled. When I introduced Ella to Freud, and she spoke a few words apologizing for her presence at this learned meeting where she had no place, the great man said with old Viennese gallantry, "But you are the pearl on this congress." She blushed, and I believe, from this moment on, she loved Freud, about whose work she then knew almost nothing.

She did not love Mrs. Freud so much. After our return from Berlin to Vienna, we were asked to tea by the Frau Professor, as we called her. It was, of course, quite informal—as you would ask a young newly married couple. In the course of the conversation, Mrs. Freud, who was a magnificent housewife, said to Ella, "You see, I always use those cups with double rims for every day." It was good practical advice for a young Hausfrau, but my wife minded it, since it seemed to her that Mrs. Freud had lectured her in the presence of her husband. A few minutes later, Ella must have said something about having been nervous the other day, because Mrs. Freud said, "Nervous? I couldn't afford to be nervous. Everything in the household has to run smoothly. Other-

wise, how could my husband do his work?" It was known in
Vienna that for many years Mrs. Freud had renounced the pleasure of attending an opera performance, because she wanted to be
present at dinner, which Freud liked to have at a certain time. Ella
did not relish the subtle reproach she had felt in the words of the
old lady. Yet, she had much respect for her. There is at least one
conclusive proof that Mrs. Freud's remark had made a lasting
impression on her. Many years later, I heard Ella say to a young
bride who visited us, "You see, I always use those cups with
double rims for every day." Where had I heard this same sentence? . . . The Frau Professor had not been Ella's cup of tea
at all, and yet . . .

Living every day with a person you love has quite a different
character from spending a few hours daily with her. The readjustment of two people to each other, one of the essential features
of wedded life, brings divergencies to light that had not been
recognized before. I was worried about the future, dissatisfied
with the present, and, paradoxically enough, often took this out
on my young wife, who looked at life much more optimistically
than I. The fact that I could not offer her more than an existence,
without comfort and devoid of pleasures, made me spoil for her
even the few and small amusements she could have. I was a joy-
killer. She was not only ready, but also happy, to share this very
modest form of life with me, and did not understand why I was
not satisfied with it. But I did not understand it myself.

I tried unsuccessfully to awaken in her an interest in psychoanalysis. Something in her personality was reluctant to see people
and human relations in such an objective light. I understood,
much later, that a certain psychological predisposition and inclination are necessary to consider men the way psychoanalysis
does. There are thousands of fine and profound minds—many of
the greatest, as Goethe's, among them—who do not want to look
at individuals and groups in this manner.

Ella was happy when I was successful in my work, and enjoyed
each sign of appreciation my early books received—but it was her
love for me, not interest in analysis, that made her feel this way.
She copied neatly and conscientiously almost all my manuscripts, but the subject matter did not appeal to her. Insensitive as

I was, I wanted to share with her my insights in this direction. I no longer think that husband and wife should necessarily have all interests in common, but I had not grasped this simple fact. Neither had I realized that my wish to share everything with Ella was one-sided. It was as if a man demanded from another: "Give me your watch and I'll tell you what time it is."

This common, everyday life let her see all my shortcomings and faults, and, looking back, I am astonished at how many of them she silently put up with. The few weaknesses and failings I discovered in her did not diminish, but rather increased her charm. They were, so to speak, only the reverse side of her many excellencies. Her way of looking at people and things, so different from mine, every small trait and detail of behavior spoke of her femininity. Her preference for human interest in art and life, which expressed itself in harmless gossip with her girl friends, her strong feeling for the poor and suffering people, her superstitions and prejudices, the attention she paid to dresses and hats—there was so much I had to understand about women.

I learned, by the great interest she took in our small apartment, that a room has for women the unconscious significance of an extension of their own bodies. Where I was sentimental, she was practical; and often where she felt moved, I looked at things realistically. Why did she cry when we left the apartment in which we had spent the first months of our married life? Did we not change it for a better and more convenient one? I could be courteous and obliging but, to speak with Goethe, she had the "politeness of the heart." There were irreconcilable differences. For me, a police officer was the personification of the law; for her, he was only a man in a blue uniform. She often appeared childish to me, and then again as if she were born older and wiser than myself. (I read, later on, what the wife of Tolstoy wrote about her famous husband, at the time when he wanted to reform the world. "Never mind what the child will try; the main thing is he should not cry.") When I was defiant and rebellious, and paced the room, saying, "I'll show them . . . !" I sometimes caught her side glance, which seemed to see in me a pigheaded, uncompromising, overgrown boy, challenging others or meeting the challenge of other boys. She was suddenly transformed into a consoling and comforting mother. A few minutes later, she was a little girl who enjoyed small things to which I had never even given a thought. She could argue well, but, at the same time, she was the most inconsistent woman, without the slightest respect for logic. The elementary truth, that a thing could not be itself and at the same time its opposite, simply did not exist for her.

So many little things she said and did gave me surprising insights into a delicacy and depth of feeling which we men do not possess. But there were, also, some little tricks which were alien to me, an indirectness of approach to a subject, a subtle way of getting around me and reaching an aim by a detour, an astonishing lack of fairness when personal emotions were in play, a kind of irrationality in things where only reason should have a voice, and not sympathy and antipathy. Furthermore, there were some days in each month when mysterious depressions and a strange wish to make order in drawers and chests appeared. A young man has so much to learn about women's ways.

There is a current misconception among young and unyoung men that to know women, you have to have many affairs. They confuse understanding women with "knowing" them in the sense that the Old Testament gives to the word, namely, to have sexual intercourse with women. In this sense, an expert on women is often considered as a man who has seduced many women, a Don Juan. But this is as if a waiter, who knows exactly what tip he can expect from the kind of customers he serves, would be considered an expert in psychology! He knows only a tiny bit of human behavior, and even this only as far as it is useful to his immediate aims! It is, I think, sufficient to know one woman thoroughly, in all aspects of her being, to understand women's character—the essence of femininity, its evanescent and its permanent features, its shallowness and its unfathomable depth.

The physicians had declared that the condition of Ella's heart made it advisable that she should not have a child. They told her that it was not certain whether she would survive the labor. But she said, "I want the child, whatever happens to me afterward." When a year after our wedding our son Arthur was born, I was often reminded of those medieval madonnas, who smilingly look at the baby on their breast. She was the kindest and gentlest mother, but she was strong, too. Patiently she could listen to the crying and shouting of the baby in the night, when she knew that nothing was the matter with him. When I could not stand it any longer, took the child up and paced the room, singing to him, she smilingly warned me that I was going to spoil him. Eleven years later, Arthur became dangerously ill with an inflammation of the leg bone and its marrow (osteomyelitis). My wife, then already seriously suffering from her heart disease, stood before the operating room. When the surgeon came out, I tremblingly asked him whether it would be necessary to amputate the leg. "That is not the question," said the physician. "We don't know whether we can save his life." Then all went black before my eyes—it was the first fainting spell of my life. It was Ella's arm that caught me as I fell.

But to return to the psychological problems of the first year of our marriage and to the comparison with young Goethe in my study, written so many years later, I had shown that the poet must have suffered from psychic impotence which he did not overcome until he approached his forties. His enthusiastic love or infatuation for so many women, Gretchen in Frankfurt, Friederike in Sesenheim, Lotte in Wetzlar, his engagement with Lilli, and finally the long, soulful, and morbid relationship with Frau von Stein—they were all affairs of the heart only. They were passionate, but they were also pathetic. None of them resulted in sexual union; each, in the flight of the lover. He used his passion in the production of beautiful poems and plays. He had, it seems, never made a serious advance toward any of these women. "His wooing was aimless," as Thomas Mann put it. Some invisible power, stronger even than his vivid sensuality, prevented him from making sexual objects out of the objects of his passion. Some mysterious fears forced him to control his desire, until he could not stand it any longer and took to flight.

Nothing of this kind can be reported in my case. Yet, there was something which could be at least reminiscent of the much more serious inhibitions in young Goethe. Was not my restraint in the seven years of clandestine engagement comparable to the inhibition which forbade Goethe to approach Friederike?

When Ella and I married, a puzzling phenomenon appeared

which cast a shadow upon our happiness of being together. We were sexually not in tune. Our physical union, so long and so ardently desired, was not successful. There was certainly no psychical impotence as in Goethe's case, but the natural development, from sexual tension to a climax, was prematurely interrupted by an untimely emission, which released it, but did not relieve it. This too sudden and too early finale left my young wife high and dry, and left me unsatisfied. What had been so spontaneous and natural in the relation with Vilma and other women, what appeared as the result of an understanding of two bodies, striving to become one, and had been taken for granted, could not be accomplished here, and filled me with the shame of failure. Artificial restraint and postponement were of no avail. Nature cannot be deceived.

This premature emission, technically known as ejaculatio praecox, appeared to me as a milder or different kind of psychical impotence. Why had such an embarrassing and discouraging experience never happened before? I had to admit to myself that it must have its psychological cause in the very relationship with my wife, whom I dearly loved. Perhaps an old sexual inhibition had been reawakened. Was it possible that the menace connected with the image of Mr. O.'s guns and revolvers continued to work unconsciously upon me, even now when we were legitimately married? There was, I told myself, the emotional aftereffect of the unnatural restraint exercised during seven years. I remembered an anecdote (was it not from *De l'amour,* by Stendhal?) about a French hussar officer who had passionately wooed a woman who did not surrender to him. Unexpectedly, she yielded and, to his shame, the officer found himself impotent. Was there also in me a trace of unconscious resentment against Ella, because of the long control? I could not discover anything of such feelings in my conscious mind, but I had already learned from Freud that you can conclude from the effects of an action or attitude (at least) one of its unconscious motives. And was not this effect that my wife remained unsatisfied? All these questions and considerations were elucidated and confirmed during my psychoanalysis with Dr. Karl Abraham, who in a relatively short time succeeded in removing this embarrassing symptom.

The thread which connects this fragment of my own story with the experiences of young Goethe becomes conspicuously thin at this point. But it is not broken, because my imperfection in sex can well be compared with Goethe's psychical impotence toward those women he worshiped. The phenomena in my own life appeared simultaneously, while those with which they could be compared in Goethe's life showed themselves in succession, following each other. I had fallen in love with Ella, as Goethe had with Friederike, and I had taken a mistress who was at least twelve years older than myself and who had a son. Only a few years after the romance with Friederike, Goethe, then twenty-six years old, found Frau von Stein, who was then thirty-three and had seven children. In the following twelve years, Goethe had been in bondage to this mother-representative, a strange and neurotic woman, who allowed him only spiritual favors.

When he then secretly fled to Italy, he felt reborn. He became a pagan, earthly in his sexual life. "Desire followed the glance, enjoyment followed desire." This is the description he gives of his Italian sex life, in his *Roman Elegies*. He gets rid of his sensitive conscience, confesses to a free sensuality; yes, boasts about it so that his friends call him "Priapus." The ladies and the gentlemen of the court at Weimar were taken aback. This whole esthetic, refined, and restrained society was shocked and shaken when the great poet took a pretty, uneducated flower girl, Christiane Vulpius, into his house and made her his bed companion. He did not give a damn about the opinion of those ladies and gentlemen, and lived in voluptuous sin for many years, with a woman who did not understand one line of *Faust*. What had taken place in Goethe's life successively had co-existed in my youthful years. The differences between him and myself were as great as those between a half-god and a human being. But on this darker and lower level, where also this immortal genius was mortal, where also this superman was human, there were, I understand now, similarities originating in unconscious emotions and secret inhibitions.

But to return to the psychological problem of impotence or its qualified, moderated form of premature emission. A great number of men can develop their full sexual potency only with women they do not respect, yes, those upon whom they look down. They fail sexually with the other group of women, for whom they feel affection or tenderness and whom they consider in the category of mother- or sister-figure. These men can enjoy all the pleasures and the deep satisfaction which sexuality gives with women they despise. They can reach the heights of devotion and idealization with the other kind of women, who appear to them untouchable and sexually unapproachable. The extreme figures in whom these two contrasting types appear to human imagination are the madonna and the whore. Between these types is erected an insurmountable wall. The one is desired with all burning passion of the flesh; the other, worshiped and elevated with all the faculty of fantasy.

Ella and Vilma represented for me, at this time, the two types. Had I not often enough compared Ella to the madonna, in my thoughts? Was she not for me the embodiment of the noblest and best in womanhood? But I paid a high price for this idealization. I could not reach full sexual gratification with her. On the other hand was the personification of the merely sexually alluring woman, for whom I had neither respect nor affection, who appeared to me "fast," a woman for all men. She could give me full physical satisfaction.

Madonna and whore—these were the two types which a student of psychology had sharply differentiated, and contrasted only a few years before, in the confused book of a genius. The older students of psychology, who had known him at the Vienna University, told me about him. The title of the book was *Sex and Character,* and its author, Otto Weininger, had shot himself in the house in which Beethoven had lived, in the Schwarzspanier Strasse. But later I learned from Freud how typical this division of love and sexual behavior is for so many men in our culture who cannot love where they sexually desire, and who do not function well sexually where they respect and idealize women. I understood, in my own analysis, how deep the roots of this division between tenderness and sexuality reach into the area of childhood and puberty impressions. Later on, when I treated neurotic patients, I understood why many men need a kind of degradation in their fantasy or in their action with women they highly appreciate or love. They have to degrade them, in order to bring them down from the elevated level which forbids the intimate physical approach. A short time after I started my analytical practice, two patients showed neurotic symptoms, which led to the conclusion that they originated in this typical attitude of men in their sexual life. The one was potent with his wife only if he called her dirty names, used extremely vulgar language before and during sexual intercourse. She had to tell him that she wanted and enjoyed sex, and had to use certain lecherous terms. The other, a serious case of obsession-neurosis, was tortured by blasphemous thoughts, which frequently occurred in church or during prayer. When he looked, for instance, at pictures of the Madonna with the Christ child, he was compelled to think of her legs lifted and straddled in sexual intercourse, in a lascivious movement. When he wanted to pray to Jesus, he often had to think, "Bastard!"

How near this kind of thought is to the threshold of conscious thinking can be recognized in two anecdotes, which Anatole France tells in one of his novels. An Italian girl sends the following prayer to the Holy Virgin: "O Thou who hast conceived without sinning, give me the grace to sin without conceiving!" Having prayed in vain for rain to Jesus, a Sicilian peasant returns to the chapel with the statue of the Madonna with the child, and says, "I do not speak to you, son-of-a-bitch, but to your holy mother!"

In these clinical cases, as in the anecdotes, a psychical counter-mechanism is operating, which tries to annul and undo the result of that isolation. This mechanism of connection tries to bridge again the abyss between the two parts that had once formed indivisible unity. Is it true that never the twain shall meet?

It became the great fashion among American psychiatrists and psychoanalysts to speak of "psycho-sexual maturity" as the most decisive criterion of individual development. It cannot be denied that almost all the greatest men whose life stories we know never reached "psycho-sexual maturity." To cite only the two titans of mankind mentioned in this chapter: Goethe had never possessed one of those women he so passionately adored. Between Frau von Stein and Christiane Vulpius was an unbridgeable abyss. The one was the real mate of his soul in whom he fully confided and whom he never touched. He shared with Christiane his bed and not much else. He was, as someone put it, "as little married as possible." Beethoven could not approach sexually any of the beautiful aristocratic ladies of Vienna. On one side is the Immortal Beloved; on the other, the slut, from whom he acquired syphilis. In Goethe and Beethoven, as in all great men, there was this deep split, this discord which had to be resolved again and again. They all felt as Faust, that

> . . . two souls contend
> In me, and both souls strive for masterdom.
> Which from the other shall the sceptre rend!
> The first soul is a lover, clasping close
> To this world tentacles of corporeal flame.
> The other seeks to rise with mighty throes
> To the ancestral meadows whence it came.

6

A few years after my return from the war, my wife showed the first symptoms indicating a deterioration of her heart ailment. It had been aggravated by the labor of Arthur's birth and by the household work without help. The slowly proceeding inflammation of the inside walls of the heart chambers frequently occurs to a heart already damaged by rheumatic fever. There appeared that zigzag fever, so characteristic of the growth of germs.* For many months my wife was in a sanatorium, wavering between life and death. The doctors gave very little hope that she would pull through. All means were applied to find and to fight the unknown germs and to strengthen the weakened organism against their fatal power. Some teeth were pulled, and her tonsils were removed because they were suspected of being the seat of the in-

* The name, endocarditis lenta, used at this time for the slowly progressing heart inflammation, is now obsolete and the currently preferred diagnostic term is subacute bacterial endocarditis.

fection. But the illness, it seemed, could not be stopped and took its slowly progressing course.

I still remember how Professor Chvosteck, perhaps the best specialist for internal diseases in Vienna, who was called into consultation, started his examination. He wanted to look into Ella's throat, and the nurse offered him an electric flashlight. But he waved it aside contemptuously and said, in pronounced Viennese dialect, "Give me a wax taper!"* (At that moment, I not only remembered that I had heard many anecdotes about this queer and magnificent physician, but also something which filled me with foreboding.) After careful examination, the famous doctor said to Ella, "I'll tell you, madam, you will recover from this illness, but it will take an awfully long time. And after that, you will have to live with a weak heart which is not compensated. I am telling you the truth. Why should you say later on that Chvosteck was an ass?" This ruthless honesty worked more favorably upon my wife than the smooth and consoling speeches of other physicians.

She told me, a few years later, that at a certain moment she had been ready to give up, that she had wanted to die. But her tired eyes followed me, pacing the room, and she was filled with pity because I looked so miserable and desperate. She decided to gather all her energy to fight her illness and to live. I know that such a belief will appear non-rational to many physicians, but I have seen many instances of serious infectious diseases, in which a strong mind showed itself victorious in its struggle with the great enemy.

But, pacing the sickroom, I did not think of myself, but of our little son who was so devoted to his mother. What would happen to him; if she should die? If I had believed in God, I would have prayed that He let her live, at least long enough so that Arthur could fend for himself. She lived longer. She saw him leave our home and marry. After many months, the fever slowly subsided, and Ella could leave the sanatorium, but treatment had, of course, to be continued at home.

I have often stated that a neurosis does not evaporate after

* He used a word which is old-fashioned, even in the very conservative Viennese dialect, namely, *wachsel,* meaning a long, wax candle.

analysis and does not disappear into thin air without any traces. What remain are scars, as after an operation, and they make themselves felt when, later on, serious inner conflicts occur and unfavorable circumstances threaten a person's security. When my wife was so dangerously ill, I felt those scars; the old wounds became sensitive in stormy weather. During Ella's illness, a new train of obsession-thoughts emerged, which I had to fight. I was again haunted by that expectancy of impending calamity. But now I had, of course, good reason to be afraid, because I had been told how dangerous Ella's disease was.

Oftener and oftener thoughts emerged which seemed to herald the catastrophe in magical connections. There were, it is true, some strange accidental circumstances which favored the recurrence of those old, consciously disavowed beliefs in magic. Here are a few of them: It was on the day after my wife and I had attended together a performance of Mahler's *Song of the Earth* that Ella had felt her first fever attack. When we left the concert hall, there was storm and rain, and my wife complained that she felt shivery. When she became very ill the next day, we thought, at first, that she had caught a cold. But it soon became clear how serious her condition was. When Mahler composed this symphony, he was already ill and foresaw that he would soon die. He shuddered at the thought that none of the great composers, Beethoven, Schubert, Bruckner, had written a tenth symphony. Each of them had died after the ninth. Mahler, who was superstitious, tried, so to speak, to play a trick on destiny and called his ninth symphony, *Song of the Earth*. He died before he could finish the tenth symphony.

I took the concert as a bad omen. The idea that some magical connection was there recurred when my wife was brought to the Loew Sanatorium, the same clinic and the same ward where Mahler had died ten years before. When Ella's physicians then suggested that Professor Chvosteck should be called, I remembered that Alma Maria, Mahler's wife, had called the same physician to Paris, when the composer returned from New York in 1910. Chvosteck had then told Mrs. Mahler that her husband was lost. But as if there were not enough coincidences: at first, Ella's disease was diagnosed as poisoning of the organism through unknown bacteria; but later the specific agent was ascertained as streptococcus viridans. It was the same as that which caused the heart of Mahler to fail. There were four incidental things: the attendance at Mahler's last symphony, the same hospital and ward, the same consulting physician, and the same disease—well, they were incidents and coincidents. Some of them could easily be explained by local and temporal circumstances, and some did not need any kind of explanation. But it was difficult to shake off the notion that there was a mysterious connection. The coincidences were unconsciously interpreted as omens that my wife's fate was sealed as Mahler's had been. These obsessional thoughts, whirling in my head, were taken very seriously, when the danger was greatest. Sometimes, they were considered only as fancies and playful caprices—quite in accordance with the character of most obsessional ideas. I had an excellent insight into the psychology of obsessional thinking; yes, I had even made a special study of it, and most of my books, until then, dealt with it. But it seemed all this did not help me much when destiny knocked on my own door. Slowly, I mastered the power of those magical thoughts. Later on, another much more serious neurotic phenomenon, which gave me a lot of trouble, took their place. I shall report it soon.

As by a miracle, the inflammation seemed, at least in its acute symptoms, to come to a standstill. In the following years, the basic cardial disease took its slow course and the bacterial growth finally occluded the kidneys. A very painful attack made it necessary to remove a kidney stone and, a few years later, the kidney—again my wife was in the Loew Sanatorium for months. When we returned home, we decided to consult different physicians. After the operation, three specialists in their field held a consultation in our apartment. I was called in, and the youngest of them said, "She is doomed. The only thing that can be done is to prolong her life by sparing her in every direction."

I had long before decided to put all my energy into this task, had given up all pleasures or distractions, and had buried my scientific ambitions. I returned to an old pattern of living. I had again condemned myself to forced labor. My *"travaux forcés"* were this time not of the kind of the Goethe compulsion. They concerned my analytic practice. I worked eleven and twelve hours daily with patients, in order to earn enough to pay all the doctors, the expensive sanatoria, cure places and medicinal baths, to secure all possible domestic help (Ella was forbidden to do any work), and, finally, to give my wife as much comfort and pleasure as possible. Besides this, I had, of course, to support her parents. This went on for many years. The words "She is doomed" echoed in my mind and, whenever I was exhausted, the reminder of the end I thought near roused me to new efforts and even greater self-sacrifice.

Strangely enough, I found in this forced labor, in this exhausting no-stop work, a kind of painful pleasure, in renunciation, a grim enjoyment, and in ruthless self-sacrifice and suffering, a concealed satisfaction. It was much later that I recognized that such a limitless suppression of all self-interest, such cruel slave-driving of oneself, deserved the name of martyrdom attitude, and that it was clearly of a masochistic character. This kind of masochism, which Freud called moral, on account of its essential psychological character, really gets gratification out of suffering, because it anticipates an appropriate reward for it. It is as if the person who has deprived himself of so much and has undergone so much suffering has acquired a claim to a fulfillment of his wishes, has earned a right to gratification of his drives. There was no doubt that my own masochistic attitude had, also, the character of an atonement and self-punishment for all my unconscious cruel and evil tendencies toward Ella, in the past, renewed and reactivated by the present situation. At the same time, my ego could unconsciously get a great advantage from such self-sacrifice and forced labor for others. It not only helped my self-respect; it made me unconsciously feel noble and kind, yes, even better than others. The more I worked and labored, the more exhausted I felt, the more hidden sweetness was in it, the greater and surer was my claim that I would, in the near future, gather the fruits of my self-torture. And self-torture it was; it was sadistic, cruel satisfaction, sadism turned upside down, turned against myself.

When I now look back at these ten years of my life, I have to say that the inner court, which condemned me to forced labor and to solitary confinement (because I was lonely), was extremely and unjustly severe in judging my thought-crimes. The punishment was not only strict. It was barbarian. When I worked like a slave and denied myself everything, like an early Christian monk, it was almost an orgy of masochism. There was, furthermore, the confusion in my mind about being kind, noble, and suffering, as if they were identical. And how much concealed conceit, how much secret holier-than-thou attitude was in this luxurious suffering! What business had I, an average man, to act like Jesus Christ? Why had I to be unhappy in order to be happy? It took a long time until I understood that I am certainly not better, and perhaps not even much worse than others.

But all this I did not know then. I discovered it at first not in myself, but in my patients during analysis. It is odd—or perhaps it is not odd—that I recognized how strong the masochistic trend in myself had been, only after I had studied, for three decades, the phenomenon of moral masochism in others; and had written about it in a book of a few hundred pages.*

Slowly, I also had to admit to myself that a change of character had taken place in my wife. It appeared first in the form of a self-centered egotism, which is so understandable in persons who are seriously handicapped by a chronic disease. But, during the following years, it took an unexpected turn. At first, it seemed as if what she wanted was only recovery. She went to Baden, near Vienna, and later to Wildungen and Gastein, to take the mineral springs. All possible treatments and cures were tried; she went from one medicinal fountain to another, to test their curative effects. It was as if she trod in the footsteps of her father, going to the same resorts and health places where he got orders for advertisements for the *Kurortezeitung*. I knew it was in vain, but who would have the heart to tell this to a person who was so dangerously ill?

But there was also an increasingly perceptible change in temperament. As if she wanted to make up for the years we had been so poor and for the war years, Ella wished now to live luxuriously—without any regard for how much I could earn. We had to rent a big cottage in the suburbs of Vienna, to buy new

* *Masochism in Modern Man*, 1941 (2nd ed.; New York: Farrar, Straus and Co., 1948).

furniture. Two maids had to be hired. When Ella felt relatively well, expensive boxes had to be ordered for first-night performances for herself, Mrs. O., and Mary. To have her parents near, I had to finance their moving from Klosterneuburg to Vienna, and to pay the rent for the new apartment. Nothing appeared to her too expensive for our son and for herself. It was as if she had, so late in life, adopted the habits and airs of her father, as if only now an earlier unconscious identification with him had come to light. I had guessed, from some remarks she had made years before, that she had once as a small girl loved him very much, but that he had deeply disappointed her on a certain occasion, in not keeping a promise. Since that time, an estrangement had taken place between Ella and her father. She obeyed him and honored him, but it seemed that her love had been replaced by an unconscious identification, which had only now become evident.

As we know from analysis of numerous patients, such latent identifications, as a substitute for love, are quite frequent, at least in childhood and early youth, when the personality is still very plastic. We often observe them in women after the loss of a love object. The lover who has deserted a girl has vanished as an external love object; the loss of the object has been apparently overcome. But his character traits have been unconsciously incorporated; the woman now appears to be changed. The old love object has become a part of herself. What once had been love has been replaced by identification and the object is preserved within the personality, which is transformed by this absorption. The observer gets the impression that the character of the woman has undergone a change, and he connects it correctly with the unhappy love affair. He fails to see that this transformation of the ego is the price for the overcoming of the failure. The object is not really expelled. It becomes part and parcel of the person. Its monument is erected in her character. Its memory is immortalized in the core of the self.

I cannot say what now brought this old identification with her father to the foreground. Perhaps Ella's disease and the organic changes in her had an influence upon this evolution. It is also true that the identification was not total and did not manifest itself in those features of Mr. O. that were hateful to me, his anti-Semitism, his narrow-mindedness, and his tyrannical and stupid self-righteousness. It showed itself instead in an urge to act the great lady, to live beyond our means, and to maintain standards which were beyond and above our situation.

There was decidedly a tendency in the direction of luxury which did not correspond with my income and which made it necessary for me to work with the utmost exertion I was capable of. Together with this trait appeared an increasing impatience and irritability, which before had been entirely lacking in my wife's character. She was dissatisfied with herself and with the people around her, with the place rented for the summer, with the food served, with her bridge partners, as well as with her maids. She was quickly annoyed and lost self-control easily, raised her voice and criticized everybody. What had become of the gentle girl I had loved? The physicians declared that such outbreaks and the whole character of impatience and irritability were significant and often met with in patients suffering from serious kidney troubles. Such moods of excitability alternated with others, in which Ella was almost apathetic and had no interest in her environment.

As was unavoidable, we had our tiffs but I can fairly say to my credit I showed an almost superhuman patience in these years, developed an affection which had its deep source in pity, and tried to fulfill every wish of my wife. I yielded to every one of her moods, and silently bore her outbreaks of anger. This has nothing to do with any innate kindness of my nature. If it would not sound funny, I would dare to say, almost the contrary. There was the persistent thought that she was so ill and had perhaps not long to live. I told it to myself ever so many times, whenever I was exhausted from overwork and thought I could not go on: She lives on borrowed time. I could not deny her the luxuries she cared for, and I worked on and on to secure them. I could not afford to argue seriously with her, because I had to think: The next week, the next month she might be dead.

Most men, after years of wedded life, ask themselves: What happened to the romance we had? And what happened to us both? Is it not possible to recapture these glorious days and months? Are they gone forever? They are. Short revivals are possible, but romantic love undergoes a change. Understanding and affection will take the place of that fancy and fantasy which is the essence of romance. This unavoidable transformation of romance also took place in our wedded life; but there was a factor which had nothing to do with this change. Ella's disease affected the situation.

Pity is incompatible with romantic love; this emotion, however noble, almost excludes the others connected with passion.* Romance means to idealize the object, to see perfection in it, to endow it with excellencies we missed in ourselves. Pity sees the object miserable or poor. In romance, one feels humble. The person we pity can be admired and loved, but, in one direction at least, one is in a better position, and the fact that the object is not considered a supreme being any more almost excludes romantic feelings. To see the romantically transfigured woman in pain will fill us with deep sympathy, but not with romance. To give her the bedpan and to render the other little services of the sickroom, the sight of pus and blood—all this prevents romance from prospering. Charity can easily overcome disgust, and so can sexual desire, but romantic love stops before this hindrance.

My deep feelings for my wife were not diminished in those many years of her illness. I took the best care of her and gave her all my affection, but romantic love yielded to pity, sometimes to the degree that I became a fellow-sufferer. And yet, it was sometimes possible for me to see her in all her charm and loveliness, as before.

When my sister Margaret and I were children, we often heard our grandfather, who was a Talmudic scholar and a very respected but strange man, say, "When a man knows, after two years of married life, what his wife really looks like, he has never been in love with her." We snickered because it sounded funny to us. A man should not know what his own wife looks like? It is true, nevertheless. He knows, of course, what she looks like, but the image he had once painted of her can extinguish the reality, and stands gloriously before his eyes, while the material

* *A Psychologist Looks at Love* (New York: Rinehart & Co., 1943).

object, the real woman he looks at, is different. This psychical
reality created by his own fantasy can be stronger than what his
eyes see. The image from the past, which he carries within himself, is separated from the reality and is indestructible and imperishable.

Here was Ella, ill and prematurely gray, with hollow cheeks
and bags below her eyes, the forehead full of wrinkles, the face
aged long before her time; I saw her clearly and distinctly. And
yet, there was—how often—the other image. . . . There are the
sights, the sounds, and the smells of a summer forenoon in a
garden. And a lovely girl of seventeen comes toward me on the
narrow path across the meadow. Her full blue skirt touches the
flowers on both sides, as in a gentle caress. She walks in beauty.
. . . Now she has seen me, and there emerges this heavenly smile
around her lips, while her eyes remain serious. And I hear an
unforgettable, gentle voice say, "How do you do, Mr. Reik?" The
present had vanished and I felt as Faust toward the image that
memory has called up:

> To this very moment I would like to cry,
> Oh, linger yet! Thou art so fair.

7

What happened in the next ten years must be presented here
in a very condensed form. I was discharged after the end of the
war in 1918. The years after my return to Vienna were happy
ones. I worked successfully in my analytic practice, continued
my scientific research, and enjoyed the confidence that Freud
showed in my future development. We lived modestly enough,
but we were able to save some money for a rainy day. We could
not know then that the rain would rain every day. We understood
each other as much or as little as a young man and a young
woman in love can understand each other, and preferred each
other's company to any other. We were now also sexually in tune.

Then came the outbreak of Ella's illness and those eight years of lingering disease, often interrupted by long phases of acute complaints. I described before that I went into a kind of forced labor which was now directed to earn enough money for the treatment. I do not want to speak of those masochistic self-tortures, but would rather describe how it came about that a repetition of old emotional experiences occurred after some years.

I do not believe that healthy and average men can for long periods remain chaste in the flower of manhood. It is well known that the ideals of the Y.M.C.A., clean thought, clean speech, clean action, are difficult to realize in those best years. It seems that the blessing of unperturbed chastity is restricted to those few whom God loves especially: to the saints and to the poor in mind. In other words: to ill persons. It should not be denied that many healthy men can live without sexual satisfaction for some time, when they are possessed by an idea. This victory of mind over the needs of the organism cannot, however, be lasting.

In these years of my wife's illness I was in the unfortunate situation of making extensive self-observations on this very subject. There I was, between thirty and forty years old, condemned to sexual abstinence or to the refuge of masturbation if I wanted to remain "faithful" to my wife, who was so ill. When the theme of masturbation is discussed in literature it is mostly in connection with guilt feelings, especially in the childhood years. I do not agree with my New York colleagues that this relationship is as direct as they present it, nor do I think that guilt feelings are the only negative reaction to masturbation. A man of, say, thirty-five years whom external or inner circumstances compel to take his refuge in masturbation usually does not feel guilty and certainly not in the sense of a boy of nine or ten years. It ain't necessarily so. In many cases this form of sexual gratification can produce other different negative reactions, for instance, shame. This means the man feels it degrading, harmful to his self-respect as a person and as a man that he, as an adult, has to regress to this infantile procedure. He feels it incompatible with his age and his maturity. It is as if the president of the Guaranty Trust Company, instead of going to the golf course, should join boys of five and six years playing marbles at the street corner.

I tried at first to live in sexual abstinence and to divert my thought to my work. Being submerged in my forced labor I had some success. But then those imperative urges could no longer be driven off. Whenever they seemed to be kept away by strong mental effort in the following months, they returned through a side entrance, interfered with the demands of the day and the sleep of the night. Their re-emergence endangered the work to which I had given myself.

In my manhood I was forced to revert to a practice of my youth, at the time of our secret engagement. I searched for casual relations with women who were willing to have "fun," to release me from the unrest and the pressure, and to help me to work again without disturbance. To tell the truth, I did not want to find a sweetheart, because I loved my wife, but merely a sexual object, a physical relationship, if possible, without emotional involvement. I was not haunted any more by scruples whether one had the right to use a decent woman in this way. Reasons of caution as well as of taste forbade me even to consider promiscuous women. But what decent girl would be content with this kind of relationship which was the only one I could offer? I had decided not to pretend to be in love, and to be as frank as possible about my intentions and my emotions. I often asked myself: What have I to offer to attract a nice young woman? I had not even time to pursue my chances, if there were any, because I had to give almost the whole day to my practice and I wanted to be in the sanatorium near my wife in my spare time.

The astonishing thing was that I nevertheless found what I searched for—a few such casual relationships lasting some months, relationships which were as little time- and energy-consuming as possible, and with women who did not resent my troubled, impatient, and irksome personality. One of my patients, who is at psychoanalysis at this time because he has difficulties in work and in his relations with women, the other day reported a casual sexual experience. "It was nothing to write home about," he said, and added humorously, "if you write home about such things at all." This is indeed the question here: whether to write about such things at all. It is, at the moment, the great fashion in American novels to give a detailed report of the sexual doings of the hero or the heroine. The main part of many contemporary novels is a sequence of bedroom and barroom scenes. I do not think of myself as prudish. In reading them I feel neither morally indignant nor sexually excited but bored. If the description is only a vivid report of sexual acts without any insight into the emotional processes, without any individual and characteristic features, why put it into a book which is not supposed to be pornographic? If it is meant to arouse sexual excitement, why not declare it as pornographic? I am of the opinion that the presentation and discussion of sexual problems deserve a large place in fiction because sex has such an important part in the lives of men and women. But it is not the subject matter itself which gives this presentation its value, but the writer's way of dealing with it.

None of those casual relations meant more to me than they were supposed to mean, and that was not much. I often thought that the game was not worth the candle, yet I thought this only after the game, or in the time between the games, never during them. Here is an instance of how an affair of this kind started and developed. It is not chosen at random, and its analysis will be significant for my emotional situation. In the pauses between the analytic sessions and after them I hurried to the sanatorium and stayed in Ella's room as long as possible. This was true, of course, also after the kidney operation, which was followed by a longer period of recovery. I could not smoke in the sickroom, but often took a walk in the hospital corridors. It so happened that, turning a corner on one of these walks, I collided with a young, pretty nurse who was hurrying to an operation. I said "Sorry, sister," and that was that.

It was not strange that I ran into this same nurse several times in the following days, because she served in a neighboring ward. There were no more collisions, but once in the attempt to let each other pass in the narrow corridor we stepped aside in the same direction. Instead of one giving way to the other, we stood thus in each other's way. We both smiled and corrected the *faux pas,* but we stepped again simultaneously to the same side. The same thing occurred the next day. I said a few words about my awkwardness and she answered humorously. Next day I ran into her again and we exchanged a few remarks. A week later the old gauche situation repeated itself, and I asked her which day she was off duty. This was the beginning of this song and what followed these first bars was the necessary continuation of the tune to its climax.

The interest of the psychologist will be turned here to the unconscious significance of the successful wrong step, to the concealed motive of the clumsy cleverness. The seeming awkwardness in stepping into each other's way, and the following turning to the same side, this finding each other in avoidance, was unconsciously stage-managed. This comedy of errors had concealed designs. In not watching one's step, one unconsciously watched one's step. We wanted to get away from each other, but something led us to each other. The wrong step was unconsciously dictated by the wish to let the other one not pass, to stay together. I must have wished to make the acquaintance of Louise—the name of the young nurse—but this wish was then unknown to me. It expressed itself only in that symptomatic action, in my clumsy movements at the encounters. The effect of those symptomatic actions speaks clearly enough for the character of the hidden impulses.

There must also have been in Louise an unconscious tendency to meet me halfway, not only figuratively, but literally. Only when her own unconscious wishes corresponded with mine did this to-and-fro make sense. She told me later on that she had observed me several times before our encounter—she knew about the disease of my wife and she felt sorry for me. I learned also that she had broken off an affair with a man a few months before and was feeling lonely.

It seems to me that psychoanalysts, submerged in the pathological problems of the neurosis and psychosis, scarcely pay attention to those little accidents and those inconspicuous symptomatic actions which are so revealing. How is it otherwise possible that their discussion does not appear more frequently in analytic literature? To prove my point, I am adding here another frequent accident which, to my knowledge, has never been mentioned or interpreted in analytic books. I mean the accidental losing of one's partner in a crowded place or street. Here is a good example from psychoanalytic practice: A patient walked

with a young woman he had known several months on the frequented Kaerntnerstrasse in Vienna, in lively conversation. The
next moment he found himself at the side of a lady whom he had
never seen and to whom he talked animatedly. He had lost his
companion in the crowd and had continued his conversation with
the stranger as if she had been his partner. The patient smilingly
reported this little incident next day in the analytic session and
denied that there was any meaning in it. His following thoughts
nevertheless gave the solution of the little psychological riddle
posed by losing his partner.

He and Sophie, his companion, had just been discussing Mabel,
a mutual acquaintance. Sophie had made some remarks which
the patient called "catty" about Mabel's superficiality and flirta-
tiousness. The man was ungallant enough to agree with his companion. It was just at this moment that the couple "accidentally"
got separated in the crowd. It was, it seemed, a moment of perfect
understanding. Why should the separation occur just then?
Should we assume that God had put asunder what men wanted
to join together?

The circumstances of the situation are revealing. During the
last months Sophie had shown my patient ill-concealed signs
of her inclination, while Mabel, in contrast to her usual flirta-
tiousness, had treated him rather coolly. (Later on it became clear
that Mabel's reluctant attitude was a clever tactical move to
attract him.) Mabel was younger and prettier than Sophie. The
patient felt more attracted to her, although he realized that she
was as coquettish and as shallow as Sophie had said.

He was just going to agree wholeheartedly with Sophie in her
criticism, when he found himself removed from her and speaking
to a stranger. It cannot be difficult to interpret the psychological
meaning of the losing of Sophie, and of my patient's confusing
her with another woman. Translated into the language of conscious thinking the hidden emotion could be expressed: "I want
to get rid of you and I would prefer to walk and talk with Mabel."
The stranger was a substitute for Mabel. When one is consistent
in one's conviction about the psychical determination of such
symptomatic actions, and when one puts the unknown woman in
the place of Mabel as in an equation solved, one arrives at the

following meaning: The patient would have preferred to tell Mabel herself what he thought of her. But this was just what the man had uttered a few days ago in an analytic session—he had been annoyed with Mabel and had decided "to give her a piece of my mind." In spite of such a critical attitude he could not deny to himself that his thoughts had been preoccupied with the pretty girl, and that sexual fantasies with her had occurred to him. Now the attraction he felt to Mabel had found an expression at the moment when he was going to agree with Sophie's derogatory remarks about her. On the other hand, his dislike of Sophie had got the better of him. The accidental loss really means: lose the person, make her disappear. In some cases I analyzed, an unconscious feeling of annoyance or irritation, sometimes only of boredom, found its expression in such a separation. The complication of the continued conversation with a stranger whom one confuses with one's acquaintance at one's side allows the interpretation: I am fed up with you; I would like to change my company. I would prefer to speak with someone else.

Although very little has been written about the unconscious meaning of such small accidental mistakes lately, their psychological evaluation appears very important to the analyst. As my acquaintanceship with Louise started with those awkward steps, indicating an unconscious wish to meet her, so the end of our relationship, a few months later, announced itself in advance by a number of mistakes which made us annoyed with each other. We misheard or could not catch each other on the telephone, and we misunderstood the place or the time of a date, so that we waited in vain for each other. Small real incidents, as unexpected professional detentions to keep a date, did not help matters and were unconsciously conceived as purposeful. The last time we got into an argument was because I waited for Louise in one cafeteria, while she thought we were to meet in another one two blocks away. All these incidents appeared as trifles, but out of them emerged cause for friction, a feeling of irksome impatience and intolerance. We did not understand each other any more.

What I had experienced, I found repeated in the lives of my patients in different forms and confirmed in its psychological evaluation. Soon afterward, I treated a patient who reported that she had wavered between two men for a considerable time. The one, Hermann, had been her first lover, had deserted her temporarily, and turned to another girl from whom he repentantly returned to her. He asked her to marry him. She had resented his infidelity, and had in the meantime become the mistress of another man, Jim, who had wooed her before. She now rejected Hermann, and promised to marry Jim. She and Jim were to meet the next day to go to the office where marriage licenses were issued. The place of their date was a subway station in London, from which they could conveniently reach the office. My patient waited one hour. Jim did not turn up. He waited, too, at the entrance of the station, while Kate stood waiting downstairs. It was due to this "accidental" misunderstanding, or rather to its emotional repercussions, that in the end Kate did not marry Jim but Hermann.

On the day after she was "stood up," Kate went to the analyst who was treating her at the time. He seemed not to pay much attention to her complaints about her "bad luck." He seemed to think that there was much ado about nothing. He considered the fact that she had waited downstairs, while her fiancé had waited upstairs, as just an accident, as "just one of those things, you know." He was therefore astonished when a few days later she announced that she had broken with Jim. I am of the opinion that the analyst should have paid more attention to the concealed meaning of that misunderstanding. He should have, it seems to me, thought then that the privilege of his patient's sex also included the possibility of changing her unconscious mind.

Those little dissonances, misunderstandings, and misconstructions which interfered with my relationship with Louise indicated an unwillingness in each of us to continue our affair. In each of us, I am sure, operated powers of unconscious conscience which interfered with what we both wanted. As far as I was concerned, I became aware of self-reproach, because the affair with Louise had, so to speak, developed under the eyes of Ella. Louise was not in the same ward, but she knew of my wife and her illness. She seemed to accept the situation, but it must have disturbed her somewhat. She almost never mentioned Ella, but she must have been in her thoughts to a great extent. There were stronger scruples in myself, although I tried to fight them. The proof of their existence and emotional effect came in the surprising form of new obsessional thoughts and doubts.

It was the subterranean work of these obsessional thoughts that brought our affair to an end. It was not the material fact of my infidelity, nor my delicate conscience in its conscious manifestations that interfered with it. I now considered sexual satisfaction a biological, or rather psycho-hygienic necessity. The conflict within me was displaced to the fact that the affair was with a nurse of the sanatorium in which my wife was seriously ill. I looked at this first not as at a thing of bad morals, but of bad taste. I showed lack of tact in picking up Louise who was nursing in the neighboring ward. But had I really picked her up; was it choice and not rather making use of the circumstances? Where had I occasion to meet a girl who would be compliant to my wishes when I spent my time in the office most of the day, and went out only to see my wife in the sanatorium? And was it not, after all, to be reasonable, a satisfactory arrangement which saved time and trouble? I tried to convince myself that it was only a question of expediency. If (I argued with myself) I have an affair at all, why should I not have one with one of the nurses in the sanatorium, why rather with some girl outside? Thus spoke the voice of reason.

But there was another voice and it presented the counterpoint: Delicacy of feeling should have prevented me from getting into an affair in this place. But why? My reason rebelled. The fact that Louise was a nurse in the same hospital did not affect Ella. It did nothing to change the fact of the affair, did not contribute a sordid or shameful note to it. Yet there was the feeling that just this fact was an offense against Ella. I tried in vain to reason with myself. Louise was in another ward, had never seen my wife, had no influence upon her treatment, and my wife had no knowledge of Louise's existence. But my feeling was more stubborn than my intelligence.

This inner argument was not brought to a decision because one of the contestants had the last word. A new voice became audible and drowned the others: an obsession-thought. It was at first vague and indefinite. It emerged in the form of a mental potentiality and was devoid of all emotion. At first, I played with the thought, but later the thought played with me. It appeared originally in the form: If I sleep with Louise, something will happen to Ella; she will get worse, or she will have a relapse. That was just at the time when the recovery of my wife made progress after the operation. From this phase of the obsession to its practical consequence was only a small step. The clear formulation of the obsessive thought which appeared, the decision of the inner oracle, amounted to a forbidding: You must not sleep with Louise any more. I rebelled against it and continued to see Louise. But my anxiety increased, and at this time all those small incidents and misunderstandings which interfered with our relationship multiplied. Finally, I decided to break up the affair. Now I was convinced that the game was not worth the candle, especially as the candle did not give as much light and comfort any more as at the beginning. I could not hide from myself that there was a kind of glow of satisfaction in my renunciation as the subtle self-torture connected with it. More important, however, was the release from the pressure of anxiety which I had carried so long. This relief is mostly felt when one obeys those obsessive commands and inhibitions.

It was easy enough to judge later on that my doubts and conflicts were of the nature of shadow-boxing, but those shadows which were cast by myself appeared fateful. I knew, of course, that my affair with Louise had no influence upon Ella's state of health, but such clear thinking had little power compared with the onslaught upon my unconscious convictions. There must be a germ of psychological justification even in the magical thought-connection I had built. Which was it?

When one traces back the obsessive thought to its origin and inserts the missing links, the hidden meaning becomes clear. As the obsession-thought first emerged, in a very abbreviated and distorted form, it did not make sense, and yet there is a good psychological sense in it. Here is the reconstructed complete text: If I have sexual intercourse with Louise (and Ella should learn of it), my wife would reproach me and despise me, which would make me very angry. In my fury I would wish her to die, and this wish would have an influence upon her recovery—she would really have a relapse and die. Deprived of the connecting links, the thought appeared in the form: If I have intercourse with Louise, Ella will get worse. My affection for my wife and the anxiety which the imagined possibility awakened in me led to the mysterious forbidding and to the end of my affair. In the sense of my magical thoughts this was a measure which protected a life dear to me.

The consideration that it was mean of me to start an affair in the sanatorium in which Ella was ill does not only concern an aggravating circumstance. It was not just the nearness itself that bothered me; but what it indicated psychologically: a special inconsiderateness, a lack of finer feeling, an absence of delicacy. The nearness appeared as an allusion to the fact that the thought of Ella's serious disease did not disturb me more in my sexual desire. It concerned the immediate and unconditional character of my sensual appetite. There was a special indecency in picking up a nurse in the same sanatorium. My sexual misbehavior or my infidelity could, it seemed to me, be judged more mildly by myself if I had taken a mistress outside the sanatorium. That it was possible that I could make a date with Louise, after I came out of the sickroom of my wife seemed indelicate, the expression of a special cynical attitude against which something in me resisted, although something in me welcomed it too.

But besides and beyond those subtler feelings, there was a magical belief, a hidden obsession-thought. It already indicated itself in the fact that Louise and I very particularly avoided mention of my wife. The subject seemed to be taboo and had to be left out of our conversation as if it were a sore spot. We could, of course, not avoid it in our thoughts, and the more we tried to exclude it from the small ground common to us, the more it recurred. It could not be entirely avoided because sometimes I could not keep a date when Ella felt badly, and Louise had to be informed about it. The obsession-thought which was going to emerge and was caught in the state of being born had this embryonic form: I was afraid that Louise would have hostile feelings against Ella and these emotions would lead to a deterioration of my wife's health; in continuation of this thought: would lead to Ella's death.

It is psychologically obvious where this flicker of an obsessive thought originated and what was the germ from which it grew. When I once told Louise that I had to stay with Ella and so could not keep a date that evening, I saw an expression of disappointment in her face. Once she asked me whether it was really necessary to stay with my wife and whether I could not postpone it to another evening. From here it is not a far cry to the half-unconscious assumption that she had jealous and hostile feelings toward Ella.

Magical fears like the one I have mentioned (scruples about Louise being a nurse in the same sanatorium, and our mutual silence about Ella) are generally at the roots of feelings of social delicacy or decency. These very obsessional thoughts are the ones which prevent us from acting tactlessly. Those superstitions and fears are perhaps the soil from which many social feelings grow. Here they develop as measures of protection against the dangers which threaten from our hostile, aggressive, and envious tendencies. The defenses against those destructive impulses acquire, later on, a solid form and establish themselves as guarantees of the society against many powerful selfish drives.

Some other relations of a similar kind followed that with Louise. In spite of my conscious decision to consider them as "so-what affairs," I always took them too seriously, and never succeeded in dealing with them in a lighthearted way. I was convinced, at the time, that those few extramarital adventures, those back-street experiences signified that I was not true to my wife, and I appeared to myself as a low kind of villain. It was as if a provincial came to New York and sat alone with a highball at the Stork Club, watching the couples dance and imagining himself to be thoroughly depraved and taking part in an orgy. Men would rather think of themselves as scoundrels than admit that they are just average men. Vanity of vanities! To think of oneself as particularly evil is also an expression of conceit. We are neither patterns of virtue nor of vice. We are not first-class scoundrels either. The sober truth is: Man is nothing first-class.

8

Ella, recovered from the kidney operation, had returned from the sanatorium. She had to avoid every physical effort on account of her weak heart, but she could now sometimes go out to bridge parties and theater performances.

The first time we were sexually together again became a terrible experience: to see my wife fighting for breath, her face bloated, the bluish shine around her lips so well known from observation on the sickbed in the last years. The fear that her weak heart, this poor heart always threatened by the uncompensated deficiency, would suddenly fail shook me to the depths. Would this heart be up to the extraordinary effort? This fear made sexual gratification impossible because it did not leave me; or, if suppressed, recurred at the critical moment. I had to admit to myself that the temptation to approach my wife sexually was associated with the vision that she could die in my arms. The most attractive image of a beloved woman melting away in the rapture of sexual pleasure was thus changed into the image of passing away. The moment supreme appeared at the last moment. The eyes, which showed the moist gleam and change of expression, seemed to grow suddenly dim. It was as if Ella had unconsciously sensed my concealed fear, because she seemed in a subtle way to encourage my love-making, but I am sure this was only under the impression that sexual satisfaction was a necessity for a man.

That panic which Goethe experienced in those nightmares in which he saw Friederike pale, ill, and close to dying, after he kissed her, those terrible pictures in which he saw her as the victim of a mysterious curse, what were they compared with my own fears and images which were not created by imagination only? The dark Angel with the bare sword stood invisible at the end of our bed, and I shudderingly felt His nearness and presence.

Here was a situation which, although so different from Goethe's fear of kissing, secured the mold from which the first vague guessing of Goethe's unconscious processes sprang. I was not aware of the emotional connection between my own expression and Goethe's when I wrote that study on the Sesenheim affair. It is, in my view, also not essential that I had this experience in reality. The only factor which matters in cases of this kind is the psychical reality.

It so happened that there was in my life a real situation which could lend itself to a psychological comparison with Goethe's because its emotional repercussions were similar to his, whose actual experience was so dissimilar to mine. Love-making appeared in its consequences as an instrument of destruction. As Goethe was afraid of the tragic consequences of his kissing Friederike, thus was I terrified by the image that sexual intercourse might endanger my wife's life. In Goethe's obsessive fear magical and obsessive motives were prominent, although some considerations of reality concerning Friederike's tuberculosis were in the background. In my own anxiety the reality justified my fears much more, but they were superstitions and obsessive thoughts hidden behind those considerations.

The fears which were brought to the surface by my wife's disease were hidden in the unconscious depths a long time before they emerged. They were dormant in the emotional subsoil, waiting for the day when they could pierce the crust and appear in the form of a thought-connection between sexuality and death. Deeply rooted in the dark emotional underground and originated in childhood impressions, these thoughts associated sexual union with one's own or the partner's death. There was a vague and superstitious expectancy of impending calamity following intimate intercourse, a thought-bridge between sexual gratification and annihilation. In Goethe's case the expression "kiss of death" was not a melodramatic phrase, but marked a psychological situation of a very definite and definable character.

I wondered for a long time why this hidden thought-connection in Goethe was not discovered previously, and recognized by the Goethe philologists and literary critics who left not a single line of the great poet undiscussed. It becomes so transparent to an attentive reader who follows Goethe's poetic production with psychoanalytic understanding. Often veiled, but sometimes very clear, this sequence of thoughts, which reveals itself psychologically as a consequence in thoughts, appears in his novels, plays, and poems. I am restricting myself here to quoting two instances from his ballads as representative of an abundance of material of this kind. In "The God and the Bajadere" it is the lover whom the girl finds dead after the night's sexual pleasures, and she desires to share death with him as she did sexual union a few hours before. In the "Bride of Corinth" the dead girl warms herself in the embrace of the youth to whom she was once promised and who will die soon after touching her.

Here are survivals of superstitions or obsessive fears of sexual intercourse, remnants of a magical fear of sexual touch. It cannot be incidental that in those two famous classical ballads the lovers are again and for the last time united on the funeral pile. It cannot be accidental that in both poems it is religion whose prejudices interfere with their intimacy:

> Sacrifice is here
> Not of Lamb nor Steer
> But of human woe and human pain.

But why refer to instances from poems, novels, and plays? The reader who follows Goethe's life story will recognize that it was this very obsessive and superstitious fear that prevented the temperamental poet from approaching a woman sexually until he almost reached middle age. For the psychologist the life Goethe lived is stranger than the fiction he wrote.

Freud was the great teacher of inner courage and sincerity to all of us young psychoanalysts in Vienna. He taught us to face the truth about ourselves. We came to him not so much for help and advice, but for insight which made advice superfluous. He also helped me in the emotional emergency situation with which this part of my story is concerned. To a psychologist who takes an objective position and observes from without, the events of the subsequent period of my life reveal an increasing pressure, a logic of their own. This became clear to me many years later. At the time I lived through those events, their deeper logical and psychological significance was hidden from me. I still consider it strange how the obvious eluded me then, and that I did not catch a glimpse of the dark emotions in myself. Yet I had good psychological insight into similar experiences of my patients and I could well explain their secret meaning. It seemed that my psychoanalytic understanding was often profound; it stopped only in my own case.

The Moving Finger writes, and having writ, stops. I am now reflecting on the extraordinary value of the experience of those days I owe to Freud. I became suddenly ill. I suffered from attacks of dizziness, vomiting, and diarrhoea. The onset of these attacks was unexpected. I remember that the first sensation of this kind surprised me one day when I left the sanatorium after visiting my wife. I suddenly felt so giddy and unwell that I had to cling to the wall of the house to keep myself from falling. In the following weeks and months these attacks repeated themselves, grew worse and became more frequent. They occurred in the middle of the street, or while I attended a theater performance, at the bridge club or at home, while I was analyzing, when I was alone, or when I was with my wife and son. The dizziness in which I found myself became so severe that everything seemed to spin around me, and I had to lie down immediately. The character of the attacks seemed to indicate a serious disease. Their onset was accompanied by an overwhelming sensation of the end, by the anxiety that annihilation was very near, as in the spasms of angina pectoris. The breast was oppressed as in those dangerous attacks, and the physicians were at first inclined to assume that my complaints were those of angina pectoris. Once I had to be brought home in an ambulance, and nothing succeeded in giving me relief. These attacks sometimes lasted only a few minutes, sometimes many hours during which I was convinced that the end was near.

As far as my emotions were concerned, I died a thousand deaths in those spasms, because I experienced the most vivid sensation of dying. I had experienced the fear of death often enough under artillery fire during the first World War, but I had never felt anything like the overwhelming terror during those attacks. The physicians, at first, thought of a heart disease, then of nicotine poisoning. I gave up smoking, and followed the doctors' orders, but there was no improvement of my health. Then, some physicians thought that the attacks, accompanied by sudden loss of equilibrium and violent dizziness together with vomiting, indicated the ear disease known as Meniere ailment. I was examined many times and treated in different ways, but the attacks continued and their stormy character increased rather than diminished. I was given calcium injections, but they did not help.

My complaints had continued quite a few months before I casually mentioned them to Freud. He said he did not believe that they indicated angina pectoris, because I was too young to have this disease. I asked Freud for help. I was now convinced that my attacks were of the nature of conversion-phenomena.

It was much later that I used the summer vacation to go to Freud, who then lived in a cottage he had rented in the suburbs of Vienna. There I saw him quite a few times. Then already an analyst of many years' experience, I found myself on the analytical couch as a patient of Freud. It was an extraordinary situation, and became an emotional and intellectual experience which I shall treasure to my last day. But I do not want to talk about the general character of these analytic sessions with Freud, of the indelible impression they made on me, and the lasting mental value they acquired in my life, but of the special theme of those mysterious attacks which, strangely enough, did not occur while I was in Vienna.

I told Freud all that had happened in my life since I had left my native city and gone to Berlin. He knew, of course, of the dangerous disease of my wife, had often asked me about her, and had always shown sympathy and friendly feelings toward her. Once before I had mentioned that I spent almost all the time I could spare near her bed in the sanatorium. I had felt his side glance, and heard him say, "Perhaps this is not so good. It might be better to stay only a short time, perhaps a quarter of an hour, then go somewhere else, and return after some time to stay with her again only a short time." I was astonished and could not figure out what he meant.

Now, lying on the couch, I followed the train of my free thought-associations, in which, of course, Ella's disease and my relationship with her played an important part. I told Freud about my fears of the dangers of sexual intercourse with Ella, about the terrifying impression of the breathing difficulties during it—all this had occurred some years earlier—and I described to him the conflict in which I had found myself later on. I had made the acquaintance of a girl who, many years younger than myself, attracted me in many ways, not only sexually. I confessed that the thought had sometimes occurred to me to get a divorce from my wife and marry this girl, but I added that I knew, of course, this was impossible: you cannot divorce a wife who is dangerously ill. And then, I knew too that Ella remained dear and near to me, although I felt the increasing attraction of this young girl who seemed to care for me. I spoke then of my forced labor in those last years, of the difficulties of earning enough to make treatment and sanatoria possible for Ella, of my reluctance to lead a life which I considered beyond my modest standard of living. I spoke of these and other things too, but from time to time I returned to the description of those attacks of dizziness accompanied by the panic of the end which had interfered with my work. I confessed that I was in mortal fear they could recur.

I spoke of them also in the last analytic session before my return to Berlin. Freud had said almost nothing during this hour. He had silently listened to my reports, my complaints, doubts, accusations, and remorse, to the confused tangle of my emotions and to the clash of thoughts which reflected the many contradictions in myself. Near the end of this last session, I heard for the first time his low, but firm voice. He said only a few words. It was a simple question, but it echoed in me long afterward. The question had followed my repeated description of those spells of dizziness, and came to me as a complete surprise. The first moment I heard it, I entirely failed to understand what bearing its contents had on my report or the train of my associations. I failed to grasp its connection with what I had spoken of during this hour. I waited as if I expected an explanation, but none came. There was only silence.

But something else happened: there was for one second—and for this second only—a sudden faint dizziness, just enough to be felt, nothing comparable to the sensation in the attacks, only an allusion to the sensation, an echo of a familiar tune. It vanished, and I then understood what the question meant. I heard myself say, "Oh, that is it?" I knew I had arrived at the unconscious meaning of these spells.

The surprising question was: "Do you remember the novel *The Murderer* by Schnitzler?" Did I remember the novel? The question was not only surprising because I did not understand its connection with the subject I had talked about just then, but surprising also with regard to its content. Freud must have known, of course, that I remembered the novel. Had I not many years before written a book under the title *Arthur Schnitzler as Psychologist** in which all the works of this Viennese writer were discussed from the psychoanalytic point of view? Freud knew my book which had been dedicated to himself. There were not many people in Vienna who knew the writings of Schnitzler as well as I. Had I not even dug out in some long-forgotten Viennese magazines a few early poems and novels Schnitzler had published in his youth, and which remained unknown to the general public, and had I not written a paper on them?** Of course, I knew *The Murderer* well. Yes, I had once spoken about it with its author.

The outline of the novel: A wealthy young man, Alfred, has a long-standing affair with a girl, Elise. Alfred slowly becomes tired of his gentle, pretty mistress. He meets Adele, the beautiful daughter of a manufacturer, and falls in love with her. Adele responds to his wooing, and Alfred looks forward to the day he may marry her. He has not enough strength of character to tell Elise about his new love, and carries his affair further, postponing the unavoidable talk with Elise. Once, he finds the girl rather tired and hears—she had kept it a secret—that from time to time she suffers spasms of the heart. The next day Alfred goes to Adele's father to ask for her in marriage. The manufacturer is friendly, but insists that Alfred should spend a year in travel abroad to test the stability of his feelings. There is to be no correspondence between the two young people during this time. If they should feel the same way about each other after this year, the father will have no objections to their marriage.

* Minden, 1912. (Not translated into English.)
** In the magazine *Pan*, Berlin, 1912, edited by Alfred Kerr.

Alfred immediately starts the journey with Elise. He hopes that during this year of waiting his relations with Elise will dissolve in one way or another. They spend many months in Switzerland and England, visit Holland and Germany, and, when fall approaches, go to Italy. In Palermo Elise suddenly has a heart attack but recovers quickly. Alfred worries about her, but when she gratefully kisses his hand, he feels a wave of hate against her which astonishes him. At the same time, a passionate desire for Adele makes him impatient.

Alfred and Elise continue their journey. The girl "did not know that it was no longer she herself who was now in his embrace, in the silent dark nights at sea, but the distant bride who was called up in all fullness of living." But then fantasy fails Alfred and he keeps away from Elise, giving as his reason for restraint a slight recurring symptom of her heart disease. Once, when he finds Elise on her bed, almost faint from an attack, he feels a dark hope awaken in him. On the way back, on board ship, Elise has several attacks, and the ship's physician admonishes Alfred, in appropriate but no uncertain terms, to spare his beautiful wife in every direction.

Alfred is inclined to obey the physician, but Elise pulls the resistant lover to her as if she wishes to reconcile him by her tenderness. But when she melts in his arms, he feels a smile come to his lips out of the deepest ground of his soul, which he slowly recognizes as one of triumph. He has to admit to himself that the realization of the secret hope would not only mean the end of his conflict, but that Elise herself—if the end is unavoidable and she has a choice—would wish to die under his kisses. Night after night he observes the signs of her blissful melting away and feels as if deceived when, grateful to him, she awakens to a new life. When he arrives at Naples, Alfred finds no letter from Adele whom he had passionately asked to write. He is disappointed and realizes that he could not imagine life without her any more. He thinks of confessing the truth to Elise, still on board ship, but he is afraid of the fatal consequences of such an open confession. Preoccupied with such desperate thoughts, Alfred walks on the seashore, "when he suddenly felt dizzy and near fainting. Overwhelmed by anxiety he sank on a bench and sat there until the spasm was dissolved and the fog before his eyes evaporated."

Schnitzler's novel goes on to tell that after this Alfred decides to kill Elise. He poisons her to make himself free for Adele. Elise dies a few minutes after sexual intercourse. Alfred returns to Vienna, finds that Adele has been engaged to another man, and hears from her own lips that she does not love him any more. The unorganic end of the novel lets Alfred be killed in a duel. He finds atonement in his last moment for the murder of the girl whom he had loved.

Before I heard myself say, "Oh, that is it?" I had remembered the essential content of Schnitzler's novel as in a flash, or rather, I had a series of quickly passing visual images which presented certain scenes of the story to my mind. But even before these images occurred, there was this moment of dizziness which signified not only the confusion in which I found myself, but the beginning of my reorientation. It marked the point where the first vague understanding of myself entered in the form of a temptation to reproduce the attack. There was, for the length of a heartbeat, the possibility of experiencing the attack instead of experiencing the insight into its origin and motivation. This fleeting sensation of dizziness must have emerged when in my thought-associations I saw the scene in which Alfred, in the garden in Naples, suddenly is overcome by dizziness, a sensation of fainting and anxiety. It was thus a moment of identification with the leading character of Schnitzler's novel, of an identification founded on the similarity of the emotional situation and of the dynamics of the psychical processes.

Freud's mention of the novel corresponds thus to a psychological experiment which worked in an indirect way. In remembering the outlines of the novel, I found an unconscious approach to understanding myself. It was as if you were shown the photograph of an unknown person who reminds you of someone, and then you realize that the subject of the photograph resembles yourself. He is not you, but a double of yours, your Doppelgänger; not yourself, but your second self. This second self is the whole of one's emotional potentialities, the personification of the possibilities dormant in us, the representation of the life we did not live but could have lived. The Schnitzler story gave a terrifying picture of a possible destiny hidden in my character. The double, the Doppelgänger, is the deed of what we only thought.

Strangely enough, facing the reality of what I had thought did not get me into a panic but quieted me, and secured this distance I had not had before. In showing me what could have happened, it convinced me that it was destined to remain a potentiality, could never have happened to me. It could never have changed from thought to deed. These shadows were always shadows, could never become substance. Just seeing them in a mirror brought the clear recognition that it was all over, that my fright and my anxiety were exaggerated. It was as if the sudden light which fell upon them let me see them as mere products of my imagination, let me recognize their true nature. A man who comes into a dark room at night can, for a moment, imagine that there is a burglar or killer waiting for him in the corner. He is terrified and fumbles for the electric switch; as the room is lit, he sees that what he took for the figure of a man is only a chest. The cruel and aggressive tendencies and impulses which are repressed in all of us acquire a specially dangerous appearance when they try to pass the threshold of conscious thinking in the area of emotional and mental twilight, where thought and deed seem to be identical. They seem to threaten to become reality, so that a new strong effort has to be made to reject them, and to ban them into the nether world.

This is what had happened to me: when I once left the sanatorium, I must have thought Ella would die, or I would find her dead, when I returned the next time. This thought, or rather this wish, must have been rejected with great power because of my conscience and the affection I still had for her. But the repression of the death wish was already a reaction to the unconscious satisfaction I had from this daydream, which must have threatened to be so vivid as to attain reality—I must have unconsciously enjoyed the image of my wife dying or dead. The dizziness signified the transition from this unconscious abandon to a secret hope for the realization of the dream. It marked the moment of awakening from the daydream to the life of the day. I became dizzy when the reality around me made me aware that I had day-dreamed and had been lost to this world of reality.

This dizziness showed that a new orientation to reality became necessary. Many of our patients have a moment of dizziness at the end of the analytical session as they get up from the couch. The change of position is not important, it supports only the more essential emotional change: for almost one full hour the patient has lived in the world of psychical reality, where there was freedom for all thoughts, emotions, and impulses, where he could give himself entirely to fantasy, where actions were carried out only in imagination. He has to get up suddenly and has to face the world of material reality, has to live again in the sphere of hard facts, conventions, rules and regulations. This transition expresses itself often enough in the passing symptom of dizziness, in the sensation of giddiness, which disappears after a few seconds. The reorientation to the real world has been achieved.

If my dizziness thus marked the rude awakening from a day-dream, what did this terrible attack of illness, this feeling of dying, mean? The symptom that I condemned myself to death for my murderous thoughts, for the imagined possibility of kill-ing. If I experienced all the horrors of annihilation, it could only mean that I unconsciously felt I had to die because I wanted my wife to die. Our unconscious life follows here the oldest and most primitive law of talion: the same unwritten law expressed in the sentence: eye for eye, tooth for tooth. The person who murdered should be killed. The man who commits a thought-murder has to punish himself with the sensation of dying. The character of the punishment corresponds to the nature of the crime. From the imagined punishment you could conclude what was the deed committed in thought.

Whenever, during the following months, I had my unconscious fantasy, or whenever the repressed wish that Ella should die threatened to become conscious, the forceful rejection was ex-pressed in the form of my attacks: in this attempt of reorientation and in the following feeling of terrifying illness. Each murderous wish was followed by the image and the sensations of dying my-self. I did not know what hit me. I only knew that, out of a clear blue sky, something let me feel that my end had come.

With such severity I punished myself for my thought-crime. I never thought consciously that my wife should die. The possibility of her sudden death had often enough occurred to me, but always accompanied by panic. My obsession-thoughts show, of course, clearly enough that those murderous wishes must have been there. My anxiety and my measures of protection prove that these thoughts were working in me, but they were always with a negative sign.

Something new must have entered the stage of emotional processes, otherwise those repressed thoughts could never have won power to approach the threshold of conscious wishes, yes, of hopes. It is easy to guess what this was: my infatuation with that young girl. The thought must have emerged: If Ella dies, my conflict will end; I could marry the young girl. From here to the thought, or rather the wish, that my wife should die was only one step. In fantasy this step was taken. It expressed itself, so to speak, in an unconscious action of will, in a thought-murder. When the thought threatened to become conscious, returning from the area of the repressed, all counter-forces of morals and of the old affection were mobilized to prohibit the thought from entering. The success of this prohibition was achieved, and only the punishment I had inflicted upon myself showed that a thought-crime had been committed.

The sentence of the Roman lawgiver *"Nulla poena sine crimine"* ("No punishment without a crime") is valid also in the sphere of unconscious thoughts. The punishment points to the criminal deed that was imagined. The thoughts, first playfully dealt with, I had disposed of in my obsession-thoughts and doubts. Now they threatened to come across the footlight of conscious thinking, pushed there by my desire for that young girl. How dangerous they must have appeared to me is shown by the serious symptoms of my attacks. All powers of mental defense were called up to fight the intruder. I thought I would have to die, because I had such intense and vivid murderous wishes against Ella, or, I thought I would prefer to die myself rather than see her die or dead. Both these interpretations of the attacks are, of course, possible: one does not exclude the other. They can co-exist; yes, the special nature of unconscious processes allows even a fusion of both in the form: the other person dies in one's own dying.

Let me add a few remarks about the psychoanalytic significance of Freud's words. He must have known a long time before this last session what was the unconscious meaning of my attacks. I must have given him enough unconscious material to arrive at a psychological conclusion which was so remote from myself. Why did he wait so long with the explanation, and why did he choose the special form of tying it in with Schnitzler's novel? I think I can guess the reasons for his analytic tactics, and I have learned not only to admire them but to follow them in my own practice.

Only the unexperienced psychoanalyst, the greenhorn in our craft and art, will yield to the temptation to tell the patient immediately what he, the analyst, has guessed and understood of the unconscious motives and origins of his neurosis. Analytic experience recommends rather to wait until the patient is psychologically prepared for the interpretation the analyst has to give him. In most cases it means waiting until the patient seems to need only a few steps to arrive at this explanation himself.

It is difficult to define when this time arrives. Certain unconscious signs, perceived by the analyst, indicate that the patient is psychologically prepared or ready to receive and absorb the explanation.* In certain cases it will be necessary—often due to external reasons, for instance, pressure of time, but more often to some factors in the emotional situation of the patient—to work with a psychical shock. That means to give the patient a psychoanalytic explanation or interpretation at an earlier moment, when the analyst's explanation would come entirely unprepared so that it is bound to have the effects of a shock. Also in these cases it will be necessary to secure at least a certain amount of preparation, or to bring to the patient the material—which will come as a surprise and will stir him up—in a form that will soften the emotional blow and soothe the discomfort.

In my case Freud postponed his explanation as long as was possible within the time we had at our disposal. If he had told me

* More about this point in my book *Listening With the Third Ear* (New York: Farrar, Straus & Co., 1948).

immediately after he understood the unconscious meaning of my attacks, "You want your wife dead so that you can marry this other girl," I would not only have been shocked, but I would not have believed him. My repeated description of my actual conflict secured, analytically, an emotional preparation which made me more susceptible.

It is a special psychological problem why words which are spoken by us have another emotional effect upon us than the same words only thought by us, but it is an undeniable fact that they work differently. It is as if pronouncing them, saying them, already secures a certain externalization, removes them from the sphere of secrecy. The words you say face you and allow you to win an emotional distance from their content. My report of the situation made the approach to the material I had repressed easier just through this effect of objectivation, of the coming into the open of something which had been caged in so long.

The surprise was also softened by the indirect form Freud chose. I would emphatically deny that this form was consciously well considered by him, "figured out," determined by conscious reasoning. It was, I think, his unconscious response to my tale. While he listened to me "with the third ear," his thoughts, stimulated by the emotional similarity of the situations, must have led him to the comparison with Schnitzler's novel. But why did it not remind me?

The unconscious motives of the leading figure in that novel and my own were of a similar character. The sole difference was that Alfred committed the crime which I only thought of. Also, the emotional reaction of Alfred and myself to the thought when it first emerged from the repressed was different only in degree. While he was overcome by dizziness and anxiety feelings only for a few seconds, my attacks often lasted several hours. The sensations of oneself dying are lacking in Schnitzler's presentation. In my case these reactions were of great violence and awakened greatest anxiety. It seems thus that Alfred experienced no unconscious guilt feelings, did not turn the murderous wish against himself, and this lack of deep reactions makes it possible for him to commit in reality the murder which remained only in the sphere of my thoughts.

The similarity of the two characters and of the conflicts was, nevertheless, strong enough to have led Freud's thoughts to Schnitzler's novel: there was the man between two women, the heart disease of the one, signs and symptoms observed during intercourse, the "kiss of death." Another factor helped to bring about this association: Freud had read my book on Schnitzler, and he knew that I had often talked with the writer whom he knew, too. It was thus not an analytic tactical maneuver which Freud performed, but a crossing of a thought-bridge which built itself in his unconscious reaction and was perceived as appropriate and helpful.

The reader who understands how psychoanalysis works will appreciate that Freud's technique in this case was a stroke of genius. One will appreciate it the more, considering that Freud dealt with the problem not in a mechanical manner, prescribed by a rigid technical conduct, but as a sovereign, following his intuition. After he had let me tell my story for some hours, and thus made me gain a certain emotional distance from my own experience, he did not give me a direct and immediate analytic explanation, but he made me find it myself. He did not accompany me the whole way to the goal, but brought me to a certain point from which I could follow the way. There was, no doubt, a good deal of trust in my intelligence and moral courage in this procedure, but he was right in not trusting them too much. If I had had sufficient moral courage, I would have faced the unpleasant truth in myself, and the neurotic escape into the attacks would have been superfluous. If I had been brave before the dangers of my own thought, if I had not shied away from them, as a horse does before his own shadow, I would have arrived at the analytic insight without his help. He acted thus as a father who does not take his little son to the door of the school but to the corner of the street from where the boy can without fear continue on his way by himself.

The question: "Do you remember the novel *The Murderer* by Schnitzler?" is also surprising, as seen from the point of view of analytic technique. I wonder how many of us psychoanalysts, now experienced, would dare to choose such an entirely unconventional approach—not to mention the ingenuity and the psychological wisdom of the choice.

The reference to Schnitzler's novel seemed not only to work as a surprise, but put a new unexpected hindrance in the way, created a stop which made a mental effort on my side necessary, namely, to remember the content of the novel. The question thus seemed on first sight to work as a diversion. Nearer and clearer seen, the deflection was in this case the best manner of attacking the problem; the detour, the shortest way to the goal which was difficult to reach otherwise. Taking this hurdle, seemingly put artificially at this point, meant winning the race; marked at the same time arriving at the goal which had been concealed but became suddenly visible. When the surprise was overcome, and the contours of the novel were remembered, I found myself on familiar ground. Remembering the plot and the situations of the novel served thus as a guidepost to self-understanding.

The indirect interpretation by introducing Schnitzler's novel brought me nearer to the solution, but in doing so produced the impression that I had found the secret springs of my behavior myself. I recognized my own image in the mirror of Schnitzler's novel, but I realized only a few seconds later that it was a distorted picture, an image of oneself comparable to those you see in convex and concave mirrors, in which you see yourself with grotesquely enlarged hands and feet. I came face to face with myself there, but almost at the same time I knew that here was not my real face, but one I imagined or feared to have. This was not myself, but how I had unconsciously conceived of myself as a ruthless murderer. This indirect interpretation allowed identification with Alfred. I saw him as a potentiality of myself, but also became aware of the distance from him, understood that he represented only the dark fringes of my personality. After I had felt how near I was to Alfred in my imagination, I recognized how remote I was from him in fact. The encounter with this double of mine whom Freud had called up for me had two phases, following each other in the space of a few seconds. The first implied the recognition that he only did what *I* wished to do. The second moved the emphasis in this sentence: He did what I only *wished* to do. The effect of the first phase was that it made clear the psychological problem. The consequence of the second was that it cleared it up.

After having said goodbye to Freud I walked out into the summer afternoon, and I wandered for a few hours in the half-rural
streets of Vienna's suburbs. I felt strangely quieted and encouraged. I had not only gained distance from my own experience, but
began to accept myself. It was an uplifting feeling such as I had only
experienced before after some achievement. But this sensation
of strength and of a new courage was not the result of any achievement, but of relief from the pressure of unconscious guilt feeling.
I understood, while I walked through the familiar streets and
over the hills of Doebling and Grinzing, what had made me the
victim of those terrifying attacks, and I knew that they would not
come again. They never did.

Strangely enough, the experience which gave me new heart let
me also see the present and the future in a more hopeful light.
I felt the strength in me to overcome all hindrances on my way,
was not any more oppressed by the thought that I would not
earn enough to support my family and myself, and was confident
that some of the aims of my ambitions were within my reach. The
future did not look as gloomy as it had in the last years. I felt
strong enough to challenge my destiny. I was, after this session
with Freud, in a mood similar to Faust's after seeing the sign of
the ghost of Earth:

> I feel the courage, forth into the world to dare,
> The woe of earth, the bliss of earth to bear,
> With storms to battle, brave the lightning's glare
> And in the shipwreck's crash not to despair.

Also experiences which are helpful and raise our spirit, situations in which we overcome our unhappiness, are not immediately perceived and understood by us as far as their emotional
significance is concerned. They too can have the character of an
emotional shock, and need time to become part of our conscious
possession. The emotional meaning of this final session with
Freud became only fully understood in later years. Although its
effect was immediately felt, its aftereffects had much more impact
for my life as a man and as an analyst. When Freud asked me
whether I remembered the novel by Schnitzler, I had been in a

momentary haze. I came out of it when it was remembered, and the words "Oh, that is it?" marked the beginning of my under-standing. But only the beginning; it was as if a hole had been torn in a dense fog. When I later took that long walk in the sub-urbs of Vienna, this opening was enlarged. The fog receded and the view became clear; but this view showed only the recent past and had no great depth dimensions.

What the truth I had learned, and had learned to face, meant to me became clear to me only later when it unfolded itself in all its aspects and depths. This truth had more than one simple reso-nance. Freud had said at the end of that session, rather astonished, "I would have thought you stronger." This sentence often re-sounded in me. Freud did not consider my hidden and forbidden impulses and the punishment to which I had subjected myself from the point of view of morals. He did not evaluate my be-havior according to the categories of bad and good, wicked or noble, but thought of it as weak and strong—whether the ego was weak or strong. If I had been strong enough, I would have faced the terrible thought squarely and would not have needed to punish myself when it recurred. I would have considered its emergence as human and natural under the circumstances. I would not have condemned myself to the death penalty, the pun-ishment for a murderer.

To stand one's ground in the face of such wicked, cruel, hostile, mean thoughts, which everybody has and of which everybody be-comes sometimes aware, to look at them with open eyes and to reject them consciously without becoming panicky, this is what Freud meant by strength of the ego. The basic conception of the strength or weakness of the ego became one of the valuable acquisitions of this session. I knew it before, but it remained just theoretical knowl-edge, was not experienced in my own life. I felt its significance when I walked around on that summer day in Doebling and Grinzing, when my breast was at last free from pressure, when I could breathe again and look forward to a future which was preg-nant with possibilities of grief and joys. I knew from books and courses what the strength and weakness of the ego was, knew that this ego-part of us has to fight a two-front battle against the intense urges of the instincts and against exaggerated demands

of the superego, that severe and punishing power of conscience. I
had often enough seen patients being punched alternatively or
simultaneously from both sides until their ego was hanging help-
lessly on the ropes. But all this had remained pale and dry, gray
theory, until I found in my own experience what it meant to be
strong or weak.

I understood it even better when I met similar situations and
reactions with my patients, when I observed how they took to
flight before some thought-temptations and produced neurotic
symptoms on account of the same weakness of the ego which often
contrasted strongly with their intellectual gifts, and initiative. I
saw men and women, who had achieved remarkable things in
their lives, break down before a terrifying thought, before a temptation which had emerged in them. They ran in wild panic into
neurotic symptoms, inhibitions, and anxieties which made them
emotional invalids. I even saw some patients give themselves into
helpless bondage out of guilt feelings toward a wife or a friend
whom they hated. I saw men who carried invisible chains on
their arms, tying them to unworthy mates because they felt an
intense guilt feeling toward them. If Hamlet had been born or
brought up in New York, he would, perhaps, have said, "Thus
conscience doth make suckers of us all." I often saw, later on,
persons of great energy and capability behave as if they were unconsciously paralyzed by such terror of their own thoughts, and
I realized why what they had planned lost "the name of action."

I had thus plenty of opportunity to examine experiences similar to my own with regard to their origin and motivation, to
compare the emotional dynamics in the cases of my patients with
the ones in my case, which had been understood long ago. But
in spite of all I knew, I believe, I could look at this knowing as
being my own only for a few years. I then treated a psychiatrist
who, among many other problems, suffered great anxiety before
entering the clinic in which he was an assistant. We soon discovered that the main reason for his anxiety was the unconscious
thought that he might learn that the professor, whose position he
coveted, had died during the night. I was astonished that this
clever man had not seen the danger from which he had escaped
into his anxieties. At the end of my analytic interpretation I

expressed my astonishment with the words "I had thought you stronger." Only afterward did I remember when and from whom I had heard the same sentence.

9

In the years when we lived in Berlin and The Hague we used to spend the summer vacations in the Austrian mountains. The beautiful village of Alt-Aussee near Salzburg was the place where we spent the summer after my visit to Freud. My wife felt relatively better at the time. She could even take little walks if she was cautious and avoided every exertion. Her mood oscillated between depression and those characteristic flutters of great irritability. She was full of discontent and felt dissatisfied with everything, with people, the cottage we had rented, and even with the charming landscape. Impatient, she sometimes picked quarrels with me and others about trifles, and sometimes turned away from me and others apathetically.

There had been no sexual relations between us for a long time. I did all I could to make life comfortable for her. I spared neither trouble nor expense to secure all comfort. She was, nevertheless, dissatisfied, and she often put my patience to a hard test. She could not resign herself to two things which deeply disappointed her. Our son Arthur had fallen in love with a Dutch girl and had told us of his plan to marry her. He had joined us here in Alt-Aussee with Judith, his bride, to say farewell to us, because he wanted to emigrate with his wife to Palestine.

Ella, whose whole love had been concentrated on our son, could not stand the thought that he could leave her for another woman, and could go from us to a country so far away. She saw herself deserted by me and him, and the certainty that her only child would leave her cast a shadow on her life, which had been so gloomy for so many years on account of her disease.

The second fact to which my wife could not resign herself was my relationship with the girl, which I have mentioned before and which had been continued now for quite some time. Sexual intercourse with Ella was made impossible on account of her heart ailment which had been aggravated in the last years. I had, of course, taken every possible precaution to conceal from her that I had searched for sexual satisfaction outside our home, but secrets of this kind have a tendency to reveal themselves and "accidents," whose psychological character are not always incidental, give them away. The discovery of my extramarital relations filled Ella with indignation and she felt deeply hurt. She could not understand why a man in the best years should not be able to live a chaste life, why he had to go to women to get relief from sexual pressure. The puritanical education of her childhood and young girlhood had left deep traces in her character.

With great distaste my wife finally accepted the fact that I had to see other women occasionally to get sexual relief. But when she discovered that this girl meant more to me than just a sexual object, Ella could not stand it. She felt humiliated. She was well aware of the saying among Viennese women: "One girl is more dangerous than many girls." Yet I never neglected my wife, never thought I would desert her for another woman, yes, in a kind of attempt to offer her every comfort for so much she had to miss on account of her disease, I worked the harder for her the more sorry I felt for her. Through many years I went to operetta performances that bored me stiff, I spent many hours with the members of her family with whom I had nothing in common, just to please her. I sat beside Ella many hours looking on at her bridge-playing, often until late in the night, fighting desperately against sleep and extreme fatigue after eleven hours of analytic work. Looking back at that time in which I never hesitated to make every sacrifice, I tell myself now that my pity for her was exaggerated and that I was then not, as I had flattered myself, a good fellow but a stupid fellow. There is no doubt that my unconscious guilt feeling toward her made me do things I would never have done otherwise, and made me carry burdens which were almost too heavy for an average man to bear.

But to return to our summer in Alt-Aussee: Ella had discovered that the girl of whom I have spoken lived near that village and that I had seen her at her place. My wife discussed this with me and reproached me severely for my unfaithfulness. She got more and more excited the less I had to say, and what was there to be said without mentioning her disease? At the end she was carried away by her fury and shouted, "You are a scoundrel." It was like a blow on the head. I left the room silently and walked into the garden that surrounded the cottage.

There had been tiffs and disharmonies between us before—as in every marriage of many years—most of them in the first years because of my impatience and intolerance, many in the later years because of her irritability originated mostly by her illness. There had never been any name-calling, never a scene like this one. I felt as in a daze. I still remember it was a beautiful summer afternoon and everything was flowering. The air was so quiet and the landscape presented its most beautiful view. The Dachstein, a high mountain wall on the right, seemed to look down on me majestically. On the left the forest sent the subtle smell of pine trees over the meadows. I walked round and round along the garden paths which encircled a large flower bed. The scenery was so harmonious. God or the artist we imagine by this name must have created it when he was in a Mozartian mood, in the same divine humor which so often filled the music of that human genius born in the city of Salzburg, not far away.

I walked around the big flower bed and there was, it seemed to me, not a single thought in my head. I did not feel depressed. There was apparently a heavy load on my breast because I could not breathe freely. It seemed nothing mattered any more. I was far away from myself, walking there, and in a kind of depersonalization, in one of these states of mind in which one is a stranger to oneself. I do not know any more how long I walked around the small garden paths automatically and unthinking, in the quietness of that summer afternoon. Suddenly I heard myself say, "I am not a scoundrel," and again and again many times, "I am not a scoundrel."

Something seemed to loosen itself within me. That pressure on my breast seemed to become lighter. And then I looked up because my cheeks were wet. Was there one of those fine thin-string rains (*Schnuerlregen*) which so often occur in the middle of a beautiful sunny day in the Salzburg region? No, I had cried and had not known it. I returned to the apartment and spoke to Ella in a quiet and very friendly way. I did not feel reproachful and I understood, or sensed, that what she had said was not meant seriously, was shouted on the spur of the very angry moment. Our conversation was friendly and it did not concern the subject of our discussion a short time before, but the prospect of Arthur's marriage and departure. We both now felt that we belonged together. There was, however, a new tone in my voice. It was gentle enough, but it was also firm, and it did not sound guilty any more as it had sounded a few hours ago.

What had happened? While I walked around in the garden I had experienced indescribable emotions, but their character and the development they took can well be guessed in retrospect. I had been unexpectedly hit and had suffered an emotional shock. I had felt guilty for a long time and now had an open and clear accusation and condemnation coming from the very person toward whom I had felt guilty. For a few minutes I must have felt cast out, utterly reprehensible, lower than the worm in the dust. I am sure when I first walked on those circular paths, I felt crushed.

I saw myself with Ella's eyes—as a scoundrel. Just when I felt lost, I had suddenly found myself. Something in me protested in passionate upsurge against submitting to the verdict that I was a heel or a rascal. This something had to do neither with thoughts of self-justification nor with reasoning or measuring. It had nothing to do with weighing my good qualities against my bad ones. The protest came from the depth of my character. I knew I had often been inconsiderate, impulsive, and violent, often perhaps impatient, proud, weak, and pulled by many drives hither and thither. I had not been a scoundrel.

I had yielded at first to the emotional temptation to surrender to the condemnation which I had heard, but then from some deeper source emerged the counter-reaction and with it strength. Freud's words had echoed in me and enabled me to stand the sudden assault. They gave me strength not to yield to the terrifying wave of self-hate and guilt feeling which towered over me. The attack had had the effect of a powerful blow, but I had regained my equilibrium and I had recuperated, thanks to some hidden resources.

I rarely thought of this summer afternoon in later years. Some incident brought the memory back to me only a few weeks ago. A patient told me that his little son Peter, three years old, had made a clumsy gesture at the dinner table and spilled his orange juice over the whole tablecloth. His mother, a kind but nervous woman, had scolded the boy and had put him to bed. Half an hour later—the young parents sat in the living room reading— they heard a loud voice from the bedroom of the child: "Peter not a bad boy! Peter not a bad boy!" and again, in passionate protest and between sobs: "Peter not a bad boy!"

After Arthur had left us to go to Palestine with his young wife, Ella felt very lonely, and every attempt to distract her failed. She could not get accustomed to life in Holland, where we thought ourselves safe from Hitler. Ella's longing for our son became stronger and finally unbearable; in spite of her weak heart, she decided to undertake the long journey to Jerusalem. She arrived safely and Arthur and Judith did everything in their power to make her sojourn there comfortable. Although under the careful supervision and treatment of excellent physicians, her heart ailment got worse. Oscillating between depression, apathy, and great irritability, and living with the newlywed couple, she did not find the peace of mind she had searched for. Her letters to me were always affectionate. There was never a trace of bitterness or complaint in them.

After several months in Jerusalem, she decided to go to Vienna to see her parents. She undertook the journey from Haifa, crossed the Mediterranean to Italy, and took the train to Vienna. She must have felt that the end was near, and she wanted to be with her parents in her last hour. On the train she became very ill. When she arrived at her parents' home in Vienna, the physician, called in all haste, saw that her life could last only a few minutes. She spoke a few sentences to her mother and father and breathed her last. Again her strong mind had proved its power over matter; she lived long enough to die at home.

Ella was buried in the family plot. At the time of her funeral I was in Holland and I have never seen her tomb. When the news of her death reached me in The Hague, it did not awaken very intense emotions. Too often, and for so many years, had I anticipated her end with feelings of anxiety and panic. Too often had I forced my reluctant imagination to face the terrible event which cast its long shadow on my life. This anticipation in thought had taken place so often that I only later understood its magical significance. It was an unconscious measure of emotional self-protection, which would prepare and harden me against the blow of destiny, but would soften it too. The basis of it was a magical or superstitious belief that I could perhaps avert the catastrophe when I imagined it and what it would mean to myself and my small son.

On the other hand, there was the expectancy that the blow would not hit me so terribly if I anticipated it. You could call this particular piece of thinking, which anticipates in thoughts the worst, magical discount. I have an obsessional patient who bets against himself in thought. He tries to convince himself that the opposite of what he really wishes will happen, so that his disappointment, if his wishes should not be fulfilled, will not be too severe and depressing. He can also console himself then that he foresaw the unfavorable outcome and obtain a confirmation of his belief in the power of his thoughts in this case of his fears.

All that is so long past, and what came afterward is separated from it by a sharp stroke; the breakdown of Europe and the second World War, and with it the collapse of the civilization in which I grew up.

While writing the preceding pages, I often wondered why I felt so guilty about mere thoughts and wishes, and why I did not feel guiltier when I was inconsiderate, malicious, rude, or even cruel in fact, as I had no doubt often been toward my ill wife. I was, it is true, a slave-driver of myself, I had subjected myself to forced labor to secure all that was necessary or only comfortable for her. But I was not really gracious and generous because I wanted the sacrifices I made to be appreciated and praised, and I often spoiled all my service by bad humor and reproachfulness. I often acted like a good cow that gives plenty of milk but afterward, lashing out, overthrows the milk tub.

All the obsessional thoughts and anxieties I had felt had evaporated, and I did not feel guilty any more of my thought-crimes, my evil wishes and impulses. There was, however, a remnant of magical thinking in the form of a special half-formed belief when I thought of my wife's death later on. I often thought that she died, so to speak, as a vicarious sacrifice for myself. The fleeting idea was that I should have really died, and that she died in my place, that destiny had taken her life in place of mine which was forfeited. The emotion accompanying this magical or superstitious thought was a mixture of guilt feeling toward Ella and affection for her. Guilt feeling because she died, so to speak, for my sin for which I should have died, affection because I felt that she would have gladly given her life to save mine. Once it occurred to me that the origin of this magical belief was in a religious ritual which I had seen as a child. Religious Jews sacrifice a chicken on the day of atonement (Yom Kippur) as a vicarious victim for their own sins, for which their own life is forfeited. My grandfather, who lived some years with us, took a chicken by its legs on this highest holiday, and waved it several times around my head, when I was a boy, saying a prayer or a formula. This formula says that the chicken was, so to speak, to take over my sins, and would be slaughtered as atonement for them in my place. My superstitious belief must have been a remnant of this childhood memory. I do not know where I originally found the impudence to think that my life was more precious than my wife's, and why hers should be taken instead of mine, but at the end of this train of thought I always felt a wave of affection and gratitude for her, and a feeling of unworthiness, as if I did not deserve so great a sacrifice.

I felt sincerely sorry because I was often inconsiderate and cruel toward Ella. But also these feelings were of a fleeting nature. It sometimes seems as if I could not feel any more those intense emotions, as if it were very difficult and sometimes impossible to remember their intensity, yes, even their existence. Has old age, and the emotional change associated with it brought this about? Have I already become so much cooler? It is as if the intensity of emotions which youth once had has already yielded to clarity, circumspection, and cool-headedness. All I experienced during those years appears as if seen from a great distance, and the figures appear sharp but small, as if looked at through the other side of opera glasses.

Yet I know, and I know it to the core of my being, what Freud and Ella, what the master and friend, and what the wife meant to me in those years I was growing and maturing. They were not just persons who had become very important for my development; they meant more to me. Meeting Freud and Ella in those years was a stroke of luck. They became primal images. Ella was not just a single girl to me, but the model of a girl, girl-hood that had become personified. Freud was not only a great man to me, but the model of a man. It was as if in his personality were combined all the qualities, I thought, a man should possess: integrity and moral courage with strength and ingenuity. What Ella and Freud were to me in those young years left deep traces in my character which remained indelible. I was not blind to their human weaknesses and shortcomings, but thinking of them, leads always to the feeling: Their memory shall be blessed.

Having arrived at the end of this "fragment of a great confession," I become aware that it covers a very small segment of a man's life, and even this little piece is unsatisfactorily presented. Childhood and boyhood were scarcely mentioned. The description was confined to a certain phase of life, and of one aspect of this period; my life in relation to my sweetheart and my wife. Other relationships with colleagues, friends, and relatives were hardly touched upon; various activities and interests not even mentioned. Also the relationship with Ella was psychologically not as completely and as precisely pictured as would be necessary for the purpose of scientific research. What is presented here is thus a fragment of a fragment of a great confession.

Why, I ask myself, is it that such confessions when spoken by an unknown person almost always awaken our interest, and why do we demand certain qualities, which we do not require in life, when they appear in a book? It seems that our human interest in the person to whose confessions we listen remains alive because we do not only hear his words, but also what is said and left unsaid between and beyond the words. We do not only listen, we also look at the person, observe him, become aware of peculiarities of his gestures, of his posture, of the movements of his body, and of his facial expressions. All these features tell a story besides and beyond the story he tells in words. We miss them in a book except when the writer has a very personal or expressive style. Confessions for confessions' sake bore us easily when we read them. When they are nothing else but confessions they do not speak to us. They must have other added traits which interest us. The great confessions of world literature fascinate us just by these additional features which, strictly speaking, are not inherent to confession as such: the *Confessions* of Augustine by the religious conflict in the writer and his zeal, the *Confessions* of Rousseau by their merciless self-observation, Goethe's *Truth and Fiction* by the incomparable plastic quality of the artistic presentation. The writer of this fragment has nothing to offer which could be likened to such excellencies. He can only hope that the interest of the reader is attracted to the psychological problems which are contained in these self-analytic pages. If this interest is lacking, nothing else recommends them to the reader.

Many psychoanalysts will find fault with the form of presentation of this fragment because many emotional processes and trains of thought are not properly labeled. They will complain that the appropriate scientific terms are not applied, that, for instance, in the description of my relationship with Ella the psychoanalytic expression ambivalence is not to be found.

I was, of course, ambivalent toward Ella, in this typical emotional tension between love and hate. But does this explain the specific nature of my obsessional thoughts and fears, does it make me understand why I felt such a sense of terrible responsibility for her and why I was filled with choking anxiety when she felt worse? We are not only tied to a person by love or by hate, or by a combination of both feelings. It would be much more to the psychological point to stress that I was then tied to Ella by unconscious guilt feeling. But I was not trying to explain what is obvious. Putting labels on psychological phenomena does not appear very important to me. The question is not whether the labels we put on things are correct or not, but whether they are essential and significant for the individual case. It is due to such psychoanalytic labels that people in most case histories do not appear as living persons, but as pasteboard figures. The psychological impact of emotions and thoughts gets lost in the wasteland of such schematic, verbalized classifications, and what was real life, vibrant with feeling, is banned into the shadow existence of technical terms, of "Psychoanalese." I am told that a six-year-old girl who was taken to the Museum of Natural History with her school was asked where she had been. She answered, "In a dead zoo." When we read descriptions of neurotic and psychotic people in many psychoanalytic books, we too could say we had been in a dead zoo whose specimens were neatly labeled but poorly prepared by their taxidermists.

I shall try to demonstrate how narrow and inappropriate, how poor and pitiful the effect of psychoanalytic terms can be, compared with emotional experience. Here is an instance from my present analytic practice. A patient, Anne, a pretty girl of sixteen years, told me that she spent some time of the past summer together with her father and his present wife, Margaret, in the country, near the Hudson River. Anne had a pleasant time there, and often sailed and swam with Margaret, whom she liked. She once suggested to Margaret, who is much older than she, that they should swim together in the nude. Margaret first hesitated, and then rejected the suggestion; Anne did not know why. Let me add to the report a few facts which are not unimportant for its psychological understanding. Anne's father had had a love affair with Margaret while he was still married to Anne's mother. He finally won a divorce and married his mistress. Anne had first taken her mother's side, and had turned against Margaret, but during the last months she had made friends with her, and had spent much time with her, especially in the summer vacations.

What unconscious meaning or motivation, if any, would the average psychoanalyst attribute to Anne's suggestion to swim together in the nude? And what to Margaret's refusal? Is there anything psychologically significant in this little incident at all? I asked several psychoanalysts; they all answered it was immediately obvious to them what Anne's suggestion meant. It was, they stated, the expression of her voyeurism and of her homosexual tendencies. At the same time, they added, the plan to swim in the nude was a manifestation of Anne's exhibitionism. In other words: Anne wanted to get sexual gratification from looking at Margaret's nude body and from showing her own body to Margaret. The homosexual component expressed itself in the wish to be in the nude with the older woman.

Does this psychoanalytic interpretation explain the hidden motives of Anne's behavior? Does it allow us to catch a glimpse of the dark stirrings within the young girl? It seems to me that these analysts looking at that phenomenon have a poor sense of color, they see only the most conspicuous differences. Are they not supposed to see and to observe the finest shades and nuances? Should they not be able to recognize the infrared as well as the ultraviolet in the prism at their disposal? Is the aspect of hidden human agents in the case here presented really caught in the words voyeurism, exhibitionism, and homosexuality? Should not psychoanalysts be able to hear more than commonplace sounds when they listen with the third ear to the voice which tells that story? But so many of them have ears and do not hear, and have eyes and do not see.

Here is another psychological aspect, one of many: When Anne asked Margaret to swim in the nude, an important unconscious motive was the curiosity of the younger girl to see the body of the woman with whom her father slept, a curiosity of a hostile kind. The gratification of this wish to see was not of a crude sexual nature, and not akin to that of a peeping Tom. It was an aggressive tendency. This has not much to do with voyeur impulses which are searching for sexual excitement at the sight of another naked body. Seeing this body meant here to observe that it was so much fatter, flabbier than Anne's own youthful slimness. If there was exhibitionism in her suggestion, it was not of the kind analysts usually associate with this term: Margaret should not see Anne's body to get sexual pleasure out of the sight, but so that Margaret should be made envious or jealous by the more beautiful body of the young girl. Analysts speaking of exhibitionism mean that the display of another naked body should sexually arouse the onlooker. They do not mean that it should make his blood vessels explode. These undercurrents were not perceived, the hidden was not sensed, the intangible not recognized, when the essential character of the incident is determined as homosexuality, exhibitionism, and voyeurism.

Margaret's reaction to Anne's suggestion should itself give a hint of its concealed character. Margaret's refusal was not the rejection of an improper homosexual proposition. It was not the expression of her chastity. It was dictated by an intuitive understanding of the hidden hostile character of the offer. It was as if delicacy of feeling made her reject it, as if she had answered: I do not want to give you the satisfaction of looking contemptuously or condescendingly on my figure. It was as if she sensed in the suggestion the concealed indelicacy of a curiosity eager to see the naked body of a rival. She did not react to it as if it were obscene or lascivious, but as if it were offensive to taste and tact, which it was. Examples like this one do not prove much; however, they show enough to lead us back to some general psychological problem, especially to the question of how we guess what goes on in the unconscious of another person, and how we can recognize what unconsciously goes on in ourselves.

It seems that it is easier for all of us to understand the emotions and thoughts of another than our own. There is no doubt that, paradoxical as it might sound, the interest in the psychological processes of other persons is older than that in our own experiences, that we are originally more curious about what goes on in other human beings. We live distantly from our own experiences.

Take the instance presented here. One day, as a psychologist, I became interested in Goethe's love experience with an Alsatian pastor's daughter. I had known the tale in *Truth and Fiction* since my late teens; I had then wondered why Goethe acted the way he had and was ready to condemn him as a faithless and heartless egotist. I began to see the unconscious motives which propelled him when I read his tale more than twenty years later. I recognized now in the flashlight of psychoanalysis certain clues, a number of seemingly unrelated things which, joined together, give psychological circumstantial evidence. When I wrote the story on Goethe I had not the slightest notion that I attempted to master emotionally an experience of my own which had certain points of contact with his. My attention was concentrated on the unconscious motives of a young poet who, one hundred and fifty years ago, had fallen in love with a charming girl, had been pursued by mysterious obsessional thoughts and fears, and had deserted his sweetheart. Ten years after I had written it, while reading my own book, certain features, especially those chapter titles, brought me to the realization that I had written my own story, and I began to understand why I had done it and what it meant. How many years I needed to recognize what had unconsciously taken place in myself! How long a time it took until I came to my own track! It seems that the core of our own experiences is as distant from our own psychological understanding as the light of some planets which needs many thousand years to reach us. Some of these stars were extinguished long ago but we still observe their light. It is such a "pathos of distance" which separates us from the unconscious meaning of our experiences.

And how long a detour we often need to come to ourselves! We have to become strangers to ourselves, and have to see ourselves as if with the eyes of other persons in order to see correctly. Goethe is right: nobody learns much about himself by direct self-observation. You have to get at a certain emotional distance from yourself if you want to see even the contours of yourself.

There is a strange paradox in the character of guessing and understanding unconscious processes. When we want to understand ourselves we have to observe others and compare them with us. When we want to understand others, we have to turn our look inward, have to take the clues from our own psychology. Is it not as if we were strangers at our own home, and as if we had to go out and return to feel really at home?

It is late. I feel weary and would like to put down the pen. Station WQXR signed off for the night long ago. The last sounds heard in this room were of Mozart's music. Yes, Mozart. . . . My thoughts begin to wander. . . . Salzburg, where he was born and grew up. . . . Alt-Aussee from where we went to the Salzburg festivals. . . . We heard there in Schloss Leopoldskron *Eine Kleine Nachtmusik.* . . . It was magnificent. . . . The musicians were in the costumes of Mozart's time. It was in the wide yard of the castle, and torches on its wall illuminated the night . . . And next day we listened to Mahler's Fourth Symphony in the Salzburg Festspielhaus. . . . The last movement is akin to Mozart's music. . . . I remember that Mahler in his last hour, already unconscious, suddenly said, "Mozart darling" (*"Mozartl!"*), as if he heard his music. . . . I think again of Alt-Aussee and now the image of Beer-Hofmann appears before me. . . . and I see myself walking at his side from his cottage along a brook near a forest. . . . I had then visited the beloved poet in his cottage and we sat in his studio on the first floor, smoking, talking, and looking at the view of Alt-Aussee which is so Mozartian—Oh, yes, I understand now what was the thought connection between Beer-Hofmann and Mozart. I must have been thinking of the beautiful *"Gedenkrede auf Wolfgang Amadeus Mozart,"* a few pages of wonderful prose which Beer-Hofmann wrote and which are as profound as they are beautiful.

I first heard the name Beer-Hofmann when I was eighteen, and shortly after my father's death I had read his *"Graf von Charolais."* I was deeply moved. Here was a poet, a real poet, of incomparable power of expression and riches of the heart. My first book, a small pamphlet, was on the work of Beer-Hofmann. I was twenty-three when I wrote it and full of pride when I showed the first copy to Ella. On the first page stood the words *"Cum ira et studio,"* because I was then full of indignation about the Vienna critics who did not give full appreciation to Beer-Hofmann, and very keen to show how wonderful the *"Graf von Charolais,"* and *"Schlaflied für Miriam"* were. That was 1911, the year Mahler died in the Loew Sanatorium in Vienna. And I remember how I, a few years before, once shyly followed Mahler on his way from the Opera, where he had conducted, to the Ringstrasse. . . . I had a crush on him like a schoolgirl's infatuation with a movie star. But I was really in the last year of high school then. . . . How I admired him, the man and the music he made, although I knew so little of him. . . . Three years later I stood in the Berggasse and talked with Freud, told him about my plans and looked fascinated into his eyes. . . . He had inherited the worship I had for Mahler and he meant so much more to me.

They are dead now, all the men who had meant so much to my youth in Vienna. The pictures of Freud, Schnitzler, Mahler, and Beer-Hofmann on the walls of my room do not greet me any more. . . . Why do I suddenly feel so lonely?

My glance falls upon the framed page which Beer-Hofmann had given me. It now hangs at the right side of my desk. This handwritten poem has inserted on it in calligraphic lines: "To Theodor Reik in memory of past days, most cordially Beer-Hofmann, Vienna 4.1.1935." I remember that I called on him; we talked about Schnitzler and Wassermann who were both his friends. He gave me that handwritten page when I left him.

I tried to translate it into English—difficult to communicate the music of the German lines and to translate those first stanzas. Perhaps:

> All the paths we tread are leading
> To the one, the lonely way.
> Never-weary hours are weeding
> All that grew once sad and gay.
>
> All misfortune and all pleasure
> Pale as in reflection shone.
> What we suffer, what we treasure
> Fades—leaves us with us alone.
>
> Was I not in dancer's round,
> And what struck, struck not me only?
> Is no hand stretched out? No sound?
> Silence looms. The road gets lonely . . .

Everything around me and within me is quiet. No strong urges, no intense emotions. . . . But there is that unpleasant sensation of pressure and tightness, the heavy breathing and a slight giddiness. . . . No sorrows about a sweetheart any more, but worry about the muscle of the heart . . . I should have a new electrocardiogram . . . Dr. Vogl said the other day I should stop smoking. . . . While I put my cigarette out, I suddenly recall a sentence sage, old Freud once said: "As soon as the soul attains peace, the body begins to give trouble."

PART THREE

The Gift for Psychological Observation

The Gift For Psychological Observation

I

1

How does a man become interested in psychology? Psychologists—that is, psychologists who, in our sense, are curious about emotional problems—are born, not made. Psychological interest and the gift for psychological observation are as inborn as a musical sense or a mathematical talent. Where it is not present, nothing—not even courses, lectures, and seminars—will produce it. The comparison with musicianship is justified in more than one sense. Musicians, like psychologists, are born; but, in order to become what they are, they must be trained and they must work long and hard. Talent alone is not enough; but work and industry alone, without talent, are nothing. Lack of psychological endowment becomes especially conspicuous when a psychoanalyst is ready to turn to creative work, to present new psychological findings in a book or paper. Nowadays we read many books and articles in psychoanalytic periodicals that are cleverly written and present interesting material of a medical, sociological, psychosomatic, or physiological nature. I do not doubt their value, but there is not the slightest trace of psychology in them.

Rossini went to hear the opera *The Huguenots* for the first time. "What do you think of this music, maestro?" he was asked. "Music—I did not hear any music," the composer answered. Similarly, the reader of certain psychoanalytic books and magazines may have read and learned many things, but no psychology. That music is essential to an opera might be a prejudice, but one we would like to keep.

The German scholar, O. Klemm, has stated that psychology has a long past but a short history. Psychology is, as a matter of fact, one of the youngest sciences. The naïve man, living under the command of his instinctual needs, is not concerned with psychological matters. He turns his interest to the external world

247

and the knowledge he acquires is directed toward mastering the world outside himself, and making it serve his wishes. He tries to conquer a piece of material reality and does not covet any other kind of mastery. The kingdom of the psychologist is not of this world, not material reality. When conflicts arose in the mind of primitive man, when his wishes remained unfulfilled, he tried to master them by projecting their power into the external world, into lightning and thunder, rain and fire. He used magic and spells. He became a sorcerer, and finally, renouncing his omnipotence in favor of his gods, he became a religious person, a worshiper of deities. He cast his passions, needs, conflicts, and frustrations into the realm of the powers of nature, as we cast a picture on a screen. He looked at these pictures and was unaware that they only mirrored processes within himself. For many hundreds of thousands of years, the unconscious projection of his own psychical processes into the outside world remained the natural way of dealing with them, of understanding them. What forced man finally to discover them in himself? The sincere answer is that we do not know.

But something must have happened to bring this change about. Paul Moebius, the German psychologist, says: "It is, so to speak, natural to direct one's look to the external world; it is unnatural to turn it inwards. We can compare ourselves with a man who looks from a dark room through a small window at a world in sunshine; outside everything is easily discernible. When he turns around, he has difficulty finding himself at home in his dark room."* The comparison helps. Only when there is no longer anything to be seen there, or when something happens in the room itself which forces him to turn around, will this man's attention be turned away from the world in sunshine.

Psychology does not begin as self-observation. It ends there. Yes, self-observation, as possibility and fact, sets a psychological problem of its own. Every scientific research demands an object and a subject—an object to be studied and a subject that tries to recognize its nature. The objects of the other sciences are facts and connections between facts in the outside world. The subject

---

* Paul Moebius, *Die Hoffnungslosigkeit aller Psychologie* (1907), p. 12.

is the observer, the research worker. In introspective psychology, the object is the investigator's own psychical processes; the subject is himself. Here, then, is an identity of object and subject that is puzzling. This fact is so extraordinary that the best way for psychologists to deal with it was to take it for granted, without wasting any thought on it. If Aristotle's assertion that research starts with wonder is true, then it must be admitted that most psychologists did not bother with this superfluous emotion.

Think of the famous inscription on the temple of Apollo at Delphi: "Know thyself." The statement was apparently simple enough. There was no mystery about one's self. What the son of Zeus meant seemed to be as clear as a textbook on psychology: Turn your attention to your own personality and know yourself.

Today, however, we seriously doubt whether such was the real meaning of the admonition of the Delphic god. Oracles were full of obscure and double meanings. Behind those two words, "Know thyself," hides another idea. They impose the most difficult task imaginable—a task which something in human nature resists. To fulfill it a man must fight against heavy odds. The Delphic words do not mark the point of departure but rather the end of psychological research. If to know oneself were so easy, it need not have been put as a demand.

William James has described the puzzling phenomenon of self-observation in the words, "The *I* observes the *Me*." It is obvious that the pre-condition for such a phenomenon—observation of one's own mental and emotional processes—must be a split within the ego. This split makes psychology possible. In fact, this split makes psychology necessary. If the ego were undivided, it could not observe itself. It would have no need to observe itself.

Self-observation is the result of a late phase of psychology. Nietzsche remarked, "The *Thou* is older than the *I*." Every child is selfish, but it is at first not interested in itself. There is not even a clear-cut self. Primitive observation is directed to the person or the persons in the environment. There is no direct path from observation of others to self-observation. The *Thou* remains for a long time the only object. The *I* is but newly an object of observation—so young that many psychologists had not discovered it as an object worthy of their attention until recently.

Your own psychical processes are inappropriate material for statistics, curves, graphs, tables, tests, and schedules.

Where is the transition from observation of others, as we see it in children, to self-observation? There must be an intermediary phase which has been neglected. Here it is: The child realizes at a certain age that it is an object of observation on the part of its parents or nurses. Stated otherwise, the *I* can observe the *Me* because *They—She* or *He*—once observed the *Me*. The attention the persons of his environment paid to the child will be continued by the attention that the child pays to itself. Self-observation thus originates in the awareness of being observed. The intermediary stage between the observation of others and self-observation is thus the realization that one is observed by others.

Where the personality is split, as in certain psychotic diseases, self-observation is again transformed into hallucinations of being permanently observed by others. In another form the phenomenon of depersonalization, in which the person complains that he does not feel but only observes himself, reinforces this point. A man gives a speech and suddenly becomes aware of peculiarities in his voice, of certain gestures that he makes, of some personal ways of expressing himself. This awareness is not independent of the fact that he sees or senses the impression his speaking or the content of his speech makes upon his audience. We have a good expression for this kind of recognition. The speaker becomes self-conscious. One does not become self-conscious only in the presence of others, although that is usually the case. The occurrence of this reaction when one is alone is much more rare, and of a secondary character.

I repeat, self-observation is not a primary phemonenon. It must be traced back to being observed. One part of the self observes another part. I assume that differences in the kind and intensity of this observation may be significant for the future psychological interests of the individual.

A little girl I know asked her mother, "Why do you always smile when a lady in Central Park smiles at me?" The child had observed that her mother smiled at another woman who looked with pleasure at the pretty little girl. Such a case shows not so much self-observation as observation of others who react to one's self.

By primitive observation the child learns early in life to interpret the reactions of his parents or nurses as expressions of approval or disapproval, of pleasure or annoyance. Being observed and later on observing oneself will never lose its connection with this feeling of criticism. Psychology teaches us again and again that self-observation leads to self-criticism, and we have all had opportunity to re-examine this experience. Add that self-observation is from its inception a result of self-criticism. This self-criticism continues the critical attitude of mother, father, or nurse. They are incorporated into the self—become introjected. Introjection, or absorption of another person into oneself, is an indispensable pre-condition for the possibility of self-observation. Without it a child cannot transform the feeling of being observed into self-observation. The process describes a circle: attention directed to external world and others; awareness of being observed, often criticized; incorporation of the observing or critical persons into oneself; self-observation.

We know that many psychologists have wondered—some did not even wonder—about the possibility that the *I* can observe the *Me*. We see now who this observant and observing *I* is. It is the object taken into oneself, the mother, the nurse who observed the child. The split, which enables one to observe oneself, comes about through the introjection of the supervising person into oneself. We make one part of the self the supervisor of the other part. The observant *I* is a survival of the observing mother or father. We are reminded at this point of the genesis of religious belief in the omniscience of God, the belief that God sees everything. A little girl was very indignant when she heard this and said, "But that is very indecent of God."

Freud once remarked that the introspective perception of one's own instinctual impulses finally results in inhibition of these tendencies. We would like to add that such self-observation of one's tendencies is already the result of a previous inhibition. If there were no memory-traces that persons in the child's environment reacted with disapproval or annoyance, with withdrawal of affection, to certain instinctual expressions, no self-observation would develop. Let us return to our speaker. When he becomes self-conscious, and if this feeling reaches a certain intensity, he becomes embarrassed. He begins to stammer, to hesitate, to make slips of the tongue, to grow uncertain. That would be the result of the impression he gets that his speech is not being received with approval, but is being met with negative criticism. To become self-conscious means to become conscious of the negative attitude of others, to realize or to anticipate that the others are critical of one.

Psychology makes the presence of two persons necessary—even if it is introspection done by a researcher in a lonely study. There is always a second person there who observes the *Me*. We know this person was originally the father (or mother) who now continues his existence within us. The seer of oneself has an overseer; he who has received a vision of himself has taken on a supervisor.

Psychoanalysis has given a name to this invisible superintendent of the self; it calls him the superego. We thought we were masters in our own household until Freud discovered this inspecting and introspective factor, the superego—the image of the father incorporated, taken into the self as a part of it. The superego is also the second person present in self-observation.

I want to avoid the impression common among many analysts that the superego is a factor that only criticizes, punishes, forbids. If this part of ourselves, this concealed roomer in our psychical household, is a survival of the father and mother of our early childhood, he cannot have only these functions. We learn in psychoanalytic practice that the superego can have pity on the individual, and we call this experience self-pity. It is really nothing but the unconscious idea: If mother or father could see me in this misery, she or he would feel sorry for me.

The superego can smile, console, and seem to say, "Take it easy; it isn't half as bad as you think it is." We call it humor. We even know situations in which the superego forgives the person who is aware of his misdeeds or sinfulness, and we call this self-forgiveness. Religion calls it grace that descends upon the worshiper. In many cases where we use words with "self" (like "self-confidence"), "self" refers to the part of the person which is the representative of the father within him. Without knowing it, we mean the superego.

The ego is primarily an organ of perception directed toward the outside world. It is unable to observe the self. The superego is the first representative of the inner world. It is the silent guide in the subterranean realm of our psychical life. Psychology started with the supervision of emotional processes by this superintendent, this proxy-parent within us. It was this factor which examined what took place in our thought and emotional life. Its attention and vigilance were directed to those tendencies and impulses that were socially disapproved. It would criticize, condemn, suppress, and finally repress them. The first discoveries in the field of psychology were made in the service of those suppressing powers. The origin of psychology can be easily recognized in our psychological descriptions and judgments. Language has immortalized this origin. How do we characterize or describe a person? We say, for instance, that he is stubborn or avaricious or pedantic or kind or friendly. Does not the voice of the superego sound in such psychological descriptions? We want to observe and describe without preconceived ideas, but our miserably poor language forces us to put an undertone of approval or disapproval into scientific statements. Psychology was for a long time in bondage to moralistic and religious conceptions, and the superego is a witness to this servitude to ideas foreign to the spirit of research. The superego knows more about what takes place in the human mind than the other parts of the ego, exactly as worldly-wise, clever priests often know more about people than people know about themselves.

Psychology, I asserted, was at first put into the service of those powers that supervise the thoughts and emotions of the individual and of the community in order to keep away forbidden impulses and ideas. The psychologist was once a censor of the human soul; sometimes a stupid one, sometimes a wise one; sometimes tolerant and sometimes severe. The best way to deal with especially rebellious and ferocious elements is to ban them, to eliminate them. Thus psychology became a servant in the service of the repressing powers. It ignored, disavowed, and disowned certain tendencies within the ego. When their existence could no longer be denied, psychology gave them other names, distorted their nature by classifying and describing them. Even when psychology apparently freed itself from the supervision of the suppressing power, its attitude of liberty was an official one only. Proud of its independence, it continued to hold on to preconceived ideas. It was—and to a great extent it still is —a situation that calls to mind the cartoon in which two men get into a furious argument with one shouting at the other, "You shut up! Don't you know that you are living in a free country?" That was the nature of psychology for many hundreds, perhaps for a couple of thousand years.

Then there slowly came a change. It was heralded not by psychologists, or at least not by professional psychologists. It took its point of departure from the discovery of the hidden, disavowed, disowned, and forbidden tendencies. They had appeared before only in the plays of Shakespeare, and other poets, in novels, and in poems. Their voices began to be heard in the writings of Montaigne, of La Rochefoucauld, of Chamfort, and other, especially French, searchers after truth. Free or freed spirits, they labored to unmask the hidden, to disenchant a world in bondage to self-deception and magic. Another part of the ego, the same that lent its power to the suppressed tendencies, helped now to remove the chains. The great turn in modern psychology began. Heralded by the French moralists, it was brought to its most significant expression by Friedrich Nietzsche (here considered only as one of the great psychologists) and reached its peak in Sigmund Freud.

Psychology started its research in the service of the censorship of the emotional life. The observing and controlling station within the ego called conscience (or social fear) examined the ideas and tendencies that should not trespass upon the land of conscious thoughts. Psychology in this phase of its development furnished a kind of alibi for these forbidden impulses. The admonition "Know thyself" was very necessary because psychology was then the best method by which to deceive oneself about oneself. Later, very late indeed, psychology realized that its task was the removal of repressing powers, the lifting of the ban of repression, the search for the forbidden forces. This was at first an underground movement. With Nietzsche and louder still with Freud, the voice of the suppressed instincts and disavowed impulses sounded from hidden recesses. The underground movement of psychology came at last into the open and made itself known.

The organ of psychological observation, and therefore of psychological research and discovery, is to be found within oneself. It is for this organ that I want to search in these pages, an organ which observes, recognizes, and discovers what happens in us. This organ is not yet found. It is unknown; more than that—it is unconscious.

2

It takes two to practice psychology, even psychological self-observation. When you want to recognize and understand what takes place in the minds of others, you have first to look into yourself. Such a searching is only possible when a division of yourself has preceded the observation. The premise for psychological interest is thus a disturbance within the person. Without it no possibility of psychological recognition exists. Moreover the emotional disturbance has to be overcome to a certain degree, the conflict almost resolved—otherwise psychological interest would not arise. When a man is very angry, he will not be inclined, nor will he be able, to observe his own psychical processes. We would thus presuppose that Freud, who was a genius at psychological observation, must have been subjected to emotional conflicts of such a nature that they made psychological interest not only possible, but also necessary.

We put aside here the problem of his special gifts and ask: What enabled Freud psychologically to make his great discoveries, to solve the riddle of the dream, to penetrate into the recesses of human motivation; what forced him to descend into the netherworld of the neuroses while so many others remained on the surface? He himself often enough described how he came to the new science: "Psychoanalysis was born of medical necessity. It originated in the need for helping the victims of nervous disease to whom rest, hydropathy, or electrical treatment could bring no relief." These are his words.* In order to help these patients he had to understand their hitherto unfathomed symptoms. This is the route by which Freud arrived at psychoanalysis. But how did psychoanalysis come to Freud?

This question remains unanswered. Up to the present it has not even been asked. What were the personal motives which impelled him? What was the conflict-situation that made this psychological interest so strong, so governing, so consuming?

The explanation Freud himself gives is, so to speak, only the official one. Is there another one besides? One need not preclude the other; they can co-exist like two rooms, in one of which a luster sheds its light while the other is illuminated only by a small candle that leaves the corners dark.

Here we are interested only in this dark room. I once compared Freud with Rembrandt. There is no artist comparable to Rembrandt for exactitude of observation, but light came to him only as a contrast to the darkness in which great portions of his pictures are kept. Freud was a confessor, an autobiographer of admirable moral courage and frankness, but at the same time he kept certain personal secrets to himself. He was a self-revealer and a self-concealer. In a certain passage he writes of the "discretion which one owes also to oneself."

This discretion was rarely breached. It was as if he felt he had to keep personal things to himself, even from those of us who were his most loyal students. In his old age he sometimes spoke to one or another of us almost casually of a fragment of his own life he had never mentioned before, as if he had suddenly tired of his secrecy. In his "Interpretation of Dreams," in the *Psychopathology of Everyday Life* and other writings, he had presented startling discoveries that he had made about himself, magnificent instances of self-analysis, forever belonging to the most precious self-revelations of great minds. All that psychoanalysts throughout the world have since written pales into insignificance beside those pages, distinguished by unheard-of sincerity, by an unequaled moral courage, and by a cool, pitiless observation that is

* In the Preface to my book, *Ritual* (New York: Farrar, Straus & Co., 1946), p. 7.

always self-searching and never self-seeking. There were, however, limitations that he imposed on himself—not because he shied away from certain things, but because he knew this hypocritical world and realized it would misunderstand or fail to understand his fearlessness before the shadows that fall on everybody. "The very best that thou dost know thou dar'st not to the striplings show," we often heard him quote from Goethe's *Faust*.

There were self-revealing reports about suppressed and repressed emotions, conflicts, doubts, fears unearthed by the analyst—by Freud himself—in many a book he published and in many a conversation with us, his students. There was always, however, a remarkable restraint and discretion about himself—a distance from himself, so to speak. In a conversation with me he once emphasized the difference between "privata" and "privatissima," between private things you talk about when there is a scientific need for it, and things so private that you do not talk about them even when it would be valuable to discuss them.

Is there no way that leads to this secret room now, after his death? Our wish to find it is not dictated by idle curiosity of a personal nature; no spying into Freud's secrets is intended. We want to discover what led him to the psychology of the neuroses. It is thus psychological interest of an important kind that makes us ask. He himself would not mind it; he often admitted that he felt indifferent to personal things after his death. He did not believe in survival and immortality, and thought with Heine that the resurrection would be a long time in coming.

What follows is, as far as I can see, the first attempt to discover what determined the intensive personal interest of Freud in the psychology of neuroses. The approach to the secret room is difficult, particularly because of his discretion. Where is it located?

Most psychoanalysts have not observed that psychoanalysis has, so to speak, two branches. One is the research into the symptomatology and etiology of the neuroses, of hysteria, phobia, compulsion neuroses, and so forth. The other is the psychology of dreams; of the little mistakes of everyday life such as forgetting, slips of the tongue, and so forth; of wit and of superstitions—including all that Freud called metapsychology.

The first branch led to the contributions to the theory of sex, to the concept of impulses, especially of the libido. It goes in the direction of biology or tries to build a bridge between psychology and biology. It is clear that these theories are the results of experiences and observations of others. Here are the most precious discoveries used for the understanding of neurotic and psychotic diseases.

The other branch concerns purely psychological phenomena, emotional processes—no connection with biology is sought—inner experiences of the individual, best observed by himself. Dreams, wit, slips of the tongue, old superstitions conflicting with our free, conscious thinking—all these and many other phenomena are analyzed by Freud mostly from instances taken from his own life.

These two branches, it is true, are not always clearly separated. They sometimes appear intertwined, and deep down their two roots must invisibly meet; but one is bent more in the direction of the pathological, and the other more in the direction of general psychology. Nevertheless, they are two clearly distinguishable branches. The future of psychoanalysis—perhaps the future of psychology—will depend upon the choice of the research worker as to which branch he considers the more important one, which of the two will bear better and richer fruits for future generations.

Freud told us many times—and he repeated it in his writings—that he had no great liking for the profession of physician. The therapeutic ambition, the need to help sick people, was not strongly developed in him, and for a long time he could not make up his mind whether to study medicine or follow his other interests. He heard a lecture on an essay of Goethe's entitled "Nature," and this experience decided his choice. Was ever a profession wooed in this humor? In Freud's case it was not only wooed but won. He considered it, he said, a personal triumph that he returned on this "detour" (the study of medicine a detour!) to his first and primary wish—to discover something new in the field of psychology. He considered himself first and last a psychologist, not a physician, and here is the line of demarcation which separates many psychoanalysts from the founder of their science, to whom they pay lip service and little else.

Their concept of psychoanalysis is basically different from his.

They consider it a branch of medicine and their memory makes them conveniently suppress Freud's explicit sentences. He emphasized that he takes it for granted that psychoanalysis is not a "special branch of medicine. I cannot understand how one can resist recognizing that psychoanalysis is part of psychology; not medical psychology in the old meaning and not psychology of the pathological process, but pure psychology; certainly not the whole of psychology but its underground, perhaps its foundation. One should not be deceived by the possibility of its application to medical purposes. Electricity and X-ray are also applied to medicine, but the science of both remains physics. Neither can historical arguments change the fact that psychoanalysis belongs to psychology. . . . The argument has been brought forward that psychoanalysis was discovered by a physician in his efforts to help patients. But this is immaterial in its evaluation."* These remarks are followed by the confession that he realizes after forty-one years of medical practice that he has not really been a physician and that he became a physician professionally only by a deviation from his original intentions. He had, he says, passed all his medical examinations without having felt any interest in medicine; external necessity forced him to renounce a theoretical career. He arrived at neuropathology and finally "on account of new motives" at the study of the neuroses.

Here is a purposeful rejection of the view that psychoanalysis is a medical science. It is, of course, possible that the majority of physicians in America know more and know better than the founder and the greatest representative of the new science what it is—but it is rather unlikely.**

There is a very clear warning to physicians not to consider Freud as one of themselves in his "Please count me out." There was more than the Atlantic between psychoanalysis in New York and psychoanalysis in Vienna. There was an ocean of difference in the conception of it.

What interests us at this moment is the question: What per-

* Freud, *Gesammelte Schriften*, XI, 387.
** In one of his last letters to me dated London, July 3, 1938, Freud sharply criticized this concept of our New York colleagues "for whom analysis is nothing else but one of the maidservants of psychiatry."

sonal stimulus led Freud to the research into the psychology of neuroses? What were the "new motives" he mentions that made him turn his attention in this new direction? It is clear that his older interest was to discover something new. He says in the years of his youth the wish to understand something of the mysteries of the world and to contribute something to their solution had become especially strong. He had never played "doctor" as a child, and his curiosity turned in other directions.

What follows now is my attempt to build the bridge of motives between what we think were Freud's earlier interests and his later intellectual preoccupation with the problems of the neuroses. The bridge is narrow enough, but, it seems to me, capable of bearing the burden. As I have said, Freud did not often speak about himself and his intimate life. My impression is that he became more confidential after his seventieth birthday; at least he then told me some things about himself which I could never have guessed. One memory is the most important. I accidentally met him one evening in the Kaertnerstrasse in Vienna and accompanied him home. We talked mostly about analytic cases during the walk. When we crossed a street that had heavy traffic, Freud hesitated as if he did not want to cross. I attributed the hesitancy to the caution of the old man, but to my astonishment he took my arm and said, "You see, there is a survival of my old agoraphobia, which troubled me much in younger years." We crossed the street and picked up our conversation after this remark, which has been casually made.* His confession of a lingering fear of crossing open places, his mention of this remnant of an earlier neurosis, made, of course, a strong impression upon me. It took me by surprise, and his casual way of telling it to me intensified, rather than weakened, my astonishment. If such a thing had been possible, the free admission that his neurosis had left this scar on his emotional life would have added to my admiration of his great personality.

The other day Siegfried Bernfeld published a paper, "An Unknown Autobiographical Fragment by Freud,"** in which he

---

* The scene must have taken place before 1928 because I remember that I saw Freud in later years only at his home.
** *The American Imago* (August, 1946), IV, No. 1.

showed that an article of Freud's on screen-memories contains a piece of self-analysis, in this case disguised in the form of a report about a patient. This analysis concerns a man of thirty-eight years "who had maintained an interest in psychological problems in spite of his entirely different profession." Freud asserts that he "had been able to relieve him of a slight phobia through psychoanalysis." Bernfeld proves by means of a careful examination of details that this unknown patient is Freud himself disguised. Freud used the same method of speaking of himself as of another person when he wanted to disguise his identity in another paper later on.* Bernfeld, when he published his paper, did not know of Freud's remark made in that conversation with me.

What interests us here is not the biographical significance of Freud's phobia itself, but the fact that it reveals the hidden missing link between his primarily psychological interests and his later occupation with the neuroses. Here is the personal motive that made necessary for him the understanding of neurotic disturbances. In addition to the wish to help nervous patients, there was the demand: Physician, heal yourself. In this case the postulate took the form: Physician, understand your own symptoms and your own disease. But such an understanding was impossible without self-analysis, which could not remain restricted to the symptoms only. From here on we can apply the explanation given by Freud of his own case as a general one. He described how psychoanalysis led away from the study of the nervous conditions "in a degree surprising to the physician," how it had to concern itself with emotions and passions, how it learned to recognize the significance of memories and the strength of unconscious wishes.** "For a time it appeared to be the fate of psychoanalysis to be incorporated in the field of psychology without being able to indicate in what way the mind of the sick patient differed from that of the normal person." In the course of the development of psychoanalysis, Freud declares, it came upon the problem of the dream, which is "an abnormal mental

* Freud, "Der Moses des Michelangelo," *Gesammelte Schriften* (1914), X, 414.
** In Freud's preface to my *Ritual,* p. 7 ff.

product created by normal people." In solving the enigma of the dream, "it found in unconscious mentality the common ground in which the highest as well as the lowest mental impulses are rooted, and from which arise the most normal mental activities as well as the strange mechanisms of a diseased mind. The picture of the mental mechanisms of the individual now becomes clearer and more complete. . . ."

Freud himself clearly realized the connection between the interest necessitated in the first instance by his own neurosis and that arising from his concern with general pathology and psychology. The dream—and certainly also wit and the little mistakes belonging to the psychopathology of everyday life—secured the bridge from one shore to the other. The analysis of these phenomena presented the clue to the secret room of his own mental life. In helping himself he brought understanding, help, and recovery to thousands of others. When he learned to recognize the meaning, hidden to himself before, of what took place behind the façade of his own conscious thinking, the meaning of unconscious processes of all people dawned upon him. He could not have discovered the most valuable secrets of the human mind had he not found them in himself first.

Everybody who has read Freud's most important works knows that these insights were reached by analysis of his own dreams, his own slips of the tongue, and so forth. They were arrived at by self-observation and self-recognition, directed by an extraordinarily fine ear for his inner voices. When, later on, observation of others and research into other minds were added, comparison with his own emotional processes helped him to understand others. Criticism of premature analogies, of conclusions too quickly reached, corrected such comparisons and led to deeper insights, made recognition richer and extended it beyond the frontiers of Freud's ego; but the first and most important source of psychological understanding remained this self-observing factor in the psychoanalysis of himself.

Here are the results to which these introductory remarks inevitably lead, results that separate me from the majority of psychoanalysts in this country: psychoanalysis is psychology. Its application in the service of the therapy of neuroses and psychoses means making use of a method that is purely psychological in origin and nature. The most important and the most valuable insights of psychoanalysis are found by self-analysis. Wherever and whenever psychoanalysis makes really important scientific progress, it will be accomplished by an experience in which self-analysis plays the greatest role. No deep insight into human minds is possible without unconscious comparison with our own experiences. The decisive factor in understanding the meaning and the motives of human emotions and thoughts is something in the person of the observer, of the psychologist himself.

The following pages will, I hope, show to what important scientific consequences our first conclusions will lead. Before that I must, however, point out what will forever separate Freud's way from that of other psychoanalysts, setting aside now the differences between a great man and mediocre minds. His discoveries were made by himself. They were therefore not only a personal experience of unique value but also a triumph comparable to that of the greatest inventors we know. They were the triumph of a mind in search of itself, which, in reaching its aims, discovered the laws governing the emotional processes of all minds. We learn these discoveries with the help of books and lectures; we make them again, rediscover them, when we are in the process of analysis—that is, when we are analyzed or when we analyze others. Our psychoanalytic institutes seem to be unaware of the fact that being analyzed cannot compete in experience value with unearthing these insights oneself. The one experience cannot be likened to the other. It remains for us a poor substitute, a second or third best. It is ridiculous to consider one's own psychoanalysis as equivalent to the original experience. One's own psychoanalysis—however important, indeed indispensable, for the understanding of oneself and others—is, of course, not comparable to the process by which Freud arrived at his results by a heroic mental deed, by a victory over his own inner reluctances and resistances. When we are analyzed by others, it is an entirely different process, induced from outside even when we ask for it ourselves. It lacks the intimacy and the depth of experience felt in discovering one's secrets oneself. Nothing said to us, nothing we can learn from others, reaches so deep as that which we find in ourselves. The most a psychoanalyst can do for the patient and for the student is to act the mental midwife or obstetrician. Everybody has to bring his own child into the world. The psychoanalyst can help only in the delivery; he can mitigate the labor pains. He cannot influence the organic process of birth—either in himself or in others.

Many psychoanalysts who train psychiatrists think that the analysis of the students is sufficient. They are so sadly mistaken that it is not even funny. As if being analyzed were enough of an emotional and mental experience to become a psychoanalyst! As if this other, more penetrating experience—to arrive oneself at psychological insight into oneself—were superfluous! Or do they really think that study, attending courses and seminars, can be a substitute for self-acquired knowledge? It is as if listening to a poem were psychologically equivalent to writing the same poem. If being analyzed is not continued and supplemented by a man's own creative experience in finding himself, without the guidance and supervision of a psychoanalyst, it remains an isolated experience, which has no deep roots in himself and bears no rich fruit. Of the psychoanalyst, too, it may be said: By their fruits ye shall know them.

I said before that I do not share the belief of many psychoanalysts that the most valuable things in psychoanalysis can be learned. They can only be experienced. I am certainly far from underestimating the requirement that everybody who studies psychoanalysis be analyzed. This demand appears to me as imperative as it does to them, my stepbrothers in Apollo. But I do not agree with them that one's personal experience of psychoanalysis is finished with this process. I would almost say it begins with it. If there is any possibility of coming even close to the neighborhood of Freud's original experience, it can only be by a self-analysis that follows the process of being analyzed, continues and completes it.

Let me explain what I mean with the help of a comparison. A young man decides to become an actor. Reading the classical authors he becomes convinced he will one day act Hamlet, Othello, Faust. He has to learn to act; he goes to the best dramatic academy and is trained by the best teachers. He is taught how to pronounce words, to achieve the right intonation, to time sentences, to speak verses, and to give them their actor's due. He learns how to move on the stage. Now when he speaks Hamlet's great monologue, when as Faust he discusses ethical and religious subjects with Mephistopheles, he knows how to apply what he has learned, how to give emphasis and theatrical effect to his acting. For all that, he may remain a bad or mediocre actor who fails to strike a chord in us, the people sitting in the theater. What must be added, if he wants to reach us emotionally, to make us believe him?

It seems to me that two more steps, one negative and one positive, must be taken. The actor should, when he walks out upon the stage, forget what he has studied at the academy. He must brush it aside as if it had never been there. If he cannot neglect it now, in the moment of real performance—if it has not gone deep enough so that he can afford to neglect it—then his training wasn't good enough. If he has to consciously think and remember how he should speak, move, make gestures, he had better give up his career.

What he has been taught has by now reached tissues so deep— and I mean this literally: his nerve tissues in both brain and body—that he can afford to act as if he had never seen the inside of a dramatic academy.

The man in the audience takes the technical routine for granted and looks for something more: that the actor recover the essential part of the emotion that made him want to be an actor in the first place. On stage, in other words, he becomes Hamlet or Faust, feels what they feel. He must be transformed into Hamlet or Faust when he acts them. There is only one way for such a thing to happen. He has to feel again and anew what he felt and experienced when he met Hamlet and Faust the first time—in a book or at the theater as the case may be. Otherwise he will never touch us; he will leave his audience cold.

Psychoanalysts are like actors applying what they have learned in the academy. I know psychoanalysts who—to continue my comparison—have not learned enough at school. And I know a second group technically perfect but with no style of their own. They are unable to recapture the zeal of their first experiences.

Finally, I know the rare psychoanalysts—the masters—who have studied their field thoroughly and behave in the manner of sovereigns, rulers of the stage whom nobody can think of as previous students of an academy.

This analogy is as valid for analytic self-recognition as for the analysis of others. No good psychoanalyst has to think back consciously to what he learned from his own analysis. Nobody can be a good analyst for whom analysis—of himself or others— has lost the value of a personal experience, of *a search* and research.

Apply this test to the field of psychoanalytic writing, and what do you get? There are papers published in psychoanalytic magazines nowadays that are as far from personal experience as Sirius is from our planet. Sterility in psychoanalytic research, its distance from men's lives, has gone so far that some of the papers look like mathematical operations—purely formalized thinking in its most abstract form. Reading such papers, I sometimes wonder if many analysts haven't taken a common and solemn vow to stay awake while reading them. It would take a wilder fantasy than any Shakespeare dreamed to imagine that the investigator got his results by way of experience. Science practiced this way remains science for science' sake; it can have no practical outcome. Nothing that does not originate in an experience can become an experience for others.

The element of personal experience can, of course, remain hidden. It may not appear, but it will be felt in the quality of the psychoanalyst's work, whether in practice or in his research. I therefore repeat: By their fruits ye shall know them.

3

The overvaluation of intelligence among cultured people in our country has reached a frightening degree. Not only our public schools and our colleges and universities but also our research institutes give the impression that the intelligence test is the only criterion of man's mental endowment. It is as if intelligence, nowadays called "smartness," were the one and only decisive factor in measuring or in evaluating a person's qualities. It is as if other gifts were not even to be considered; as if imagination, moral courage, creative faculties were of no importance. I am convinced that Beethoven had a lower I.Q. than a bank director, but I am willing to exchange all bank directors for the one Beethoven. One is inclined to believe that Mozart's I.Q. was not equal to that of many college graduates. It was, I am sure, even lower than that of most psychoanalysts.

This general, silly overvaluation of mere intelligence has led to a misconception about the origin of psychoanalysis or about Freud's way of discovering it. The first is that this new research method was discovered by hard and penetrating thinking, by a great intellectual effort. Freud in his incomparable sincerity denied it energetically. He emphasized again and again that he was led to his most important discoveries by a prejudice, a preconceived opinion. He used the German *"Vorurteil,"* which really means "pre-notion" or "pre-judgment." What he really meant can be better expressed by the English word "hunch." What is a hunch? It seems to me that it is an impression reached by intuition, a kind of foreknowledge—sensing something rather than knowing it or judging it by means of reason. The birth of psychoanalysis out of a hunch—that is perhaps not a comfortable idea for us scientific minds, for us psychoanalysts. But the birthplace of an idea is not the decisive factor. Jesus was born in a stable and his idea conquered the world.

As a matter of psychological fact, many of the greatest discoveries and inventions originated as hunches, as every textbook on the history of science reveals. Freud stated again and again that he gained his best insights by trusting to hunches. He did not agree with the accepted opinion of the scholars that the dream is only a physiological process, but with the average man and woman on the street that it has a secret meaning and can be interpreted. He had another hunch: he did not accept the official view of the physicians who explained hysteria as a physically determined disease, but thought of it as resulting from emotional conflicts. He felt that the generally valid theory of psychiatry did not explain the genesis and the nature of the neuroses, but he preferred rather the concept of the uncultured masses who considered neurosis as an emotional disturbance. He generally preferred concepts in the field of psychology that nobody took seriously. He was not afraid to remain in the minority, and his strong will as well as his moral courage enabled him not to give a tinker's damn about what the majority of his professional colleagues thought of him and his new views. For us psychoanalysts it is hopeless, of course, to try to emulate Freud's genius and mental endowments. We should, however, at least wish to emulate him with regard to his fearlessness, his moral courage, his readiness to suffer for his convictions and to remain lonely. Alas, I see very few signs of such a wish among psychoanalysts today.

The technique of psychoanalysis as we know it at present was born as a hunch about the essential nature of the dream and the neuroses. The simple and leading thought, which seems to be so near now and was so far from the minds of Freud's contemporaries, is that men reveal themselves—all their emotional secrets —when they talk freely about themselves; not just when they talk about their secrets, but about everything concerning themselves. They give away what bothers them, disturbs and torments them, all that occupies their thoughts and arouses their emotions—even when they would be most unwilling to talk directly about these things.

Freud has said that mortals are not made to keep a secret and that self-betrayal oozes from all their pores. The ego has built mighty defenses against the forbidden impulses that drive and push to gain some measure of expression. They are pressed into oblivion, into the dark abyss of rejected and condemned emotions and thoughts. They are disavowed, banned, and outlawed, and live in the netherworld, never to be mentioned. In panic fear of their power, man has rolled obstacles as strong as the Rock of Gibraltar before the door to prevent their return. They betray themselves, nevertheless, and give notice of their subterranean existence and activity in little, unsuspected signs, words, and gestures. They give themselves away in spite of shame and fear. The old Negro spiritual knows it:

> . . . . I went to de rock
> To hide my face,
> De rock cried out, "No hidin' place,
> Dere's no hidin' place down dere."

Here are the roots of that basic rule of psychoanalytic technique, the only rule which the student or patient need promise to follow. At first hearing it sounds simple enough. Yes, one cannot easily imagine that there could be anything simpler than to say just what occurs to you. But how difficult it is! How much training, what a long will-training will be necessary, not to reach, but merely to approach this aim!

The basic rule is known by the name of free association. Modern writers like to speak of the "stream of consciousness." The comparison is not without merit, but it has its demerits too. The stream sometimes changes into a sea that threatens to drown the person. Sometimes it degenerates and declines into a trickle and it often seems to run dry. It is, it seems, a peculiar kind of stream.

What course this stream takes was, of course, recognized by psychology and formulated in the shape of laws of thought-association long ago. We are following certain laws when we think of an apple, a garden, blossomtime, or of an apple and apple strudel in succession; when we look at a portrait and think of the person who posed for it; when we smell something and think of a certain dish. We are as obedient to these laws of association as when we think of cold-hot or low-high. Freud had a hunch that this stream had undercurrents to be investigated that determined its course to an even greater extent perhaps than the factors then known to psychology. These undercurrents are the unconscious impulses and interests, the repressed emotions of men. Free associations are only free on the surface. They are dictated by a power behind the throne of reason.

Freud followed his hunch. He asked his patients to say whatever occurred to them without any exception and without using the censorship to which we submit our thoughts otherwise. In general we try to follow a certain direction in speaking. We tend to speak logically and to the point (the effort frequently fails, as the speeches of our senators show). The patient in psychoanalysis should say what occurs to him without such order and restriction. He should jump about in his thoughts.

We might contrast the different types of mental activity thus: Thinking is like marching on the beaten path of custom to a certain aim; saying what comes into one's mind is like walking about without any destination. But are not the two ways of mental activity mutually exclusive? Certainly not; there is room enough for both in our psychical life. They take place in different layers. It is possible that on the fourth floor of a building a pianist is practicing a Clementi sonata, while another artist in a room in the basement is playing a Beethoven sonata. They do not disturb each other as long as they do not hear each other.

It is obvious that the two ways of thinking have separate realms, with a border between them that neither may cross without creating disturbances of one kind or another. A corporation lawyer would reach no satisfactory result were he to follow every fancy in thinking about a difficult legal problem. A poet, on the other hand, would write a very poor poem if he were to examine each metaphor in his love poem to see whether it met the tests of strict logic. One way of thinking is not appropriate in the first case, the other would have no place in the second. The lawyer will do his work best when he thinks and concludes logically and uses all the reason at his disposal. The poet cannot write his verses after long reflection and mature consideration. If he should meditate and ponder about the expression of his feelings, they would lose all spontaneity. The French poet, Paul Valéry, said that thinking or reflecting means to lose the thread, *"perdre le fil."* The lawyer thinks he has lost the thread if he follows a capricious idea, a whim, while working on his brief. One man's meat is another man's poison.

Is it not easy simply to tell what occurs to you? Should it not be very easy to speak without order and logical connection, to say everything that flashes through your mind without rhyme or reason? No, it is rather difficult; it is more like a steeplechase than a flat course. Every minute a new obstacle blocks your way. You will be surprised by the kinds of thoughts that occur to you. You will not only be surprised; you will be ashamed and sometimes even afraid of them. More than the conventions of society has to be thrown overboard when you want to say everything that occurs to you. Fear and shame, which is perhaps a special kind of fear itself, have to be discarded before you can succeed. Thoughts and impulses concerning sexual and toilet activities and needs are not easy to utter. Mean, aggressive, and hostile tendencies—especially against persons near and dear to us—are difficult to admit.

It would, however, be erroneous to assume that those tendencies are the only ones that are hard to confess. An analyst often makes the surprising discovery that a man is more ready to talk about a perversion than about a tender feeling he has had. In one of Zola's novels a defendant is willing to speak in a matter-of-fact way about a lust murder he has committed, but is hindered by shame from admitting that he once kissed the stocking of a woman. Often a petty or trivial thought is much harder to tell than a mean deed. The psychoanalyst finds men are often more ashamed to speak about ideas they consider stupid or superstitious than about impulses that they condemn as criminal or antisocial.

But why enumerate and evaluate all the hindrances and obstacles in the road, when a simple experiment can convince the reader how difficult the task is? The experiment, it is true, is not equivalent to the real psychoanalytic situation; but it has some of its elements and it has the advantage that it can be made here and now. The reader is invited to take paper and pencil and to write down whatever occurs to him during the next half hour. He should eliminate all censorship of his thoughts while he writes, take no consideration of logic, esthetics, or morals, and concentrate only on jotting down what occurs to him, lost to the social world that at other times dictates his train of thought. If he is sincere with himself and overcomes all tendencies seeking to prevent him from writing down all his thoughts, whether they are clever or silly, conventional or indecent, important or trivial, without bothering about their order, aim, and connections, without selection or censorship—just as if they had been dictated to him by another person—he has done a good job. He should then put the written sheets into a drawer and leave the room. When he takes them out the next day and carefully reads them, he will meet a person there who reminds him of himself in many ways but is in other ways an unknown man. Was it he who thought all that? Here is a new *I* to whom he gets introduced.

Today the experiment can be considerably improved, thanks to an instrument that modern invention has provided. This instrument is called the dictaphone. When one speaks all that one thinks into a dictaphone for an hour under the conditions just mentioned and disconnects the instrument, one has the possibility of listening in comfort to one's thoughts the next day, as one might listen to a third person. The advantages compared with writing are clear. The road from thought to speech is shorter than from thinking to writing. It is really a return to the original, because what we think is only what we say within ourselves without pronouncing the words. Everybody has observed that many people make mouth movements as if they would speak when they read and even when they write. The spoken words have an emotional quality different from the words that have only been thought. The Catholic church does not recognize a confession which is only thought or written down. The confession must be *vocalis*, spoken; is must be articulated, vocalized. A comparison between written and thought words shows that the effect of articulate speech is different not only upon the hearer but also upon the speaker himself. I know a girl who said, "I never know what I think until I hear myself saying it." The advantage of the dictaphone is that one can "hear oneself think." Such experiments can, of course, never replace the psychoanalytic situation, but they can convince the skeptic that he has thoughts and impulses that are unknown to him. There are hidden roomers that live in his mental house without being registered.

There are certain other conditions necessary; certain requirements have to be fulfilled before such experiments can even approach an elementary self-analysis, but one thing is clear: a person has to become at least capable of making such an experiment before he can hope to "analyze himself."

Anybody who tries the experiment will soon realize that one quality is more important than any other in psychoanalysis: moral courage. This quality and this alone enabled Freud, as he once emphatically stated,* to make his most valuable discoveries. Many psychoanalysts think that their intellectual endowments qualify them especially for their profession. The truth is that every psychoanalyst with a long experience has had patients who were intellectually his superiors by far; and every psychoanalyst will be ready to admit that to himself. I have had the good luck to treat and to help men who were famous as writers and scientists, and I have often had the opportunity to admire their genius. Two factors render the analyst in the situation in the consulting room an authority. The first—his knowledge and experience in psychology—could be acquired easily by every one of his gifted patients. The other factor is the moral courage that enables the psychoanalyst to face in others as well as in himself unpleasant and repressed thoughts and tendencies, which the patient in his present situation avoids. To help the patient stand his ground before these impulses and ideas is the most important part of the analyst's task. The analyst plays the role of the midwife in helping to bring those unborn thoughts and impulses to the daylight of conscious processes and to convince the patient that they have a right to exist and to be considered.

The psychoanalyst himself is subject to the same dangers as his patient: to disavow and repress thoughts and impulses he does not want to realize in himself, to play hide-and-seek with himself. Every analyst should put himself to the test periodically to determine how sincere he can be with himself. Such self-analysis will teach him a lesson he will remember whenever he is inclined to become impatient with the patient's resistance against recognizing some unpleasant truths. Such self-managed experiments will remind him that he has much to learn and recognize about himself long—in many cases even a few decades—after he was analyzed by another. Only superficial and shallow thinking can make an analyst believe that he knows himself thoroughly and that he does not need any added analysis to become acquainted with himself. He will experience some surprises whenever he faces himself. Meeting oneself is rarely a pleasant experience even for the psychoanalyst.

* Freud, "Josef Popper-Lynkeus und die Theorie des Traumes," *Gesammelte Schriften*, XI, 297.

Every experience of this kind will bring him new insights and added psychological knowledge brought up from the deep wells of his emotional life. At this point I hear a voice saying, "It is easy enough to give advice that one is unwilling to take oneself."

I accept the challenge and interrupt my writing to subject myself to the experiments.

What are my thoughts at this moment? I see the pussy willows on my bookcase . . . a prehistoric vase . . . spring, youth, old age . . . regrets . . . the books . . . the *Encyclopedia of Ethics and Religion* . . . the book I did not finish. . . . My eyes wander to the door. . . . A photograph of Arthur Schnitzler on the wall . . . my son Arthur . . . his future . . . the lamp on the table. . . . What a patient had said about the lamp once when it was without a shade . . . the table . . . it was not there a few years ago . . . my wife bought it . . . I did not want to spend the money at first . . . she bought it nevertheless. . . .

These are my thoughts as I should tell them to a person in the room to whom I have to report them the moment they occur. It is clear that most of them are determined by the objects I see; the connections between them seem to be made only by the sight of the objects and by thoughts of the persons they remind me of. Some, as for instance the two sequences, *Encyclopedia of Ethics and Religion*—the book I did not finish and pussy willows—spring—old age—regrets, do not follow the same laws of association, it would seem.

But are they really my thoughts? Aren't they rather abbreviations, clues to my thoughts, not the thoughts themselves? As such, they give nothing but the most superficial information about what I was thinking. If I want to tell what I really thought, I shall have to fill the gaps between these clues, put flesh on this skeleton. Here is what I really thought (and not all, not by a long shot, but enough to make me realize what occupies me at this moment).

I see the pussy willows on my bookcase . . . they are in a prehistoric vase that I brought with me when I came from Austria . . . the flowers remind me of my youth in Vienna . . . I am getting old . . . I regret that I have not enjoyed my youth more . . . I remember a joke I heard from Dr. S. when I last saw him:

"When one is six years old, one thinks the penis is there for urinating; when one is sixty, one knows it." . . . unpleasant thoughts about impotence, which threatens with old age . . . return of the regrets that I have not enjoyed my younger years sexually . . . a French proverb: *"Si jeunesse savait si vieillesse pouvait"* ("If youth but knew, if old age but could") . . . I try to console myself . . . I worked, I achieved something . . . I wrote many books . . . how many? Twenty? Thirty? . . . the *Encyclopedia of Ethics and Religion* reminds me of the second volume of my *Psychological Problems of Religion* which is not finished . . . without saying it I promised Freud to continue the studies . . . the door . . . leaving . . . dying . . . the photograph of Arthur Schnitzler . . . I remember him and I see him as I took a walk with him in Vienna on the Sommerhaidenweg . . . we lived in the same street and my son was named after him . . . I once wished that Arthur would become a writer like Arthur Schnitzler, whom I loved. . . . Schnitzler was once a physician but he left his practice because he preferred writing . . . I hoped my son would study medicine; that was in Holland, but he had to break off his studies and preferred to become a bookseller . . . perhaps he would not have finished his studies even if the Nazis had not come . . . a slight disappointment, because I wanted him to have a brilliant career . . . will he succeed in his profession? . . . the son of Arthur Schnitzler occurs to me . . . his name is Heinrich. . . . Like my son he is now in this country. I have not heard anything about him for a long time. Perhaps he is in Hollywood. His father may have wished another career for his son, too. I am sure he did not like Hollywood. I remember his blue eyes, his gray beard . . . the story I heard in Vienna when Heinrich, Arthur Schnitzler's son, was in the first grade of public school. The teacher had asked the boys whether they knew who Goethe was. No one knew, but little Heinrich said, "I am not certain but I believe he is a colleague of my father." . . . Clever saying of my son Arthur when he was a child. Once after listening to a concerto by Mozart, he asked his mother, "Is he not called Mozart because his music is so *zart?*" (German for "gentle, fine, delicate") . . . affection for Arthur . . . his passionate interest in music. . . . It used to worry me, he seemed too interested.

Grillparzer (the great Austrian poet) said about his sweetheart, "She gets drunk on music as another on wine." . . . I once hoped Arthur would become a composer . . . he showed a great musical gift but like myself was too lazy to study an instrument . . . I remember that as a small boy he sang tunes from the symphonies of Mahler . . . he loves this composer as I do . . . the lamp on the table . . . it is a big lamp with curves . . . once the shade was broken and the bulb was visible . . . a lady who was a patient of mine at the time said, "The lamp looks so nude." . . . the table on which the lamp stands was not there . . . my wife suggested that we buy a table for this place near the wall . . . I thought it unnecessary and did not want to spend the money . . . we have so little money . . . my wife did not argue, but a few weeks later the table was there and the lamp stood on it . . . she got around me . . . am I henpecked or indulgent? . . .

Here are my thoughts, and not all the thoughts at that. Many I have skipped because, as Freud once said, one owes discretion even to oneself. There are other associations that do not appear here because I owe discretion to my wife, my son, and other persons who would otherwise be mentioned in this report. It also does not put my train of thought to good account because it considers only what takes place in the center of my mental activity. It does not take the marginal thoughts into account and does not consider the fringes of my thoughts. I would have to write many more pages if I wanted to report them too. When I thought of Arthur, for instance, a memory flashed through my mind. In a moment the image of his mother, whom he resembles, occurred to me. I remembered a conversation we had when he was a small boy. I had even then expressed my ambitious hopes for his future, but my wife said she wished only for his happiness. Here my thoughts turned in the direction of the contrast of fame and achievement with happiness. Arthur Schnitzler was not happy although he was very famous at the time my son was born and named after him.

Such thoughts really belong to the essential psychical process and should not be excluded from this report, especially since they touch a problem that has occupied me in the last few years (see the regrets about my youth which is gone).

How does the name Mahler occur in this train of thought? Apparently only on account of the fact that my son, when only a small boy, was able to remember many tunes from Mahler's symphonies. Between the reported associations there were at least two other connections that I have neglected to give here; one superficial and the other reaching into deeper layers. First the other photograph, beside the one of Arthur Schnitzler, that hangs on the wall is that of Gustav Mahler. This association seems to correspond with the laws of association which W. Wundt and other psychologists follow. Not so the second association: both men lived many years in the Vienna of my youth without having met, until Schnitzler expressed what a deep impression Mahler's Sixth Symphony had made upon him. My son Arthur and I attended a performance of this symphony together in Vienna.

Here we meet the factor of over-determination of associations. This means that many threads connect one thought with the preceding and the following ones. As a matter of fact, no description can give a full account of this over-determination because it is not possible to describe the simultaneous interplay of thoughts moving on different levels. One must change simultaneousness into succession, and the dimensions of surface and depth in the psychical process can only be hinted at.

It is also difficult to give an adequate impression of the rich life on the margins and fringes of the thoughts. I shall give only one instance: at a certain point in my thoughts the name Goethe appeared (little Heinrich Schnitzler said in public school that he thought Goethe was a colleague of his father). But this was not the first time a memory of Goethe occurred in my train of thought. It was there before, although only on the fringes of the process: When I thought of my son's not continuing his studies, I thought also that his engagement to a Dutch girl and his early marriage had a share in his decision; and mysteriously a half-forgotten line from Goethe's *Hermann and Dorothea* occurred. There the mother of the son wishes that he would marry "so that the night will become a beautiful part of thy life." Here, connected with Goethe is an allusion to the sexual motive of marriage. The other obvious thread to Goethe is the name of Schnitzler's son. Heinrich is the name of Faust, the hero of

Goethe's tragedy, whose verses accompanied my own youth. From this point thoughts branched off to my psychoanalytic study of Goethe, to my ambitions and hope that Farrar, Straus will publish the book in an English translation in 1949, when the nations of the world celebrate the two hundredth anniversary of Goethe's birth . . . doubts whether I will live so long . . . my heart ailment . . . Schnitzler died of a heart disease.

There are further precursors and lingering notes in the train of thought that are not considered in my report above. On the walk on the Sommerhaidenweg in Vienna, Schnitzler and I had talked about marriage. He had married a girl who was much younger than himself. Here thoughts went forth to my second wife, whom I married after my first wife, Arthur's mother, died. But this same road, the Sommerhaidenweg, plays a part in Schnitzler's *Der Weg ins Freie* ("The Way into the Open") a novel which discusses the Jewish problem. It was partly the influence of the Nazi danger that made my son decide to leave Europe—here is the Jewish problem again.

There are further thoughts—connections that I have not given their psychological due because the explanation would take too long, psychologically important and informative as they are. I can give only two instances. I remembered Arthur's bright remark about Mozart; then followed my thought that my son is too interested in music; and then Grillparzer's words about the passionate love of his girl friend Kathi for music. The associative threads seem clear enough; the links are all there. But to appreciate the inner operations of the mind, one should follow the connections between the names Mozart and Grillparzer. Grillparzer appears here, in his characterization of Kathi Froehlich's enthusiasm, almost as an opponent of music, as I myself am opposed to my son's overfondness for this art. But Grillparzer was himself a music lover. He played the piano excellently, worshiped the great classical masters, often talked with Beethoven, for whom he prepared a libretto for an opera. He wrote the speech that was spoken at Beethoven's grave, over which he wept with many another Viennese.

It must be psychologically determined that Grillparzer appears here as a contrast to Mozart, whom he adored. The justified criticism of Kathi Froehlich's musical enthusiasm is not sufficient to make a bridge between Mozart and Grillparzer. The bridge was prepared in my thoughts long before this particular train of thought. It was not built on the spur of the moment; it has been there since my youth. Like all boys who attended college in Vienna, I read most of Grillparzer's plays and knew much about his life. To tell the truth, I never liked the man, although we were educated to see in him the great poet of our Austria. As an expression of this concealed dislike, I discovered in my college years an inclination to forget the year of his birth, and I once got a bad mark in an examination on account of it. But an accident helped me keep this date (1791) in memory with such certainty that I know it even now, many years later. My dislike for Grillparzer was not greater than my love for another Austrian, Mozart, who died in the year Grillparzer was born. By a simple mnemonic device that coupled the disliked date, which one is inclined to forget, with another that reminded me of a loved personality, I succeeded in retaining 1791 as Grillparzer's birth year.

My second instance of a marginal association was a visual image. Remembering Schnitzler, I recalled suddenly a caricature of him that appeared in a Vienna newspaper on the occasion of his sixtieth birthday. The cartoon, teasing rather than malicious, shows the writer comfortably smoking his cigar. The rings that the smoke makes seem to transform themselves into seductive faces and bodies of beautiful women. The writer of *Hands Around* looks thoughtfully at these rings as if absorbed in enjoyable memories. The caption expresses his thoughts: "Oh, my, those were times!"

Clearly the memory of the cartoon, which I saw only once almost twenty-five years before (Schnitzler was sixty years old in 1922), did not occur merely because my glance had fallen on his photograph. If the reader will again follow my previous thoughts, he will meet ideas about my own age, then regrets about my youth and some unpleasant thoughts about the threat of sexual impotency. Here are the highly personal associative threads. In the memory of the caricature with its delicate reminder of fading youth and sexual power, there is an echo that resounds and re-echoes subterraneous thoughts about myself, which have built a bridge of associations to the writer because I am now myself near the age he was when we were friends.

I have given here the main thoughts that crossed my mind in those few minutes of the experiment, which was made on the spur of the moment. It was, of course, impossible to give the reader even a vague idea of the emotions that, distinct or vague, diluted or concentrated, accompanied this train of thought. Words like "regret over my youth, which is gone," "memory of my wife, who died," or "tenderness for Arthur when he was a small boy" are hints at those emotions rather than expressions of their nature.

If I had these thoughts during an analytic session, my psychoanalyst would certainly get an impression of what these emotions accompanying my thoughts were. Intonation, changes of my voice, the rise and fall of the sentences, as well as pauses and other signs would betray not only what I think but also what I feel. If he were a psychoanalyst worthy of the name, he would guess or sense what emotions came alive when I remembered Schnitzler or when I felt sorry that I did not finish the book that I wanted to write because I had promised Freud I would. The most personal factor of these emotions, the intimacy of the inner experience is, it is true, not sayable, but its reflex will communicate itself like a song without words and express emotions that the listener in his turn will sense.

Besides and beyond such impressions, this succession of thoughts, ostensibly so unconnected and meaningless, would give any analyst an excellent idea of what occupies me at this time. Following my train of association, he could not fail to know that I have some thoughts about getting old, worries about sexual potency, and that I try to console myself for my lost youth with satisfaction of another kind. He would realize that I must have been a very ambitious person in my younger days and that I tried to displace this ambition onto my son and was as disappointed with him as with myself, and so forth. All these and many other thoughts and feelings emerged from dark recesses to the surface of my associations, like moles crawling out of their hills between the lights. In such experiments hearing is believing.

When we express what occurs to us, we do not always know

what we are saying. But when we read or listen to our words later on, they are, oddly enough, not odd any more. We did not know what we were saying, but even so we did better than many people who do not know what they are thinking about.

I believe that exercises in thought-association in self-analysis have a value beyond their immediate, practical use for understanding what is one's own psychological situation at a given time. They renew and deepen the experience of the analytic process, make it a living experience again, one which is part of one's life. There is always a danger that the psychoanalyst, who every day sees nine or ten patients, will consider his work a "profession," that he will see himself as an "expert" on the heights and depths of psychical life, and that psychoanalysis may become for him a standard operation procedure. He is not forever "analyzed" after he has once been analyzed.

The psychoanalyst as well as his patient must renew the impression that it is impossible to speak absolute nonsense when one sincerely expresses what has crossed his mind. What emerges from *unconscious* depths has an order, a continuity, and a reason of its own. The analyst has plenty of opportunity to observe how little sense it makes when some people say what they *consciously* think.

4

On the street or in parks you sometimes notice people talking to themselves. These persons, who seem to be carrying on such stimulating one-sided conversations, are not necessarily drunk or insane. I once asked an acquaintance who had this habit about his motives. He answered jokingly that he occasionally liked to hear what an intelligent person had to say, and to feel that he was talking to an intelligent listener. Such a high self-evaluation may be correct in some cases and wrong in others. More important is the fact that in dialogues with oneself one is more sincere than in conversation with others. The speaker is less inhibited and less conventional and will say what he really thinks, while his audience is more tolerant and more willing to listen, not only to reason, but to unreason. Certainly many matters that are never or rarely mentioned in talking to others are freely discussed in conversations with oneself.

Self-analysis is comparable to a conversation with oneself with the difference that its character is not just chattering, but discovering in oneself something which has hitherto been unknown. Self-analysis for its own sake is usually as barren as *l'art pour l'art*. Occasion for self-analysis arises only when we are surprised by our thoughts, when we find in ourselves feelings that seem strange, or when we are amazed over actions and inhibitions we did not suspect in ourselves. Such opportunities occur much more frequently than one might think.

More than a hundred years ago a Viennese satirist wrote: "I believe the worst of everybody, including myself, and I have rarely been mistaken." The remark is certainly justified but necessarily one-sided. Self-analysis reveals that there are not only unsuspected vices and horrid impulses hidden within ourselves but also friendly and even generous feelings never dreamed of or only dreamed of. This kind of deep-sea diving brings to the surface not only strange monsters but also unlooked-for treasures. Many surprises beyond good and evil await the diver there on the bottom, if he glides down at the right moment.

The following paragraphs present no more than a fragmentary analysis of mood, a frame of mind of my own, which I did not understand until some months after it had passed.

Like many of my colleagues I had left the decaying Vienna of the postwar years to live in Berlin, where the new Psychoanalytic Institute was showing a promising development. I had built up a satisfactory psychoanalytic practice in Berlin when, one day, I received from Vienna a request for an appointment. The man who wrote was unknown to me but said that he had a special recommendation from Freud. At the appointed hour the man appeared for a consultation. He was a middle-aged and very wealthy American with a well-known name. He described his nervous symptoms, giving me a good picture of his psychological situation. For many years he had been suffering from a severe obsessional neurosis that necessitated his protecting himself against innumerable imaginary and magical dangers by means of many complicated safety measures. Both because of his nervous troubles and for family reasons, it was not possible for him to come to Berlin for psychoanalytic treatment. Freud had suggested his coming to me because I had treated many similar cases in the past. The patient made me the following proposition. If I would return to Vienna to treat him and be at his disposal for just one hour daily, he would not only be responsible for my living expenses but pay me a fee much larger than the total earnings from my Berlin psychoanalytic practice. After a brief consideration I accepted his offer. Having brought some of my analytic treatments to an end and transferred other cases to colleagues, I returned to Vienna in November, 1932. In spite of the many social and cultural advantages Berlin possessed at that time, I had not been overfond of the capital of the German Reich. When I arrived at the Vienna station, I felt like a son coming home to his mother. All during the journey I had been happily anticipating the prospect of the life ahead of me. I would be free from all financial considerations and would be able to devote most of my time to scientific research. I would be able to see my family and friends as often as I wished. This wonderful opportunity would permit me to see Freud and to attend the weekly meetings of the Vienna Psychoanalytic Association, whose secretary I had been in past years. Altogether it seemed like a fairy tale come true.

The ensuing months brought the realization of these daydreams. Released from the necessity of spending ten hours a day in psychoanalytic practice, I worked on the two books I had planned, saw much of my family and friends, visited with Freud, and regularly attended the meetings of the Vienna Psychoanalytic Association. I enjoyed the first days of my return to the utmost. It made me happy just to walk in the morning through the familiar streets of my native city on my way to the university library.

The apartment my patient had taken for me was, like his own, in the Hotel Bristol, which, in splendor and dignity, was comparable to New York's Waldorf-Astoria. I still remember how I could scarcely believe my good luck when I awoke the first morning and looked about me at the magnificently appointed rooms which were now my new home. Humming a Strauss waltz, I went

down to breakfast at my usual hour. Of course there was no one in
the dining room to serve me—it was not yet seven. As I passed the
night clerk at his desk, he looked up at me with a startled expression as if I were some ghostly apparition in the middle of the
night. It dawned on me that guests in such a place as this would
scarcely be expected to appear for breakfast much before eleven
o'clock. I took breakfast and lunch in more modest establishments.
At the door of the Bristol dining room that evening, I was met
by a headwaiter who looked like a duke at the very least and who
accompanied me ceremoniously to my table. The waiters at once
appeared to hear my wishes. I looked about me and realized with
some embarrassment that I was the only person in the great shining room not dressed in evening clothes.

For some days I continued to dine at the Bristol. I was now
appropriately attired but I dislike having to shave again every
evening and changing into my dinner jacket. Besides, the lordly
headwaiter, his three attentive assistants, and the elaborate ritual
of the meal made me uncomfortable. The luxury of the place
somehow oppressed my spirits. Every morning I left the hotel
early to get breakfast at a little coffeehouse in a near-by side street.
I slunk past the night clerk and was annoyed with myself for being embarrassed when he noticed me. It was really absurd. Why
did I feel almost guilty about going to breakfast at seven o'clock
in the morning? I must confess that I even began positively to dislike the headwaiter and his three helpers when I thought of how
they walked to my table with a stateliness that suggested a procession of high dignitaries. I gave up the Bristol dining room and
enjoyed my dinners in less sumptuous surroundings, ruefully admitting to myself that I simply could not feel at home in my
magnificent domicile. Gradually it became clear to me that I
actually preferred less grand and formal living arrangements. A
feeling of not belonging walked with me through the gleaming
corridors of the Bristol.

Another factor worked unfavorably upon my spirits. My patient, for whom I had reserved a fixed hour daily, did not show
up. True, he had prepared me for this during our talk in Berlin
when he had said that perhaps he might sometimes be unable to
come at the appointed hour. As it turned out, I saw him in the

next three months only a few times. Then he came just once for one hour. After that I did not see him or hear from him again. When we had made our arrangements in Berlin, he had asked me not to write and not to call him on the telephone because that would arouse his fears relating to certain magic ideas. He expected me to stay put until he needed me. Since I had agreed to this, I was bound by my promise now. As the weeks went on I learned that it was disturbing to me to be paid so much money without working for it, without really earning it.

I urged myself to be patient and told myself that I was by no means lazy. Did I not work hard every day? Had I not written one book and done preliminary work on another? Did I not study all the new literature in psychology and psychiatry? Evidently I considered these activities pleasure rather than work. Often I caught myself ashamed at the thought that I, in the prime of life, was not earning my living. This was paradoxical enough since I was "earning" more than I ever had before. This too easy life without duties and obligations was uncomfortable. I even began to feel a resentment against my patient whom, in all reason, I should have considered my benefactor. How often in the past, tired from my ten hours of analytic work, had I daydreamed of an easeful life, free from financial burdens, which would permit me to devote myself to the realization of my research plans? And now when kind destiny had made me a gift of just this situation, I could not enjoy it.

I tried in vain to shake off the strangely unhappy mood that had taken possession of me and grew worse as time went on. Again and again I asked myself what kind of odd discontent it might be that, precisely when I had every reason to be satisfied with my lot, prevented me from enjoying it. Measured by my own modest standards, I was now almost wealthy. I was getting a great deal of money without working for it. (A few years later, of course, Hitler took all my savings.) My life had every possible amenity and I was home in Vienna where I wanted to be—what the hell was the matter with me? The explanations I found were such obvious pretexts and pretensions that I could not consider them valid. A cloud darkened the most beautiful holiday. It was mysterious that I was so often restless or sad without reasonable reasons. To be sure my dark mood left me for hours at a time, but only to return at an unforeseen moment. I recall that it overtook me once after I had walked home from a delightful conversation with Freud, and again while I crossed the street coming home to the Bristol from the opera house, where I had enjoyed *Der Rosenkavalier*. It was with me again as I returned from hearing Mahler's Fourth Symphony. I was still under the spell of the last movement, which is full of gaiety and childlike happiness. Walking in the winter night, I sang it over and over under my breath, when suddenly I felt depressed. I had known moods of this sort before, but none so persistent as this. My unrest and dissatisfaction increased, although I put up a good fight against them.

Finally I could bear it no longer. I wrote to my patient expressing my thanks and my regrets that it had not been possible for me to be of greater use to him. Without giving reasons—for I had none—I asked him to excuse me and then packed my trunks. The next morning as the taxi took me through the streets of Vienna on my way to the station, I felt wonderfully lighthearted, as if I had thrown off a heavy burden. The air of the radiant spring morning was delicious, and I looked with friendliness into the faces of the people in the streets. My farewell to Vienna was not sad but full of tenderness. It was like taking leave of a sweetheart whom one will never forget.

Many weeks later I began to understand what had happened to me between arrival and departure. I became aware that I had been discontented, not in spite of my good fortune, but because of it. Much later still I recalled just when the first shadow had fallen across my days in Vienna. One afternoon I had by accident —but was it accident?—passed the house in which I was born and had spent my childhood years. My father, who was in the Civil Service, had often been worried about money and had had difficulties in making ends meet on the meager salary of an Austrian official. As I walked along, childhood memories crept up from shadowy corners and I saw again the worried faces of my parents. A sudden sadness had come over me by the time I reached the Bristol. From then on the mood only left me for brief hours at a time. Its full psychological significance only became clear to me much later.

It was as if I could not permit myself to enjoy my rich surroundings, my too comfortable life, or the money come by so easily but not felt as deserved for work done. The childhood memories had brought back to me the poverty in which my parents had spent their lives, the sacrifices they had made to give us children educational advantages. Here in the same city, only a half hour's walk from my childhood home, I had lived in luxury. A slight discontent had already appeared at the Hotel Bristol prior to this incident, but I had explained it to myself as being due to the fact that I was unaccustomed to so much elegance. My mood had continued and had become worse, the longer my carefree life continued.

It was not possible, finally, to avoid the psychological conclusion that my depression had originated in an unconscious guilt feeling arising from the fact that I was living in abundance and that my parents had lived in so much poorer circumstances. They had deprived themselves of all the pleasant things and had lived in sadly pinched circumstances in order to give their children advantages. It seemed that I might allow myself a certain modest comfort, but that a mysterious factor within, called conscience, forbade my enjoying extraordinary luxury or much money, unless it had been earned by hard work, and opulence that was undeserved. It was as if I had not the right to live sumptuously where my parents had suffered so many hardships. My attempt to adjust to a comfortable, luxurious life had failed.

Later on I admitted to myself that I had been a damned fool but also that I could not then have acted otherwise. When I told Freud the story some months later, he laughed at me cordially (I loved it although the joke was on me), and, if memory does not fail me, it was on this occasion that he expressed the wish that I might "acquire a sclerotic conscience." I hope that since then I have secured this "hardening of the conscience." Alas, I was never given the opportunity to find out whether, after this one experience, I might behave differently in a similar situation. I am afraid that destiny does not have another chance in store for me—it will have to hurry to reach me—but I rather think that I would take to some comfort and luxury much more kindly today.

Recently a playwright, a former patient of mine, wrote me a

letter in which he told me how much he was enjoying a fabu-
lously luxurious life in Hollywood. Engaged to write scripts for
one of the big movie companies, he has been drawing an enormous salary for many months, without as yet having written one
line for his employers. The young man relishes the high life and
his leisure in Hollywood without unnecessary scruples and superfluous moral considerations. He already has the "sclerotic conscience" I lacked.

Later during a brief visit to Vienna, I saw the Hotel Bristol
again. Something prompted me to enter the lobby of the hotel,
the scene of my triumph and my defeat. I just looked about for a
moment, glanced at the guests lounging in their deep chairs, and
left. Out again on the Ringstrasse, I heard myself thinking (the
expression will be explained immediately), "Those people have
just too much money."* The sentence was banal; obviously only
very rich people could stay at the Bristol. Why had I thought
that? It had been thought, or rather almost said, with a certain intonation and in a Viennese dialect that, though familiar to me,
I myself seldom use. It had been thought or said as if not I had
been the speaker, but some other person, a long way back. It was
like the delayed echo of something heard long ago. I do not recall having heard my father say this sentence, but the pronunciation and the intonation were his, not mine. The note of disapproval in the words that came to mind so surprisingly must have
been the determining factor in the genesis and development of my
discontent while I stayed at the splendid hotel. It was as if I myself had been one of those people who "have just too much
money," one of those people of whom my father had spoken so
disapprovingly.

It seems that the severity of our unconscious conscience lessens
as we grow older or after we have paid for our thought-crimes by
suffering. The above presentation would be incomplete without
tracing the genesis of my strange mood back in still another
direction. It would perhaps be more flattering to one's ego if one
could assume that an unconscious reaction of conscience emerged,
but it would be neither honest nor correct.

* The sentence in its original form: *"Die Leut' hab'n halt zuviel Geld."*

Intellectual integrity demands the confesion that such a strong moral reaction could not have taken place without having been preceded by a feeling that was unconsciously considered as guilt. What happened may be easily reconstructed. I must have been too proud of my good luck at first. There must have been some feelings of haughty presumption in me, as if it were because of my superior achievements that I could now live in the finest hotel in town. Painful though it may be, it must be acknowledged that there must have been at first some mood of triumph or conceit, that I prided myself on having become so much more successful than my poor father and brothers. The depression which followed was, of course, of a moral kind, as if such pride and presumption were a crime in thought. All the characteristic traits of my ensuing sadness show the opposite of the unconscious tendencies.

Curiously enough, a few moments after leaving the hotel another memory occurred to me, a children's poem that I am almost sure I had not thought of since I was a boy. The verses came back to me as suddenly as if they had popped up from a trap door on a stage. This folk poem that the public-school children of Vienna used to recite is called "The Little Tree That Wished to Have Different Leaves." It tells the story of a small fir tree that stands among trees of other kinds in the forest and is ashamed because it has only prickly needles. It wishes to have leaves like the other trees. It receives such leaves, but a goat comes along and eats them up. The little tree then wishes for leaves of glass, but a storm destroys them. The tree now wishes for itself leaves of gold; a peddler sees them, picks them, and carries them off in his bag. The disillusioned little tree now only wants its old needles back. It was immediately clear why the forgotten poem had emerged from its long oblivion. I was making fun of myself and my insatiable wishes. Certainly it is significant that the two isolated memories, the sentence heard from my father, and the poem learned in grammar school, both occurred to me within a few minutes. I must have originally heard both when I was about seven or eight years old. They belong, so to speak, to the same geological stratum of my past. They not only served as an indirect confirmation of the psychological analysis here sketched but also convinced me that the moral teachings and codes of my childhood were deeply rooted and continued to live a sub-terranean life within my personality in the years of late manhood.

Self-analysis of this kind originated in the need to obtain insight into my own moods, thoughts, and impulses as they appeared in everyday life. It brought some surprising revelations concerning my personal peculiarities and information about my character and emotional development. I learned to understand why an enemy or a group of enemies are among my emotional needs, why I cannot imagine myself as a member of a political party, why my ambition goes in one direction and not in another. I learned, too, why I always wish I had written a book or a paper when I admire it, which proves that my admiration is usually accompanied by envy. (Strangely enough, I can read whole volumes of the *Psychoanalytic Quarterly* without the slightest trace of such envious feelings.) Self-analysis has given me these insights and a hundred more, many of them painful and unflattering, a few that are pleasant, all uninteresting to others but of considerable interest to me as a psychologist and as a person.

II

1

I T IS not difficult to show how a psychologist arrives at insights from careful self-observation. But how can I give my readers a concrete idea of the processes that enable us to conjecture and comprehend the inner processes in others? They are by no means so simple as they appear to the layman, and it is the more difficult to describe them because they are, in part, incapable of expression in words. I propose to begin by dividing the process of conjecture and comprehension into three sections, although I know how artificial this division is, and how misplaced it must appear in face of the living current of the psychical act.

The first section of the way, thus artificially divided, leads from the conscious or potentially conscious perception of the subject matter to the point where it dives down into the unconscious mind of the psychologist. The second would then represent the unconscious assimilation of the observed material. The third stretches from the re-emergence into consciousness of the data so assimilated to the point of their description or formulation. Of the middle of these sections we can say nothing except that we have no direct access to it and that it interests us most of all. The other two sections are more accessible. True, we cannot fix the moment in which a perception dives down below our consciousness. No more can we state precisely the time of its re-emergence. For the rest, it is not only in respect of time that we are liable to error in this matter.

The actual process is only partially accessible to introspective observation. The act of slipping down into the unconscious region, the assimilation there, and the re-emergence into consciousness, may best be compared with the passage through a tunnel. For each of the two sections there is a different degree of light. Whether we can depict them depends upon the brightness of that light.

The first section begins in the clear daylight of consciousness. Let us call to mind the analytic situation that presents itself to us daily. The subject speaks or is silent, and accompanies his speech or silence with "speaking" gestures. We see the play of his features, the variety of his movements. All this communicates to us the vital expression of what he is feeling and thinking. It supplies the psychical data, which the analyst then assimilates unconsciously during the period that we have called the second section.

But is this really the whole of the psychical data that he has at his disposal and uses? If we recall the course of an analytic session, do we not feel that something is missing in this account, something important, nay, decisive? Our feeling is right. *In truth, we are incapable of dissecting into all its components parts the process by which we recognize psychological fact.* The data presented to the analyst must be more extensive and differentiated than appears to him during or after the treatment. His field of observation must be wider. It appears that I have committed errors even in my description of the data at his disposal. What the analyst

is able to perceive and comprehend consciously is probably only a
selection that he makes retrospectively, after the event. What his
conscious memory supplies him with is only a small portion of
what he actually uses. In other words, the analyst knows only a
part of the data on which his judgment is based, that such and
such processes are going on in the unconscious mind of the person he is observing. Our apprehension of the other personality is
not restricted to our conscious perceptions.

The individual inner life of a person cannot be read in the features that psychology has hitherto grasped and been able to grasp.
Of course I know that there is little that is new in what I am
now saying. It is the unconscious mind of the subject that is of
decisive importance, and the analyst meets that with his own unconscious mind as the instrument of perception. That is easy to
say, but difficult to realize. Psychologists can hardly conceive the
notion of unconscious perception. For psychoanalysis the notion
presents no difficulty, but to understand the peculiar nature of
unconscious perception and observation is not so easy.

For the moment we will turn from the theoretical consideration of the problem, and proceed with the help of any casual
example from daily practice. One is as good as another. A patient
told me how on the previous day he had had a violent quarrel
with his girl (he had been having a sexual affair with her for a
considerable time). At first the conversation turned upon the
girl's health; she had been feeling weak and poorly of late. She
had remarked that she was afraid of tuberculosis; she weighed too
little and must put on flesh. The young man, my patient, did
not think that necessary. He opposed it on aesthetic grounds.
How did the analyst suddenly perceive that the quarrel centered
unconsciously upon the question of a child? Nothing in the
young man's account pointed that way. Looking back, I discern
that my sudden idea must have carried me back at one bound to
something my patient had told me about a year and a half
earlier. About two years previously the girl had become pregnant
and, at his urgent entreaty, had procured an abortion. She had
offered no great resistance to the suggestion of abortion, and had
undergone the operation, which proved difficult owing to special
circumstances, with real heroism. Subsequently she had seldom

mentioned the incident, and that only in passing. And my patient had seldom thought of the subject for a year and a half.

Now was it the words "putting on flesh" in his story that roused the memory? How else could the latent meaning of the lovers' quarrel have revealed itself to me? I could not tell, even though I were to repeat the story with the accuracy of a gramophone. It must have declared itself somehow or other, in spite of the fact that the girl's fears, according to the patient's account, sounded entirely reasonable and justifiable. In spite of her perfectly well-founded plea, he must have detected some note of secret reproach in her words—a tone must have conveyed to him that the girl had never got over her loss. What psychoanalysis tells on the subject is that my own unconscious mind had acted as an instrument of perception and seized upon the secret meaning of the quarrel, a meaning hidden, moreover, from both principals. It is good to know that, but is it enough? My unconscious mind is able to conjecture a hidden meaning only through given signs. It requires tokens in order to detect something. Now, I have deliberately chosen a primitive example. This is a case of cryptomnesia, people will say. A memory no longer present in my consciousness was responsible for my recognition of the latent meaning. The unconscious remembrance of that long-past incident, emerging suddenly during the story, set me on the track.

Let us take an example that is only a little more complex and has to do with a like conflict, but in which no such memory of heuristic value can be traced. A young girl under psychoanalysis evinced an extraordinary fear of marriage. She repulsed any man who made approaches to her, and shrank from any chance of marriage or sexual intercourse. The reason she always gave for her attitude was her exceptional terror of the dangers of childbirth. She was convinced that she would not survive the pain, and would die. At the mere thought of childbirth, she was overcome by violent terror. She brought up the fact that many millions of women survive childbirth without injury and mentioned the possibility of preventive measures, but she nullified both factors by stressing the uncertainty precisely in her own case.

Now, she had spoken of this fear of hers several times without my understanding more of the nature or mental origin of her emotion than any other observant auditor. How was it that on a new occasion I suddenly recognized that, apart from all other mental determinants, a profound fear must be at work, over-shadowing all other feelings, that she was incapable of bearing a child and that any man must be unhappy with her? Of course I did not give expression to this idea about the suppressed nature of her fear, but waited till the astonishing surmise had been confirmed again and again. I cannot detect in myself any memory of a previous communication, emerging suddenly from the un-conscious and helping me to find the connection. Nothing in the girl's statements, so far as I could remember then or have been able to recall since, pointed to her being dominated by an un-conscious fear lest she be unable to bear a child. This fear I was subsequently able to trace to apprehensions based upon long-con-tinued masturbation. I had listened attentively to her lamenta-tions and her story without dreaming of any such thing, when suddenly this idea entered my mind, giving me my first and most im-portant means of approach to an understanding of the case. Here, then, there was no memory, or—to put it more cautiously—none traceable. Nevertheless, there must have been something in the patient's words, or something to be read between the lines, that pointed in that direction, something in her utterances, verbal or mimetic or otherwise, that suggested the connection.

Here we are faced with a whole series of questions. The idea must have arisen from something. Why did it arise just at this juncture, since we had talked of her fear previously, since, in-deed, she had often told me about it? What went on within my mind, on what mental processes was the idea based, and what preceded it? But is it not erroneous and unjust to lay special stress on this side of the problem? Is it not better to assume that my idea must have been based upon some factor not hitherto grasped, that is to say, that it must ultimately be traced back to some sense perception? In that case, unnamed impressions be-come the means of communicating psychological knowledge. That brings us back to our starting point, to the nature of the data at our disposal. It appears to me that it is here that we must begin, if we want to discover the foundation of the psychical comprehension of unconscious processes. If Kant begins with the statement that cognition arises from experience, that true dictum must be supplemented by the statement that experience has its origin in our sense perceptions, that nothing can be in our intellect which was not there before in our senses. (*Nihil est in intellectu quod non prius fuerit in sensibus.*) This statement is also true for a psychologist who seeks to grasp the unconscious processes in others.

Psychical data are not uniform. We have, of course, in the first place the considerable portion that we seize upon through conscious hearing, sight, touch, and smell. A further portion is what we observe unconsciously. It is permissible to declare that this second portion is more extensive than the first, and that far greater importance must be ascribed to it in the matter of psychological comprehension than to what we consciously hear, see, etc. Of course, we seize upon this, also, by means of the senses that we know, but, to speak descriptively, it is preconscious or unconscious. We perceive peculiarities in the features and bearing and movements of others that help to make the impression we receive without our observing or attending to them. We remember details of another person's dress and peculiarities in his gestures, without recalling them; a number of minor points, an olfactory nuance; a sense of touch while shaking hands, too slight to be observed; warmth, clamminess, roughness or smoothness in the skin; the manner in which he glances up or looks—of all this we are not consciously aware, and yet it influences our opinion. The minutest movements accompany every process of thought; muscular twitchings in face or hands and movements of the eyes speak to us as well as words. No small power of communication is contained in a glance, a person's bearing, a bodily movement, a special way of breathing. Signals of subterranean motions and impulses are being sent silently to the region of everyday speech, gesture, and movement.

A series of neurodynamic stimuli come to us from other people and play a part in producing our impressions, though we are not conscious of noticing them. There are certain expressive movements that we understand, without our conscious perception really being at work in that understanding. We need only think of the wide field of language. Everybody has, in addition to the characteristics we know, certain vocal modulations that do not strike us; the particular pitch and timbre of his voice, his particular speech rhythm, which we do not consciously observe. There are variations of tone, pauses, and shifted accentuation, so slight that they never reach the limits of conscious observation, individual nuances of pronunciation that we do not notice, but note. These little traits, which have no place in the field of conscious observation, nevertheless betray a great deal to us about a person. A voice that we hear, though we do not see the speaker, may sometimes tell us more about him than if we were observing him. It is not the words spoken by the voice that are of importance, but what it tells us of the speaker. Its tone comes to be more important than what it says. "Speak, in order that I may see you," said Socrates.

Language—and here I do not mean only the language of words but also the inarticulate sounds, the language of the eyes and gestures—was originally an instinctive utterance. It was not until a later stage that language developed from an undifferentiated whole to a means of communication. But throughout this and other changes it has remained true to its original function, which finds expression in the inflection of the voice, in the intonation, and in other characteristics. It is probable that the language of words was a late formation, taking the place of gesture language, and it is not irrational to suppose, as that somewhat self-willed linguist, Sir Richard Paget, maintains, that the movements of the tongue originally imitated our various actions. Even where language only serves the purpose of practical communication, we hear the accompanying sounds expressive of emotion, though we may not be aware of them.

There are, besides, nuances of smell and peculiarities of touch that escape our conscious observation and yet enter into the sum total of our impressions. They accompany the coarser or stronger conscious sense perceptions as overtones accompany a melody. In a state of hyperesthesia we may even consciously observe these variations of tone, glance, or gesture, the minutest facial movements, and muscular twitchings; but that is exceptional. In a general way it is only the grossest of these accompanying movements, tones, and smells, that reach our consciousness and are consciously used as psychological data. The others appear as part of the total impression. They do not emerge separately in our perception. There can be nothing wrong in likening these unconscious perceptions with the minute sense stimuli that psychology teaches us need only be added together or multiplied in order to become accessible to conscious perception. Each of these minute stimuli, then, must have contributed something to the sensation. We know that technical science has devised apparatus to bring within our grasp these natural processes, which we should otherwise be unable to perceive. And here I call attention to the important fact of repression, which greatly restricts our capacity for perceiving tiny signals of this kind.

Perhaps we shall do well to draw a distinction between this part of our psychical data and another, even though the distinction may prove at a later stage to be purely descriptive. It is true that the facts with which we have just been dealing are unconscious, but they do undoubtedly fall within the group of sense perceptions of which we have knowledge. I should like to draw a distinction between these data and certain other data, also unconscious, helping like the former to shape our impressions, but such that their precise nature can only be surmised. That is to say, we receive impressions through our senses that are in themselves beyond the reach of our consciousness. The assumption that these sense perceptions have no place in human consciousness, or have lost their place in it, is supported by certain facts and rendered exceedingly probable by others. I mean especially the fact of sense communications, having their origin in the animal past of the human race and now lost to our consciousness. The sense of direction in bees, the capacity of birds of passage to find their way, the sense of light in insects' skin, the instinctive realization of approaching danger in various animals, all bear witness to sense functions with which we have almost no human conceptions to compare. Of other sense functions that resemble those of the animals, it may be said that our perceptions are much vaguer, weaker, and less certain. It is easy to detect in them the rudiments of originally keen and well-developed senses. We need only compare the large part played by the sense of smell among dogs with its small significance in our own lives.

Freud has established the probability that the importance of the sense of smell has been greatly diminished in man through the development of his upright gait. The fact that the sense of smell tells dogs of things no longer accessible to us may serve as an example of the diminished importance of a number of sense functions in the life of the human race. Certain senses are reduced to rudimentary remnants because they have been less and less used. Do we not say, "I smell a rat" when we are suspicious of evil and concealed motives behind X's behavior? Is it accidental that we can use such a figure of speech as if we were still olfactory creatures? I am of the opinion that there are more of these rudimentary senses, tracing their origin to the evolution of prehistoric man, which, though not, indeed, totally lost, have lost their significance.

In addition there are other senses of which we have completely lost consciousness and which yet retain their efficacy, that is to say, are able to communicate unconscious impressions to us. A comparison with the sense perceptions of animals—for instance, the way certain insects can receive and communicate perceptions —points to the supposition that like senses may survive unconsciously in ourselves. I have in mind such a thing as the means of communication among ants, described by K. Frisch, and the signals ants give with their antennae, which the research of Forel, Wismann, and others has explained. Assuredly, there is a significant language in the animal kingdom and means of communication not ours, or no longer ours. The biologist Degener, in his study of simple animal societies, has assumed a kind of telepathic communication. A minute stimulus given by a particular species of caterpillar to a single individual within a large group caused a simultaneous palpitation throughout the whole group. Degener speaks of a hyperindividual group soul in these animal societies. Freud, too, has pointed to the possibility of such direct psychical communication. With reference to the common will in the large insect communities, he thinks that this original, archaic means of communication has been replaced in the course of racial evolution by the superior method of communication by signs. But the older method may survive, he thinks, in the background and human beings revert to it under certain conditions.

It will be observed that, in assuming a direct psychical communication through these archaic, rudimentary surviving senses, we approach the complex of problems known as telepathy. I believe that in the special case of communication between two unconscious minds called by that name, these neglected senses, favored by the weakened action of the others, do really come into action. Such telepathic communication is not supersensory. It makes actual those senses that have become alien to our consciousness. By using as signals the expression of stimuli that do not cross the threshold of our consciousness, and calling them in to supplement or correct our normal sense perceptions, it gives rise to special psychical apprehensions. The conversation between the unconscious of the one and the other mind does not proceed in a vacuum. It is served by certain means of communication comparable with those which we have assumed in the lower animal societies. They are not so much supersensory as subsensuous phenomena, that is, information conveyed by means of ancient, ordinarily discarded senses. The return to these unknown senses, which must formerly have played a far greater part in the activities of living organisms, may sometimes give rise to the impression that telepathy involves no sense perception at all.

We have here, not mysterious powers of divination, but rather an interruption of the customary working of our psychical machinery to make way for older methods, not otherwise applied. Thus the unconscious perception passes the bounds of communication received through our known sense organs. We have ears, and hear not with them alone; we have eyes, and see not with them alone. Possibly these unknown senses work faster than those we know, can communicate their perceptions to the unconscious faster than the senses developed later, and so seem to act through the air. And it is further worth observing that this action upon secret feelers of which we are unconscious belongs mainly to the realm of instinct, so that we may speak rather of instinct-reading than of thought-reading. The suspension of customary functions thus renders our less keen senses hyperesthetic —by way of comparison we may recall the greater intensity and subtlety of the sense of touch in people who have lost their sight —and long-forgotten senses recover the power of functioning. The enhanced effectiveness is, therefore, caused by the neglect of the mind's ordinary methods of working.

We have long been aware that the acknowledgment of telepathy as a psychical phenomenon does not imply that higher powers are substituted for the dynamics of mental action. It is not necessary to assume supernatural happenings because some small fragments of what goes on in the world are still unexplained. We need not give ourselves up to magic because the cause and effect of some process is unknown to us. We must confess that our knowledge is not adequate to explain the phenomenon. It does not become more explicable if we refer it back to some greater unknown factor. When we want to drink a glass of milk, we have no need to buy a cow. The psychological valuation of the efficacy of unknown or little known senses has brought us here to the limits of our subject.

While we have thus been reminded of the prehistoric past of sense perceptions, we may now cast a hasty glance in the opposite direction. The advance of civilization has caused certain senses to perish, and others to become more specialized and differentiated. In general we may say that the development of civilization has reduced the importance of sense perceptions, has challenged the exclusive dominion they originally held over the life of the individual. The aim is to manage with a minimum of sense perception and to leave the subsequent process of cognition to the intellect. With the advance of civilization sense perceptions are more and more markedly degraded to despised acts preparatory to the intellectual mastery of phenomena. We may cite as a sign of this weakening our mistrust of the data with which they supply us. The development of civilization brings a weakening and stunting of sense impressions that may be compared with the loss of keenness in our sense impressions in old age, deafness and far-sightedness, which, however, are due to biological causes.

There are reasons to support the hypothesis that refers this diminished significance of the senses to the advance of the age-long process of repression. The concepts "sense" and "sensuality" are not merely loosely associated in speech, but there is an inner connection that gives us an insight into certain psychical processes. The pleasure of the senses really is a pleasure arising from the tension and relaxation of the sense organs. Sense perception, the significance of which is more and more restricted with advancing civilization by the intellectual processes, particularly memory, is closely associated with the satisfaction of organic and elementary instincts. As memory develops, it comes to represent a substitute for the fading strength of sense perceptions. It might be argued that the loss of intensity and significance in the senses is a mark of diminishing vitality in the human race since it is associated with a weakening of sexual instinct.

Perhaps the retort might be made that it is precisely civilization that has greatly increased the keenness of our sense perceptions through the instruments it has created. It enables us to see things through the microscope and telescope that were not formerly visible; enables us, by means of appropriate instruments, to hear sounds formerly inaudible; and communicates sensations of touch and vibration otherwise beyond the reach of our consciousness. That is true, but it is not in contradiction with the previous statement. In part, these instruments serve to correct the very evil caused by civilization—for instance, eyeglasses—for the rest, their efficacy has certainly nothing to do with processes that are of vital interest to the human organism. Undoubtedly, they are of great importance, but it cannot be denied that they are artificial expedients, offering a poor substitute for the direct data communicated by organic sense perception. Perhaps we may venture to regard memory itself, which with advancing civilization challenges the importance of sense perception, as a disposition to feel the strength and immediacy of sense perceptions over again.

Let us return from this digression to our main argument. We have sought the special significance of sense perception in psychology in a different direction from that pointed out by modern sense physiology and psychology. We have grasped how varied and differentiated psychical data are when we set about to investigate them from the point of view of sense perception, but also how hard to differentiate. Besides the main path, they can use a number of side paths, subterranean passages, secret ways. In addition to our conscious sense perceptions, we receive communications through other organs of perception which we cannot consciously call our own, although they are within us. We can treat these signals like any others. We can attend to them or neglect them, listen to them or miss them, see them or overlook them. There is a very natural temptation not to attend to them or observe them. (A frequent part of our capacity for unconscious and pre-conscious perception is the observation that something is lacking, the subterranean awareness that something is not there.) It is certainly right and useful to sharpen our powers of conscious observation of things perceived, but we should not overlook the value of unconscious perception. We must not reject what makes itself felt by other means, even if it fails to make itself felt in consciousness at once.

A psychoanalyst must aim at bringing into the field of consciousness those impressions which would otherwise remain unconscious. Undoubtedly individual differences will excercise an influence upon his efforts. The practice and sensitiveness of the individual will vary; the readiness to trust to tiny stimuli and the capacity to register these tiny impressions are not possessed by everybody to an equal extent. And so we should pay attention to the first, hardly noticeable impressions that we receive of a person, however much they may soon be drowned by other, more insistent impressions. Without doubt, first impressions are of importance. First impressions may not be right, but they often contain true apprehensions in a distorted form.

These signals do not convey clear information. They are nowise comparable with modern signposts, upon which destination and distance are precisely indicated, but rather with old milestones whose lettering is weather-beaten and half legible. Many of the gaps and errors in our psychological comprehension must be attributed to our inattention to these unconscious signals. They may be blurred and their import difficult to determine, they nevertheless supplement conscious perception. In certain cases they alone enable us to discern its significance or correct the significance we mistakenly ascribe to it. It is true that psychological investigation meets here with much that is imponderable and difficult to grasp. Research must not ignore these factors. The best that we owe to the psychology of the unconscious is the result of prolonged observation, without premises. But it would be a mistake to assume that this observation is purely conscious. Not until we have learned to appreciate the significance of unconscious observation, reacting to the faintest impressions with the sensitiveness of a sheet of tin foil, shall we recognize the difficulty of the task of transforming imponderabilia into ponderabilia.

In fact, our psychological impressions are the result of the joint assimilation of conscious and unconscious perceptions. And here the conscious perceptions act, in a sense, like the last fragments of day, to which something different is attached, behind which something different lies concealed, something deeper than daytime thoughts. If we thrust aside the doubtful communications from the unconscious, as being unreliable, indefinite, and contrary to our conscious judgments and prejudices, we shall, it is true, seldom be deceived, but then we shall seldom attain surprising knowledge. Indeed a special kind of keen scent is no less essential than acumen for a psychologist who wants to grasp the unconscious processes.

If we survey our psychological data once more in all their variety and over the whole field, from the strongest expression of emotion to the imponderabilia, we become aware that we are treating them as if they served no other purpose but to tell us something about the inner life of another person. That is certainly not exclusively the case, and yet it is the case. I mean to say that they aim, among other things, at communicating to us something about the hidden processes in the other mind. We understand this primary endeavor; it does serve the purpose of communication, of psychical disburdenment. It has, therefore, a sound function in the economy of the inner life. We are reminded of Freud's view that mortals are not so made as to retain a secret. "Self-betrayal oozes from all our pores." I believe, moreover, that these words indicate the organ that was the sole medium of self-betrayal in the early stages of evolution. Originally most likely it really was first and foremost man's bodily surface, the skin, that showed what was going on within. It was the earliest organ to reflect mental processes. Blushing and turning pale still betray our feelings, and perspiration still breaks out when we are afraid. All self-betrayal makes its way through the pores of the skin. That statement clamors for a sequel. What sequel may easily be guessed when we reflect that we react to the unconscious with all our

organs, with our various instruments of reception and comprehension. *The self-betrayal of another is sucked in through all
our pores.*

2

The last chapter spoke of communications for which conscious
perceptions have only the function that relays have in telegraphy.
It would, of course, be nonsense to assert that this language of
the unconscious is understood only by psychoanalysts. (Sometimes
it would seem that it is least understood by analysts.) As a matter
of fact, these interchanges of impulses goes on between all human
beings, and analysis only evaluates them as psychological indications. Psychoanalysis is in this sense not so much a heart-to-
heart talk as a drive-to-drive talk, an inaudible but highly expressive dialogue. The psychoanalyst has to learn how one mind
speaks to another beyond words and in silence. He must learn to
listen "with the third ear."* It is not true that you have to shout
to make yourself understood. When you wish to be heard, you
whisper.

What can an analyst teach his younger colleagues in this direction? Very little. He can speak of his own experiences. He can
report instances, which have the value of illustrations only. And
he can—above all else—encourage the younger generation of analysts to unlearn all routine. We speak of routine only in the
gathering of unconscious material through observation, not of the
use which the analytic technique makes of it. We have to insist
that in the area of observation he keep fancy-free and follow his
instincts. The "instincts," which indicate, point out, hint at and
allude, warn and convey, are sometimes more intelligent than our
conscious "intelligence." We know so many things that "aren't
so" but, we must admit, we guess many things that seem to be
impossible but "are so." Young analysts should be encouraged to
rely on a series of most delicate communications when they collect their impressions; to extend their feelers, to seize the secret
messages that go from one unconscious to another.

* This phrase is borrowed from Nietzsche, *Beyond Good and Evil*, Part
VIII, p. 246.

To trust these messages, to be ready to participate in all flights and flings of one's imagination, not to be afraid of one's own sensitivities, is necessary not only in the beginnings of analysis; it remains necessary and important throughout. The task of the analyst is to observe and to record in his memory thousands of little signs and to remain aware of their delicate effects upon him. At the present stage of our science it is not so necessary, it seems to me, to caution the student against overvaluation of the little signs or to warn him not to take them as evidence. These unconscious feelers are not there to master a problem, but to search for it. They are not there to grasp, but to touch. We need not fear that this approach will lead to hasty judgments. The greater danger (and the one favored by our present way of training students) is that these seemingly insignificant signs will be missed, neglected, brushed aside. The student is often taught to observe sharply and accurately what is presented to his conscious perception, but conscious perception is much too restricted and narrow. The student often analyzes the material without considering that it is so much richer, subtler, finer than what can be caught in the net of conscious observation. The small fish that escapes through the mesh is often the most precious.

Receiving, recording, and decoding these "asides," which are whispered between sentences and without sentences, is, in reality, not teachable. It is, however, to a certain degree demonstrable. It can be demonstrated that the analyst, like his patient, knows things without knowing that he knows them. The voice that speaks in him speaks low, but he who listens with a third ear hears also what is expressed almost noiselessly, what is said *pianissimo*. There are instances in which things a person has said in psychoanalysis are consciously not even heard by the analyst, but none the less understood or interpreted. There are others about which one can say: in one ear, out the other, and in the third. The psychoanalyst who must look at all things immediately, scrutinize them, and subject them to logical examination has often lost the psychological moment for seizing the fleeting, elusive material. Here—and only here—you must leap before you look; otherwise you will be looking at a void where a second before a valuable impression flew past.

In psychoanalysis we learn to collect this material, which is not conscious but which has to become conscious if we want to use it in our search and research. That the psychoanalyst immediately recognizes the importance and significance of the data brought to his attention is a stale superstition. He can be content with himself when he is able to receive and record them immediately. He can be content if he becomes aware of them. I know from conversations with many psychoanalysts that they approach this unconscious material with the tools of reason, clinical observation, meditation, and reflection. They approach it, but that does not mean that they even come close to it. The attempt to confine unconscious processes to a formula like chemical or mathematical processes remains a waste of intellectual energy. One doubts if there is any use in discussing the difference between the two types of processes with such superior minds. The Austrian poet, Grillparzer, and the German playwright, Hebbel, lived at the same time (about one hundred years ago) in Vienna, without meeting each other. Grillparzer was reluctant to speak with Hebbel, who was inclined to reflection and brooded over many metaphysical problems. Grillparzer admitted he was too shy to converse with the prominent, meditative playwright. "You know," he said, "Mr. Hebbel knows exactly what God thinks and what He looks like, and I just don't know."

It seems to me that the best way to guess something about the significance of "insignificant" data, the way to catch the fleeting impressions, is not to meditate, but to be intensely aware of them. They reveal their secrets like doors that open themselves, but cannot be forced. One can with conviction say: You will understand them after you have ceased to reflect about them.

No doubt, the third ear of which we often speak will appear to many not only as an anatomical, but also as a psychological, abnormality—even to psychologists. But do we not speak of hearing with the "inner ear"? What Nietzsche meant is not identical with this figure of speech, but it is akin to it. The third ear to which the great psychologist referred is the same that Freud meant when he said the capacity of the unconscious for fine hearing was one of the requisites for the psychoanalyst.

One of the peculiarities of this third ear is that it works two ways. It can catch what other people do not say but only feel and think; and it can also be turned inward. It can hear voices from within the self that are otherwise not audible because they are drowned out by the noise of our conscious thought-processes. The student of psychoanalysis is advised to listen to those inner voices with more attention than to what "reason" tells about the unconscious; to be very aware of what is said inside himself, *écouter aux voix intérieures,* and to shut his ear to the noises of adult wisdom, well-considered opinion, conscious judgment. The night reveals to the wanderer things that are hidden by day.

In other words, the psychoanalyst who hopes to recognize the secret meaning of this almost imperceptible, imponderable language has to sharpen his sensitiveness to it, to increase his readiness to receive it. When he wants to decode it, he can do so only by listening sharply inside himself, by becoming aware of the subtle impressions it makes upon him and the fleeting thoughts and emotions it arouses in him. It is most important that he observe with great attention what this language means to him, what its psychological effects upon him are. From these he can arrive at its unconscious motives and meanings, and this conclusion again will not be a conscious thought-process or a logical operation, but an unconscious—I might almost say, instinctive—reaction that takes place within him. The meaning is conveyed to him by a message that might surprise him much like a physical sensation for which he is unprepared and which presents itself suddenly from within his organism. Again, the only way of penetrating into the secret of this language is by looking into oneself, understanding one's own reactions to it.

The reader is asked to think this over. A little known and concealed organ in the analyst receives and transmits the secret messages of others before he consciously understands them himself. And yet the literature of psychoanalysis neglects it. There is one word that may make claim to being a rarity in psychoanalytic literature (with the exception of Freud): the word "I." With what fear and avoidance does the analyst write about his own method of coming to conclusions, about his own thoughts and impressions! The devil himself could not frighten many analysts more than the use of the word "I" does in reporting cases.

It is this fear of the little pronoun of the first person singular, nominative case, that accounts for the fact that reports of self-analysis are such a rarity in our literature. The worship of the bitch-goddess objectivity, of pseudo precision, of facts and figures, explains why this is the only book that deals with this subject matter, or which insists that the subject matters. In our science only the psychical reality has validity. It is remarkable that the unconscious station which does almost all the work is left out of analytic discussions. Imagine discussing the science of sound, acoustics, without mentioning the ear, or optics without speaking of the eye.

Nothing can, of course, be said about the nature of those unconscious impressions we receive as long as they remain unconscious. Here are a few representative instances of some that became conscious. They concern the manner, not the manners, of persons who were in the process of psychoanalysis, little peculiarities, scarcely noticed movements, intonations, and glances that might otherwise have escaped conscious observation because they were inconspicuous parts of the person's behavior. People generally tend to brush aside observations of this sort as immaterial and inconsequential, little things not worthy of our attention.

In the hall that leads from my office to the apartment door is a big mirror beside a clothes tree. Why did I not observe that a young, pretty woman patient of mine never looked into the mirror when she put on her coat? I must have seen it before, but it came to my attention only after the fifth psychoanalytic session. I was aware that she spoke without any emotions about her marriage or her family, and I became suspicious that her remoteness and coolness were expressions of a schizophrenic disease. Walking behind her to the door, I observed that she did not even glance at herself in the mirror, but I did not recall perceiving this trait before. I must have perceived it before without noticing it and, when I paid attention to it now, I did so because I saw it as an additional symptom. I had seen the patient walk to the door in front of me five times, and I knew now that, unlike other women, she never looked into the mirror. Now I also became aware of how carelessly she treated her hat, that she threw it on rather than put it on. It gained significance now—why not before?

Why did I recall only then what I had often said before, namely, that men who treat their hats with great care are usually not very masculine and women who do not pay attention to their hats are, in general, not very feminine?

I am choosing this instance as representative of many others in which we become aware of a slight divergence because we miss a certain detail of behavior. Experience in psychoanalysis teaches us that we are inclined to overlook the absence of a usual bit of behavior, although it is often a valuable clue and can become a part of the psychological circumstantial evidence we need. That something is not present where we expect it, or that something is not in its usual place or order, is less conspicuous than the presence of something unusual. Only when the trait appears important or when it is missed immediately will it become conspicuous by its absence. Otherwise, we generally ignore what is not there. Sometimes, just the observation of the absence of such little features leads to understanding. The other day I read a mystery story in which a murder is committed during a theater performance. The audience is searched and the fact that one man has no tie yields a precious clue.

In contrast to the case mentioned above, I observed very soon after the beginning of an analysis that a patient, a middle-aged man, spent a long time before the mirror in the hall, smoothing his hair before he put on his hat, and so forth. This trait came to mind when the patient reported that almost every night through the window of his darkened bathroom he spied on women undressing and that the sight often made him masturbate. My peeping patient was also potentially an exhibitionist. Later on it became obvious that he identified himself in his unconscious fantasies with the women he watched.

Perceptions of such a vague character, impressions that almost elude us, support us in reaching certain stations on our road to insight. We appreciate their value when we have learned to control our impatience and when we do not expect immediate, but rather intermediary, results from these trifles of observations. The smell of a perfume, a gesture of a hand, a peculiarity of breathing, as well as articulate confessions and long reports, give away secrets. Sometimes an observation of this kind scarcely deserves the name of observation but proves important none the less. Sometimes a transient impression remains unnoted until it occurs often. Only its repetition makes us realize its presence. Peculiarities of voice, of glancing, often reveal something that was hidden behind the words and the sentences we hear. They convey a meaning we would never have guessed, if we had not absorbed the little asides on the fringes of the stage that accompany the main action. Men speak to us and we speak to them not only with words but also with the little signs and expressions we unconsciously send and receive. Observation of these signs begins with our isolating them from the total pattern of the behavior. When we succeed in doing this, we can make the impression clearer and stronger by repetition. Their psychological evaluation and interpretation occur sometimes to the psychoanalyst immediately, sometimes later on as we follow the trail. In the process of "catching" these elusive signs we must trust to our senses and not follow the voice of "reason" which will try to brush them aside. The psychologist who approaches this valuable field as sober as a judge will not capture many data because he will also be as unimaginative as a judge. Only he who is fancy-free and opens all his senses to these impressions will be sensitive to the wealth he will encounter.

The trail uncovered by first impressions sometimes leads to insights that could otherwise be obtained only after a long time and by dint of hard psychological digging. A young graduate student at Harvard started his analysis in a very low voice. His manner of speech appeared deliberate and considered. I asked him to speak louder. He made an effort to do so, but after two minutes dropped back to a low tone that became almost inaudible. At first I had the impression that he was shy or timid and that it was difficult for him to speak of the serious conflicts that had disturbed his childhood. This impression could not explain his manner of speaking because his voice was not only low but also exceptionally deep, and it was as if he chose his words very deliberately. Whatever his reasons, whether shyness, disturbance, or emotions that had to be controlled, you cannot analyze someone without hearing what he has to say.

After trying my best to catch what he mumbled, I decided to

interrupt what seemed to be a monologue that excluded an audience. My first impression had given way to another. His manner of speaking was much more significant for his personality than what he had to say to me in this first session. Neglecting everything else, I entered into a discussion of his low-voiced and controlled way of speaking and insisted that he tell me all that he knew about it, at the same time asking him again to make himself heard. We soon arrived at the insight that his low voice and dignified manner were a late acquisition that had developed as an expression of his opposition to the shrieking, high, excited voices of his parents, especially of his mother. There was a story in that, a story we meet frequently in American-born children of East European immigrants. In this case it was further complicated by the neurotic conflicts of the young man. His parents had retained the behavior and manners of the old country when they came to the United States. They spoke loudly and with vivid gestures. They were highly temperamental and made no effort to control the expression of their emotions. Entirely Americanized, the boy began to feel ashamed of his parents and developed this characteristic manner of low speaking and overcontrolled dignity as a counter-action to the temptation to speak and act like the members of his family. He acquired, so to speak, a second personality superimposed on his originally passionate and excitable nature. Early conflicts, especially with his mother, intensified and deepened this reaction-formation whose external signs were his way of speaking and similar traits. Analyzing these features, we soon arrived at the core of his neurotic conflicts.

In this case a practical necessity of the analytic situation forced the analyst to turn his attention to a special trait of personal behavior, which, if it had been less clearly developed, might have remained unobserved. The first analytic session thus started with the discussion of this special characteristic, an exception that proved justified as well as useful.

The analyst can achieve some psychological insight into a patient even before the beginning of treatment if he will only trust his impressions as soon as he becomes aware of them. A young woman made an appointment to consult about the possibility of continuing her psychoanalysis with me. She told me she had broken off her analysis with Dr. A. some months ago. I listened to the story of the conflict that was making it impossible for her to return to her first psychoanalyst. She rapidly sketched the difficulties in her marriage, her social relations, and her pofessional life. There was nothing, it seemed to me, unusual in what she told me; nothing an analyst does not meet with in many patients. She seemed to be intelligent enough, sincere, and friendly. Why did I feel a slight annoyance with the patient after she left? There was nothing in our conversation that could explain such a feeling. As my attention turned to other patients, I brushed aside the vague impression.

When the patient telephoned two days later, I did not recognize her name and did not remember that she had promised to call me. Now I was forced to follow the rule: Analyst, analyze yourself!

I remembered feeling slightly annoyed, but I had not become aware of any reason for this feeling. It was certain that I had not disliked the patient, and certainly she had not done or said anything during the consultation that could have annoyed me. Well, there was the conflict with Dr. A. I had the impression that the analyst had lost patience with his patient at the end—perhaps after she had provoked him many times—and that she could not take what he had told her about herself. She had definitely rejected my suggestion that she return to Dr. A. and try to continue the analysis with him. But that could not possibly have annoyed me. She was entitled to decide that herself, and I scarcely knew Dr. A.

What was it then that made me displeased with her? Now it slowly came back to me. There were two things she had said the unconscious significance of which I had not realized but had nevertheless sensed. At the end of our conversation she had asked me if I would continue her analysis. Before I had time to answer she had wondered whether I would advise her to go to Dr. N., another psychoanalyst, whom she did not know. The question was asked rather casually, but it had left some trace in me of which I now became aware. It seemed strange. The young lady had consulted me about her neurotic troubles, had asked me whether I would bring her analysis to its end, and then whether she had not better go to Dr. N. instead. I had advised her, of course, to go to Dr. N. Now over the telephone she said that Dr. N. had no time for her and that she wanted to continue her analysis with me. Her question concerning Dr. N. during the consultation appeared at first quite natural and not in the least conspicuous, a question just like any other. Looking back at it, however, it took on another character. I remembered that she had looked at me with a leer, and I understood now, much later, what her sidelong glance and her question meant. It was a provocation of a teasing or malicious kind.

I want to make this element clear. Compare this situation with similar ones. What would we think of a patient who asks to be treated by one physician and then during the consultation asks whether he ought not to go to another physician? It did not make sense, and yet I had to assume that there was some concealed sense in it. When you go to a shoemaker to have your shoes repaired, you do not ask him whether you should take the same shoes to another shoemaker. You do not ask a girl to dance and then wonder aloud whether you should not rather dance with another girl.

When I suggested that she go to Dr. N., I must have been reacting unconsciously to the unconscious meaning of her question. I was not surprised or annoyed, as might be expected. On the contrary, I reacted as if her question were the most normal thing. Only later did I realize that it was extraordinary. I reacted not only to the question but also to the look with which she asked it, as if to say: "If you doubt whether to come to me or to Dr. N., please go to Dr. N. I do not want you as a patient." I reacted as if I had understood the meaning of the glance while I did not even notice it consciously. I had been aware of a slight annoyance after her visit, but not of what had annoyed me. My unconscious reaction then (in my answer) and later (not remembering her name and our agreement) showed that I had somewhere, hidden even from myself, understood well enough that her question was really a provocation.

After that I remembered that the sidelong glance had appeared again at the end of the consultation. The patient had casually mentioned reading a rather unfavorable review of one of my books in the *Psychoanalytic Quarterly*. As far as my conscious thoughts went the review did not affect me. But that is not the point here. Why did she mention it? Where was the need to say it? It seems that I felt annoyed, not at being reminded of the criticism, but by her intention in reminding me of it, which I sensed. Well bred and well educated, she would certainly not say to a stranger she had just met at a dinner or cocktail party, "Oh, I read an unfavorable review of your last book just two days ago." Why did she do it just before leaving my room and why this sidelong, expectant glance? Considering her otherwise excellent manners, there must have been an unconscious hostile or aggressive tendency in her remark.

What was gained by my insight, what was the advantage in catching these imponderable expressions that had appeared incognito? There was more than one advantage—besides the satisfaction of the psychological interest. That side glance was revealing. It not only observed; it was observed; and for a fleeting moment I caught the real face behind the mask. The situation was like that of a masquerade at which a person has the advantage of seeing a lady who believes herself unobserved, without her mask. Later, when he meets her again in disguise, he will know her identity. This early insight proved very useful later on. It was a promising beginning and it helped me in the difficult situations that merged in the later phases of analysis. It was much easier to understand the masochistic provocation to which the patient resorted again and again. And it was easier to convince her finally that some unconscious tendency in her forced her to make herself disliked. I had, of course, overcome my initial annoyance quickly after I understood its reasons and, forewarned and forearmed by my early insight, I could tolerate the provocations much better than my colleague, who had yielded to the temptation to become angry with her.

The discussion of this case and the many others that follow seems to present a good opportunity to inject a few remarks about the psychoanalyst himself. What kind of psychoanalyst, some readers will ask, can feel annoyed or impatient? Is this the much-praised calm and the correct scientific attitude of the therapist? Is this the pure mirror that reflects the image of the patient who comes to psychoanalysis with his troubles, symptoms, and com-

THE GIFT FOR PSYCHOLOGICAL OBSERVATION 315

plaints? Is this the proper couch-side manner? The question is easily answered. The psychoanalyst is a human being like any other and not a god. There is nothing superhuman about him. In fact, he has to be human. How else could he understand other human beings? If he were like a block of wood or a marble statue, he could never hope to grasp the strange passions and thoughts he will meet with in his patients. If he were cold and unfeeling, a "stuffed shirt," as some plays portray him, he would be an analytic robot or a pompous, dignified ass who could not gain entry to the secrets of the human soul. It seems to me that the demand that the analyst should be sensitive and human does not contradict the expectation that he should maintain an objective view of his cases and perform his difficult task with as much therapeutic and scientific skill as is given him. Objectivity and inhumanness are two things that are frequently confused, even by many psychoanalysts. The sensitiveness and the subjectivity of the analyst concern his impressionability to the slightest stimuli, to the minute, almost imperceptible indices of unconscious processes. It is desirable that he be as susceptible, as responsive and alive, to those signs as a mimosa is to the touch. He should, of course, possess the same sensitiveness to, and the same faculty for fine hearing of, the voices within himself. His objectivity, his cool and calm judgment, his power of logical and psychological penetration as well as his emotional control, should be reserved for the analytic treatment. He will not feel the temptation to express his own emotions when his psychological interest outweighs his temperament. He will be able to check and control impulses that he has in common with his patients when he remembers that his task is to understand and to help them. It is ridiculous to demand that an analyst, to whom nothing human should be alien, should not be human himself. Goethe has expressed it beautifully: If the eye were not something sunlike itself, it could never see the sun.

The instances reported above contrast with others—alas, so many others—in which I remained unaware of those trifles, of those little revealing signs, or in which I observed them much later, sometimes even too late. It does not matter how much or how little too late. It makes no difference whether you missed your plane by only a few minutes or by a few hours. In every one of those cases my lack of sensitiveness was punished by additional work, an increased intellectual and emotional effort that would have been unnecessary if I had been more impressionable or observant. In almost all of them there was also a hindrance in myself that blocked me or dulled the sharpness of my observation. Here is such a case, one of many:

A young man had come for psychoanalysis because he wanted to rid himself of many nervous symptoms and some serious difficulties he was encountering in his private and professional life. I succeeded in a relatively short time in freeing him of his most oppressive symptoms, but the other difficulties remained. They seemed to be stationary and did not improve. I often told myself that something in me hindered my deeper penetration into that secret. But I could not find the road that led to it. The young man had obliging, open manners and showed brilliant intelligence, wit, and humor. What a pity that all these gifts remained sterile and displayed themselves only when he talked! His intellectual endowment and his emotional alertness made everything he said interesting whether he talked about his own symptoms, about his complicated relations with relatives and friends, his past emotions and experiences, or of the present, of a sexual adventure, or money matters. He knew how to tell a tale about himself or others. He was stimulating as well as stimulated. Nothing changed, however, in his inner situation after he had lost his most serious symptoms.

One day he told me that his sweetheart, who had listened to his stories for a long time, had smilingly asked, "But, John, why do you make such an effort? I am not a girl whom you met yesterday." My eyes were suddenly opened wide by this remark of a third person. I had really overlooked the fact that the young man had not talked to me, but had entertained me in the last weeks. The girl was right, so absolutely right. He dazzled people. He bribed them with his reports, which were always very alive and vivid, vibrant and interesting. In speaking of himself, however, he did not give of himself. He spent himself, but he did not surrender. He figured in his reports like the storyteller in a modern novel narrated in the first person—a story by Somerset Maugham.

In talking about himself, ostensibly quite freely, he was hiding himself. Listening to him with sharper ears, I now received a new impression of his inadequacy feelings, which made it necessary for him to conquer all people anew whenever he met them, to use his endowments to win them over and thus overcome his deep sense of insecurity. I had let myself be bribed like so many others by these great, ever-recurrent efforts. Then along came a young girl whose psychological knowledge did not surpass that of other students of Vassar or Smith and gave me a lesson I would not forget. She hit the target easily and casually, reminding the young man that he need not exert himself. She had said, "I am not a girl whom you met yesterday," and with these nine words she had shown the path for which I had searched in vain. I took my hat off to this unknown Vassar girl and felt thoroughly ashamed of myself. Who had taught her the fine art of psychological observation and discernment? You do not learn such things in the psychology department at Smith or Vassar. I was ready to believe that the girl was smart enough, but it was not her intelligence that had spoken like that. It was her heart that had told her.

Experiences of this kind (I could tell many more) make us psychoanalysts modest about our psychological endowment—or should make us more modest. There was I, who thought myself a trained observer, and I did not recognize what was so obvious. "What is a trained observer?" I asked myself. He is a man who is trained to pay attention to certain things and to neglect others. He is a man who overpays attention to features he expects to see and remains in debt to others that escape his notice.

3

Nobody can get a good hold on the essential discoveries of psychoanalysis without a certain measure of suffering. The truth lives among us unspoken, and someone should come out with it, whatever effect it will have on our student analysts. It sounds simple enough, and yet it is calculated to stir up debate—even among analysts. In every society there are some things that are taken as a matter of course. Yet we need only utter them in order to make them the subject of serious differences of opinion.

I chose the word "suffering" intentionally. I might very well have said "pain" instead. But my object was to denote the most vital and significant element of that pain, the very element that is associated with the acquisition of the most important analytic experience, and for that I know of no other name than suffering. It may be prudent not to call things by their frequently alarming names; but it is not equally truthful.

What? Can the knowledge of objectively valid truths, of definite laws demonstrable by everyone and to everyone, of typical conditions, be dependent upon the observer or learner suffering under them? It will be said—and often has been said—that a condition of so subjective a nature is unheard of in scientific investigation. People will say it recalls the way religious doctrines of salvation are learned, that it is calculated to endanger verification of the objective facts, that no such condition has ever been attached to the acquisition of psychological knowledge, and so on. Unable to meet such a shower of arguments and unschooled in dialectics, I shall not attempt to put together what can be said in reply to these objections. I will only remind the reader that the conditions upon which we can acquire certain knowledge do not depend upon the teacher's will, but first and foremost upon the nature of the knowledge to be acquired.

It is the peculiar nature of the knowledge that justifies my statement, and not only of the knowledge but also of the experiences that must be acquired. The most important analytic knowledge cannot be acquired in its full significance without the removal of repressions. And here we strike upon a central conception. The motive and purpose of the repression was nothing but the avoidance of pain. The removal of the repression must cause pain—taken here in its broadest significance. But the removal of the repression, the conquest of the resistance against certain ideas and emotions becoming conscious, is the inescapable condition of acquiring the most important analytic knowledge. Assuredly it is not only the individual's sensibilities, his pride and his vanity, that are touched by analysis, but other things besides. Our dearest illusions are brought into question; dear because their maintenance has been bought with particularly great sacrifices. The views and convictions that we love most fervently analysis undermines; it weans us from our old habits of thought. This new knowledge confronts us with dangers that we seemed to have mastered long ago, raises thoughts that we had not dared to think, stirs feelings from which we had anxiously guarded ourselves. Analysis means an invasion of the realm of intellectual and emotional taboo, and so rouses all the defensive reactions that protect that realm. Every inch of the ground is obstinately defended, the more ardently the more trouble its conquest once cost us. But where analysis penetrates to the deepest and most sensitive plane of our personality, it can only force an entrance with pain.

There is nothing misleading in saying that the man who really wants to understand analysis must experience it and its effects on his own person; but it is a vague assertion that paraphrases the position rather than describes it. It is correct to say that the analyst's most significant knowledge must be *experienced* by himself. But it is even more correct and approaches nearer to what is essential to declare openly that these psychological experiences are of such a nature that they must be *suffered*.

What we have to do is to throw light on the problem in its obscurest corners; perhaps the subjective capacity to suffer or, better, the capacity to accept and assimilate painful knowledge, is one of the most important prognostic marks of analytic study. It seems to me that we have no right to withhold from learners the fact that the deepest knowledge is not to be had if they shrink from purchasing it with personal suffering. And this capacity is assuredly not one that can be learned. Suffering, too, is a gift; it is a grace. Let me make my meaning clear. Among my patients at the moment is a talented playwright. His craftsmanship, his dramatic sense, his stylistic endowment are beyond dispute; he is smart, witty, observes sharply, and knows the world. What makes him fail? Goethe gives the answer: he says the poet is a person to whom God gave the gift to say what he has suffered, what we all have suffered. My young playwright would have the ability to say what he feels. The trouble is that he does not feel suffering.

He always chooses the easy way out of conflicts; he will not stand his ground in the face of unavoidable grief, sorrow, despair. We analysts often cannot spare our patients pain. In order to make an omelette, you have to break eggs.

But how can an analyst understand others if he has not suffered himself? We return here again to the statement that qualities of character are more important than intellectual ones for the making of an analyst.

Now does not a good deal of psychological knowledge get through to the patient painlessly? Certainly, I was speaking here of the most significant part of analysis, the most important both in theory and practice, which starts from the problem of repression and remains dependent upon it. But a deeper comprehension of these questions presupposes a clarification of the analyst's own conflicts, an insight into the weakest and most endangered parts of his own ego, the rousing and stirring of everything that slept deepest in him—if it slept. That knowledge can only be purchased at the price of staking his own person, of conscious suffering. Before sitting down on the chair behind the couch, the analyst should have stood up to life.

In this sense the reading of analytic literature and attendance at lectures on analysis only mean preparation for the acquisition of analytic comprehension. They certainly do not give the penetration that alone deserves the name of comprehension; they remain on the surface of intellectual comprehension, and show little power of resistance. But why do I lay stress upon just the suffering? Doesn't anyone who wants to understand the depths of human experience also have to feel pleasure, joy, happiness? Certainly; but a person who has once experienced deep suffering need not be anxious about his power to comprehend other emotions. That intellectual freedom, that profounder psychological insight, that clear vision that come from the conquest of suffering, can be attained by no other means.

To spare ourselves pain sometimes involves sparing ourselves psychological insight. The unconscious knowledge that I have so often spoken of springs not least from the reservoir of our own suffering, through which we learn to understand that of others. Not unhappiness, not calamity, not *malheur* or unfortunate ex-

periences produce it. It is true that misfortune teaches us pru-
dence. But suffering, consciously experienced and mastered,
teaches us wisdom.

Before I conclude this contribution to the discussion, I will
return once more to the theme of inner truthfulness, which appears to me as one of the essential psychological conditions for
the investigation of the unconscious. It is a quality that will not
only prove of value in the conquest of unexplored regions of the
mind; it is also needed in order to stand out against a pseudo
rationality that declares it superfluous to range the distant realm
of the unconscious when the good territory of the conscious lies
so near at hand. In our analytic work we soon feel the temptation
of yielding to that admonition, for the forces of our own conscious habits of thought will influence us to reject at once an idea
about the psychological data that seems absurd or scurrilous. And
we must consider that the data, emerging rapidly, often vanish
and are lost just when they are received. But if we recall one of
these ideas later, it often seems not only senseless and in bad
taste, but without tangible connection, farfetched. Although the
idea as such has not then been drawn back into the unconscious,
its matrix in the conditions of the psychical situation has.

The voices of those around him, to whom he tells the strange
idea or impression, will then sound to the analyst like an echo of
what resists the surprising perception within himself, and will
sometimes drown other voices. Everyday considerations will
mount up, ironical reflections will block the way, sophisms will
appear to check the action of reason, and the jugglery of consciousness will prevent penetration into the region of repression.
In the external world ancient wisdom will unite with modern
cocksureness to lure the analyst away from the blurred trail. And
it needs moral courage to hold aloof from obvious "explanations."
For if the budding analyst, deaf to the seductions of exalted reason, cleaves obstinately to the track once found, like a hound set
on the trail that is not to be turned from it by strangers calling
him, he will get no encouragement from society, even if the trail
brings him nearer to what he is seeking. He will feel the desola-
tion, chill, and gloom of the man who dedicates himself to intellectual solitude and is soon alone. The comfort remains to him

of the knowledge expressed in the proverb: *"Se tu sarai solo, tu sarai tutto tuo."* And this is the blessing of such loneliness: he who is always listening to the voices of others remains ignorant of his own. He who is always going to others will never come to himself.

Rejection by our neighbors and the absence of outward success, joined to our own doubts, is harder to bear than we like to admit. But if we have the hope of illuminating obscure mental relations, these reactions of society may make us lose our temper, but they cannot make us lose courage. That danger is nearer when the way we are seeking seems to lose itself in the darkness ahead or in the far distance, while other people seem to have reached the same goal long ago along the broad highway.

The line of least resistance in psychological cognition does not simply mark off the general opinion from the analytic point of view. We shall find it in our own camp, nay, in each one of us. We, like other people, are exposed to the temptation to try to comprehend obscure psychological relations rapidly and according to formula. Indeed, there is one factor that occasionally brings the temptation nearer: analytic theories are no less susceptible to hasty and false application than other scientific assumptions. We must warn young people not to make short work of the intellectual processes that precede the spoken word, and train them to postpone judgment and put up with doubt. Knowledge too hastily acquired assuredly does not imply power, but a presumptuous pretense of power.

I take it as a good omen of the scientific quality of an analytic worker who has only been practicing for a few years, if the explanation of unconscious processes does not come easily to him when he finds himself confronted with the confusing wealth of psychological data. Thus a young psychoanalyst lamented to me not long ago that he had failed to comprehend a relation in, or to grasp the peculiar psychological character of, a case he was observing. I advised him to wait and not yield to impatience. If a thing is very easily comprehended, it may be that there is not much to comprehend in it. He said hesitantly that from his school days right on into the years when he discussed problems of his science with academic friends, he had envied people who rapidly and easily discerned intricate relations and could solve a problem with ease. His case may permit of a few remarks on something beyond the special circumstances.

Very many of us know these moods well. At congresses or meetings of analytic societies when somebody has boasted how easily he had found the solution of a psychological problem, how deep he had penetrated into the structure of a case of neurosis, and how soon he had discerned all its psychical conditions, I have felt nothing of calm assurance, but sometimes a strong sense of my own inadequacy. While I had not yet really grasped where the problem lay, the other man had solved it long ago. I looked enviously upon a facility, a rapidity of comprehension that I could not hope to attain. My intellectual inferiority seemed to be confirmed by the harsh—and still more by the mild—verdict that contrasted my own dullness and slowness of grasp, my "long-distance transmission," with the other person's ease and rapidity of comprehension. I thought then that the intellectual rating of an individual was essentially determined by these qualities. Scientific psychology had worked out, in its tests, methods of making these conditions appear the only important and unchangeable ones.

And then as my youth slipped away and I subjected this much-lauded ease of comprehension to closer examination, my respect for it was considerably diminished. Was it, perhaps, experience that taught me to be suspicious? I do not think so; experience as such teaches us hardly anything, unless we want to learn from it. But that requires a coincidence of certain psychological conditions. The truth is that I learned to mistrust all that is intellectually glib and slick, smooth and smart. I often recognized it as a mark of shining and worthless superficiality, a "phony," to use the slang expression. I began also to mistrust the rapid power of "understanding" and I remembered what they used to say in Vienna about an Austrian statesman: his grasp of things and persons was always quick, but always false. I acquired the ability to resist the great defensive power of other people's experience, for the experience of others often enough prevents us from gaining any of our own. On occasion it is the downright protector of tradition and the purveyor of false assumptions handed down to us.

I do not speak here of those cases in which such comprehension amounts to the acceptance of the opinions of predecessors or authorities that have come superficially to our knowledge. Such cases are, indeed, of the utmost importance to the rising academic generation. I am discussing the comprehension that comes after we have examined the facts and found a reasonable and sufficient explanation. The temptation that is perhaps the most difficult to recognize as such, and to which we therefore so readily yield, is that of accepting an explanation because it is plausible, rational, and comprehensible. This easy comprehension is often the sign of intellectual haste, let us say, the expression of an intellectual avidity that is content with the first intelligence that offers, instead of thinking the best obtainable just good enough.

In analytic psychology we have daily illustrations of how liable we are to this temptation. There is, for instance, a wholly logical connection between two elements in the manifest content of a dream; but it is only a shadow bridge across a hidden gulf. We hear a very reasonable inference, a logically unassailable reason for certain personal peculiarities, and yet it forms only a well-camouflaged super-structure in the system of a serious compulsion neurosis. All that and much more besides is only external, a logical façade, intellectual mimicry, and camouflage, set up in order to lure research away from more important things and keep it away from its real objects. Anyone who interprets a slip of the tongue as the absent-minded substitution of one letter for another or the dropping of a sound need not go on with research. Anyone who regards the compulsion of a nervous patient to wash simply as an expression of intensified cleanliness has allowed himself to be led astray by the logical tricks of a compulsion neurotic. If we once abandon ourselves to deceptive logic and yield to the obscure urge to comprehend rapidly, then we cannot stop. We are soon convinced; it must be so, and nowise else. With less and less intellectual resistance, we shall then comprehend everything on the basis of false assumptions—strictly logically. Everything proceeds swimmingly; single contradictions and omissions are passed over, rifts unconsciously bridged. Any detail that does not fit is pushed and pulled into place, and conflicting elements are guilelessly forced into a new artificial system. The advice that we must give to young psychological investigators must be: Resist the temptation of understanding too quickly. (*"Principiis intelligendi obsta."*)

We hear the boast made on behalf of psychoanalysis that, behind the mental phenomena that have hitherto been regarded as absurd and senseless, it has discovered a secret meaning, a hidden significance, and brought it to light. Confronted with this mighty achievement, which has opened the road to the comprehension of the unconscious mind, I fear that we have too little appreciated the other achievement that preceded it, without which, indeed, it would not have been possible. Psychoanalysis has resisted the acceptance of mental associations simply because they were reasonable, or, indeed, because they were "the only reasonable explanation." It has refused to recognize a chain of cause and effect in the inner life as the only one solely because it seemed plausible and there was no other in sight. The theory of physical stimuli seemed capable of explaining the phenomena of dreams; puberty was thoroughly accepted as the beginning of sexuality. In these matters nature herself offered the obvious explanation. Several physiological phenomena clearly indicated the etiology of hysteria, of phobias, and compulsion neuroses—everything was plain, there were no further problems to be solved. To hold these reasonable and sufficient explanations inadequate, to renounce easy and convenient comprehension of psychical facts—that could hardly be called eccentricity—it was obviously either want of sense or else scientific conceit, *hubris.*

It must be stated more than once—it must be said three times—that not to understand psychological relations represents an advance over superficial comprehension. Whereas such comprehension amounts to arriving in a blind alley, all sorts of possibilities remain open to one who does not understand. To be puzzled where everything is clear to others, where they merely ask: "What is there to understand?"—to see a riddle there still—need not be a mark of stupidity; it may be the mark of a free mind. Obstinately not to understand where other people find no difficulties and obscurities may be the initial stage of new knowledge. In this sense the much-lauded rapid apprehension, including that by means of psychoanalytic theories, may be sterile since it touches only the most superficial levels. Regarded thus, a mediocre intelligence, an intellectual mobility, and capacity to be on the spot, which places, classifies, and establishes every phenomenon as quickly as possible, may have less cultural value than apparent intellectual failure or the temporary miss, which is sometimes the forerunner of deeper comprehension.

In the inner world, too, there are situations in which the cosmos, the ordered, articulated universe, seems, so to speak, to be turned back to chaos, yet from which a new creation emerges. We think, perhaps, that we fully understand such and such a psychical event, and then it suddenly becomes incomprehensible. We had worked our way to the opinion in question and made it our own. And then all of a sudden it is lost, without our knowing how. We had tested and examined everything and decided that it was all right; and then everything became uncertain again. In the midst of light we saw obscurity. Problems solved long ago become problematical again.

Questions answered long ago show that there was something questionable in the answer. Surely everybody has had the experience of a carpet pattern seeming to change under his very eyes. Gradually or suddenly we see it seem to lose the familiar form; the lines, combined so significantly and pleasantly in figures or arabesques, suddenly part, tangle, and try to follow their own strange ways, darker than those of the Lord. As long as we have known the carpet, we have seen that arrangement of lines in it, one figure. Our eye is used to tracing the threads that make the memorable form. We never expected to see anything else. And then one day the accustomed order of the lines is dissolved, the old pattern is blurred and hazy. The lines refuse to combine in the old way. They arrange themselves in new, hitherto concealed figures, in new, hitherto unnoticed groupings. A like surprise, in ceasing to recognize something to be transformed later into the light of new knowledge, may be the lot of many investigators. What has long been classified, arranged, judged, and clearly known may suddenly become incomprehensible to an individual pioneer. That means that the conception hitherto current, according to which everything was clear, no longer seems to him worthy of the name of comprehension. The investigator in question might then say, "I am beginning no longer to comprehend."

It would seem that one of the most important conditions of this non-comprehension is an uncommon measure of intellectual courage. I do not mean here the courage to confess we have not understood something that is as clear as daylight to everybody else. That kind of courage would denote something more external, something of a secondary character. What I mean is rather the courage in the world of thought that is able to draw back from what is universally comprehensible and reasonable, and not to join the march into the region of the plausible. It takes courage to mistrust the temptation to understand everything and not to be content with a perception because it is evident. It takes courage to resist the wave of general comprehension (in the sense of superficiality or common sense). It requires inner truthfulness to stand out against our own intellectual impatience, our desire to master intellectually and to take associations by storm. This, too, is a form of belief in the omnipotence of thought, and it requires courage to reject it—not to take the path of least intellectual resistance, of speedy and effortless comprehension.

Assuredly it is not true, as a group of scientific nihilists tell us, that man will have nothing to do with truth. On the contrary, I believe that mankind has a great thirst for truth. The greatest hindrance to the advance of knowledge is rather of a different nature; it is that people think they have long been in possession of the truth, the whole truth. The realms in which the human spirit will make new and surprising discoveries are by no means only those hitherto unexplored, but also those of which we have very accurate and reliable maps. It is the problems already "solved" that present the most numerous and difficult problems to the inquirer. If we want to attain new knowledge, we must look around among the old, familiar questions, just as Diogenes sought men in the crowded market place of Athens. But we need a measure of intellectual courage to raise and solve these problems. It is this courage that will, sooner or later, overcome the resistance of the dull world.

PART FOUR

Psychoanalytic Experiences in Life, Literature, and Music

Psychoanalytic Experiences in Life, Literature, and Music

I

1

AFTER more than forty years of theoretical and practical occupation with psychoanalysis I still consider those insights
most valuable that come as a surprise to me. An insight into
human beings that is only figured out, a psychological understanding that is obtained only by reason, can have but intellectual
fruits. Here are some inner experiences leading to a few new
concepts and insights into unconscious emotions. Observations
and impressions obtained in everyday life and in analytic sessions
often echo the inner experiences shaped by a great writer. Those
echoes are memories of character or situations read in a book or
seen on the stage. Yet such fleeting and half-forgotten impressions
are often the hidden sources from which the "intuitions" of the
psychoanalyst flow. His unconscious knowledge and understanding—what else is "intuition?"—are acquired not only from the
experiences of life, but also from their reflections in literature
that mirrors life. We do not often relate the psychological insights of great writers to our analytic work in our daily wrestling
with the demons of the consultation room. But these insights
pervade the atmosphere nevertheless. The invisible can sometimes be strongly present. Under favorable internal circumstances we are sometimes able to grasp these insights and to put
their content and character into words. I should like to present
an example of such an exceptional experience, of the re-emergence of impressions otherwise subterranean, to show what an
important part they play in our work. It is a strange experience
to meet in everyday life the very counterpart of characters or
situations which once were conceived in the imagination of a
perceptive writer.

Here is a dream of my patient, Tom, who is thirty-one years

old: *"Bill and I sit together and he tells me that his father died a few days before. He laughs while he tells me this and I am surprised."*

Bill is an acquaintance of Tom's who often spends the evening with him. The two young men had dined together the night before Tom's dream occurred, and at this time Bill had, in reality, spoken warmly of his "old man," whose character he praised and whom he described as being still vigorous and hard-working. Tom got the impression that Bill and his father are on excellent terms. In his analytic session the following day, Tom reported first this conversation and then his dream. We do not hesitate to guess that the conversation with Bill functioned as a day remnant for the dream, and that thoughts or emotions awakened during the evening were its source.

There were no associations helpful in penetrating the secret meaning of the dream. Its interpretation, at least in its essential content, emerged in a sudden flash, facilitated by my knowledge of the dreamer's life story, and by the insight gained into his character during several months of psychoanalysis. When Bill had talked so affectionately of his father, there must have been in Tom some feeling of envy and some longing for his own father, who had died twenty-one years before. Tom felt an impulse to speak of this father whom he had lost when he was ten years old. The dream originated in the thought: "If Bill should ask me about my father, I would say . . ." The reversal of roles in the dream appears more plausible when we understand that Tom would, in actual life, speak very much as Bill did in his dream. Tom likes to hide his strong emotions behind a casual and somewhat cynical front. He makes fun of himself and others, and in many analytic sessions spoke in a flippant and sarcastic manner of things that were painful to him.

The concealed meaning of the dream becomes clear when one reverses the roles and transforms a thought possibility into a real situation: "If I now talked about my father, I would say that he had died a few days ago and then I would laugh and Bill would be surprised." Such behavior would be quite in character for Tom, as he had frequently demonstrated in the past few months. Besides his need to hide his emotions and to make fun of himself, his temptation to startle and impress people, to act a part, is very powerful.

Tom did not react to my tentative interpretation of his dream. He neither confirmed nor denied it. He remained silent for a moment, and then spoke of a slip of the tongue he had experienced a few days before. It was as if he wanted to turn to another subject and avoid discussion of the dream. But the character of the mistake he now related confirmed, in an indirect manner, my interpretation of the dream. "I made a funny slip of the tongue the other day. Paul [another acquaintance] and I were in a bar and we were pretty high He asked me about my father, and I said, 'I died when I was ten years old.' " In saying, "I died," instead of, "He died," Tom gave his genuine feelings away. The loss of his father marked the turning point of his boyhood. It was as if he had died himself when his father was killed in a car accident.

We have learned that there is a secret communication between the unconscious minds of two persons engaged in a conversation such as this. When Tom spoke of his slip of the tongue, he continued the theme of the death of his father, and what he said amounted to an unconscious confirmation of my dream interpretation. However, his thoughts had a further unconscious meaning. The story of his slip was, so to speak, his own contribution to the interpretation of his dream. This contribution was not consciously intended and was not perceived by him as such.

My attention was turned to an important feature of the dream that had been neglected in my interpretation: his father had died a few days before instead of twenty-one years ago. This detail of the manifest dream content had not been considered in my interpretation, which therefore left out one of the most essential meanings of the dream. In his slip of the tongue ("I died when I was ten years old"), he had made a mistake concerning the personal pronoun. But does this slip not say, "I still feel the terrible loss today as I did when I was a boy of ten years . . ."?

The dream element that his father "died a few days ago" must have a similar concealed meaning. We sometimes say, "I remember as if it had happened yesterday," when we speak of an event that occurred a long time ago but has made a lasting and vivid impression upon us. Such a meaning is not manifest in the wording of the dream feature, but it can easily be guessed.

The following paragraphs not only reveal this missing interpretation but go beyond this to demonstrate again that a most important part of analytic understanding emerges from unconscious processes of the psychoanalyst.

The fact that the patient told me about his slip of the tongue had turned my attention to the one still neglected element of the dream. But if this was the effect of his report, was it not also its unconscious purpose? When his reaction to my original interpretation was neither to agree nor disagree, but, instead, to tell me of his slip of the tongue, there must have been an unconscious connection in his mind between the dream and his mistake. The very succession proves that there were threads running from the first to the second subject. The content of his slip points in the direction of that concealed connection. It says, in effect, "I was only ten years old, but it is as if it happened yesterday and as if I had died myself."

Shifting now from the patient's thought processes to my own, I shall try to describe as precisely as possible on which interesting detour the understanding of that neglected dream element was reached. It was as if the report about the slip of the tongue had acted as an unconscious stimulus and was used for the interpretation of the still unconsidered detail. The hint was unconsciously grasped by me as if it contained a further clue until then missing.

At this point the name "Hamlet" emerged suddenly into my thoughts. Tom's slip of the tongue had become connected in my mind both with the dream element ("my father died a few days ago") and with some memory-trace of Shakespeare's play—as if the dream wording awakened a familiar echo. I became aware that the purposeful absurdity of "a few days ago" reminded me of some similar, grimly distorted and bitter lines spoken by the Danish prince.

Suddenly the scene of the play within the play came vividly before my mind's eye: the King, the Queen and the Lords in the royal castle at Elsinore; the wide hall illuminated by torches; Ophelia sits beside the Queen, and Hamlet asks the girl whether he may lie with his head upon her lap. I did not then remember the exact words, but felt there must follow some sentences that Hamlet's father had died the other day. No, not a few days ago as in Tom's dream; a few hours ago . . .

After Tom had left, I looked the scene up (Act III, scene 2). Here is the passage:

> Ophelia: You are merry, my lord.
> Hamlet: Who, I?
> Ophelia: Aye, my lord.
> Hamlet: O God, your only jig-maker. What should a man do but be merry—for look you, how cheerfully my mother looks and my father died within's two hours!
> Ophelia: Nay, 'tis twice two months, my lord.
> Hamlet: So long? Nay, then, let the devil wear black for I'll have a suit of sables. O Heavens! Died two months ago and not forgotten yet? Then there's hope a great man's memory may outlive his life half a year, but, by'r Lady, he must build churches then . . .

The bitter mockery expressed in Hamlet's joking is not unlike that in Tom's dream. This parallel awakened my preconscious memory of the play. The dream and the scene from *Hamlet* were linked in my thoughts not only by the similarity of the emotions but by the resemblance of their expression—as in the pretended shortening of time passed since the father's death. This echo made me understand how much method and madness were in Tom's dream, as in the behavior of Hamlet.

For a moment the shadow of the Bard had passed through the consultation room of an analyst and had helped him to penetrate the concealed emotions of a disturbed mind.

2

"If Hamlet's father hadn't been murdered—" When that odd thought occurred to me—it was in the middle of an analytic session three years ago—I brushed it aside, of course. First because it was utterly silly, second it had nothing to do with the patient, and third one is a rational human being who should not think such foolish stuff. Thoughts must not run around wildly as dogs do in the traffic of the city but should be kept on a leash. What would the world come to if there were no rules and regulations concerning trains of thought? Chaos would come again as at the dawn of creation before God said, "Let there be light!"

The first time the idea emerged, it had the innocence and naïveté of all silly thoughts. It just crawled into my brain like an insect into one's sleeve. One becomes aware of an unpleasant sensation that something is creeping on one's arm before discovering it is an ant. I was at first astonished, then I became indignant at the intruder, and finally I felt ashamed of myself. What would people, for instance my colleagues, say if they knew what kind of ideas occurred to me! "The thought-company he keeps!" they'd say. I ordered that interloper to shut up. But it didn't and I slowly yielded to it. Why shouldn't a man have silly ideas occasionally? Is there no such thing as intellectual recreation, as a playground for thoughts? I am a law-abiding, tax-paying citizen, a psychoanalyst, which means I have a more or less honest profession. I am as entitled to have foolish ideas as the next man. This is a free country. Remember (I said to myself, said I) the many stupid, even moronic thoughts expressed at the sessions of Congress, at the conventions of the Republican party, at the meetings of psychiatric associations! No one there is ashamed of having stupid thoughts. They all get a hearing, they are even advertised and publicized. People are proud of them, all kinds of people, congressmen, lawyers, doctors. They fill the official publications of the government, the law journals, the scientific books, the newspapers and magazines of the nation.

Then—of all things—the basic rule of psychoanalysis occurred to me. Don't we ask our patients to say all that comes to mind, however stupid, silly, insignificant or immaterial it may appear to them? And don't we believe that just those thoughts to which the patient refuses entrance bring most valuable material to light? We assume that these intruders from the dark underground are the offspring of ideas, intimately connected with the vital problems of the patient. A "silly" obsessional idea, interpreted and analyzed, leads into the core of neurotic difficulties. A thought gone astray makes sense when we can reconstruct its origin and evolution. Following those silly thoughts might lead us to a new insights, might even result in an original concept. "Give me your tired, your poor, your huddled masses yearning to breathe free!" These displaced, suppressed thoughts should enter.

Why should we analysts not follow the same rule when silly thoughts occur to us? What intolerably pompous and conceited fools would we be, if we believed that our thought processes are different from those of our patients, who are often superior to us in intelligence, imagination and in many other qualities!

That half-formulated idea occurred to me again during an analytic session a few days later. It then came to mind in the middle of Rank-Olivier's production of *Hamlet*. It came quite impudently into the open during the movie and behaved as if it were a reasonable and respectable thought, not self-conscious at all among some quite sensible ideas about *Hamlet*. It was here at least appropriate to the occasion. However queer, at least it was not a displaced idea any more, not a refugee thought. It was still intellectual flotsam and jetsam.

The odd thought appeared here in the middle of critical voices that drowned my admiration for the *Hamlet* picture. Am I allowed to report those negative impressions and put aside the many things I enjoyed? The first impression that astonished me was the sight of the castle of Elsinore. It deserves to be included in the list of miracle buildings of the world beside the Pyramids, the Indian temples, and the Empire State Building. One can boldly assert that so many stairs do not exist anywhere else. They are perhaps meant to be symbolic, but no other single building can boast of so many stairs. There must have been master-builders in Denmark at the time, architects who worked on the difficult problem: Is there no other place in the castle where stairs could be installed?

I was, of course, impressed by Olivier's acting, by the scope of the emotional expressions of his face, his voice and his gestures. The trouble with his performance was that this Hamlet had read Freud's and Ernest Jones's explanation of his conflict and personality. Had read it? More than this, had accepted and absorbed it—not wisely but too well. I consider the analytic interpretation

of Hamlet as correct, but I do not believe an actor should act
the part according to this or any interpretation.

Take the scene between mother and son in the third act. Hamlet, who fiercely denounces and accuses the Queen, passionately
embraces her. He is her lover, not her son; or better, her son-
lover.* "Come, come, and sit you down here. You shall not
budge," sounds, accompanied by those gestures, as if it were an
invitation to a petting party. The Prince again clasps his mother
in his arms. Less would be more. He says to the woman, "would
you were not my mother!" In this performance she isn't, or only
in a biological sense. But for the incestuous barrier which
threatens to disappear before our eyes, she is his sweetheart. Does
not the Prince admonish the actors they should not "tell all"?
Olivier's Hamlet does. He leaves no doubt in his audience's mind
that he has studied Freud.

The adverse impression was strengthened by the fact that
Olivier's Hamlet appears to be too old, compared with his
mother, acted by Eileen Herlie. Not by the stretch of a Shakespearean fantasy can you imagine this very pretty young woman
to be mother of this son. Not even when you concede that make-
up can rejuvenate the appearance of middle-aged ladies. We, too,
have heard of your painting. "God hath given you one face and
you make yourselves another"—but the actress did not succeed
in making her own that other face of a middle-aged woman.

How old is Hamlet? I asked myself. Well, Yorick's skull has
lain in the earth three and twenty years and "he has borne me
on his back a thousand times" and has been kissed by the boy
"I know not how oft." The child was old enough not only to
understand but also to appreciate Yorick's jokes. The Prince is at
least twenty-seven years old, if he is not thirty or more. How old
is the Queen, his mother? At least in her late forties. In this performance the ages of mother and son appear almost reversed. While
I looked at the couple in the Queen's chamber, a song occurred
to me—is it not by George M. Cohan?—and parodistically accompanied the scene: "An old guy like me and a young girl
like you."

* As early as 1922 the "Freudian implications" (reviewer's expression) of the
closet scene were rendered obvious in John Barrymore's performance.

A few moments later—exactly when the ghost appears—that foolish idea re-emerged, this time in the form of an incomplete conditional sentence. The silly thought was not vague or disguised any more. It appeared among serious reflections on Hamlet's conflict, like the fool at the Court in one of Shakespeare's plays. Here is the text of the odd idea, the line the fool in my thoughts speaks: *If Hamlet's father hadn't been murdered, but had died a natural death, and if the Queen hadn't remarried—*

Here the thought broke off in mid-air as the sentence of a drunkard or of a fool. That same evening I tried to follow the idea wherever it would lead me. Don't the fools in Shakespeare's plays often say wise things, putting them in an odd way? I did not get very far in the pursuit of that elusive thought. It was late in the night and I was very tired. I repeated the absurd sentence in my thoughts and tried to find a continuation. Mysteriously the phrase began now with the added word "Even." It now ran: "Even if Hamlet's father hadn't," and so on. What followed were a few words, a kind of fragmentary continuation in the form of a question or a doubt like "wouldn't Hamlet . . . ?" What he wouldn't or would, I did not find out because I fell asleep. The last words I thought before I dozed off were a greeting to his figure: "Good night, sweet Prince!"

When I awoke, the funny thought had vanished as had the King's ghost when "the morning cock crew loud." The "demands of the day" had driven it underground. I did not think of it again until late that afternoon during the analytic session with Tom, the same patient in whose analysis the thought had first occurred to me. Tom spoke of his childhood and of a letter he had received from his mother. When now that odd thought came to mind again, I understood that, however silly, it had its roots in a sane mental soil. I still didn't know what Hamlet wouldn't or would have felt or done, if . . . but I had an inkling of what had made me think of such an unimaginable possibility, that would remove all the premises of Shakespeare's plot.

Tom is the patient whose dream I interpreted in the preceding paragraphs. A similarity of Tom's emotional attitude with that of the Prince, manifested in the wording of the dream, must have awakened the memory of some bitter lines Hamlet speaks while he listens to the players acting in the play within the play. I had not consciously thought then of another concealed factor facilitating the thought-connection between the Prince and Tom. It was the idea of murder. As I reported before, Tom's father had died in a car accident when the boy was ten years old. The accident occurred on a business trip when the chauffeur drove the car into a ditch. Tom's father was immediately killed, the driver suffered only a few light wounds and bruises. So far there are no similarities between the older Hamlet's death and the fate of Tom's father, but some can be found in the boy's thoughts afterward. When the tragic news was brought to the house, Tom, who loved his father, began to suspect foul play. There was not the slightest reason for such suspicions in the external facts, but many in Tom's mind. His father had been a very successful banker who had acquired a fortune in a relatively short time. Many people in his home town and in the country had envied him, and he had made several enemies. When the accident occurred, the boy, who had learned much from conversations he had listened to and who suspected more, must have thought that one or the other of those enemies might have had a hand in the accident—for instance, a competitor with whom the father had a quarrel not long before. The investigation of the accident brought no reason for such suspicions, but Tom nourished them because he felt hostile toward some relatives and business competitors of his father. The boy did not utter any of those doubts,. which slowly lost their power over him, but ·they reappeared during his analysis when he returned in his memories to the years of his childhood and to the death of his father. There were again the serious suspicions that his father could have been murdered and did not die in an accident for which no one was responsible.

Here is the emotional similarity: Tom's father was not murdered, but the boy suspected that he was. He must have been in the same mood as the Prince who suspected foul play before he had any evidence from the lips of the ghost. "O my prophetic soul!" cries Hamlet.

It dawned upon me during this analytic session that the puzzling sentence must have had its origin in a preconscious comparison of Hamlet's and Tom's attitude to the father's death. In the one case the father was really murdered, in the other the son thought that there had been murder. In Hamlet's case material reality, in Tom's only psychological reality. Tom's suspicions were well "in character" with his personality. He often projected his own unconscious impulses onto other people and suspected them in a paranoic mechanism of hostile and aggressive intentions he himself unconsciously felt.

There was another factor that facilitated the comparison between Hamlet's and Tom's stories. Many suitors had wished to marry Tom's mother who was still young, pretty, and rich, but she remained unmarried. Soon after his father's death Tom felt increasingly hostile toward his mother, who adored him, and his resentment against her continued to work in him until his analysis slowly mitigated it. During his analysis he did not tire of attacking her behavior, and for a long time it seemed as if an inner reconciliation with his mother would not be possible. There was no doubt that his hostility against her was later on displaced and generalized to all women. He was homosexual.

The material here reported shows which elements made the thought-bridge between Hamlet and Tom possible, and which threads ran in my unconscious associations from the life story of my patient to the destiny of the Prince. Tom's father was not murdered, but could have been killed. His mother did not marry again, but the boy thought she would soon. Here were potential destinies living a shadow life beside the realities. My thoughts went beyond them in that formulation: Even if Hamlet's father had died a natural death, and so on. Here is the other end of the possibilities founded on the analogy Hamlet's father—Tom's father.

The if-sentence had, however, not been finished. The idea did not deserve that name because it was broken off before it reached the shape and dignity of a complete thought. It had been nipped in the bud by the white frost of reason that forbids the growth of fanciful productions of the mind.

That missing condition of the sentence was found when I tried to analyze the emotional reactions of another patient whose father died during his son's analysis. The old man had been very sick in the hospital for some weeks, and the family knew the end was near. It came when the son was alone with the heavily breathing father, whose wife was at the time in the corridor of the hospital. When she was called, she cried and sobbed, and my patient felt that her mourning was exaggerated and hypocritical. This impression repeated itself at the funeral and in the following weeks, especially when relatives and other visitors came to the house. The son felt a wave of hostility against his mother whom he accused in his thoughts of not having treated the old man well and of not having taken enough care of him. In all external aspects, he behaved toward her as an affectionate and attentive son would in the time of mourning and tried to console and support her, but he had to make an effort to conceal his increasing hostility. He was haunted by the memory of the scene of his father's death and suffered for some months from insomnia, restlessness, and stomach symptoms.

I shall add only a few representative instances from many years of analytic practice of similar attitudes of sons toward their mother after their father's death. In another case the father had died when the son was eighteen years old. His mother fell into pathological mourning which was akin to melancholia and which lasted a few years. She did not leave the house, neglected her household duties, and showed no interest in her children. The son's resentment against the mother increased to such an extent that he had violent outbreaks of anger against the poor woman whom he accused of selfishness and self-indulgence. He felt that she had no right to neglect everything and was jealous of the intensity of her mourning for his father. At the same time he often longed for the deceased and repented many occasions when he had caused grief and worry to him.

Another case provides us with an interesting variation: the father did not die, but left the family. The son was six years old, when his parents divorced. He saw his father only rarely in the following years. On these occasions the boy felt an overwhelming pity for his father who was shabbily dressed and gave the impression of a beggar, while the mother lived very comfortably. The boy's critical and hostile attitude against her increased when she went out with different men in the years following the divorce. Most of these men were friendly to the boy, showed interest in his play, his attempts to build a radio, and so on, but he very rarely returned their cordial feelings. On various occasions when the mother talked to one of her suitors on the telephone, the son was told not to speak because Mother did not want the man to know that she had a child. The boy resented this bitterly. He had already stammered before the divorce, but he traced his speech defect to those times when he was cautioned not to betray his existence when Mother spoke with a man on the telephone. His stammering was especially bad when he was asked by other boys where his father was. He felt ashamed that his parents were divorced. The estrangement with his mother continued until the middle of his twenties. His relationship with her improved only in analysis. The case is interesting because here the father did not die, but left the home, and yet after a short time the same reactions can be observed as in the other cases in which the son lost his father through death.

The complete sentence then is: *Even if Hamlet's father hadn't been murdered, but had died a natural death, and if the Queen hadn't remarried, wouldn't Hamlet have felt hostility against his mother?* This sentence is neither grammatical nor elegant, but English grammar will never be one of my strong points (English is not my mother tongue and I am often wrestling with the genius of this language as Jacob with the angel of the Lord without being blessed). The sentence is, at least, intelligible. It expresses a valid, if not a valuable, possibility. It asserts that the Prince would perhaps have felt resentment against his mother even if the premises of the situation were much nearer to everyday experience.

It was not accidental that the odd thought first emerged during the analytic session with Tom. The comparison of the emotional situation of his childhood with Hamlet's destiny built a slight and rocking bridge in my thoughts. What had happened at the castle of Elsinore remained in the area of thought possibilities at the cottage in Knoxville, Tom's home. From here is only one small step to the idea: What if the events in Denmark were also only a grandiose production of Hamlet's imagination, like the apparition of the King? The thought following this tentative assumption then led back to the psychological problem that had occupied me in Tom's case: that of resentment against his mother after his father's death.

Considering this underlying problem which must have lingered in my mind some time during Tom's analysis (and before it), the question emerging from the unconscious loses much of its fantastic and fanciful character. It amounts then to a kind of psychological reflection which brings the Shakespeare plot near to the emotional reality of everyday life.

I do not apologize for the quality of my idea, because thoughts need no apology. You are as responsible for their intellectual quality as for the timbre of your voice. I am, of course, aware that my thought went astray here and oscillated for a moment between reality and fantasy. I am also ready to admit that the question in my mind had the characteristics of a flirtation with an idea. The mental situation has a resemblance to that in which the farmer-father asks a boy whether he has honest or dishonest intentions toward his daughter and the boy says, "Have I got a choice?" But then it seemed that I had no choice, the flirtation was replaced by a serious interest.

Looking back at the emergence of that question, I can add a few facts which facilitated the comparison. The boy Tom compared his mother's suitors very unfavorably with his dead father whom he idealized. In the scene in the Queen's chamber Hamlet speaks in glowing words of his father and puts a caricature of Claudius before his mother's eyes: "O king of shreds and patches." Tom resented it that his mother saw men visitors so soon after his father's death and contrasted in his thoughts the violent outbursts of her grief with her occasional cheerfulness shortly afterward. Hamlet's:

> A little month or ere those shoes were old,
> With which she followed my poor father's body
> Like Niobe, all tears—

In his analysis Tom remembered that he once looked with misgivings at his mother who sat on a chair talking with a lawyer visiting her. She had her legs crossed and her skirt was raised so that the man must have seen her knee. In this little antagonistic observation is a trace of the same emotions that led to the violent outbursts of Hamlet against Gertrude's sensuality. In the case of the other patient whose mother went out with men soon after her divorce, the son bitterly resented her infidelity to his father. Tom who was of a rather gentle nature (Gertrude calls her son "sweet Hamlet") had in his late teens and early twenties bitter scenes with his mother who led a blameless life. He transferred his critical attitude from Mother to other women, as Hamlet does to Ophelia, but in contrast to the Prince he confessed that man delighted him.

It was, of course, far from my thoughts, however whimsical they must have appeared to the reader, to compare Tom who was an average neurotic young man to the personality of the Danish Prince. Hamlet is, as far as I know, the only character in any play whose genius is immediately recognizable to everyone in the audience. Any man or woman who has listened to him will agree with Ophelia's opinion of what a noble mind is here o'erthrown. Imagine a playwright who wanted to make Beethoven or Rembrandt or Einstein the leading character in a tragedy. He would have to make the audience listen to a symphony, or look at the "Nightwatch," or follow the logic of the theory of relativity in order to show the genius of the character. Hamlet works upon us by his personality only. But we do not deal here with the witty and wily, passionate and melancholic personality of the Prince, but with certain typical emotional reactions of a man after his father's death.

I shall sketch the emotional situation that became analytically transparent in the case of Tom and other patients, so unlike that of Hamlet in many directions and so resembling his in others. Besides the mourning for the beloved or admired father in all these persons antagonistic and sometimes even aggressive tendencies against the mother emerged, whether they were unconscious or, as in the cases here reported, reached the state of conscious awareness. The usual attitude of the son in this situation is, of course, that of increased consideration and affection for his mother. He will try to console her, to give her as much moral support as possible, and to replace the head of the family as far as responsibilities are concerned. In a certain type of man intense mourning for the father will be coupled with an emotional withdrawal from the mother, even with a certain antagonism and antipathy against her. If this psychologic observation is correct, we can for a moment really put aside such dramatic and unusual events as murder of the father and hasty marriage of the mother with his killer. Traces of the emotional reaction here reported must be observable also in cases in which the father died a natural death and the mother did not remarry—just the situation emerging in my surprising question.

But what would be the psychologic motives of such a puzzling reaction? How could it be brought in accordance with what we know from other analytic experiences about the emotions of the son after the father's death?

A careful observation of the symptomatic manifestations of that reaction, to which the discovery of a gap and its filling has to be added, leads to the analytic explanation of the puzzling phenomenon. To put the development of the process in simple terms: Father's death has realized one half of the unconscious wishes the child once had. It has removed the superior rival for Mother's love. By the death itself, those repressed infantile wishes become for a moment actualized again. They threaten to emerge from the submersion into which they had once been banned. Here is the occasion to take the place of Father, not only as head of the family, but also as the lover of Mother. Old wishes, long caved in, push to the light of the day.

According to all psychologic laws known to us, there must be a moment of unconscious triumph. We have to assume that Father's death brings about the emergence of victorious or triumphant feelings of promise and fulfillment, of freedom and of the lifting of an unconscious barrier. This upsurge can last only a second and is in most cases unconscious. Here is the gap that analytic reconstruction has to fill, because, even in the cases in which those emotions touch the threshold of conscious perception, they are immediately and most energetically repressed and will be forgotten and disavowed later on.

What follows and becomes recognizable to our observation is the expression of an intense reaction-formation to these fleeting unconscious emotions. This reaction is the stronger, the more urgently the rejected tendencies demand entrance into the realm of conscious impulses. By the power of this reaction the grief about the loss will be most vividly felt, the figure of the father will be elevated and even glorified, and the longing for him intensified. The other side of that reaction-formation concerns the mother. She who could now become the object of old desires, will in the reactive reversal awaken antagonism and resentment as if the son unconsciously protects himself from the temptation of a break-through. In this defense the re-emerging positive trends change their sign into the negative. The unconsciously renewed attraction is turned into antipathy and criticism.

It is easy to guess that the factor responsible for this emotional reversal is the unconscious guilt feeling of the son. It is as if those old disavowed wishes had brought about the death of the father, as if he had died a victim of omnipotent thoughts the boy had once experienced. It is as if something has now become reality which one could once only dare to think—and often not even dare to think. The violent reaction to this reality brings about not only renunciation of the old love object but also the reversal of unconscious desires into hostility. It is as if she were responsible for Father's death—which she is, as far as the unconscious thoughts of the son are concerned, because the attraction to her was the main psychological reason for the emergence of the infantile wish to remove the successful rival.

The hostility against Mother increases the more it becomes necessary to defend oneself against the unconscious temptation to take Father's place with her. In Tom's case, the reaction went so far that he was frightened by murderous thoughts against his mother. But also Gertrude becomes afraid of "gentle Hamlet" when he violently accuses and threatens her. Unconsciously aware of the intensity of his wrath, she thinks for a moment he really wants to kill her.

> What wilt thou do? Thou wilt not murder me?
> Help, help, ho!

As the last consequence of this psychologic insight, one arrives at the assumption that in certain cases the unconscious temptation becomes very strong, and the inner tension between triumphant, desirous impulses and unconscious guilt feelings in the son becomes intolerable. In these cases the reaction, here sketched, is not sufficiently effective and the ego wards off the forbidden tendencies with the help of another more primitive, dynamic mechanism. It tries to project them into the external world, to persons outside, and thus finds a certain emotional relaxation, a relief from the unbearable tension. The psychologic formula for such an unconscious process could perhaps best be put this way: not *I* wanted to murder Father, but *he* (another man, thought of as Father's rival)—not *I* desire Mother (but *another* man). Arrived at this point, the distance of the emotional situation of any son to the one Shakespeare envisions in the tragedy of *Hamlet* can be measured. This distance does not appear as great any more. My original question was senseless only in the most rationalistic, which means, here, in the most superficial "sense."

Still another mechanism of disavowal and defense can be observed in the case of Hamlet and of Tom. It can be brought into the psychological formula: I did not want to murder my father—on the contrary, I want to revenge his death and—I do not desire my mother—on the contrary, I dislike her and I attack her. The extension of this reactive feeling leads the Prince to scorn for all women and to the fierce onslaught on them in the scene with Ophelia.

At this point my thoughts join the analytic interpretations of Freud, Jones, Rank, and others. In the last years many contributions in which analytic insights were used to deepen the understanding of Shakespeare's play were added to earlier ones. The literature on the Hamlet problem has been enriched and enlarged to such an extent that no single person can with certainty assert that he has read all about the subject. As far as my knowledge goes, no book or article has dealt with the aspect of the problem here presented, and with its universal psychological scope.

From the beginning emphasis was put on the question of Hamlet's relationship with his mother, but even this is not the point of departure for my train of thoughts. It emerged at the Hamlet problem in a whimsical and questionable form. It landed there only by accident, if we allow accident to play a role in the field of intellectual problems. The train of thought was originally stimulated by psychological reflection on the case of Tom, and did not deal with the plot and conflict of the Danish Prince. When it touched this problem, so to speak, in an excursion on the spur of a fanciful moment, it still did not follow in the tracks of so many literary critics or psychoanalytic scholars. On the contrary, it removed all essential premises of the actual situation in Shakespeare's play as a thought-possibility ("Even if Hamlet's father hadn't been murdered" and so on).

The figure of Hamlet had thus come to mind in a roundabout way, as a thought aside. It was, so to speak, a tentative fantasy, an exciting experiment in thought in order to test a possibility that had remained unconscious. The comparison of Tom's experience with Hamlet's tended to an area beyond both cases, into the field of general psychological insights.

It is not without significance that the line my capricious thought followed was not from literature to life, but the other way around, from living experience to a work of art. I must have unconsciously wrestled with the psychological problem of whether there is not something typical or even general in the emotional turn against Mother after Father's death. Otherwise put: I was unconsciously searching for the solution of a psychological problem which had not yet been discovered and which eluded me. Hamlet's destiny offered itself to my thoughts as the extreme manifestation of this problem. Tentatively following the psychological consequences of his case, I brought it in my thoughts to the level at which all human inner experience is the same.

If this discussion can be considered at all as an original, analytic contribution to the Hamlet problem, it may deserve that title only as a by-product of the curiosity of a psychologist who sometimes goes astray in his thoughts when he explores the yet undiscovered recesses of the human mind.

3

As I consider, in retrospect, the various ways and byways, the many detours and turns through which my thoughts wandered to their destination on that particular evening, it seems to me that we all of us marvel too little at our own mental processes. We are not astonished enough at the wide circle of our own thoughts. We speak most casually of unconscious emotions and impulses and are not ready to admit that the area of the repressed is a state within a state, an underground in which movement and power can be felt and in which continual life and productivity can be observed. Without such an astonishment, psychoanalysis is reduced to a science without human interest, with technology as its medical application.

As I look back at the meanderings of my thoughts, I am inclined to agree with the sentiment expressed by a patient the other day. This clever man, who had gained insight into his own bizarre obsessional ideas, said, "The mind is an insult to the intelligence." Yet, in my own case, there were no such obsessional thoughts or any other extraordinary mental phenomena. Nothing of this kind; no conspicuous pathological speculations or ideas. Just an everyday train of thought and a fairly average slice of human experience.

It is, of course, necessary to sketch the external situation from which my train of thought emerged. Tired after a long day of psychoanalytic sessions, I relaxed on the couch after dinner. My daughter, Theodora, whom we call "Thody," came into the room and said, "Good night, Daddy." "Where are you going?" I asked. "I have a date." "Don't come home too late. Good night." I knew better than to ask her with whom she had a date. It seems she does not like such questions. Well, she is seventeen years old. . . . In my time children were not so independent. What does it matter with which boy she has a date? She is no longer a child. . . . She will be in college very soon. . . .

I turn my attention in another direction . . . to the analytic sessions of today. My patient Bill comes to my mind.

Bill is a young man from a southern state. He came to analysis because he had tried in vain to overcome his inclination to excessive drinking, and because of his inability to make any sustained effort. He is homosexual, snobbish, and in other respects a typical playboy. His amiability and a concealed shyness seem to enable him to win friends.

While I thought of this patient, I saw, so to speak, in a mental image, his face which shows little expression. . . . His voice has no rise and fall when he speaks well-considered sentences. . . . He is rather rigid and shows that remoteness and flatness of emotions characteristic of schizoid personalities. . . . He has not done a stroke of honest work for years, and, it seems, he lives on a strict diet of dry martinis. . . . His therapeutic chance is not too good, but I shall, of course, do my best.

In his analytic session this afternoon he had spoken of Paris where he spent some months a few years ago. He had spoken of his wish to get the leading role in a play soon to be performed on Broadway, and of his friends, one of whom is an actor. I no longer remember how he came from there to the subject of race discrimination, but I believe he mentioned that another of his homosexual friends was a Jew. He had then said that, in contrast to most citizens of that southern state in which he was born and bred, he did not feel any race discrimination. But a few minutes later he had spoken contemptuously of "niggers" and Jews. He had said that an art dealer whom he knew had tried to take him in the day before. The man had tried to sell him an antique piece of furniture for which he asked a preposterous price. The patient, expressing his indignation and his dissatisfaction with his acquaintance, had added, "Once a Jew, always a Jew."

The recollection of these remarks became the point of departure for my free associations which on a strange detour led me to a new interpretation of a Shakespearean play, and in a surprising digression back to a personal problem. While I rested on the couch, smoking cigarettes, I followed this train of thought with, so to speak, impersonal interest. I swam comfortably with the "stream of consciousness" until a certain point was reached at which my thoughts became objects of self-observation. To continue the comparison, it was as if the swimmer had become aware of the kind of waves and of the direction in which they were carrying him. After this point was reached, I came across some odd associations whose sequence and meaning I did not understand. I decided to follow them, to investigate them, to find out what they meant and why they emerged from unknown depths. I had become aware of undercurrents in the stream.

I then got up from the couch, took a pencil and paper from the desk, and jotted the train of thoughts down together with what occurred to me while I wrote. I regret I did not look at the clock nor did I pay attention to the time that this process took, but my impression was that not more than a few minutes had elapsed since my daughter had left the room. In a psychological experiment, precise data concerning time and other external factors are, of course, indispensable in the interest of scientific precision. However, my self-observation and self-analysis was not in the nature of an experiment. It had rather the character of an inner experience.

While I remembered what Bill had said that afternoon and while I thought of his emotional disturbance, I was wide awake. The following associations emerged when I felt increasingly sleepy, without, however, yielding to the temptation to fall asleep. The fact that these associations occurred while I was only half awake may have had a bearing upon their character and the rapidity of their succession. I became aware that one thought or word quickly followed the other, as if they crowded the threshold of consciousness. There was, so to speak, a traffic jam at the door.

The words that emerged and astonished me, because I did not understand what they meant and why they occurred to me, were: *Jones . . . Jericho . . . Jephthah . . . Jessica . . . Jehovah . . . Jesus.*

Jones . . . I do not know anyone by this name. . . . Oh yes, of course, Ernest Jones. . . . I have known him for more than thirty years. I remember him when he was in Vienna. Did I not also meet him in Holland? I had talked to him at several psychoanalytic congresses, and, of course, we had been invited to lunch at his home when we were in London . . . I have not heard from him for twelve years. . . . I read his essay on *Hamlet* again a short time ago. . . . I looked something up in his paper on a religious problem. . . . I do not remember what it was. . . . He was already at the time of our visit in England (was this 1929 or 1928?) the most prominent psychoanalyst in the English-speaking countries. . . . I teased him. I said he was the King of the English analysts. . . . Emperor Jones. . . . Of course, the play by O'Neill. . . . What a strange connection! I started from

Ernest Jones and arrived at Emperor Jones. . . . Are there any trends besides the name? Perhaps primitive religions with which Jones deals in his *Collected Papers?* . . . I now remember the play. I recall the scene in which the Negro becomes terrified in the forest and how he finally succumbs to the demoniac power of the old tribal gods in which he did not believe and which he had repudiated. The thread leading from the analyst to Emperor Jones was the thought of Negroes. . . . But my patient Bill had spoken of Negroes and Jews.

When I turned my attention away from him, the subterranean continuation of his remarks must have led to Emperor Jones. Even the detour over Ernest Jones must have been significant. But how? Perhaps the study on *Hamlet,* a play such as *Emperor Jones,* and then I had called Jones the King or the Emperor of the English analysts. . . . I liked Ernest Jones, but this comparison itself shows some latent hostility . . . why? Jealousy of the older and superior man? The green-eyed monster? . . . That is from *Othello* . . . The Moor of Venice. . . . Again the Negroes.

I am turning to the following associations. They are, of course, all names—names from the Bible. I must have thought first of Negroes, then of Jews as the patient associated them together in his remark. But each of those names must have its unconscious determination and must have meant something definite in my thoughts. . . . Even their sequence must have a meaning and some psychological significance. . . . I must find why each of them occurred to me. . . . Is there something they have in common besides their being biblical names? . . . The initial sound, the first syllable. . . . Are they only "sound associations," that means thoughts determined by *Klang,* as the German would say, joined together by the same sound at the beginning of the words? This first syllable . . . I remember that the common first syllable Je is perhaps the abbreviated Hebrew word for God. Je means His ineffable name, otherwise known as Jahweh or Jehovah. . . . Does not Jesus mean "God helps" or "Salvation by God"? . . . But I am suspicious of myself, for this first syllable could not have the same significance in Jericho and Jessica. . . . And is it true that Je is always the abbreviated name of the God of the Israelites? I become aware how much I do not know about those things. . . . Over there is the *Encyclopedia of Religion* on my bookcase. I could look up Jehovah and Jericho, but I am too lazy to get up from the couch. Even if I did find what that syllable and each name means, of what importance would that be for the psychological significance of my thoughts? The objective meaning of the names is of no interest, only the meaning I connect with those words is now of consequence. *Jericho* . . . that is, of course, the biblical city. . . . Was I in Jericho when I visited Palestine in 1937? . . . That is nonsense. . . . The ancient city of Jericho does not exist any more.

Suddenly I remember a movie I had seen a few years ago in which a man has the nickname of Jericho. . . . The story of the French film *Les Enfants du Paradis* comes vaguely back to mind. The play takes place in Paris about a hundred years ago. Its milieu is that of the demimonde, theater people, actors, audience, and hangers-on. The leading character is a young man whose misfortunes are presented from the time he acts as a clown to the period when he becomes the celebrated tragedian of the Parisian stage. It is a play of passion and destiny with a tragic ending. There is a girl whom he met in his boyhood and with whom he fell in love. When he meets her later in life, she always eludes him. It is as if a malicious destiny or that incognito traveling fate, called accident, blocks his way whenever he approaches her. Like Romeo, he is a fool of fortune.

Now the face of the actor who has the part of the leading character appears in my memory. A thin, strangely masklike face, unexpressive and unemotional, but with large luminous eyes. The contrast of this lack of facial expression with his emotional experiences lends the personality of the actor a puzzling kind of interest. . . . What was his name? . . . I now remember: Jean-Louis Barrault. It is not incidental that the movie shows him first in a pantomime in which only automaton-like movements and gestures indicate his feelings, while his face does not change at all. The actor's body has the utmost elasticity, while his personality seems rigid, almost frozen. There is a dullness of effect, even in his love of the beautiful girl. No free flow of emotions. A withdrawal from reality and something like a paralysis of will which explains better than external factors why his love object always eludes him or prefers other men, although she is attracted to him. When I saw the film, I got the impression that here was a schizoid type or even a schizophrenic.

At this point I recognized that there were concealed connections between the first subject of my thoughts and their present theme. Did I not think that Bill, my patient, was perhaps schizoid? He spoke of Paris and of plays he had seen there. *Les Enfants du Paradis* takes place in Paris. Bill wants the leading part in a play. His face must have reminded me of Jean-Louis Barrault's.

Jericho is the name of an episodic figure in *Les Enfants du Paradis*. He is an old Jew, doing shady business among theater people, a thief or receiver of stolen goods. I see his crooked nose, his unkempt hair, and his pointed gray beard. This old fence is an acquaintance of the actor during his early Bohemian times. He, surprisingly, appears whenever there is a decisive turn in the destiny of the leading character. He seems to know beforehand what will happen, seems to anticipate the future. Yes, he appears to be omniscient. He warns the hero, yet he sometimes seems to bring about the bad fate of this actor. Is he perhaps omnipotent too? This fence, who cheats, whose business shuns the light, has neither wife nor child, but he likes children. He has another nickname: *"couche seul"*—he sleeps alone.

I do not know how and why I thought that this old Jewish criminal presents the disguised God of the Jews, Jehovah, in a degraded form as he would be seen through anti-Semitic eyes. Is it possible that the script-writer unconsciously shaped in the episodic figure the reduced Jewish god, a malicious demon—a god who is vengeful and deceiving, associated with crooks and thieves?

The anti-Semitic remark of my patient comes back to mind. Negroes and Jews. . . . In the film there is also a Negro. . . . Oh yes, the actor plays the part of a Negro. . . . Of course, he is presented as Othello, the Moor of Venice. . . . There is a scene in which the actor comes into conflict with a high aristocrat, the same man who is his more fortunate rival in the love for the girl. . . . This snobbish character speaks of Shakespeare as an inferior, barbarian playwright who cannot hold a candle to Corneille and Racine. There again appear the threads between my patient's remark and the film. . . . The Negroes and the Jews. . . . Jericho and Othello.

But how does Jephthah come into my train of thoughts? . . . For the life of me, I do not know how the figure of this judge from the Old Testament wandered into my associations. . . . How did just he drift into them? A penny for my thoughts? But even this seems overpaid, because nothing occurs to me . . . Jephthah. . . . Jephthah and his daughter. . . . Did not Jephthah make a vow when he went out to fight the enemies of the Israelites that he would sacrifice the first person he encountered after his victorious return from the battle? And did he not meet his daughter, whom he then had to sacrifice to the cruel god of the Hebrews?

I am trying to reconstruct what I had thought before that. . . . The Negroes and the Jews. . . . The aristocrat who speaks derogatorily of Shakespeare and Othello. . . . Is Jephthah or his daughter perhaps mentioned in *Othello?* . . . For a moment I thought it must be there, but, no, it can't be. . . . There is some memory stirring within me that Jephthah's daughter is mentioned in one of Shakespeare's tragedies. . . . No, not in *Othello.* . . . Perhaps in *The Merchant of Venice?* . . .

I overcome my laziness, I get up from the couch and get the concordance of Shakespeare's work in order to look it up. . . . There it is. . . . Neither in *Othello* nor in *The Merchant of Venice.* . . . (The Moor of Venice and the Merchant of Venice— is this the common element between the plays? Oh no, it must be again the race discrimination. Negroes and Jews, Othello and Shylock.) The passage is in *Hamlet,* says the concordance, Act II, scene 2. . . . Ah, here! Hamlet runs into Polonius and says:

"Oh Jephthah, judge of Israel, what a treasure hadst thou!"
The old courtier asks:
"What a treasure had he, my lord?" and the Prince answers:
"One fair daughter, and no more,
The which he loved passing well."

Polonius, who is convinced that Hamlet's love for Ophelia has driven him crazy, thoughtfully remarks, "Still on my daughter . . ." And Hamlet asks, "Am I not i' the right, old Jephthah?"

thus identifying the pompous old courtier with the biblical judge.

Jephthah—Jephthah's daughter . . . Jessica. . . . Jessica is the daughter of the Jew Shylock. Here then is the connecting link with Jephthah's daughter . . . Jephthah loved his child and had to kill her. Shylock loves his daughter and yet he curses her when she elopes with a good-for-nothing fellow. . . . More than this— he wishes to see her dead at his feet when he learns that she squanders the money for which he has toiled and slaved so long.

I remember having read in the book of some Shakespeare commentator or critic that this trait adds to the repulsive picture of Shylock's character. How could a father wish to see his daughter dead merely because she throws money away? Yet, these good people do not understand that it is the Oriental temper, which still lives in the Jews of late times, which bursts forth in Shylock's rage. . . . Such wishes, as well as Jephthah's vow, are expressions of that excitable temper that flares suddenly up and is often enough followed by intense remorse and severe self-punishment. There are hateful outbreaks against objects very much loved, loved not wisely but too well. . . . Yes, those ancient Jews were afraid of themselves and of the intensity of their passions. They had to protect themselves in their love objects. . . . They were so afraid that they had a solemn religious formula in which they asked God to consider oaths spoken in moments of rage as invalid. They anticipated such outbreaks in themselves, and asked God not to oblige them to keep those vows and to forgive them. That formula or prayer is called Kol Nidre and is recited on the High Holiday, Yom Kippur or the Day of Atonement. In it all such oaths and vows taken in the year just beginning are declared invalid. I published a paper on this subject in my book the *Ritual*.

How did I become interested in the Kol Nidre? I am an infidel Jew. . . . Do I have the same inclination to swear away the life of dear persons when I am very angry? Have I some of that hot temper; do I know such sudden flareups and outbreaks as Shylock's? I suddenly feel the urgent wish to read those scenes in *The Merchant of Venice* where Shylock curses his daughter and wishes to see her dead at his feet.

I had tried first to search below the surface for the meaning of those associations and names. I did not get very far, because as soon as I caught a glimpse of the significance of the names of Jericho, Jephthah, and Jessica, my interest became deflected and turned in a new direction. Investigating those first associations took only a few minutes, and now it was late at night. I wanted to look up some passages in *The Merchant of Venice*. I did that, but then read the whole play again and spent a few hours in thinking about it, daydreaming and pondering about it, following ideas that took me far off. While I read the familiar scenes of Shakespeare's play, I went astray in my thoughts, pursuing fleeting images and impressions. Embryos of ideas, snatches of new thoughts emerged. They were brushed aside, but they recurred and would not let themselves be rejected. These new thoughts all concerned the contrast and conflict of Shylock and Antonio. There was something in the opposition of these two antagonists which I sensed but could not grasp.

This mysterious something transgressed the narrow limitations of the plot about a loan and about a legal argument and counterargument. Something there is unsaid but conveyed. Some concealed meaning is allluded to, but eludes the search of logical and conscious thinking. Shylock and Antonio are, of course, not only this money-lending Jew and that Venetian Merchant, in spite of all individual traits and typical features. They are even more than types, more than the kind and noble Gentile and the malicious son of the old tribe. That intangible and elusive element seems to overlap into an area beyond the individual and the typical. It shatters the frame of the two characters and reaches to the sky. In reading the play, Antonio and Shylock grew in my thoughts to gigantic figures standing against each other silently. I did not know what this transformation meant and I first tried to solve the problem by means of conscious analytic interpretation. It was as if a fisherman casts out a net into the deep sea. He brings something up from the depth, but it is certainly not what he wanted and hoped to get. What he tried to bring up to the surface slipped through the meshes of his net.

I am certainly not the first analyst who interpreted Shylock's terms, namely, the condition that he can cut a pound of flesh "in what part of your body pleaseth me" as a substitute expression of castration. When later on in the play it is decided the cut should be made from the breast, analytic interpretation will easily understand the mechanism of distortion that operates here and displaces the performance from a part of the body below to above. Only one step is needed to reach the concept that to the Gentile of medieval times the Jew unconsciously typified the castrator because he circumcised male children. Circumcision is, as psychoanalytic experiences teach us, conceived as a milder form of castration. The Jew thus appeared to the Gentiles as a dangerous figure with whom the threat of castration originated. Consciously, to Shakespeare and his contemporaries (as to many of our own time), the Jew appears as a money-taking and -grasping figure who takes financial advantage of the Gentiles. Unconsciously, he is the man who threatens to damage them by cutting off the penis. Because his tribe performs the archaic operation of circumcision, the Jew represents an unconscious danger to the masculinity of the Gentiles. The unconscious factor has to be added to the strange features of his different religious rituals, to the unfamiliar dietary customs and the divergent habits of the foreign minority. If Shylock insists upon cutting out a pound of flesh from Antonio's breast, it is as if he demanded that the Gentile be made a Jew if he cannot pay back the three thousand ducats at the fixed time. Otherwise put: Antonio should submit to the religious ritual of circumcision.

The application of the analytic method is really not needed to arrive at this conclusion. It could be easily reached on another route. At the end of the "comedy" Antonio demands that Shylock should "presently become a Christian." If this is the justified amends the Jew has to make for his earlier condition, it would be according to poetic justice that the Jew be forced to become a Christian after he had insisted that his opponent should become a Jew. Such a retaliation corresponds to the oldest law of the world, to the *ius talionis* that demands tooth for tooth, eye for eye.

That bit of insight into the concealed meaning of Shylock's demand remained an isolated and trifling scrap of analytic interpretation until it was blended with other impressions. The first impression concerned the character of Shylock. I remember that

I once talked with Freud about what constitutes that quality we call character. He said that in his opinion character is signified by the predominance of one or a few drives over others. While all the drives are, of course, present and operating, one of them is distinguished and superior in intensity. We say, then, that this person has character, a quality we do not attribute to others in whom all drives seem equally developed. While I read the play, Shylock's thirst for revenge impressed me more than any other feature of the man. At the same time half-forgotten lines from the Holy Scriptures began to sound in my mind, fragmentary sentences, snatches of lines. . . . "The Lord will take vengeance on His adversaries" . . . "They shall see My vengeance . . ." "I will not spare them on the day of vengeance," and others. Yes, the God of the Old Testament is a vindictive God. He has perhaps not only the virtues, but also the vices of the worshipers in whose image He is made.

At a certain moment I was, it seemed, carried away by a fancy or an impression that had gained power over me. It seemed to me that the figure of the God of the Old Testament, Jahweh Himself, looms gigantically behind "the Jew that Shakespeare drew." The mythological figure of the old God reduced to the size of a human creature, diminished and dressed up as a Jewish moneylender? Jahweh, the Lord, who came to earth on the Rialto? But the impression quickly evaporated. It was as if I had, for a moment, seen an apparition in the delusive light of that evening. It reappeared, however, later on.

I then became more interested in another impression that surprised me because it had not been there when I had previously read and seen the play: the lack of characterization of Antonio. If there is a leading character in any Shakespeare play who is less of a personality, is less colorful and less equipped with distinguishing individual traits, I would like to know of it. There is no doubt that Antonio is the leading character. His is the title role of *The Merchant of Venice,* although his opponent steals the show.

What do we know of Antonio? Only that he is kind, loves his friends, is generous to the extent of self-sacrifice and that he is sad. . . . He is kindliness itself, personified. . . . He loves his friends, he wants to give his life for his friends. . . . He is eager to make the supreme self-sacrifice. Greater love hath no man. . . . He not only suffers, he *is* suffering, grief, sorrow themselves. He is sad. Why? Nobody knows, least of all himself. Is this a shortcoming on the part of the greatest playwright of the world or is there something hidden here, unknown even to the Bard?

The play opens with Antonio's entrance and these are his first lines:

> In sooth, I know not why I am so sad:
> It wearies me; you say it wearies you;
> But how I caught it, found it, came by it,
> What stuff 'tis made of, whereof it is born,
> I am to learn;
> And such a want-wit sadness makes of me,
> That I have much ado to know myself.

His friends try in vain to explain his sadness, but he denies that he thinks of his merchandise at sea and answers with a sad "Fie, Fie" when Salarino suspects that he could be in love. He is, to all appearances, sad without reason. I now remember that I have read in the book of a Shakespeare commentator that Antonio has "the spleen." It seems to me that this concept is too British. . . . While I still ponder over Antonio's mysterious sadness, a line runs through my mind. "He was despised and rejected of men, a man of sorrows and acquainted with grief." And then: "He hath borne our griefs and carried our sorrows." . . . But those are passages from the Holy Scripture! . . . How do they now emerge? It occurs to me where and when I heard them last. A friend let me have the records of Handel's *Messiah* a few days ago.

In Act IV, Antonio says:

> I am a tainted wether of the flock,
> Meetest for death.

Actually, he does not awaken interest and sympathy by the person he is, but by what happens to him; not by his personality, but by his destiny. He is, he says, a tainted wether of the flock, destined to die. He is, rather, a lamb. . . . From somewhere the phrase *"Agnus Dei qui tollit peccata mundi"* comes to mind. Is this not from the Vulgate, the translation of the New Testament? Immediately a passage from the *Messiah* emerges, the passage of "the Lamb of God that taketh away the sins of the world."

Antonio's sadness . . . the man of sorrow . . . the Lamb of God . . . destined to die. . . . He was wounded for our transgressions. . . . He was bruised for our iniquities. . . . The scene before the court at Venice. . . . The readiness to die for others. . . . Did He not state, "Greater love has no man than this that a man lay down his life for his friend"? . . . No, I am not the victim of a delusion. Behind the figure of Antonio is the greater one of Jesus Christ. Again the motif "He was despised and rejected" emerges as if the tune wants to confirm my thought, as if the line from the *Messiah* announced that my concept is correct.

Again there is the image of Antonio and Shylock standing opposite each other, the one all charity and the other no charity at all. . . . I know now clearly what was in the background of my mind while I read the play, what were the vague impressions that crowded upon me until they became condensed into one leading thought. I am turning the leaves of the volume, and my glance chances upon the lines of Shylock in Act I, where he speaks directly to the noble Venetian merchant:

> Signior Antonio, many a time and oft
> In the Rialto you have rated me
> About my money and my usances.
> Still I have borne it with a patient shrug,
> For sufferance is the badge of our tribe.
> You call me misbeliever, cut-throat dog,
> And spat upon my Jewish gaberdine,
> And all for use of that which is mine own . . .

Here is one of the few occasions in which Antonio shows temperament and hate in contrast to his otherwise gentle and weak attitude. . . . Not a trace of charity and loving-kindness here. Not very Christian, as a matter of fact. This seems to contradict my concept that behind the Gentile merchant the figure of his God is concealed.

But then it occurs to me that this feature does not contradict my thesis. It rather confirms it. Did He not go up to Jerusalem when Passover was at hand and abuse and whip the money-changers and drive them all out of the temple? Did He not pour out their money and overthrow their tables? Behind the treatment Shylock gets from Antonio the features of the primal pattern of the Holy Scripture become apparent.

I do not doubt any more that behind Antonio and Shylock are hidden the great figures of their gods. Here are two small people in Venice, but the shadows they cast are gigantic and their conflict shakes the world. There is the vengeful and zealous God of the Old Testament and the milder Son-God of the Gospels who rebelled against His father, suffered death for His revolt, and became God Himself, afterwards. The two Gods are presented and represented in this play by two of their typical worshipers of the playwright's time.

Shakespeare wanted to present a Jewish figure as he and his contemporaries saw it, but the character grew beyond human measure into the realm of the mythical, as if the God of the Jews stood behind the stage. Shakespeare wanted to shape the destiny of a Gentile merchant who almost became the victim of a vengeful, evil Jew, but the unconscious imagination of this writer shattered the thin frame of his plot. The myth-forming fantasy of this man William Shakespeare, his *imagination complète,* as Taine says, reached so much farther than his conscious mind. It reached beyond the thoughts and designs known to him, into the region where the great myths and religious legends of the people are born and bred. He wanted only to write a comedy with a plot about the curious case of a Jew who was outjewed. Unconscious memory-traces made him shape the conflict of the two Gods, the holy story as he had absorbed it as a boy. Invisible threads connect *The Merchant of Venice* with the medieval passion plays.

He took the two plots from many sources, the story of the three caskets and the tale of the merchant who got a rough deal from a malicious Jew, and alloyed them into a play. Thus William saw the Jews as the Toms, Dicks, and Harrys of his time saw them, despised them, and mocked them, and hated them. But something greater than his conscious thought gave that Jew a voice of his own, a rancorous voice that speaks in icy sarcasm, biting and accusing, a voice full of sound and fury, rising in passionate protest and ebbing in utter despair. The creative and re-creative imagination of this man Shakespeare poured into the trivial plot of the three thousand ducats something of the stuff the great myths of people, the dreams of mankind, are made on. He added the figure of Antonio, who was to be cut and mutilated, to the mythical figures of Attis, Adonis, and Jesus Christ, who were torn to pieces. Only small inconspicuous traits, little features overlooked and neglected, invisible or only visible under the microscope of psychoanalytic scrutiny, reveal that behind the trivial figures of the comedy are hidden Jehovah and Jesus, that the real *personae dramatis* are overdimensional.

In the battles between the Danai and the Trojans, as Homer describes them, the gods of Olympus fought in the skies above the heads of the combatants. In the fight between the Gentiles of Venice and the Jew Shylock, the greatest conflict of the world is presented in a courtroom scene. I am toying with the plan to publish this new concept. Perhaps in a literary magazine. . . . And why not in a psychoanalytic journal since it is the result of psychological evaluation of small inconspicuous traits in the classical manner of analytic observation of trifles? . . . Perhaps I should entitle the paper with the sentence *"Et hic dei sunt."* Also here are gods.

When I arrived at this concept—or should I say rather when this concept arrived at me?—I felt that glow of thought known to all explorers who first recognize a secret connection, that burning felicity of discovery. It was, to be sure, only a small thing, a trifling contribution to the interpretation of a Shakespearean play, only a little bit of a new construction, yet . . . The inscription I had often seen on old Austrian cottages, when I was a boy, occurred to me: *"Klein, aber mein."* (Small, but my own.)

It is, I thought, only a trifle of an idea, but it is original. And then came the doubt as to its originality. I had the feeling that I had had this very thought before, a long time ago. . . . Yet, I knew it had occurred now, when I reread *The Merchant of Venice.* . . . Is there a phenomenon analogous to the sensation of *déjà vu* in the area of thinking, a feeling of *déjà pensé?* . . . Perhaps I read it once and have forgotten it, and now I think of it as an original idea of my own. . . . I am trying to remember what various critics and historians of literature wrote on *The Merchant of Venice*. . . . No, there is nothing comparable to my concept. . . . Yet, I know this thought from somewhere. . . . When it occurred to me, I nodded, so to speak, to it as you do to all old acquaintances whom you run into on the street and whom you have not seen for many years.

When did I first see *The Merchant of Venice?* It was when I was sixteen or seventeen years old, in Vienna. . . . Wait! I admonished myself. Let me think. . . . I have forgotten who acted —a thin man with an iron-gray wisp of beard, a dark gaberdine, and the little black cap of the orthodox Jew. His too vivid gestures and his expressive voice that ran the gamut from cold logic to embittered passion and spoke the verse of Shakespeare with a Yiddish modulation which was not at all ridiculous. . . . That was in 1904 or 1905.

The play occupied my thoughts for a long time. . . . I was a boy, and another still younger boy lived in Vienna then whose name was Adolf Hitler. . . . At this time, when I was sixteen, I did not love Shakespeare, but Heinrich Heine. . . . By God, Heine. . . . That is it. . . . I read then the splendid prose of Heine, and among his writings the paper *Gods in Exile*. In this essay the writer imagines that the ancient gods of the Greeks did not perish when Christ triumphed and conquered the world. They became refugees and left their country. They immigrated, went underground. They disguised themselves and lived anonymously in exile a pitiful or comfortable life. They tried to get jobs, incognito, of course. They drank beer instead of nectar. Apollo, who had once led the cows of Admetos to pasture, became a shepherd in Lower Austria; Mars became a soldier, and Mercury a Dutch merchant who was quite prosperous. Bacchus became Father Superior of a monastery. . . . I must have read that very picturesque fantasy of the vicissitudes of the ancient Greek gods before or at the time when I first saw *The Merchant of Venice* in the Burgtheater. . . . Sometime and somewhere the memory of those pages of Heine's *Gods in Exile* must have merged with vague ideas and impressions about the figures of Antonio and Shylock. . . . The two thoughts met and coalesced. The result of their mixture was the concept, then only dimly perceived, that Shylock and Antonio, too, are disguised figures of gods, reduced to very human size, reappearing in the earthly shape of a noble Venetian merchant and of an old vengeful Jew. . . . This paper by Heine, therefore, is the birthplace or the source of my "original" concept or, at least, it stimulated its genesis. Yes, Heinrich Heine. . . . I suddenly remember that the same great German writer wrote another short essay on Shakespeare's "Maiden and Women." . . . I had, of course, read this paper too, perhaps about the same time I read "Gods in Exile." The coincidence facilitated perhaps the meeting of the two thoughts in my mind after the performance of *The Merchant of Venice.*

I walk over to my bookcase and I take the volume of Heine's collected works. Here is the essay on Shakespeare's women . . . and here are the passages on Jessica. I begin to read and again I am under the spell of Heine's magnificent diction as I once was when I was a boy.

Heine writes about a performance of *The Merchant of Venice:* "When I saw this play at Drury Lane, there stood behind in the box a pale, fair Briton who at the end of the Fourth Act fell a-weeping passionately, several times exclaiming, 'The poor man is wronged!' " The poet thinks of this lady when he visits Venice later on: "Wondering dream-hunter that I am, I looked around everywhere on the Rialto to see if I could find Shylock . . . But I found him nowhere on the Rialto, and I determined to seek my old acquaintance in the Synagogue. The Jews were then celebrating their Day of Atonement. . . . Although I looked all around the Synagogue, I nowhere discovered the face of Shylock. I saw him not. But toward evening, when, according to Jewish belief, the gates of heaven are shut and no prayer can then obtain admission, I heard a voice, with a ripple of tears that never were wept by eyes. It was a sob that could come only from a breast that held in it all martyrdom which for eighteen centuries had been borne by a whole tortured people. It was the death rattle of a soul sinking down dead-tired at heaven's gate, and I seemed to know the voice and I felt that I had heard it long ago; in utter despair, it moaned out, then as now, 'Jessica, my child!' "

In these lines, written more than one hundred years ago, Heine has touched the most vulnerable spot of Shakespeare's Shylock. The picture of the old man who has broken down and moans, "Jessica, my child" has the gloomy grandeur of the biblical paintings of Rembrandt.

It is strange that Heine has so little to say about Jessica with whose personality this piece should deal. She is for him just a pleasure-seeking, egocentric female. But he had quite a few things to say about those Venetian young men who are friends of the noble Antonio. He sees them with a critical eye and he is right in looking down on them. Bassanio is a fortunehunter who adds debts to debts to make a luxurious trip, and who does not hesitate to risk the life of his best friend in order to impress Portia by his elegance. How low can you get? There is Lorenzo who elopes with Jessica and lives on the money and jewels she has taken from her father, lives sumptuously, throwing Shylock's money around. There are those other playboys, irresponsible, flippant, crude and conceited, shallow and out for fun only—such charming people!

Is Shylock not right when he looks down upon those noble Venetian young gentlemen and speaks aside:

> These be the Christian husbands. I have a daughter—
> Would any of the stock of Barrabas
> Had been her husband rather than a Christian!

I have two daughters and, considering these young noblemen, I feel as he does. . . .

And Jessica falls in love with one of those guys who talks big and is an empty shell. He will be fed up with her very soon, will soon throw her over, and will look down on her because she is Jewish. And the girl herself? She is ashamed of her father, calls herself daughter of his blood, not of his heart. She robs him and leaves him alone and in despair. Farewell, she says:

> And if my fortune be not crost,
> I have a father, you a daughter, lost.

I begin to wonder how I came to all these thoughts and I am curious. How did I arrive from thinking of an alcoholic patient to an analytic contribution to Shakespeare's play? I fail to recognize any connections in my associations. . . . It is really puzzling, and I would like to find out on which ways my train of thought wandered. I want to discover the truth about them, and about myself, the truth, fair or foul. . . .

I first remembered the remark of my patient Bill, who is a playboy and drunkard, about Negroes and Jews. Then only words came when I was half asleep. Only names: *Jones, Jericho, Jephthah, Jessica, Jehovah, Jesus.* . . . Oh yes, there were thought-connections: Emperor Jones, Jericho, that Jewish peddler in the film, who appeared to me as a kind of degraded Jehovah, Jephthah, who had to sacrifice his own daughter, Jessica, the daughter of Shylock. And then Shylock himself as a human representative of the God of the Jews, reduced and despised in his earthly shape, and Antonio, a small-sized edition of the Nazarene. . . . The trial as a miniature of the great conflict of the old and the new God . . . "Gods in Exile" . . . Heine . . . and Heine's words about Shylock and Jessica.

But what was there before I thought of that patient and of his anti-Semitic remark? . . . Nothing occurs to me. . . . There is a blank. I think only that I am very tired and that I should go to bed. . . . It is long after midnight. Thody is not home yet . . . Thody . . .

All of a sudden I recognize with full clarity where the whole train of thought started and why it took this direction and what it means. I am amazed, and it is at this point that I repeat wholeheartedly that sentence of my patient, "Our mind is an insult to our intelligence."

When Thody came into the room to say good night and went out for a date, I must have thought some uncomfortable thoughts. I brushed them aside and tried to run away from them. I turned my attention to the analytic sessions of the day and thus arrived at the thought of my patient and his remark about Negroes and Jews. . . . It started there and now all comes back to me, also the thoughts I tried to escape from. . . . Thody's date must have awakened a dormant fear that she could get infatuated or even fall in love with one of those worthless New York playboys, one of the ilk to which my patient Bill or Lorenzo in *The Merchant of Venice* belongs. It occurred to me that she will be eighteen

years old next year and that she could take the funds I saved for
her education and for which I toiled and worked so hard so many
years. She could elope with just such an immature young fellow
and give him her money. . . . She could elope as Jessica did . . .
and the young ne'er-do-well would use her and the money and
would shortly afterwards throw her over and abuse her.

I know, of course, that none of those fears is justified. Thody
is not infatuated with any boy and, even if she were, she is quite
intelligent and, although she is temperamental and impulsive, she
has a lot of common sense. How do I come to have such vain
fears and nonsensical thoughts? They must have originated in
fleeting impressions I have received lately. The other day Thody
expressed her discontent with our very modest apartment. She
seems to be ashamed of it and hesitates to invite her girl friends
to her house. She is sometimes impatient with my old-fashioned
views, and—who knows?—perhaps she is somewhat ashamed of me.
She is also dissatisfied with me, it seems, because I am always
working and I do not explain things to her that she wants to
know. The other day, when I had no time to explain some psychological terms, she said angrily, "I could just as well be a shoemaker's daughter." She is dissatisfied with her home, its atmosphere, and also in other directions. . . . And girls in such moods
are sometimes tempted to elope with the first boy with whom they
get infatuated.

But this is nonsense, idle fancy, and vain fears! . . . I am not
Shylock and my daughter is not Jessica. . . . Even if she should
want someday to elope with such a playboy and give him the
money I saved for her college education, I mused, what could I,
an old codger, do? . . . Have I the right to do anything? . . .
You cannot teach another human being how to live . . . not
even your own child. . . . Perhaps especially not your own child.

It is strange how the idea, or the fear, I ran away from followed
me. I tried to escape from it and it pursued me. In my associations
I went off on a tangent and was led to the center of the problem
that unconsciously preoccupied me. My alcoholic patient took in
my thoughts the place of the imaginary playboy who is the future
suitor of Thody. From there I drifted into speculations on Shylock, Jessica, and Antonio and then went into a psychological

analysis of the secret background of *The Merchant of Venice,* of the second concealed compartment of the play.

How did I come to the new idea? Certainly not by conscious logical conclusions. If there were any, they followed the concept I had already reached. It was an intuitive insight that suddenly emerged. . . . Out of the nowhere into the here. . . . But such intuition is only the sudden perception of an earlier intellectual experience which had remained unconscious and surprisingly reached the threshold of conscious thinking with the help of new impressions. Could I not later on remember some parts of those old thoughts, recognize in retrospect the raw material out of which the new concept was made?

Looking back at the process, I still wonder how the thought about my patient suddenly turned to those names: *Jones, Jericho, Jephthah, Jehovah, Jesus.* Chaotic and yet following their hidden laws, my associations arrived by a detour at their destination. There is a psychological resemblance between this disjointed way of thinking and the "flight of ideas," to be found in manic states and in the "word salad" of the schizophrenics. The pathological flight of ideas is perhaps also not a flight toward certain things, but a flight away from a pursuing idea. The old German expression *Ideen-Jagd* is more appropriate. From casually progressing associations, my thoughts increased their tempo, began to chase each other. It was as if they first were comfortably pacing and suddenly went into a gallop, like a horse that shies away from its own shadow. Then they changed their pace again when I drifted into those thoughts on Shakespeare's characters. I really reached the phase of objective study, and the origin of my thoughts, their personal sources, were forgotten or submerged. Here is an alloy of aim-directed logical and rational thinking and hidden irrational and emotional thoughts directed by unconscious drives. As far as I know, psychiatry has no name for such composite processes, which are logically progressing but governed by invisible emotions and forces.

While I thus reviewed my own mental process, I felt no emotion except the curiosity of the psychological observer. I asked myself: Did I feel any emotion during the whole process? Oh yes, there was this moment of glow when I discovered traces of the old myth in the plot of *The Merchant of Venice,* but nothing else. Even when I reread the play, there was no strong emotion. Nothing of the cathartic effect Aristotle recognized, no purification of emotions through fear and pity.

But that impression must have been self-deceiving. I grinned to myself ironically: this is certainly not a deep observation. Nothing penetrating about it. . . . Of course, there must have been emotions that directed the course of my thoughts. There was, no doubt, jealousy of my daughter, also possessiveness, fury against the unknown young man who will take her away from me. I sense how intense the rage and revengefulness against that imaginary young man must have been, because it emerged in the substitution displacement of the trial scene between Shylock and Antonio, in the Jew's insistence on cutting a pound of flesh from his opponent. Also an intense anger against my daughter can easily be conjectured, because the thought of Jephthah appeared. The scene in which Shylock wishes to see his disloyal daughter dead at his feet was vividly recalled. There were, I am sure, also love for my daughter and the awareness of my helplessness, if and when a certain situation might endanger her safety, and quite a few other emotions.

But all of them are only suggested by psychological reasoning. All this is only theoretical insight. I don't feel any of those emotions. They are only guessed and not experienced.

But then, all of a sudden, I know that they are there because I hear my own voice moaning, "Thody, my child!"

4

On the little table beside my bed are a few books (I have kept since my childhood the bad habit of reading in bed), amongst them *Anatole France en Pantoufles* and *Itinéraire de Paris à Buenos Aires* by Jean Jacques Brousson and *Conversations avec Anatole France* by Nicolas Ségur. I had read them when they were first published, shortly after France's death, but I return to them, from time to time, because of my love for the old Sage of the Villa

Said, for his melancholic wisdom and his critical intelligence, his lucidity and his subtle wit. He really lived without illusions, and yet knew that living without them is impossible. He was at a certain time the most celebrated writer of the world, surrounded by admirers, loved by beautiful women, honored by the intellectual elite of his era. Yet he confided to J. J. Brousson that he had not been happy a single hour of his life. He asserted that only the poor in mind are happy; that he himself lacked the wonderful gift of self-deception and that he had always felt *"les mélancholies de l'intelligence."*

Why is it that reading books by Anatole France makes me serene, quiets and consoles me? It cannot be only his magnificent style, his wisdom or his wit which affect the reader in this manner. Something of his personality, of his voice that comes through the lines, gives relief and relaxation, removes the *Erdenschwere,* as Goethe would put it, alleviates the oppression of living on this planet. To show that every human relation and institution is transitory and founded on illusions is in itself a triumph of a melancholic mind over the shabby and unsatisfactory matter.

Turning over the pages of the three books out of which the voice of old, wise, and witty Anatole France speaks, reading some paragraphs here and there, I chanced upon two anecdotes that brought my thoughts back to analytic sessions of the same day. The two anecdotes which the old master recounts appeared suddenly like analogies or counterparts of certain situations whose detailed report I had heard only a few hours before in analytic sessions with a woman and with a man patient.

Jane is a young widow with two children. As a very young girl she had fallen in love with a man more than ten years older than herself. The gentle, scholarly man began to pay attention to her and wanted to marry her. Overcoming the resistance of his family to his marriage with a girl who was so much younger and comparatively poor, the couple got married and lived happily ever after. It was for the girl as if a fairy tale had become real. Living in comfortable, later on even in wealthy circumstances, the two people who shared many interests found satisfaction in each other's company and realization of their hopes in their life together. They enjoyed their social as well as their sexual life for ten years. This

happy time came to its end when the husband became ill. The diagnosis of the physicians was brain tumor. The husband died soon
afterwards, and the young widow whose happiness had been
broken off so suddenly was inconsolable. A few weeks after his
death she found among his papers, which she had to examine for
some legal purpose, a concealed bundle of notes, diaries, and photographs dating from the last years. These papers left no doubt
that her adored husband had lived a double life, had had many
affairs, including a long one with her best friend, and had also
indulged in certain perversions during those years of their marriage which had been sexually very satisfactory. The young widow
was deeply shocked. She tried to master her indignation and confusion, but she suffered from depression and insomnia and became
emotionally ill. She tried in vain to find diversion in journeys,
theaters, and so on. Her thoughts invariably returned to the
shocking discovery she had made.

In the analytic session of that afternoon she had told me of an
incident that had taken place shortly after her husband's death a
few years before. A terrible forest fire had broken out near the city
in which she lived. It destroyed whole villages and left hundreds
of families homeless and destitute. The young widow drove
around in her car with food, clothes, and money and did all she
could to help these people. In touring the devastated places while
the fire was still raging nearby, she was stopped at one point by a
young State Trooper who warned her that bands of loiterers made
the villages and roads unsafe. The officer offered to accompany the
young lady on her tour in the neighborhood to protect her. She
accepted, and they drove together along the forests. After a few
hours the young State Trooper made a timid pass at her. She
quickly yielded to him and they had sexual intercourse the same
evening on the border of the blazing forest. The sudden surrender
of the well-bred woman to the unknown officer only a few weeks
after her husband's death was certainly determined in part by her
emotional reaction to the deeply disappointing discovery of her
husband's infidelity. She told me that the sight of the tumult and
riot of nature, of the forest in flames, had sexually excited her. It
was as if the elementary forces around her reflected the emotions
she herself experienced.

Nicolas Ségur in his book of memories gives a lively report of one of the evenings at the salon of Madame de Cavaillet at the Avenue Hoche. There were many guests, among them Anatole France, who was always in the center. The topic of conversation was China and the Yellow Peril, and the old master commented on the subject in his usual ironic and brilliant manner. The gracious mistress of the house asked him to tell a certain Chinese story. He protested, asserted that everybody knew it, but finally obeyed the soft command of Madame.

The place of the story is a cemetery in China. In the middle of this locality a charming young woman is seen as she is bending over a grave, ceaselessly waving her paper fan over the freshly turned mold. A student of philosophy, coming by chance upon the strange sight, stops and addresses the lady in the most polite and respectful manner, asking her what she is doing there. He explains that it is not idle curiosity that makes him ask this question, but that he is a philosopher, eager to inquire into the causes and effects of things, and he would like to make an entry concerning her activity in the little scroll of paper he always carries in his girdle. The lady just glances at him and stammers a few unintelligible words while she continues to fan the grave. The woman servant standing beside her bows to the philosopher and speaks to him. She explains that the young lady at the grave is the widow of a great mandarin who had died a few days before. Her love for her husband had been equaled only by his for her. He had been inconsolable when he realized that he had to die. His wife called heaven and earth to witness that she could not survive him. She vowed that she would die, too, when his soul left his body, that she would shut herself up in a convent of Buddhist nuns, that she would never marry again or even look at another man for the rest of her days.

The dying husband assured her that he did not wish her to bind herself by any such vows. He merely asked her not to forget him till the earth on his grave was dry. She, of course, took this oath. Her grief after his death was so great that it almost killed her. She shut herself up in her house, wept and wept and could not be consoled in her mourning. She would, no doubt, have still been weeping, had not the dead man's youngest pupil come the next day to express his condolence and sympathy. He had talked at length about her husband's excellent qualities, but then he had talked about herself and himself. He told her that he loved her and that he could not live without her. He informed her that he would come again soon to see her. He was very handsome, well proportioned, and well spoken, and the young widow was greatly impressed by his appearance and his fine manners. It is for this reason, the servant explains, that her mistress spends her time fanning the earth on her husband's grave with her fan. "It behooves her," she adds, "to lose no time in drying it, else there might be some risk that she might break her vows."

The threads running from this anecdote to the report of my patient of the same day are obvious: the great love of the woman for her husband, the deep grief after his death, the turning to another man after a short time. The accompanying melancholic tune was composed by Verdi: *"La donna è mobile."*

My thoughts, however, were not directed to this eternal and always actual theme. They went off on an analytic tangent, to the significance and the contrast of fire and water in the two stories. The two elements have, of course, only a marginal part in the report of my patient and in the Chinese anecdote. The forest fire in its grandiose power represents, as it were, only a mirror or a mirage in which the concealed desires of the young widow are reflected. In the mixture of the still painful disappointment with her husband and of the sexual desires suppressed since his death, the sight of the flames around her play only a subsidiary role. Their uproar corresponds to the power of this desire breaking through all barriers. The sexual wishes of the young State Trooper, soon perceived by her, flash across to her and set her own lingering desires ablaze. The uproar of nature puts a model to her. The sensual excitement of the officer beside her adds fuel to her own fire smoldering under the ashes.

One can scarcely speak of an unconscious symbolic significance of the forest fire in this case. The poets use expressions like flames of passion, burning desire, and so on, but in her report of the incident it appears rather as if this metaphor has returned to the place of its origin.

But how about the other case? There is certainly a symbolical significance in the condition of the dying husband that his widow should think of him till the earth on his grave is dry. The earth as a symbol of the female body was not discovered by psychoanalysis; man had been aware of it many thousand years before Freud, who found it only again in the dream. ("Mother Earth," the Earth goddesses in Chinese, Babylonian, and other mythologies.)

If the earth is unconsciously a symbol for the female body, the new vow the dying Mandarin demands from his wife can have only the significance: I expect that you will be faithful to me at least till the lubrication from sexual intercourse with me has dried up. The grave in which he rests is thus compared with the living body of the woman, and the humidity of the earth upon it with the lubricated quality of her vagina. The other possible interpretation would be that the humidity is put equal to that caused by the man's semen. The concealed significance of the vow the dying man demands would thus be: I want you to be faithful to me till my semen in your body has dried up.

It is interesting that the opposite elements of fire and water have a sexual significance in the report of my patient and in the Chinese story. Fire represents the passionate, as it were the masculine quality of sexual desire, here in a woman. In the anecdote of the cemetery in China the feminine side is emphasized. The lady should wait until the living traces of her husband's sexual desire have vanished from her body.

In both cases the sexual wishes of a younger man awakened the dormant desires of the widow soon after the beloved husband's death. It is, however, not accidental that the shock and indignation about the deceased's infidelity facilitated the sexual breakthrough of my patient, while the Chinese lady had only to deal with what she considered the demands of respect and decency to the ghost of her spouse. The thought of the sexual trends of the husband to which those papers bore such shocking witness helped to kindle the fire in the young widow. The masculine note is here apparent in the urgency, immediateness, and suddenness of the emergent sexual desire. The Chinese woman is not less eager to forget her dead husband, but her more feminine nature endeavors to obliterate the memory of his love before she yields to the wishes of her new suitors. The contrast of fire and water represents the difference of a more masculine and feminine quality in the sexuality of the two women. It is the same differentiation which seven centuries ago St. Francis of Assisi expressed in that hymn: "Praised be my Lord for our brother Fire" and "Praised be my Lord for our sister Water."

The comparison between the two stories was, of course, stimulated by the similarity of the situation of the two young widows, but the interest of the psychoanalyst was more concerned with the contrast of fire and water on the margin of the stories, so to speak, with the stage set of the show.

The other case to which my thoughts returned, stimulated by another passage in a book of memories of Anatole France, had quite a different character, and, accordingly, my attention followed another direction. The young lawyer I had seen at noon of that day had had what is popularly called a nervous breakdown a few years before and had spent a long time in a psychiatric hospital. He had been treated with electric shocks, and his doubts and fears had disappeared for a short time under the influence of this "therapy." He had adjusted himself to the routine life at the hospital, in which he felt safe. Until his doubts reappeared, he had been able to do some work in the office of the hospital's manager. Such temporary adaptation to the isolated area of the hospital, and a relative feeling of security as long as the retreat from society lasts, is not rare with patients of this kind. Robinson Crusoe was neither shy nor afraid of people as long as he was on his island.

The chief psychiatrist recommended psychotherapy to the patient. His long and careful psychoanalysis with me led to a full success. His main neurotic symptoms disappeared. He regained his self-confidence, mastered certain character difficulties, and began to work. During analysis he had fallen in love with a girl whom he married at its end and who proved to be a good mate. The patient decided not to return to his law practice. He bought a farm not far away from New York and raised poultry, doing some real-estate business on the side.

From time to time, perhaps once a month, he came to New York and saw me for an hour to discuss some actual emotional difficulties. They were, however, never very serious and could be conquered without great efforts. Also, in the session of this noon, he had given me an almost humoristic report of some obsessional doubts he had experienced in the past weeks, faint echoes of the serious obsessions that had been all-pervasive and had governed his life before psychoanalysis.

Most of those doubts originated in everyday situations in which he felt uncertainty. He had, for instance, an appointment with a lawyer about some real-estate business. While he waited until the lawyer had finished a conference with another client, he had felt an urgent need to move his bowels. Should he go to the toilet and let the lawyer, who would perhaps be free in a few minutes, wait? What would the lawyer think of him when he was absent? The very busy man would perhaps call in one of the other clients waiting for him. After that he might have another appointment or even leave the office. In this case my patient's business affair could not be taken care of on this day, and he would have to drive from his farm to the village another day, and by the delay lose precious time much needed for his work with the poultry. After he had tentatively decided to visit the toilet (in these rural surroundings, an outhouse), he remembered from previous occasions that there was never toilet paper around. Unfortunately, he had thrown away the local newspaper which had come in handy on previous occasions. Should he now ask one of the clients waiting at the office to let him have a section of the newspaper he was reading? But there was no possibility of returning it after it had been used the way he intended to. (He laughingly added that it was the only way it deserved to be used.) Asking the lawyer's secretary for some paper was excluded for several reasons. Modesty forbade that he tell the young girl the purpose for which he needed the paper. What would the young woman think if he whispered his delicate request into her blushing ear? No doubt, she would be severely shocked. But could he use a pretext and ask her for some paper to write a letter during the time of his waiting? Here he was uncomfortably reminded by unpleasant sensations within himself that he had hardly time to wait any more. There was, furthermore, the possibility that the girl would give him a single sheet, and this would not do. He could not ask for several sheets, yet, he needed perhaps as many as her boss might use for the first draft of a legal brief. (At this point, the patient's low opinion of the lawyer becomes very obvious in the displacement.) Wouldn't the secretary mind letting him have several sheets of the expensive office stationery? And would it not be conspicuous if, after receiving the saving sheets, he should get up from his chair and disappear without explanation, instead of writing a letter as he was expected to do?

The patient and I laughed together when he gave me this vivid report of the emergency situation. I could not help smiling when he told me of a minor dilemma in which he had found himself a few days before: It was early in the evening and he had fed only part of the chickens, of which he had several thousands on his farm. Just when he turned to the other, large group of birds, his young wife called to him that dinner was ready. What should he do now? Mary did not like to wait for him for dinner. If he continued to feed the chickens, she would be annoyed, she would resent his letting the steak get cold. If he asked her to wait until he had finished his work—perhaps more than half an hour—she would be hurt. But if he interrupted the feeding and followed her call and had dinner then, wouldn't he hurt the feelings of the several hundred chickens that had not yet been fed while the other members of their community had had their meals? He saw himself in a difficult situation, caught in a dilemma and unable to decide what was the right thing to do.

Reporting these instances of the problems which occupied the patient's thoughts and which he recounted that day, I wished to show the kind of minor obsessional thoughts that remained as remnants of the severe neurosis that had kept him in the hospital for two years. In these doubts and dilemmas are, of course, reflected the great problems of his life. They represent displaced details and trifles, his vital interests as in a diminishing glass. In the state of tapering off, those symptoms cannot be compared with regard to their scope and importance to those before analysis. Hit by his intense drives from one side and by his social and inner demands from the other, his ego had been helpless at that time, clinging to the ropes like a punchdrunk boxer, while he now put up an energetic and brave defense against the fleeting and obsessional thoughts that occasionally bothered him.

The patient had broken down or, as he put it, had a "blackout," when he could not solve his sexual problem. Brought up in an extremely Puritan family of a southern state, he had a furious and desperate fight against the temptation of masturbation in his puberty years. He had then been convinced that masturbation was not only sinful but also extremely dangerous and that one could become "crazy" by indulging in it. When, in his early and late twenties, sexual desires appeared in their full power, he renewed his fight with all the energy at his disposal. Too shy and too moralistic to approach women with sexual intentions, he fought with the sensual wishes that attacked him as desperately as any of the Christian saints of the fourth century in the Thebais of Alexandria. In the time before his mental breakdown, he sometimes yielded to the terrible temptation to masturbate. He found an ingenious way to rationalize and justify these occasional indulgences. He had read many books on sexuality, also on the danger or innocence of sexual gratification. While his intelligence told him that there is a biological necessity of sexual expression, his emotions were "agin it." When the desire overwhelmed him, he used the following rationalization: He would experiment with his sexual drive and find out whether masturbation was permitted if he performed it only to relieve his nervous tension without allowing himself to get any pleasure from it. Being a lawyer, he applied a legal term in his thoughts to the procedure. He thought: I have to yield to the temptation, but I shall withhold my consent. He referred, thus, to certain legal cases in which a person is not responsible for a criminal deed if there is no "intent" of it.

He masturbated but withheld his consent, and this experiment in thoughts worked for a short time. As was unavoidable, serious doubts about the legitimacy of his experimentation caught up with the procedure, and his rationalization threatened to break down. He often had to interrupt his sexual activity and to investigate whether he was now merely experimenting or felt pleasure, whether he really only wanted to get rid of the physical tension or whether he also enjoyed the process. In the long run, it became impossible to maintain the conviction that he withheld his consent. Even when he succeeded in overcoming the interfering thoughts and in reaching a sexual orgasm, he was terrified later on at the thought that he had enjoyed masturbation. He frequently brooded about whether he had withheld his consent during the whole act or only at its beginning, whether he had been still experimenting at this or that point of his excitement or had already felt pleasure, yes, even whether he really handled the problem from a strictly legal point of view or not, and so on. From here he arrived at re· flections about certain cases he had studied in his law practice and at doubts as to how far a person is legally responsible if he with· holds his consent, etc. Most of his obsessional doubts at the time circled around the problem of how much of a single masturbatory act could be attributed to the purpose of experimentation and how much to the aim to get pleasure from it. In pursuing these se· rious questions, he often found himself in a mental blind alley. At a certain point of his obsessional thinking, the world appeared to him like an alien place. He did not know any more where he was and lost the feeling of his identity. This was the "blackout" that landed him in the psychiatric hospital.

While I read the books reporting conversations with the late Anatole France, my thoughts returned twice to the patient I had seen this noon. Nicolas Ségur reports in a passage of his memories that the *"bon maître"* once made the statement that Christianity does not oppose the sexual act in itself, but only the pleasure con· nected with it or in it. Christian morals are, he asserts, not against sexual activity as such, but they condemn its enjoyments. He quotes many instances from theology and from the history of the Church and her saints in which the performance of the sexual act is even considered as meritorious. One example is St. Mary of Egypt who unhesitatingly offered her virginal body to the ferry- man so that she could continue her pilgrimage to the sacred places where our Saviour had preached and suffered. France points out that the Church does not condemn prostitutes. They don't have sexual intercourse to get pleasure from it but to keep themselves alive. But life has to be preserved to fulfill the demands of the Church and to praise the Lord. While I enjoyed the inimitable wording of France's remarks, my thoughts returned to my patient and his fine discrimination between experiment and pleasure in his sexual activity. Here was a religious analogy to his differen- tiation.

Turning to the other book on the table beside my bed, I chanced upon a passage that secured a much more impressive analogy of the individual with a collective phenomenon. It is an especially beautiful instance, which demonstrates the psychological parallelism between theological and obsessional thought-processes, as had been shown so often by Freud and myself. In this book Anatole France is portrayed on his lecture tour to South America. The old man liked to chat with his young, trim, and correct secretary, J. J. Brousson, who accompanied him. In casual conversations he often told the young writer of some material he perhaps intended to use in stories to be written. The anecdote he once recounted belonged, no doubt, to this kind of material, told in the informal manner of a rehearsal. At the time of the wars of succession, the Portuguese had taken the part of the Archduke and had turned against King Philip. They besieged Madrid in 1701, and the city was in great danger. The courtesans of the capital decided to save their beloved city. Those who were most certain they were infected dressed up and perfumed themselves. In the dusk they went to the outskirts of the enemies' camp. The ardent women did their work with such great zeal that within three weeks more than sixty thousand Portuguese were in the hospital, where the greater part of them perished of the pox.

Later on the problem was raised as to whether these women had committed the sin of fornication. Many of the most enlightened theologians examined the case of the Madrid courtesans. Some pronounced their action as sin, others declared them innocent because their intentions had been honorable: they wanted to save their country. The learned doctors remarked that in time of war it is not only permitted but even commanded to massacre enemies and to employ the most atrocious means to destroy them. Why should one neglect the pox? It is God who gives the victory, but He uses primary and secondary means, and the pox belongs to the latter category. One has furthermore to consider the feelings of the Madrid women. Did they share the enthusiastic sensations they inspired in the enemy? Obviously they could not behave like marble statues if they wanted to succeed in their patriotic task. There is, however, a professional limit to their behavior. The question was whether they were propelled only by love of the fatherland or by lechery in every individual case. The problem was carefully investigated, but only God who plumbs the depths of heart and of loin can decide whether the Madrid courtesans followed only the call of their patriotism or whether they also experienced some pleasure in the fulfillment of their heroic task.

Thus spoke Anatole France. If he had written the story, he would, no doubt, have introduced the learned theologians and their sagacious arguments and discussions of the difficult case of the Madrid women. The historic anecdote would in his elaboration be comparable to some chapters of his *L'Ile des Pingouins.* His necklace was so rich that he could easily afford to throw some of its pearls away in conversation.

A few supplementary remarks on the comparisons between the cases of my patients and the figures of Anatole France's anecdotes are here appropriate. What led my thoughts from France's story about the Chinese widow to my patient Jane? There is the resemblance of the external situations of two women who were recent widows, but this external connection is hardly sufficient to explain the comparison of the symbolic role of fire and water.

Here is the missing link in my thoughts: Some weeks before Jane told me of her experience with the State Trooper during the forest fire, the analytic situation had changed its character. Jane had shown distinct signs of a positive transference to me before that, which means she had an attitude proving that she had transferred feelings and reactions, originally tied to the figure of her father, to the analyst. She now spoke freely of her love for me and told me about sexual fantasies with me. When she expressed her disappointment because I did not respond to her feelings, I had to explain to her the significance of the transference love. I told her that her emotions were only new editions of old forgotten feelings that had once been directed to her father. They had been reactivated by the process of analysis and had nothing to do with me personally. I was only a reincarnation of her father in the development of her affectionate and sensual desires, and the figure of the analyst in the process is comparable to that of a frame for a finished picture. Jane insisted, however, that her love for me was genuine. Later on I tried to explain to her that the emotional mastering of her transference love would help her to overcome certain old conflicts and would prepare a more mature attitude toward her future love object. Mr. Reik, I said, serves only as a herald of Mr. Right. In an attempt at explanation, I used a comparison I had once heard in a play. In Vienna before the first World War modern drying processes were unknown. The landlords of new buildings rented the still damp apartments to poor people, who paid little and spent the winter in them heating the rooms. When this aim was reached, the provisional tenants had to leave and other families, the permanent tenants, moved in, paying the regular rent. A figure in a comedy by Raoul Auerheimer I had seen more than twenty years before in Vienna compares the place of a certain group of young men in the life of women with those provisional drying tenants. Those young men take girls out and provide pleasant company and harmless flirtation for them, but the young women do not think of marrying one of that group. They function, so to speak, as drying tenants who, in due time, will be replaced by the permanent possessors of the apartment. In my explanation of the transference situation, I compared the preparatory and provisional role of the analyst with the function of those drying tenants.

This comparison came to mind when I read France's anecdote of the Chinese widow who fans the damp earth on the grave and brought this woman in associative connection with Jane. The character of the connection is obvious: the drying tenants inhabit the apartment only as long as the walls are still damp and have to leave when they become dry. The Chinese widow has to wait until the grave of her husband dries out before she can grant her favors to the new suitor. The symbolic significance of the apartment (or the grave) as substitute of the woman's body and of the moisture as the state after emission is clear.

It is psychologically interesting that the role of fire, neglected in this interpretation, lingered in my thoughts. It followed me even after making the comparison of my other patient's doubts with the theological reflections of the priests concerning the Madrid prostitutes. My thoughts turned to the Holy Inquisition, which in Spain longer than in other countries found and punished heretics and condemned many thousands of people to be burned alive. The fate of those unknown men was shared by Savonarola, Hus, and other well-known historic figures who died as witnesses of their religious convictions. The moral courage of those martyrs and their modern successors who sacrificed themselves in the service of political ideas is certainly admirable. One might wonder about the absolute faith they had in the correctness of their opinion, wonder why they thought that they alone were in possession of the truth. There is a lack of modesty in the exclusion of any doubt, and a fanaticism that insists that oneself is infallible, a fanaticism which almost equals that of their persecutors.

At the end my thoughts returned to old, wise Anatole France, who once wrote the wonderful sentence: "There is some impudence in letting oneself be burned at the stake for a cause." ("*Il y a quelque impudence à se laisser brûler pour une cause.*")

II

1

THE HISTORIANS of music tell us that the original form of the overture was a fanfare whose purpose was to command silence and to make an end to the noisy conversation of the audience. It was originally not a transcribed, but an improvised piece. Later on it became an introductory composition that attempted to prepare listeners for the character of the opera. In later phases of its evolution, it contained some musical themes that would appear in the work itself.

Like the old type of overture, this introductory material starts from a fanfare-like question which, so far as I know, has not yet been raised: Why does music play no role in the work of Freud, which was to the greatest extent based on impressions received by hearing? In the fifteen volumes of his collected writings music is only mentioned three or four times. In his psychoanalytic practice, his own musical associations or those of his patients were scarcely noticed. This question has a considerable bearing on the problems we shall deal with, because the musical aspect in analytic work has been neglected by almost all analysts.

Personal characteristics of Freud were responsible for the lack of interest and attention paid to musical impressions. It is certain that he heard very little music in the first four years he spent in the little town of Freiburg in Moravia. We know how important the impressions of those early years are for the development of musical sensitivity and interest. Then, besides this factor, there were in Freud's case psychological reasons that prevented the development of a love of music. He himself gives significant information about those reasons in a passage whose psychological and biographical importance has been overlooked. He declared that works of art, especially those of literature and sculpture, had a strong and lasting effect on him.* He tried to comprehend them in his way, that is, to understand why they worked upon him: "Where I cannot do that," he says, "for instance, in music, I am almost incapable of enjoying them. A rationalistic or perhaps an analytic trait in me struggles against my being affected and not knowing why I am so and what it is that affects me." The word "almost" in this interesting statement should be well considered. The very wording of that statement about his restricted capability for enjoying music proves that there was an emotional reluctance against this art operating in Freud. He fought against the effects of music because a rationalistic, or perhaps an analytic, trait in him could not tolerate not knowing why he was affected. The most important part of this statement is the admission that he is or was affected by music. One assumes that he turned away from the emotional impressions of music and that the explanation of his attitude, the pointing to a rationalistic or analytic trait, is a secondary one—we would say, itself a kind of rationalization. It is likely that this turning away, this diversion was the result of an act of will in the interest of self-defense, and that it was the more energetic and violent, the more the emotional effects of music appeared undesirable to him. He became more and more convinced that he had to keep his reason unclouded and his emotions in abeyance. He developed an increasing reluctance to surrendering to the dark power of music.

* "Der Moses des Michelangelo," *Gesammelte Schriften*, Vol. IX.

Such an avoidance of the emotional effects of melodies can sometimes be seen in people who feel endangered by the intensity of their feelings. I know a man who, at least on the surface, became almost insensitive to music after a phase in which he was too much subjected to its effects. He told me that he began to avoid listening to music because it induced daydreams and awakened fantasies of grandeur and victory, evoking vague but intense longings and desires in him. When the music ended, he always felt disappointed. He began to build a wall of protection against that very unpleasant reaction of disillusionment, to erect barriers of defense against the effects of musical impressions because he hated to be duped by the influence of melodies. In this avoidance of the state of emotional unbalance into which music could bring him, he avoided listening to symphonies and finally became almost insensitive to their power. It seems to me that Freud built up similar defenses and later on hardened himself against the emotional appeal of music. There are other intensified reactions of a similar kind.

In the first years of my psychoanalytic studies, I wrote, besides analytic papers and book reviews, a great number of literary and general articles for Viennese newspapers and magazines. Influenced by French and Austrian writers, I perhaps immodestly felt that I had acquired a considerable facility of presentation. In a conversation—it was perhaps in 1913 or 1914—Freud spoke pleasantly of my literary talent but surprised me by asking whether or not I could suppress the stimuli for literary production of this kind. He felt I could perhaps develop as a writer to the rank of A. P. (he mentioned a well-known Viennese novelist), but that the renunciation of cheap literary laurels would greatly benefit my psychoanalytic research work, which he considered more important. I followed his advice and have never regretted it, but did not understand the mental economy and dynamics of his advice until later, when I recognized that he himself had made a similar renunciation. Wilhelm Stekel reports in his autobiography that Freud told him that he had once wanted to use the material his patients provided in the writing of novels of his own. He sacrificed literary ambition of this kind in the service of scientific research, but an echo of it is sometimes noticeable, especially in the case histories he wrote. He says occasionally, "I have been brought up with strict science and I cannot help it if my case histories sometimes sound like novels." Traces of the emotional reaction against that earlier tendency can still be found later in the form of rejection, as in that exclamation, "Don't put me into literature!" in his discussion of lay analysis.*

There are other instances that show Freud, sometimes forcefully and purposely, resisting tendencies in himself which he recognized as opposed to the goals he wished. Such reactions seemed to take the form of an energetic and sometimes even over-emphasized turnabout. He himself mentioned several changes of this kind in his writings. He reported, for instance, that he had developed an inclination for the exclusive concentration of his work on one topic or problem, much in contrast with the diffuse nature of his studies in the first years at the university. This "turn" came after 1882, and he remained true to it. He renounced also his original speculative tendencies because he did not wish them to interfere with his objective observations. He relinquished earlier interests in favor of psychoanalytic research, etc.

The psychological expectation in his advice to me was that to sacrifice my facility in writing would benefit my research interest and enrich and enlarge my analytic studies.

Is it unlikely that Freud turned determinedly away from music because he felt too deeply affected by its power at a certain phase of his life? Do not his own words show such an emotional reaction when he says that something in him struggles against his being affected by music? It is furthermore very probable that his reaction was intensified by the impression of the musicomania of the Viennese, which in the years between 1890 and 1910 reached its climax.

The denied and rejected tendencies against whose influence Freud built up such strong defenses did not disappear, but left traces in him and found different and distant expressions. Some of them, for instance, speculative inclinations and interests in early history, worked their way, in his old age, from the depth into which they were banished to the surface.

Freud's confession that he did not often respond to music does

* *The Problem of Lay Analysis* (New York, 1927).

not mean that he was insensitive to its message, but that he fought against his own sensitiveness. He had unconsciously foregone being subjected to its lure and language, and this voluntary sacrifice benefited his fine ability to hear the unconscious processes, helped him to develop the sense for the rhythm of subterranean movements of the mind.

In a passage of his writing* he discussed the teaching of G. Jung and of his school, and stated that here a new religious-ethical system was created that had to reinterpret, distort, or remove the actual results of psychoanalysis. He develops this idea: "In reality one had heard a few cultural overtones of the symphony of the world and had again missed its all-powerful melody of the drives." A man that hath no music in himself could not have thought of this magnificent comparison. Freud had heard that forceful melody of the world symphony and he wrote its score in his analytic books.

Do we not all sometimes feel, as Freud did, a certain reluctance to the compulsion of music that affects us and does not let us guess what affects us and why? We surrender to an adagio from a Beethoven symphony, yet we cannot say what it was that transported us with emotion. Here is a message which everybody understands, but nobody can translate. It is easy enough to explain what a musician playing upon his instrument does, but very difficult to find why the *dolce* of the strings in the adagio sways us, to define its special expressive value or even the precise nature of our emotional response. Yet we hear in the language of music "the secret history of our will," as Schopenhauer said; of our drives, as we would say today. The affinity of music to the other expressions of the unconscious, the kinship of this art with the dreamlike and intangible element, with the night aspect of our emotional life is of a special, not easily definable kind, because music itself cannot be defined except in the superficial terms of a dictionary. Bruno Walter tells of a young New York enthusiast who asked many well-known musicians, "What is music?"** The

* "Zur Geschichte der psychoanalytischen Bewegung," *Gesammelte Schriften*, Vol. V.

** "Von den moralischen Kräften der Musik" (Wien, 1935), p. 8. (This lecture given in the Kulturbund in Vienna was not translated into English.)

answers he received appeared to Bruno Walter either false or un-satisfactory, but he confessed that he felt incapable of answering the question himself. He admitted that he could not say to this day what music is, in spite of a long search after appropriate definitions. One is unable to grasp its nature with the clarity of reason and cannot give it an abstract verbal expression. "Music," says Bruno Walter, using a beautiful comparison, "is like a seraph in the temple of the Lord and covers its eye with two of its wings."

The intimacy of musical experience in which the pulse beat of a composition becomes our own cannot be caught in the paltry net of the words we utter. Bernard Shaw once said, "I could make musical criticism readable even to the deaf." This is believable; it is a question of style. But can Shaw or anyone else convey the meaning music has for the individual? Can he communicate the experience he had when he heard a Mozart sonata?

Language develops more and more in the direction of objective communication, denotes things and acts. It becomes simultane-ously impoverished as an expression of emotions. Music is the language of psychic reality. Music does not name objects and events. It can, at very best, conjure them up. There is much con-troversy about the meaning of words; a discussion of the meaning of music is condemned to fail before it starts. The rigid "tyranny of words" is contrasted with the sweet compulsion John Milton attributed to melody. Words have strings, but songs have wings.

Music is the universal language of human emotion, the expres-sion of the inexpressible. The composers articulate "subtle com-plexes of feeling that language cannot even name, let alone set forth."* This book does not deal with problems of music, but with a problem of psychology, namely, with the question of the significance of musical recollections within the flow of our thoughts. We do not speak here of music as an actual emotional experience. What can be said of it that could come close to its immediacy and intimacy? We speak here rather of musical recol-lections in the middle of other associations. No attempt is made to describe or transcribe the emotional response. Wherever reac-tions to musical experiences are mentioned, words are function-

* Susanne K. Langer "On Significance in Music" in *Philosophy in a New Key* (Harvard University Press, 1942), p. 222.

ing only as guideposts leading to the threshold of the domain where melodies live. In our musical associations the impressions tunes once made upon us are renewed in their effect. They resemble the bush Moses saw, the bush that burned with fire and was not consumed.

Among the physicians who practice psychoanalysis, there are quite a few who are excellent neurologists, of high intelligence, men and women well trained in psychiatry, well meaning, hardworking, and entirely out of touch with the unconscious process. Caught in the tangle of theoretical sophistication, filled with terminological labels and thought clichés, their minds move in the psychoanalytic groove without a trace of insight that they are in the wrong profession. What could you tell those who have spent so much energy, time, and money on a study for which they have all the external, but none of the inner qualifications? Beethoven said, in a similar situation, to a young man who played to him, "My dear fellow, you will have to practice a long time before you recognize that you have no talent."*

Fortunately, the majority of the young people who are trained in psychoanalytic institutes have that native gift that is the most important psychological premise for understanding of unconscious processes. There is nothing wrong, but there is something lacking in their training. Also, the native talent, in various degrees present in them, has to be developed. Psychoanalysis can be taught as far as it is a craft and cannot be taught as far as it is an art. Its methods, its means and instruments can be demonstrated to the student in the same manner as a carpenter can show his apprentice how to put boards together to make a table. All other aspects of analysis can be acquired by a gifted student, but they cannot be taught. He has to learn them in studying the examples that the masters show in their work. To teach a student the technique of psychoanalysis is possible only to the same extent it is possible to teach a musician the technique of composition. Arnold Schönberg once said that if there were ateliers of composition, as there are studios of painters in which the students watch the masters at work, the theoreticians of music would be superflu-

* Reported by Wilhelm Rust in a letter to his sister Henriette (July 7, 1808). Published in *Monatshefte für Musikgeschichte* (1869), p. 68.

ous.* "The training that would educate an artist could in the best case consist in helping him to hear himself. . . . He who hears himself acquires that technique." (Also, Freud's comparison of the analytic technique with the "fine art of the game of chess" emphasizes that the endless variety for the moves defies description. The gap in the instructions "can only be filled in by the zealous study of games thought out by masters.") **

The basic, most important rule of the psychoanalytic investigation of others and ourselves, the procedure of free association, is best expressed in the words of Rudyard Kipling: *"If you can think—and not make thoughts your aim . . ."*

Self-observation can teach each of us that such "aimless" conscious thinking is much rarer than we would assume. We demand a license from our thoughts and are afraid to let them run loose. Not only our patients, but also we analysts hold our thought on short reins. The main psychological premise of the success of free associations is moral courage alongside the conscious decision to follow one's thoughts without distortions and censured misrepresentations. Lies and pretenses to ourselves are more dangerous and harmful to self-confidence than lies and pretenses toward others.

Besides those emotional and intellectual hindrances which psychoanalysis calls resistance, there are others not based on inner objections, but determined by the inadequacy of human communication. The words we think and the words we say, the sentences we have in our minds and those we utter would not be the same even if they were phonetically identical. Our language emerges from a subsoil in which sounds, fleeting images, organic sensations, and emotional currents are not yet differentiated. Something gets lost on the way from the brain, which senses, feels, and thinks, to the lips which speak words and sentences. The most essential part of that loss and lack is, of course, emotional, or rather the specific and differentiated quality of our emotions; one could say the personal and intimate note or the emotional

* *Harmonielehre* (3rd edition, Vienna), p. 2.
** "Further Recommendations in the Technique of Psychoanalysis," Collected Papers, Vol. II.

significance of what we want to express. Language is at its poorest when it wishes to grasp and communicate nuances and shades of feelings—in that very area in which music is most efficient and expressive. Even in the language of poetry not much of the secret life of emotions comes across. Music, so poor in definite and definable objective and rational contents, can convey the infinite variety of primitive and subtle emotions.

In the flow of free associations, snatches of tunes are interspersed at certain significant points. Their perception and analytic evaluation are part of the analytic technique of finding concealed and unconscious processes. To be aware of their emergence, not to exclude them from observation, is imperative "if you can think and not make thoughts your aim." It must have psychological significance that not words, but a musical theme occurs to you. Why is it that your thought process is not expressed in imagining and planning, but in "inward singing," to borrow a term of Eduard Hanslick?* It must make a difference whether a sentence from a speech, a line from a poem, or a tune emerges in your train of thoughts. If a melody from a Mozart concerto occurs in the midst of clear, aim-directed ideas, the psychoanalytic investigation could perhaps discover not only what is on your mind without your being aware of it, but also what's in your heart. A musical passage flowing through your brain perhaps indicates your mood, expresses some feelings unknown to you, besides thoughts. Its emotional significance cannot be translated in words, but can be communicated to yourself or to the listener who knows the composition. It is certainly meaningful when a sentence, heard or thought, pursues you, and a psychoanalyst could perhaps have discovered the unconscious significance of those words that haunted Mark Twain: "A blue trip slip for a three-cent fare." Yet not only lines, but also melodies that run through your mind, phrases from a Schubert symphony or from a *Divertimento* by Mozart may give the analyst a clue to the secret life of emotions that every one of us lives. In fleeting tunes whose wings have fluttered away into the unknown as in a melody that has a hold on you and will not release you for hours, that life, con-

* *Vom Musikalisch Schönen* (Vienna, 1876), p. 75.

cealed from yourself has sent messages to the mental surface. In this inward singing, the voice of an unknown self conveys not only passing moods and impulses, but sometimes a disavowed or denied wish, a longing and a drive we do not like to admit to ourselves. The theme that is stirring deep inside you imposes itself on you, interferes with rational thoughts, and obscures the swift, straight line of logic. But the recurring tune may announce in its compelling and compulsive pressure the working of an unknown power in you. Whatever secret message it carries, the incidental music accompanying our conscious thinking is never accidental.

Sensitivity to the almost imperceptible is present in most psychoanalysts. Not many turn a deaf ear to the emotional undertones. What is neglected in the study program of psychoanalysts is, to use the musical term, *ear training:* the development of a higher sensitivity to musical phenomena of all kinds—for instance, to minute distinctions in tones. Some psychoanalysts are too eager to recognize and to define those undertones, or are unwilling to pursue them in their variations and combinations after they have acknowledged them. The comparison with musical phenomena can here be followed up even to the terms. In the development of a composition, the latent possibilities of a theme are unfolded by means of melodic, harmonic, or contrapuntal variations. Development is also called working out, which is identical with the Freudian term *(Durcharbeiten)* used for a certain phase of the analytic process. To continue the comparison of the analytic procedure with artistic creation: Schönberg, listening to the composition of one of his pupils, sometimes said, *"Das ist nicht ausgehört,"* meaning that the musical idea was not heard to its end by the composer inside, was not thought and experienced to its last and decisive consequences. It remained in its first phases, in its early form.

It is not enough to introduce a new instrument or to improve an old, forgotten one. You have to demonstrate how it can be used. This is best done by examples. There is an abundance of such examples in the mental lives of the patients we treat as well as in our own, but this material has remained almost unnoticed and unused, its psychological significance unrecognized. The other day a patient reported that a trivial tune had occurred to him together with the line:

Did you ever see a lassie
Do this way and that?

He did not know what this banal tune wanted to convey, but when it recurred, he became aware that it was accompanied by memories of a recent sexual experience and of visual images of the responsive movements of the woman during sexual intercourse. Is it without significance that another patient cannot get rid of the second part of a children's ditty in his thoughts?

Ten little, nine little, eight little Indians,
Seven little, six little, five little Indians,
Four little, three little, two little Indians,
One little Indian boy.

A few minutes before the patient had spoken of his brothers and sisters. It was easy to guess that the unconscious desire to remove his siblings and to have the position of an only child had found its expression in that ditty.

2

Music expresses what all men feel much more than what they think. Its language is an esperanto of emotions rather than of ideas. It does not emerge from the flow of conscious thought, but from the stream of preconsciousness. The following are cases where tunes appeared either as still unformulated thought germs or as heralds of thoughts that were still on the preverbal level.

Let me begin this potpourri with the story of an intelligent patient of mine. In her rather stormy married life with a musician, she observed a recurrent trait of her husband's behavior. After an argument or quarrel with her, he often sits at the piano and improvises some music, mostly popular tunes. After a few bars he regularly begins to play a tune the patient knows: "Glad to be unhappy." She remembered a line of that inane lyric: "I'd rather be blue thinking of you." The patient interpreted this habit of beginning his improvisation with this tune as "musical confession," and told me that her husband often provoked marital scenes by nagging about some trifling thing in the apartment and that he seemed to get some masochistic satisfaction from feeling unhappy later on. The other day when he again played that tune a few hours after a sharp argument, he turned to her and said, "I don't know why I always play that trash." She was too clever to enlighten him, but she felt some satisfaction when he immediately began to play the title-song of *I Married an Angel*. The husband does not have the slightest notion why he plays that song on such occasions, but it is obvious to the patient that he expresses his regrets or remorse in this musical form.

Here are a few of my own experiences that cast light on the determining factors that decide about the preconscious selection of emerging musical ideas and their function as announcing conscious thought. I was present at an amateur performance of Strauss's opera *Salome*. A young lady of my acquaintance sang the part of the Princess. I didn't like the way she sang it, but I was, of course, not competent to have an opinion about her artistic qualities. A few days later she asked me about my impressions. Put on the spot, I felt embarrassed because I could not praise either her singing or her acting. At this moment a fleeting impression of the opening bars of the opera occurred to me, and I answered, "I entirely agreed with the first sentence of the score." The first words are sung by a young Syrian soldier on the walls of Jerusalem: "How beautiful is the Princess Salome tonight!" In avoiding giving my acquaintance insincere praise, I had said something complimentary that was also true: she had indeed looked beautiful that evening. The first bars of the opera came, so to speak, "handy" to my mind.

In a conversation I was trying to give some American friends an idea of the character of old Vienna and, since the last war was mentioned, of the Austrian army in co-operation with German divisions in Russia. It was difficult to present the mixture of the resolute, military, and disciplined conduct of Viennese sol-

diers on the parade ground and their avoidance of every real
effort during the last war. How can one describe the contrast of
showy militarism with the easygoing and deeply unmartial nature
of the soldiers of my native city? While I speak of the good-
natured and jovial manner of the Viennese, a few bars of a Schubert *Ländler* (slow waltz) are dimly in my memory, to be immediately replaced by the *Deutschmeistermarsch*, the forceful military
march of the Austrian infantry regiment No. 4, whose soldiers
were all Viennese. As if the intertwining of the two tunes had
opened a door, an anecdote that well characterized the attitude
of the Austrian infantry came to mind. During the war a cannon
got stuck in the Galician mud, and ten soldiers of that regiment
were ordered to free it and to put it into motion again. The
soldiers put their shoulders on the gun, counted, "One, two,
three," many times, and shouted "Ho!" and "Go!" but the gun
did not move. A lieutenant in command of a Prussian company
chanced to march along. The officer scolded the Viennese for
their sloppiness and ordered some Prussian soldiers to put the
gun into motion while the Austrians had to stand by. He commanded in sharp and determined tones, "One, two, three!" and
the cannon was moving. The Deutschmeister were not impressed
and said, "Naturally, if you use force!" The emergence of the
march of the regiment together with the easygoing Schubert tune
in my mind paved the way for the memory of that well-known
anecdote.

Other musical echoes from the war intruded into different
trains of thought. A young, beautiful woman confided to me that
she now had a lover. A few minutes afterward, while I was still
talking with her, a tune came to mind which I could not identify.
I had heard it a long time ago. Only after I heard it in my mind
again, I remembered what it was: a song I'd heard our soldiers
sing when we returned from exercise marches:

> *Was nützet mir ein Rosengarten,*
> *Wenn and're drin spazieren gehen?*

> What use is a rose garden to me,
> When others are walking in it?

The regret expressed in such symbolical language was, at the moment when the tune occurred, not consciously felt, but following
its emergence in the very next moment.

On another occasion belated regret that I had not enjoyed my
youth more came to surprising expression. In this case, also, the
emotion was consciously felt only after a melody had heralded
it. A memory from the years of my military service was present,
and I had no doubt as to the origin of the melody, but its emotional significance became conscious after it was put into the context from which it was taken. In a conversation I had spoken of
a relatively free and gay phase in 1916, during which our troops
were garrisoned in a city near the field of battle. I was a young
officer then and I enjoyed going out on horseback every morning.
It felt good to pass from a trot to an easy canter after one had
gone beyond the suburbs and had reached the open country.
Thinking of those carefree months, I imagined the sounds of the
hoofbeats and that rhythmical tone went over into a well-known
melody: the hard C Major marching rhythms from the *Song of
Beauty* in Mahler's *Song of the Earth*. These sounds imitate
onomatopoetically the noise of tramping horses.

It was not astonishing that these rhythms came to mind. It is a
musical portrait of riding, but there are many other expressive
motives of this kind: Schubert's *Erlkönig*, Liszt's *Mazeppa* and
some ballads by Karl Löwe, the names of which elude me at the
moment. (Rereading this page, I remembered another song in
which the trotting of horses changes into a waltz melody. It is the
Fiacre Song by Gustav Pick, a popular tune in the Vienna of my
youth.) Why just the C Major tune from Mahler's work? The
sounds of the horses galloping from Schubert's lied are there for
a moment, but they immediately give way to the C Major march.
And then it comes to an abrupt end. The tender Andante that
follows appears in my memory together with the image that is
called up by the Chinese poem for which the tune was written.
Young beautiful girls plucking flowers near a stream in which
their figures are reflected; a group of young horsemen storming
by. And then the stormy scales of the strings are replaced by that
melody of the contralto voice, accompanied by harp and violins:

And the loveliest of the maidens
Sends the rider glances of yearning,
Her haughty bearing is no more than feigned.
In the sparkle of her wide eyes,
In the darkening of the eager glance,
Ascends the plaint of the passion in her heart.

While the flageolets of the harp and the flutes die away, a visual memory comes to mind. On those morning rides I often saw a young, beautiful girl in a meadow and sometimes felt her glance following me when I galloped by, but I was too shy even to speak to her. How young and stupid I was!

The other day an old tune occurred to me in the middle of a conversation. A lady with whom I am on "teasing" terms appeared at a party in a dark dress and a necklace of black pearls with a cross. The lady is Irish Catholic, her husband Jewish, but he wishes her to go to church and bring up their children as Roman Catholics. It was perhaps this thought that made the tune *Silent Night, Holy Night* appear in my memory. The solemn melody was immediately followed by the memory of an anecdote they told in old Vienna. A little Jewish girl once asked, "Mum, have Gentiles Christmas trees, too?" The emergence of that Christmas hymn (by the Austrian composer Franz Gruber) preceded and announced the thought expressed in that anecdote.

This example has some psychological interest because the thought implied in the anecdote led to a remark that indulgent listeners might call witty. Glancing at the big crucifix hanging from her necklace, I said teasingly to the lady, "You have to be careful at this party. Some people might think you were Jewish." In contrast to the preconscious thought, heralded by that melody, the thought was for a moment submerged and left to elaboration in the unconscious—the dynamic process that results in the production of wit.

The following are instances of melodies occurring in the middle of work. I am choosing as a representative example a musical phrase that came to my mind while I was writing a psychoanalytic paper that is connected with my "witty" remark mentioned before. Almost twenty years ago I wrote an analytic article, "The

Intimacy of Jewish Wit," that attempted to study certain characteristics of Jewish humor.* I pointed out that its warmth and
intimacy are expressions of an unconscious affectionate attitude
on the part of Jews toward their fellow people, of a love of
mankind, as it were. One of the cases I wanted to mention in this
context was an anecdote heard before the outbreak of the First
World War. A Jew mistakenly came into territory near the Russian frontier where a soldier stood guard. At his approach the
sentry raised his gun and shouted, "Halt or I shoot!" The Jew
replied indignantly, "Are you *meschugge* [crazy]? Put your gun
away! Don't you see that here is a *Mensch?*" While I smilingly
jotted down that anecdote, expressing a sublime and utter lack of
belief in the possibility that one human being could really want
to kill another, the solemn melody of the final movement of Beethoven's choral symphony occurred to me. *The Ode to Joy* proclaims the same theme as the Jew's words in that anecdote: the
conviction that all men should become brothers.

The tunes occurring to the analyst during sessions with patients
are preconscious messages of thoughts that are not only meaningful, but also important for the understanding of the emotional
situation of the patient. It would be an analytic mistake to brush
them aside or to take them on face value, and to dismiss them as
chance musical reminiscences. They not only convey contents unknown to the analyst's conscious thinking, but also communicate to
him something of the hidden emotions that he has not yet been
able to catch while he listens to his patient. The tunes stand in
the service of the agents responsible for the communications between the unconscious of two persons. These melodies present
themselves clearly or dimly to the mind, but what they have to
convey becomes comprehensible only when the analyst listens
"with the third ear." There is a considerable psychological difference between those "chance" tunes and quotations from poems
or sentences from novels or plays that sometimes emerge in the
thoughts of the analyst during a therapeutic session. A quotation
from a poem can be fraught with meaning and can allude to
something that had remained dark or unknown to the analyst; it

* Published in a book *Nachdenkliche Heiterkeit* (Wien, 1933). (Not translated into English.)

can carry an emotional quality of which his conscious thinking had not been aware. The melody that occurs to him while he listens to his patient is perhaps not as meaningful as lines from a poem in the intellectual understanding of the case, but it induces a recognition of its emotional qualities. The poetic line or the sentence from a play is perhaps more "telling." The musical phrase can say more in its sound allusion.

An example may be helpful in comparing the two effects. At the Highland Hospital in Asheville, where I spent some vacation months as consulting psychoanalyst, I had to interview a young man. While talking with him, I had the impression that he was withdrawn from reality, involved in fantasies or daydreams. He was there physically, but his mind was wrapped in thoughts far away, from which my questions could scarcely call him back. He was polite, but certainly not interested in finding out anything about himself. His lack of co-operation did not have the characteristics of negativism, but rather that quality of absent-mindedness which is a form of concentration on something else. While I tried with little success to pierce the glass curtain that isolated him from the external world, a melody sounded in me which I quickly recognized as the first bars of *"Ich bin der Welt abhanden gekommen"* by Gustav Mahler. The slow melody of tender resignation, akin to the Adagietto of Mahler's Fifth Symphony, expressed better than the words the emotional character of the song:

> I am lost to the world
> With which I have wasted so much time before . . .

People will perhaps think that the artist is dead:

> I cannot object to that
> Because I really died to the world.

He rests in a quiet area and lives only in his thoughts and songs.

The emergence of the Mahler song heralded the diagnosis of schizophrenia that was consciously made a few minutes later on. If the rather pallid, intellectualized verses by Friedrich Rückert, whose poem Mahler used as text for his song, had come to mind without the fine melody, they would have certainly announced the same diagnosis at which I would have arrived, at all events, without verses and music. But the moving melody conveyed something more of the emotional atmosphere in which this patient lived.

Let me describe another instance of this kind. At the same psychiatric hospital I treated a young woman who had intense anxiety attacks with many psychosomatic symptoms. Her anxieties occurred mostly when she was alone in her house, on a farm in Kentucky. The first approach to the analytic understanding of the case was secured by her complaints about her sexual life. Her husband, a salesman, was, it seemed, of weak or capricious sexual potency and could not satisfy her. It was guessed that she had unconscious fantasies that a tramp could enter the house while she was alone and rape her, and that she reacted with extreme anxiety to the unconscious wish in these fantasies. Later on this guess had to be replaced, or rather modified, by the insight that her anxiety attacks were reactions against the temptation to masturbate when she was alone. When she again complained about the sexual inadequacy of her husband, a simple ditty I had heard another patient in the hospital sing on the evening before, resounded in me. The words followed immediately:

> Three blind mice,
> Three blind mice,
> See how they run.
> They all ran after the farmer's wife,
> Who cut off their tails
> With a carving knife.
> Three blind mice. . . .

The thought was, of course, the precursor of the recognition that my patient was unconsciously partly responsible for the sexual failure of her husband, that she frustrated him by her attitude and castrated him in her fantasy. (The three mice as representing the male genitals in its three parts, the farmer's wife cutting off the tails.) If the words of the ditty alone had occurred to me, they could, of course, have contained the same unconscious idea. What did the simple tune contribute to it? Nothing to the content but something significant to the characterization of the patient. It was not "just music," but the just kind of music. The young woman, when she did not have her anxiety attacks, behaved very cheerfully and was easygoing, speaking of her husband's sexual inadequacy as if it were a negligible weakness. There was not the slightest conscious notion of her own hostile and castrating tendencies toward him. The contrast between the cheerful tune of that ditty and its pathetic content reflects the other contrast between the gay and gleeful behavior of the patient and her sinister and hostile attitude against her husband, whom unconsciously she would like to have emasculated while she complained about his lack of virility.

The modulation or the cadence of a ditty of such a kind often remains astonishingly long in one's memory, sometimes much longer than its lines. That alone proves that it has a psychological significance beyond the text that is never a literary achievement. Drawing analytical conclusions from the material a patient had presented during the therapeutic session, I expressed the conjecture that she, the patient, might have experienced a scene in childhood in which she had felt very ashamed and was made fun of by other children because she had soiled herself. The patient could not remember anything of this kind and considered such a scene very unlikely. On her way out, waiting for the elevator, a ditty from early childhood occurred to her and she remembered other children singing it to her: "Shame, shame, I know your name."

Psychology asserts that tone images are grasped earlier than word images, and that the memory for the first is more tenacious than for the latter. It is likely that this is one of the factors responsible for the fact that our memory frequently retains a melody after we have forgotten the text of the song. The emotional value might be responsible for the partiality we show for the melody compared with the text. Even where the text is maintained in our memory, we use it to call up the forgotten melody. It is much rarer that we make use of the melody of a song or of an aria to remember its lines. The libretto of an opera lives in our memory by the grace of the score. With most of us, also, the visual impression of a performance of an opera is less vivid than its melodies.

Here are a few instances from psychoanalytic practice as evidence for the priority of the tune. A patient has a dream: *She is in the bath and is worried because she has forgotten to take off her watch which could be ruined if it gets wet.* There were no helpful thought-associations to the dream. In the pause between her report of the dream and the following sentences she spoke, a long-forgotten tune came to my mind. I recognized it later as the opening bars of a song by Karl Löwe I had not heard since childhood. The title is *The Watch,* and the first lines, remembered only after the analytic session, are:

> *Ich trage wo ich gehe*
> *Stets eine Uhr bei mir.*
>
> Where'er I go, I carry
> A watch with me always,
> And only need look
> Whenever I'd know the time of day.

The watch meant in Löwe's song is the heart. Only after I had remembered those lines did other associations help to interpret the dream. The Viennese girls used to say, "With me it is punctual as a watch," referring to the regularity of their monthly period. I remembered a proverb I heard the Serbian peasants quote during World War I: "With a watch and a woman there is always something to repair," alluding to troubles of the genital region.

At her next analytic session, the patient returned to her dream and said she had forgotten to put the diaphragm in when she had taken a bath before going to bed, and she was worried because she might have become pregnant the last time she had sexual intercourse.

As in this case where the mentioning of a watch awakened musical memories followed by associations to the dream interpretation, in another case a melody was suggested by the idea connection—hair, hairdresser. Marion, a young woman, began her analytic session with reproaches because I had kept the patient preceding her a minute overtime and her own time was shortened by my preferring the other girl. What had that blond hussy got that she, Marion, hadn't got? There followed a critical comment on the physical shortcomings and possible intellectual weaknesses of the other patient. An attack on me and my partiality leads easily to suspicions and doubts concerning my capabilities as an analyst. The rest of the analytic session was to a great extent filled with a discussion of Marion's troubles with her lover, who pays attention to other girls when he goes with Marion to a party, often looks at other women when he is with her at dinner in a restaurant, and so on. Near the end of her session Marion reported that yesterday she had been very annoyed with Henry, the hairdresser at Caruso's. He had done her hair badly and she compared the attention and care he shows toward other customers with work he does for her. What have those dolls got that she hasn't? There followed an extensive description of the appearance and manner of the blond young woman in the neighboring booth at Caruso's. The pattern is, of course, clear.

What does it mean that, after Marion left, an old tune occurred to me of which I had not thought for several decades? I recognized it as the "Lorelei," the poem by Heinrich Heine, composed by Friedrich Silcher. What has Marion to do with that beautiful minx on the rock on the Rhine? I tried to remember the lines. Oh, of course, the fairy sits on the rock and combs her golden hair with a golden comb and sings a sweet song, bewitching boatmen on the Rhine. The comparison was suggested by the thought-association —hair, hairdresser. I did not remember the final stanza of Heine's poem. Only the slow sentimental melody returned to my mind as if it wanted to be heard. Only then the content of those lines was recalled: that at the end the waves engulf boatmen and ship, and that the Lorelei has cast an evil spell over the men who, enchanted, look up at her, sitting on that rock and singing. Not the lines, but the music with its sad finale told me the story and brought the concealed message to me of the meaning of Marion's behavior. Her unconscious hostility against men, concealed behind her passionate pleading for more attention and consideration, and her hidden destructive trends became clearer to me with the help of that old tune.

This is perhaps the place to report another instance that shows image and tune in competition, where the musical memory proved, though more fleeting than the picture in my mind, more helpful to analytic understanding. My patient Charles, a lawyer in his late thirties, showed unusually intense resistance during a certain phase of his analytic treatment. He fell into long silences and declared that nothing occurred to him. Pressed to say whatever he thought, he uttered some trifling sentences and relapsed into silence and sighing. During an analytic session that was characterized by that negative pattern, he interrupted his silence for some minutes to mention a thought that had just occurred to him. It was a memory from the war, in which he had served as a commander in the Navy. He recalled the exhaust of the engines of the ship and that in some weather it escaped in a certain direction. I guessed then that he must have fought with flatulence and that he thought I would smell the "exhaust." That did not explain the nature of his resistances, but it alluded to it. When I had recognized the concealed meaning and hint in his thought-associations, I remembered a picture I had once seen in a book on Felicien Rops, the Belgian painter. The reproduction of the etching showed a nude young woman, crouching in the grass, her beautiful behind raised in the air. In the distance a windmill is merrily revolving. The artist has entitled his picture with a sentence from the Gospel of John: *"Spiritus flat ubi vult"* ("The mind waves where it wishes").

In the pause provided by the continued silence of my patient, I could give myself freely to my thoughts: for a fleeting moment a phrase from the Bacchanale of the Böklin Suite by Max Reger occurred to me. I had heard the piece only once, and that theme now occurring was in the next moment gone with the wind or rather with the wind instruments that had played it in the performance. In the next moment a little story I had heard about it popped into my mind. The princess of a Middle German state attended the first performance of this suite and was very impressed by the polyphony of the orchestra. She had paid special attention to the themes of the fagots in the bacchanale movement and asked the composer later on whether the musicians had produced those strange tone figures with the mouth. With great seriousness Max Reger replied, "I would very much hope so."

The memory of that passage from the Böklin Suite paved the

way for the return of the story, but the meaning of the story was already implied in the mental reproduction of the musical phrase. When the psychological moment came, I could tell my patient not only that his resistance during the session was determined by his effort to control the impulse to expel gas (the association of the "exhaust" of the ship was a hint in this direction), but also what the unconscious expression of this impulse meant. In contrast to his respectful and even sometimes admiring attitude toward me, the impulse to pass wind expressed feelings of unconscious contempt and disdain. His silence was his defense against the temptation, against the wish to let go. He was afraid I would hear the noisy demonstration of these tendencies. I could meet his doubt by pointing out that in our society an indulgence of this kind is considered indecent, and the company reacts to it with indignation and rejection, as if it conceived of it as an expression of contempt for those present.

The affinities of certain melodies to some unconscious or preconscious emotions, as in those cases mentioned, were observed and well described by Marcel Proust in his *Remembrance of Things Past*. "The little phrase" from the andante movement of Viuteuil's sonata for the piano and violin* had become merged with Swann's ideas in an inextricable whole: the sorrow and charm of *la petite phrase* speak to him and remind him of Odette. The memory of it haunts him, evokes the image of his lost sweetheart and brings about her magic presence. Those floating chords become a kind of national anthem of their passion (*"une sorte d'air national de leur amour"*). Hearing the fugitive phrase, emerging for a few moments from the waves of sounds, has for him the significance of an actual idea. Musical phrases occurring to us in this manner may not be as significant as other associations, but they are as worthy of special psychological attention as immediate emotional expressions. And, for the psychoanalyst, heard melodies are sweet, but "those unheard" are not only sweeter, but also more meaningful.

* French musicians thought that the phrase can be found in Saint-Saëns's Sonata in D Minor for violin and piano.

3

My memory, otherwise reliable in such things, sometimes threatens to fail me when I want to remember who composed the two *Liebeslieder Walzer*. I have heard those graceful melodies often enough, and I know, of course, that Johannes Brahms wrote them, but it needs a little effort to remember his familiar name as their composer. There is a kind of small mental pause before the name is called to mind. Yet the character of that uncertainty is not the same as in other cases when I try to remember: "Who wrote this?" It is rather the conquest of a doubt or the expression of some disbelief. When this weakness of my memory occurred, I decided to find out what caused this special failing. Such a decision can be compared to making up one's mind to clean a neglected drawer. The analytic method lends itself rather well to the service of a mental vacuum cleaner in cases where emotional dust prevents our memory from smooth functioning.

The first attempt at free thought association revealed that my doubt or disbelief hung somewhere on the word *Liebe,* as if I were doubting that those waltzes really express genuine feelings of love, as if it is hard to believe that Johannes Brahms could have been deeply in love with a woman. My subjective concept of the composer is that of a shy, remote, and inwardly cool personality, unable to express his emotions freely except in music. This impression is, of course, not based on knowledge of his life history, of which I know but little, and I wonder about it. I argue with myself: What about that deep and lasting affection for the widow of Robert Schumann? If this intimate and tender emotion for Clara Schumann for so many years was not love, what else was it? But the countervoice makes itself heard: In spite of all intimacy, of all protestations of love and of passion, he never approached her sexually. He loved and desired her in his mind only. . . . What in Heaven's name kept him back? . . . She was fourteen years older and had, if I am not mistaken, seven children. . . . They were both free, loved each other—why did he not possess her in those many years? . . . There were, I am sure, caresses, something of what is called "heavy petting" today, but nothing else. . . . *"Tout excepte ça,"* say the Parisians: "all but that." She was perhaps a mother-representative figure to him and as such sexually untouchable, while he satisfied his sexual needs by relations with degraded objects, streetwalkers. As a matter of fact, the latter point is detailed by the biographers of the composer,* but I know it from more direct sources.

The image of my Aunt Resi (Viennese abbreviation of Thérèse) appeared in my memory. I remember Tante Resi as an old woman, but she was perhaps middle-aged when she died, and I was eight or nine years old. She lived in the Wieden, a quarter of Vienna that appeared suburban to us children at the time, in a small apartment on a narrow side street. She had been a widow for many years, living on a small pension. She kept her rooms immaculately clean and neat, and I still remember how carefully we children had to wipe our shoes before we were allowed to enter her apartment. There we had to sit quietly on the couch and were forbidden to touch any of the numerous pictures, knick-knacks, and whatnots which stood on little tables. We did not like to visit Aunt Resi because we had to be on our best behavior with her, but our mother took us there every Saturday. In my family they frequently told the story of how Aunt Resi promised my little sister to leave her a golden bracelet in her will, and that my sister asked her immediately after arriving for the weekly visit, *"Wenn sterbst du schon?"* ("When are you going to die?").

Tante Resi spent many hours of her day sitting at her window and observing all her neighbors. She knew a lot about each of them and she liked to tell what she knew. Otherwise put, she was a gossip and, if one could trust family hearsay, of a malicious kind. My sister Margaret and I listened, of course, to what our aunt had to say to my mother about her neighbors.

In my thoughts, Aunt Resi is connected with my early recognition of some facts of life and with Johannes Brahms. It seemed that my aunt's pet hate was a pretty young woman whose windows faced hers in the apartment across the street. Aunt Resi

* Dr. Edward Hitschmann described this characteristic division of Brahms's love life in a paper "Johannes Brahms und die Frauen," *Die Psychoanalytische Bewegung* (1933), No. 2, Vol. V.

knew quite a few things about this neighbor whom she could see when she leaned out her window. If one believed our aunt, "that woman" was no good, she slept till noon, was lazy and sloppy to a scandalous degree, and she saw "men" in her apartment. . . . Aunt Resi mentioned that a Herr von Brahms used to visit this lady regularly and then added something in a lower voice. This Mr. Brahms appeared to me as someone a little lower than a criminal as he kept company with that woman, whom our aunt sometimes called a *Hur* (whore). This was the first time I had ever heard this expression—it was certainly before the age of kindergarten—and I asked my mother on the way home what the word meant. My mother was shocked and forbade me ever to utter that bad word. She gave me no information about its meaning, but even at the time I must have sensed what it signified. Some of that foreknowledge about sex, so regularly met with in children, must have told me why the unknown Herr von Brahms used to visit that woman.

The second time I heard the name of Brahms was not long after Aunt Resi's circumstantial gossip. On a walk with my father we met a stocky old man with a long gray beard. My father took his hat off to him, and the man did likewise to my father. "That was Herr Brahms," said my father. "You know he is the man who wrote many of the lieder Mother sings. He has written beautiful music." I turned around and looked after the man, who walked in a very dignified manner. I remembered that Aunt Resi had spoken of this man, and also in what connection, but I did not tell Father. In spite of her report, it was difficult to imagine Mr. Brahms as a lover—he was old and dignified—but I had to believe Aunt Resi's words.

His name had come up in the meantime because Mother had sung some of his songs, accompanying herself on the piano. I did not like all of them, but some, like the vivid and tuneful *Vergebliches Ständchen*, I could soon hum. When Mother once mentioned the composer's name to a lady visitor, I had asked whether that was the same man who used to visit the lady across from Aunt Resi's house. Mother answered, "Yes."

I understood the text of *Vergebliches Ständchen* in a vague and childish manner. I realized that the song is a dialogue between a lover who pleads with a girl to let him come to her in the evening and that she refuses him and finally sends him away. I also knew that the title of the song *Vergebliches Ständchen* meant, in effect, a disappointed or futile serenade. In a naïve manner I brought the text in intimate thought-connection with the personal life of the composer about whom I knew only what Aunt Resi had told my mother. I imagined that "that woman" had once refused to let Mr. Brahms come to her room and that he complained about this misfortune in his song. It seems I did not give much thought to the fact that such behavior on the part of the lady would be in contradiction to her attitude on other occasions when Mr. Brahms spent the night in her apartment, according to Aunt Resi's report. I assumed that the lady once rejected him for reasons of her own.

My mother sang the *Vergebliches Ständchen* occasionally in later years. As a matter of fact, I heard her sing it after I was in my adolescence. The title and the content of the song had, in the meantime, taken on a new and secret meaning for me.

I had then acquired not only an adequate knowledge of what adults do in sex, but also a rich, if vulgar, vocabulary for sexual activities. The boys in school and on the playgrounds were good teachers, and the gutter was an excellent school for a boy curious about the facts of life. The vulgar word for the erection, the upright position of the penis, in Vienna is *Ständer*, a derivative of the word "stand," comparable to the American vulgar expression "hard-on." *Ständchen* could be interpreted as a diminutive of "stand," and would then mean a small or modest erection. The title of the Brahms lied *Vergebliches Ständchen* would, thus understood, mean futile small erection, that is, a state of sexual excitement of the male without release. In that phase of boyhood the fantasy was filled with sexual images and the interpretation of the song and of its title is not as astonishing as it now sounds. The lascivious fantasy of the "naughty" boy transformed the disappointed serenade into the picture of an erection not brought to its organic end, a sexual excitement that was frustrated by the cruelty of a girl.

In later years, also, when I read about the relationship of the composer and Clara Schumann, the thought of that lady of easy virtue, Aunt Resi's neighbor, sometimes appeared. It was so persistent that it emerged when I heard the *Vergebliches Ständchen* again. In spite of what mental and emotional maturity I could muster in the meantime, the suspicion remained that the *Ständchen* was futile or the sexual performance of poor Brahms. So stubborn was this impression from boyhood that this thought sometimes emerged disturbingly when I passed the impressive monument to the great composer that stands before the Technical College at Vienna—not far from the street where Aunt Resi and her blond young neighbor lived.

Remnants of that old doubt of Brahms's capabilities as a lover were, it seems, displaced to his authorship of the *Liebeslieder Walzer* as if I were not certain that the master was able to love a woman. Later on there was the puzzling problem of how it was possible that Brahms was so much in love with Clara and yet could regularly visit that slut in a back street of Vienna. I still remember that, during junior high-school years, I read the shocking sentence Gustave Flaubert once wrote to the effect that a young man can worship a certain woman and in spite of it run every evening to prostitutes (*"Un jeune homme peut adorer une femme et aller chaque soir chez les filles"*). But many years had to pass before I found, in Freud's psychoanalytic writing, an explanation of that division in the love life of many men.

Returning in thought to the *Liebeslieder Walzer,* one remembers that the North German Brahms spent most of his life in Vienna, and Johann Strauss was his contemporary. The two composers knew each other well and often met in Vienna and in Ischl, the lovely summer resort near Salzburg. Brahms admired the melodic invention of the Waltz King. Asked to autograph the fan of Alice Strauss, he wrote the first bars of the *Blue Danube* waltz and beneath it: "Alas, not by Johannes Brahms."

This enchanting waltz came to my mind the other day in another connection and with it another memory of young years. It deals with a different aspect of the sexual problems.

The other night before falling asleep I skimmed through the pages of two books I had read before: *Anatole France en pantoufles* and *Itinéraire de Paris au Buenos Aires* by Jean Jacques Brousson, the master's secretary. The wit and the wisdom, the mordant skepticism and the penetrating insight of Anatole France delighted me again. In a certain passage, the old master of the Villa Said alludes, in conversation with his young, alert secretary, to Remy de Gourmont's *Physiologie de l'amour* and praises the snails as masterpieces of creation because they are male and female simultaneously and can try now one sex and then the other. Their sexual union lasts five or six weeks. Anatole France remarked, "That would be worth while indeed," and added that for us poor humans the pleasure lasts but the time of a lightning flash.

He reminded Brousson of the Capuchin friar, Barbette, who thundered to his audience from the pulpit a few hundred years ago: "You give yourself up to frivolous living and to fornication, you poor people, you are nothing but fools. The game is not worth the candle! In your ecstasy you touch the seventh heaven, but how long do you remain there? If it lasted seven years, seven months, seven days, seven hours only! But it lasts only a moment and in a trice you are already in hell!" The old master certainly imitated the pious indignation of the Capuchin father who tried to convince the faithful that the short duration of sexual pleasure, followed by hell-fire, is, so to speak, a bad investment. Anatole France regretted with Father Barbette the transitoriness of sexual pleasure and pointed out that the snails who are ugly and repugnant animals have some advantages over human beings: they are hermaphrodites, their loves last six weeks and they have an exitatory genital instrument with a long point. "Yes, my friend," Anatole France added, "just this is worth an immortal soul."

The secretary gave a detailed and intimate report of France's lecture tour in Latin America. On board ship, the writer, now almost sixty-five years old, began an affair with a French actress. He admitted to Brousson that she was no youngster—as a matter of fact, she was fifty years old—and that her face had many and marked wrinkles, but the rest of her: "Ah! youth itself!" In the meantime, Madame de Cavaillet, his mistress of so many years, sat alone in Paris in despair because the news reaching her left no doubt that Anatole France had made a fool of himself. Brousson reported in his books many witty sayings of his genial master who still did not believe in "pure love." France amused his serious Provençal secretary in elaborating on and embroidering the story Seigneur de Brantôme told in his *Mémoires* in 1650: that he met an old man whom he had once known as a young, gallant, and handsome fellow and as a favorite of the ladies. He had become a druggist and now manufactured all kinds of excellent drinks. Brantôme visited him, surrounded by his vials, and congratulated him. But the old man confessed to the young one that all his liquors, however excellent, were not as valuable as the wonderful liquid which he had once used and enjoyed so much and of which old age had deprived him.

Did not Schopenhauer praise old age because the sexual desire ceases with it? But it is not true, only the sexual power ceases. A clever German woman, Alice Berend, once wrote that the bad thing in getting old is not that one becomes older, but that one remains young. The French writers are not only more worldly-wise but also more sincere and courageous in sexual matters than the writers of other nations. They candidly state that it is not the desire that is wanting in old age, but the performance. They do not play hide-and-seek with themselves, and they assert that the sexual pleasure is one of the greatest that human life has to offer. What other satisfaction can be compared with it? Achievement, fame, social recognition? Zola's Pascal Rougon, sixty years old, looks back on his life and often feels like cursing his science which he accuses of having stolen from him *"le meilleur de sa virilité."* In Maupassant's *Bel Ami,* an old writer speaks to a younger one in the same vein as Anatole France spoke to young, alert Jean Jacques Brousson, who flattered and envied the famous master: "What use is the goal, fame, if I can't enjoy it any more in the form of love?" And he adds the wonderful sentence: *"Encore quelques baisers et vous serez impuissant."* France himself calls the impotence of old age *"la première mort."*

Yes, the French writers have the courage and the candor to express a high evaluation of sexual satisfaction, and they do not shrink from presenting the sexual misery of old age whose desire is mostly in the mind. There is a lot of talk, serious and flippant, about sexuality in American literature, but what writer speaks as clearly and definitely and in such matter-of-fact manner of certain aspects of sex as the French?

They are neglected or brushed aside even in psychoanalytic literature. Only Freud courageously turned against the moralistic hypocrisy of our society that looks at sexual pleasures condescendingly at best. In some passages of his writings, he speaks of the high evaluation of sexual satisfaction in contrast to a conventional and hypocritical attitude that treats it as if it were secondary and really dispensable. He reports, for instance, that the Turks in the Herzegowina evaluate sexual pleasure above all others and that sexual disturbances make them fall into despair that strangely contrasts with their fatalistic resignation when facing death.* A Turkish patient told his doctor, "You know, sir, if that does not function any more, life has no value."

While I was pondering on such a high evaluation of sexuality as is expressed by Zola, Maupassant, France, and that Turkish patient, I felt increasingly sleepy and I was gliding into that state between being awake and falling asleep which is favorable to a looser way of thinking. On the threshold of sleep the first bars of the Strauss waltz *On the Beautiful Blue Danube* were suddenly heard by the inner ear. I wondered from where these bubbling rhythms emerged. The face of Johann Strauss appeared in my mind, as I have seen it in photographs and on the monument in the Stadtpark in Vienna: a grand seigneur of music, surrounded by beautiful women. Some memory connected with that monument was stirred up, but I could not grasp it. I was too tired to think. The tune of the *Blue Danube* waltz accompanied me into sleep.

A few weeks later I invited a lady to have dinner with me at Fassler's Viennese Room on Fifty-first Street. On the walls of that restaurant are pictures of different places and houses in Vienna, and on the tables are wind-protected candles as at the *Heurigen,* those little restaurants in the suburbs of Vienna, and there is music, too: a piano player and a violinist as well as a singer. Behind the piano is a life-sized bronze bust of Johann Strauss, illuminated by light from above. For a moment you can have the illusion that you sit again at a *Heurigen,* listening to the old

* In *On the Psychopathology of Everyday Life* (New York, 1914).

familiar melodies. Now the piano player begins to play, the violinist joins him, and there it is: the *Blue Danube* waltz.

That tune in my ears and the bust of Strauss, shining in the candlelight in the corner, brought back in a flash the memory for which I had searched in vain the other day. It had not been really forgotten; it was only that I had not thought of it for many, perhaps for forty years. There was the distinct image of the alleys and meadows of the Stadtpark and of that monument of the Waltz King on the right side.

Quite clearly I see the figure in my mind's eye, his face, the full head of hair, the mustache (he dyed both when he became old). The violin under his chin, the bow in an elegant pose. At the right, at the left, and on the high arch above the composer's figure are beautiful dancing women whose dresses seem to flow into waves at their feet, the waves of the beautiful blue Danube.

And now that scene comes distinctly back to mind, as if it had been yesterday and not forty-five years. . . . Ah, I was twenty-two years old and it was early in the summer, the time before the last examinations. . . . When we did not have to attend lectures, we took our books to a public garden to study there. Once I sat in the Stadtpark on a bench facing the monument of Johann Strauss. I had the psychology books by Wundt and Ziehen with me and made a determined effort to cram as much knowledge of physiological and psychological facts as possible. There was an old man sitting beside me, comfortably smoking his cigar and sometimes looking into his newspaper. I rarely glanced up from my book. When I once looked after a pretty young girl who had just passed the bench, I felt that the man smiled at me. He said in a broad Viennese dialect, "Quite good-looking, isn't she? . . . I bet you would not say no, if she would ask you to, would you? . . . Yes, it is nice to be young. . . . You will understand that much better when you become old."

I must have made some inane remarks to the effect that to be old had some advantages also, because the man replied in a vivid manner, "Oh, don't say that, my young friend! Look over there, yes, to that monument." He pointed to the statue of Strauss.*

* Here is a mistake of memory: Strauss's monument was erected a few years later.

"They called him King Johann the Second because his father who was a conductor was also called Johann. You know, I am a violinist and I played in his orchestra many years. . . . I quit only after he died. Back in 1894—you were a child—they celebrated his fiftieth jubilee as an artist. There was a week of concerts in his honor, a brilliant torch parade, all the streets were full of banners and decorations. The Emperor and the Court congratulated him, and thousands of cables arrived from all over the world to pay homage to him. Verdi and all the great composers wrote and praised him. I shall never forget how he conducted our orchestra on that day in the Theater an der Wien. We played, of course, the *Blue Danube* waltz and all those beautiful tunes. Each of us came over to him and paid his respects. He pressed my hand and he took me aside. And you know what he said? "Look, my dear fellow, what's the use of fame and all that? . . . I *can't* any more, don't you understand, I *can't* any more." The old musician wanted to tell me more about his beloved master, but I had to hurry to a lecture at the university.

"What were you thinking of?" asked the lady who was my dinner guest. "You smiled the way you do when you think of a delightful anecdote." I told her that I had returned in my thoughts to old Vienna and to the time when I was twenty years old. I spoke also of Johann Strauss whose bust glimmered in the candlelight over there and whose sparkling *Blue Danube* waltz the musicians had just finished playing. I told her about his anniversary at which he was celebrated by the Viennese like a god. But I did not tell her of the conversation with the musician in the Stadtpark nor of what Johann Strauss had said at his jubilee.

4

It has often been said that "music and mathematics go together," that composition and mathematical creation have a sturdy stem in common from which they branch in opposite directions. The most fundamental of the arts and the most fundamental of the sciences show in their best creations the necessary conditions of inevitability, importance, and economy, the same logical progression from one stage to another.* The interest in music that appeals to emotion and in mathematics that appeals to intellect often coexist. Many mathematicians and mathematical physicists from Pythagoras to Einstein feel very attracted to that art, and quite a few composers have occupied themselves with mathematical problems. It seems to both groups possible to turn with relief from one interest to the other. We are not astonished when we learn that musical associations sometimes stimulate mathematical research work.

Nothing of such an affinity is known between music and scientific psychology, although the one speaks the language of emotions and the other explores them. The urge of imaginative expression on one side and the special curiosity that leads to scientific inquisitiveness do not often meet. The preceding chapters presented many examples in which tunes appeared in the mind of the psychoanalyst or the patient during analytic sessions or in connection with them. It was pointed out that they fulfill a certain psychological function and that the analyst has to listen to the whisper of their meaning while until now he did not give them a second thought, if he gave them any. In this chapter, an example will be presented in detail which, I hope, will prove that musical associations also have an unconscious purpose in abstract psychological research.

My restricted reading does not allow me to state that there are no statements or reports on whether and how musical associations have influenced scientific work, interfered with or advanced the mental task of research. It would be very interesting to know what influence musical impressions had on the thought processes of Theodor Billroth, to whom modern surgery owes so many new methods, and who was a friend of Johannes Brahms and very interested in music.** Were the profound reflections on physics of Albert Einstein, who was an excellent violinist, sometimes interrupted by melodies?

Cautious questioning concerning the emergence and influence of musical associations was neither encouraging nor conclusive.

* Guy Warrage, "Music and Mathematics," *Music and Letters* (Jan., 1945), Vol. XXVI, No. 1.
** Dr. Billroth published a book *Wer ist musikalish?* (Vienna, 1896.)

Some scientists could not remember that their research work was ever influenced by musical ideas. Others stated that some melodies had occasionally occurred to them during their research work, but they treated such emergence as a pleasant diversion which had nothing to do with the intellectual task that occupied them. A few attributed a vague stimulating effect to tunes that had come to mind, or considered them as expressions of good or sad moods. Two physicians told me that they liked to listen to music while they pondered on possible diagnosis of cases. A chemist said that he had caught himself humming a phrase from Beethoven's Sixth Symphony while he considered a certain succession of biochemical experiments, but that he was irritated when he heard piano playing while he worked in his laboratory on experiments that demanded precision and undivided attention.

Even when inquiries are restricted to the group of researchers who love music, the danger of glib generalizations has to be considered. The emotional situation of the investigator while he is working has to be taken into account as well as the nature of his specific work. It is less likely that the solution of an equation, some logarithmic calculation, or the search for a chemical formula is accompanied by a musical association than an abstract speculation about some mathematical or chemical process. It might seem that a purely mechanical occupation, let us say a laboratory experiment in the pursuit of a research project, favors the emergence of some tune, but we run here into the psychological problem of attention. It is very possible that the mind of the chemist who is performing the experiment, just because his work is at the moment of a mechanical nature, is occupied with some complex problem.

Our mental activity is a mixture of goal-directed, logical, and rational thinking and of loose, imaginative, fantastic, and irrational thought-processes. The ratio of mixture in each individual thought-act is different, and in our thinking as a whole variable. We say "sober as a judge," and mean that the opinion of the judge is as much as possible unbiased, devoid of emotional interferences, and governed only by logical and rational conclusions and considerations. But we cannot know to what extent irrational, prejudiced emotional factors enter even into what we like to call "our considered judgment." It seems that melodies express that emotional and loose, fantastic component of our thinking and manifest that part of our thought-productivity which results more from our imagination than from logical operations. The information I was able to get from quite a few researchers and scientists seems to confirm this conjecture, at least in the majority of cases.

As a kind of psychological circumstantial evidence, the following observation, reported by different scientists, can be considered: The hearing of a symphony or of some chamber music, far from interfering with the intellectual work, had an indefinite, but distinct stimulating effect upon the research as long as the scientist did not pay more than casual attention to the music and was concentrated on his research problem. Whenever he became more attentive to the melodic texture or the harmonic structure of the composition, he felt that his interest in the research problem was receding. It did not vanish, but it moved into the background and reappeared only after that other musical interest flagged. A psychiatrist, occupied with a theory on schizophrenia, reported that, while considering the physiological and psychological factors of that psychosis, he could listen to the Fourth Symphony of Brahms in the described aloof manner. He enjoyed the theoretical speculations about the nature of that psychotic disease at the same time as the melodies of the symphony. His trains of thought, directed to the relation of somatic and psychogenic factors in schizophrenia, were interrupted by the memory that he had once read that this Brahms symphony had been called the Oedipus Symphony. The name, meaningful to the psychiatrist, interfered with the pleasure of scientific daydreaming as well as with the enjoyment of music.

In another case the thought-process of a chemist, directed to the possibility of finding a new antitoxin, was interrupted because he followed a certain musical motive through a Mozart quartet. Before this moment he was well able to pursue his ideas while listening to the composition. When he began to pay attention to that motive, when he, so to speak, waited for its reappearance within the movement, his attention was deflected from the chemical problem. I can add a self-observed experience to these examples: While thinking of a psychological theory on the differences of the sexes,

I listened to the *Siegfried Idyll* by Richard Wagner. When it occurred to me that the composition celebrated the birth of Wagner's son, my thoughts moved from the psychological subject to my own son Arthur and to memories of his birth, to my wife, to Vienna where he was born, and so on. While listening to a symphony or to chamber music in many cases does not interfere with and sometimes even favorably influences theoretical and abstract thinking, it is difficult, if not impossible, to follow ideas or reflections of this kind, if, for instance, the attention is directed to the words of a song or to the text of an opera aria. The indefinite and wide-spaced character of the melodic, rhythmical, and harmonic development of a symphonic movement does not interfere with the thought-process, while the words of a lied or of an aria compel the turning of the listener's attention in a certain direction.

The bits of information gathered in the preceding paragraphs are in no way appropriate to fill the gap in our knowledge about the influence of music, especially of musical associations, on abstract and scientific thinking. They cannot satisfy our hunger for understanding because they are too unsubstantial and light. They do not provide enough food for thought, but rather whet our appetite. They are more comparable to hors d'oeuvres served before a meal than to its regular courses.

Since there is such a lack of information and a complete absence of appropriate instances, any contribution, however trifling, should be welcome. The following presents an instance that attempts, for the first time, as far as I know, to demonstrate the way in which a musical association can enter the area of theoretical scientific thinking. In giving a precise description of the origin and the evolution of the intellectual process up to the point where the melody emerged, I hope to make obvious the psychological meaning and function of its appearance and how it differs from other associations. Needless to say that the theoretical part of the research here considered is of secondary importance. It has, nevertheless, to be accurately described and minutely presented in order to define at which point the musical association intruded the area of scientific hypothesis. The patient reader will thus bear with a detailed presentation of the psychological problem of re-

search which is followed by a shorter discussion of the significance of the tune that surprisingly emerged in the middle of attempts to come to conclusions. The subject matter of the research
was as remote from the area of music as possible. It concerned
the psychology and psychopathology of obesity, especially its emotional factors. I shall try to show what the emerging melody
meant, but, more than this, that its occurrence within a certain
train of thought gave me a new angle on the problem and marked
progress on the way to its solution.

The evolution of psychological theory does not take place in a
vacuum remote from the experiences of everyday life. It is a result of many impressions and insights that have to be verified and
checked many times before they reach the first and still vague
shape of a tentative theory. From where I, as psychoanalyst, sit,
namely, on a chair behind the patient, human emotions, thoughts,
and impulses look one way, while they have a different appearance when you look at them from your desk, alone late at
night, trying to abstract their general character from the individual cases and formulate their essential qualities apart from the
particular and personal traits. The different phases in the evolution of a theory require different talents of the researcher. For
the first phase originality of observation is, it seems to me, the
most important requirement, while for the following the
capability of seeing phenomena in a general, abstract way is
indispensable.

The following concept is taken from the transition phase between observation and the first shaping of a new theory. During
the analysis of several cases, I had received certain impressions,
condensed by accumulation, about the emotional dynamics of
aggressive drives in obese and overweight persons. Certain behavior traits of patients seemed to point to a common pattern,
however different their personalities were. The representative
instances considered in this period of the formation of a theory
germ were two men and two women.

Jack, a man in his late thirties, had some emotional difficulties
with his boss in the office. He often felt insulted and humiliated
by the criticism of the older man, who was a father-representative
person for him. Jack had many revenge fantasies and often day-

dreamed that he would give his boss "a piece of my mind." The samples he presented in analytic sessions were filled with abuses and curses of the vilest kind. Jack's vivid imagination went beyond scenes in which he cursed his superior to fantasies in which he added cruel injuries to unprintable insults. Jack's aggressiveness exhausted itself in those fantasies. He realized that in real life he was unable to inflict any harm on his antagonist. He complained that he could not be a heel and a villain as he would like to be, and daydreamed that he might just once become a ruthless and reckless character, able to walk over the corpses of his enemies. He was sometimes desperate because he behaved in a quite friendly way toward a man whom he hated and whom he wished to destroy. He sometimes had short-lived flare-ups of temper, but was soon reconciled by a few friendly words. The complaint he expressed several times during an analytic session sounded almost pathetic: "If I only could be a son of a bitch just once, I need not be a son of a bitch any more." It is conspicuous that in moods of indignation or rage he sometimes ate much more than usual. On some occasions he indulged himself in a moderate kind of eating orgy—for instance, taking dinner twice within an hour. Jack was stout and will perhaps become fat in progressed middle age.

The case of Alice was distinctly different in all essential traits. She had been a very fat child and continued to be plump until her late twenties when she reduced under an energetic regime of diet, drugs, and exercises. When, ten years later, she became my patient, she had a perfect figure according to the present fashion. She wanted to keep it because she wished to remain attractive, but she had an intense craving for food to which she occasionally yielded with subsequent regrets and remorse. Her attitude to food was also influenced by various neurotic fears; for instance, by hypochondriacal alarms. She suffered periodically from the fear that she had tuberculosis, cancer, and various infectious diseases, and attacks of these fears sometimes reached the degree of panic. Many of them could be traced back in analysis to reactions on aggressive impulses against persons of her family. She was, for instance, afraid that she might take a knife and cut the throat of her daughter or in a moment of absent-mindedness poison her husband.

The connection between this kind of obsessive thinking and her hypochondriacal symptoms became obvious on many occasions. One instance will serve as representative. She had cocktails before dinner with her husband with whom she chatted amiably. When she went to the kitchen to get something, she suddenly had the suspicion that her husband would use her absence to put some poison into her cocktail glass. Shortly after dinner she felt very ill and "unswallowed," the refined expression she used for vomiting. The operating of a paranoid projection mechanism became obvious on many occasions of this kind.

The patient's attitude to her appearance was dependent on her emotional situation in more ways than one. On the whole, she felt satisfied with her youthful figure when she looked at herself in the mirror. But sometimes her slimness became the very reason for hypochondriacal fears, and she anxiously asked herself: "Is anything the matter with me? I am perhaps ill without feeling pain." She remembered having seen some cases of cancer in which the patients rapidly lost weight, and she became terrified at the thought that she could have various forms of the dreaded disease. She then detected several symptoms of carcinoma in herself and became the victim of intense anxieties anticipating the agonies and the inevitable end. To assuage her fears, she began to eat compulsively until she looked too fat and started a strict diet again. During the analytic treatment, this cycle could be observed several times. It was interesting that Alice's temperament seemed also to be affected by it. When she ate too much, she appeared amiable, well meaning, and affable, good-tempered and inclined to do favors for people. When she kept a strict diet and became slim, she was often sharply critical and sarcastic, suspicious, remote, and cautious in social intercourse.

The third case is that of Victor, a writer, forty-one years old. The center of his emotional difficulties was formed by his attitude to his father, stepmother, and his brothers. He had considerable swings of mood, reaching from depressions in which he was almost apathetic, to hypomanic states in which he made himself the butt of many, sometimes excellent, jokes. He described his emotional situation as a battlefield of opposite forces, and felt best when those antagonists in him had arrived at an armistice. The well-read patient described those peaceful phases in theological terms; for instance, in those of the German mystics as Eckhart, Boehme, Tauler, and others. He spoke of those periods as of "states of grace" in which he was neither under the compulsive power of intense drives of hatred and sexual desires nor subjected to overpowering feelings of guilt and shame. He oscillated in his emotions from those of a sinner in despair and atonement to those of a saint who feels superior to others, and but rarely succeeded in reaching the state of a person ready to make compromises between his own impulses and the demands of society.

The change from depression to an almost humorous self-mockery was sometimes immediate. During a progressed phase of his analysis, when he had been lying on the couch in a kind of apathy for a longer time than usual, he interrupted his silence with the following sentence: "I don't know why I am punishing myself so cruelly. All this because I have killed a few people in my thoughts? When you think of the millions murdered during the war, the number of persons I killed does not even need consideration." This kind of sorry humor in which he looked at his troubles and emotional difficulties from a bird's-eye view also appeared in his writings. He was able to deprive himself of food when he felt in the mood of atonement and to go on a "binge" of eating when the severity of his self-accusations diminished. The following action appeared to me very significant: He once appeared on a Sunday morning at the apartment of his family, ready to make peace with his father and stepmother. When, unannounced, he entered the living room, he saw among the things laid out on the breakfast table a big coffeecake. His relatives who were unaware of his arrival were in the next room, and he overheard some unfavorable comments they made about him. Seized by a sudden rage, he took the coffeecake destined for the whole family from the plate, and tiptoed to the door without revealing his presence. While he hurried home through the streets, he ate the whole cake in an attack of voracious fury.

The last case to be considered in this context is not as colorful as the previous one. Margaret, a woman in her late thirties, had divorced her first husband and had married a man much younger than herself. She discovered some years later that her husband had resumed an earlier affair and recognized that she could not hope to win back his love. After a time of stormy scenes in which she expressed her rage and despair, she glided into depression bordering on a melancholic state. She neglected her appearance and started to eat excessively. In a relatively short time she was transformed into an overweight matron of stout figure, double chin, and excessive bust and hips. She neglected her household duties and dedicated most of her time to playing rummy and gossiping. Margaret appeared phlegmatic and egocentric, although friendly and good-natured. While her mood was in general depressive, she had moments in which a kind of resigned and even lovable humor broke through the clouded atmosphere of her life.

The first impression these representative cases of obese personalities make is that the patients have reacted to an emotional frustration, or rather to several frustrations, by oral regression—that is, by returning to an early phase of development in which the gratification of food is most prevalent. The excessive intake of food has the function of consolation and compensation for those emotional frustrations among which unfulfilled desire for love and social recognition has the first rank. The consolation in these cases would be basically the same as in the case of a child to whom a wish is denied and who forgets his unhappiness when he gets a lollipop. This impression or psychological hypothesis is accepted by the majority of psychoanalysts who have investigated many cases of obesity and consider it as the result of a personality disturbance in which excessive bodily size becomes the expression of an emotional conflict.*

That general impression becomes qualified by the study of compulsive eaters, a type that contributes most cases to the group of overweight persons. These patients admit that they are not hungry, but that they cannot resist the craving for food. Almost all analysts can report cases of men and women who after a rich dinner sneak to the refrigerator and eat all within their reach. The psychological concept of this, as of all compulsions, is that

* The analytical literature on the problem has recently been enlarged by contributions by Hilde Bruch, Gustav Bychowsky, Alfred Schick, Eduardo Weiss, and many other investigators.

it generally appears as a defense against a danger or a threat from within—originally from without, but later internalized and transformed in o a part of the ego. The earliest and most primitive form of such a danger in the cases here considered would be that of starving. Compulsive eating would, thus considered, amount to an exaggerated defense to ward off the anxiety of starving. Compulsive intake of food and the resulting obesity are determined by the dread of famishing which is met by the tendency to stuff oneself. That elementary fear can be put into the formula: Eat or you will starve. Nothing or almost nothing of such a primitive menace reaches the conscious level. It is mute, yet able to express itself in the language of neurotic symptoms.

Thus far, this presentation has followed the line of most psychoanalytic theories on obesity. At this point it branches off in a new direction: at the roots of that primitive fear there must be something still more elementary and more intimately connected with the struggle for existence than expresses itself in the return to oral satisfaction. It is to be assumed that this unknown impulse does not belong to the early history of the individual, but to his prehistory or even to the prehistory of the race. Speaking in comparison, the elementary drives and the collateral fears are not to be traced back to the era of the earliest Egyptian dynasties, but to the ancestors of Neanderthal Man. The most primitive forms in which those impulses are expressed live only in remnants with the cannibalistic tribes of Australia. Other traces are to be found in distorted forms of neurotic symptoms and in ancient myths and fairy tales. The alternative in the tale of "Hänsel and Gretel" appears in the shape: to eat or to starve. But when the children arrive at the house of the witch, the situation is changed. Through all tranformations and distortions you will find below the superstructure of those old myths and fairy tales the cannibalistic drives and cannibalistic dreads. Hänsel and Gretel are afraid of being eaten up by the witch. But at the end they are pushing her into the oven, we have to add, to be cooked and eaten. Even before that they are eating from the witch's gingerbread house, which is a symbolic substitute of her body. Behind that fairy tale is the alternative to eat or to be eaten. That was then the question.

At this point the clinical pictures before described and others not here recorded led to the budding of a little analytic contribution. Its original form attempts an answer to the question: Why are obese and overweight people supposed to be harmless, realistic, and not malicious or, otherwise put, what happens to the cruel and aggressive drives of those persons?

The germination of that tiny theory was favored by the re-reading of the famous book *Körperbau und Character* by Ernst Kretzschmer.*

Otto Fennichel considers Kretzschmer's attempt to co-ordinate certain types of character with body structures "not very attractive to the analyst."** That, of course, is a question of taste. The fact that Kretzschmer's work is not analytic in its point of view does not exclude that it is of great importance. It is very attractive to this analyst, especially because its thesis was intuitively anticipated by great writers and because its basic view of characterological types coincides with my own observations and experiences. In spite of its obvious shortcomings, Kretzschmer's differentiation of schizoid and cycloid personalities and the characterological distinction between them is a valuable and valid contribution to the recognition of human temperaments. Kretzschmer attributes to the schizoid type a slim body build and a cold, remote personality, and to the cycloid type a rather stocky or stout physique and a warm, conciliatory, and realistic personality.

The German psychiatrist considers those types as extreme ones and differentiates many mixed forms, alloys, and so on. In the description of the cycloid type, mostly found in well-nourished or obese persons, Kretzschmer points out different basic groups of temperaments: sociable, good-natured, and genial people; another, he characterizes as cheerful, humorous, and jolly and soft-hearted. In general, obese people are friendly and sociable, tolerant and affable, compared with the thin, sharp-featured schizoid type which is often fanatic, idealistic, introverted, philosophically inclined, systematic, often sarcastic and scheming, of a cold and remote personality.

The aggressiveness of fat people is not of a cruel and sadistic

* English translation (2nd ed.; London, 1925).
** *The Psychoanalytic Theory of Neurosis* (New York, 1948).

type, but rather characterized by primitive orality. It is more directed to incorporate their object than to tear it to pieces. Fat people are more inclined to eat their object than to bite it. The clinical papers of Karl Abraham divide the oral development of the child into two stages, an early suckling phase and a later biting one.* According to this differentiation, obese or overweight persons either remained in their development on that earlier phase or returned to it under the influence of frustrations. In contrast to the lean and hungry type, they are less inclined to be aggressive, biting, tyrannical, and argumentative.

Kretzschmer remarked that the Devil usually appears in the fantasy of the people as lean, with a thin beard growing on a narrow chin. He should have added that God, in contrast to the Evil One, is mostly imagined as an old, stout man with a bushy white beard.

The analytic continuation of Kretzschmer's theory would lead to the assumption that the cycloid type is characterized by a regression to the first phase of orality. In this return, the aggressive and cruel, sadistic drives are to a great extent replaced by oral tendencies. A finer distinction would perhaps differentiate another group within the cycloid one which has built a kind of oral defense against the danger of retribution for his aggressive and cruel drives. Otherwise put: this type is afraid of the intensity of his own aggressive and hostile drives and therefore regressed to an earlier phase in which there were no serious and dangerous conflicts with the external world. The energy, otherwise used in the pursuit of aggressive, hostile, and sadistic strivings, becomes redirected to protect the self that is afraid of the consequences of its repressed aggressiveness. The mechanism is thus a defense against the threatening retribution and at the same time a regression to the phase of an infantile pleasure-ego, an early organization of the individual in which the world is "tasted," orally tested as to whether it tastes good or bad. That defense would manifest itself not only in a lack of aggressiveness and cruelty that could endanger the self in the form of retribution, but also generally in avoidance of dangers, risks, and bold adventures, and in the last consequences in physical caution and even cowardice.

* In *Selected Papers on Psychoanalysis* (London, 1942).

The four clinical pictures presented before show, in various forms and variations, those emotional dynamics or their results. Jack is full of rage against his boss, but his vengefulness is expressed only in curses and abuses, and his conscience or his caution does not allow him to transform his fantasies into deeds; he cannot even give his boss a piece of his mind. In his reflections he oscillates between expressions of his impulses and those invisible counter-tendencies and his imagined enterprises lose in this way "the name of action." His sentence "If I could be a son of a bitch just once, I need not be a son of a bitch any more" is, so to speak, a Hamlet reflection in Brooklynese. The case of the patient who vacillates between her craving for food and her hypochondriacal fears shows the suggested process in flux. She protects herself against the dreaded retribution for her murderous impulses in the form of eating. The nature of her fear points in the direction of the menace of being eaten up from within (cancer). Her anxiety when she sees herself becoming thin reflects the elementary dread of starving. Margaret's obesity is the result of excessive intake of food after her frustration and disappointment in her marriage. At the same time it marks her resignation and renunciation of her aggression and rage against her husband and her rival. Her regression to oral gratification replaces her violent outbursts and is her defense against their repetition. Her depression seems to show that she still has to fight against guilt feelings. Victor's symptomatic action, the eating of the breakfast coffeecake, is almost a manifestation of a certain phase of that process, in which aggressiveness expresses itself in a purely oral form. As such, it marks a transition from a progressed stage of aggressive action to an infantile level.

This theory—better, this onset of a theory—went a few steps farther beyond the area here sketched in the investigation of the vicissitudes of aggressive drives of obese personalities. It attempted to conceive of the swings of moods, so conspicuous in the cycloid types, in terms of their oral attitudes. It is daring, but not nonsensical, to compare the hypomanic mood or phase with the emotional attitude of enjoyment of a meal and with the mood of saturated appetite, and the depressive phase with the time of unsatisfactory or unpleasing digestion. Putting aside all intellectual cautions for a moment, one could venture to assert that the elation or the manic phases manifest the enjoyment of food (licking one's lips!), while the depression would indicate that the meal did not agree with the person.* To evaluate this psychological alternative, one has to regress in one's ideas to the most elementary level. The elation, thus considered, would mean that an incorporated object was well digested, and the depression would signify that the incorporation was not very successful. The proof of the incorporated object is in the eating, or rather at some time after it. At the highest level such disagreeing of food would find its emotional correlation in depression or guilt feelings. Following the two possibilities of elation or mania and of depressions, the investigator who has picked up a trail has gone the limit of a working hypothesis, from the earliest phase of primitive incorporation to the last in which all is in the mind.

The preceding theory was no more than an attempt to make understandable to myself the lack of aggressiveness, cruelty, malice, and grudge in obese or overweight persons. It was freely admitted that the hypothesis at which I arrived had not matured enough to be validated or voided. It had scarcely progressed beyond the phase of conjectures and suggestions and had not jelled enough to deserve the name of an analytic theory, merely that of an outset of theoretical reflections.

I do not share with my fellow-psychoanalysts the worship of science, and I do not kneel down before science which has been enthroned in the place left by God in the modern world. A respectful bow to scientific research is, to my way of thinking, enough. This lack of awe might explain, but perhaps not excuse, why I did not pursue the theoretical possibilities sketched before nor test and reexamine them by verification. I left the idea in suspense. It was at this point not a conscious decision, but a kind of indifference that left the future of the budding thought to destiny. I could have tossed a coin: heads I stick, tails I quit. Instead of trying that popular modern oracle, I let my thoughts wander into some sort of scientific daydreaming.

* These tentative psychoanalytic assumptions were jotted down long before Bertram Lewin's book *The Psychoanalysis of Elation* was published (New York, 1950). Dr. Lewin's interesting contribution does not mention Kretzschmer.

The continuation of Kretzschmer's thesis took its point of departure from observations of clinical cases. It moved from there to psychological assumptions and logical conclusions near the point where it should be formed and formulated into a scientific theory. Before it was crystallized, my attention was deflected and turned in a new direction. The process may well be compared to walking to a certain goal. On his way the wanderer becomes interested in something on a bypath and turns his attention to this new impression, forgetting for the moment his original goal. One is not always master of one's interests. Sometimes one does well in following one's inner voice rather than one's considered intentions. The destination that we had in mind can be quite remote from the place to which destiny sends us.

In the second part of his scientific work, Kretzschmer occasionally refers to proverbs and sayings of the people who seem to have anticipated some of his typological findings and who bring body build and character into intimate connection. He could have quoted many more and have added the sentences of writers who some centuries before his book confirm his opinions. There is, however, one greater authority he quotes. Shakespeare, speaking with the voice of Julius Caesar:

> Let me have men about me that are fat;
> Sleek-headed men and such as sleep o'nights;
> Yond' Cassius has a lean and hungry look;

In spite of what Antony has to say in praise of that Roman noble, Caesar remains unconvinced:

> Would he were fatter!
> . . . He loves no plays
> As thou dost, Antony; he hears no music;
> Seldom he smiles, and smiles in such a sort
> As if he mock'd himself and scorn'd his spirit,
> That could be moved by smile at anything
> Such men as he be never at heart's ease,
> Whiles they behold a greater than themselves,
> And therefore are they very dangerous.

While following Kretzschmer's typological considerations with great attention, I had been thinking coherently and rationally, but at this point my mind slipped away to all kinds of random thoughts. I can only guess that it was the memory of my patient Jack whom I had seen the day before that led my thoughts to the subject of vengeance in connection with Shakespeare's figures. Jack had again uttered wild curses against his boss and had sworn bloody revenge, which, I knew, he would never take. In contrast to him, the figure of Shylock and his terrible revengefulness came to mind. I imagined the Jew of Venice, a thin, sharp-featured older man, full of nervous energy and aggressiveness, a distinct schizoid-paranoid type. There is no superfluous flesh on his body, and his mind does not know a moment of leisure. The similes and terms he uses with regard to that bond are not accidentally taken from the area of food: "I will feed fat the ancient grudge I bear him." The question of what good a pound of flesh would do him is answered in the same vein: "To bait fish withal. If it feed nothing else, it will feed my revenge." Shylock is starving in this voracious hunger of vengeance and he does not allow himself much food. The sentence Heinrich Heine once wrote about an antagonist could be applied to Shylock: "He would not be so biting if he had more to bite." His sarcasm is bloody and its effects correspond to the sense of the Greek word which means tearing the flesh to pieces. His insistence on that pound of flesh from Antonio's body is a substitute for a cannibal craving. He seems to be a personification of that second sadistic, cannibal phase of orality as it is sketched in Karl Abraham's psychoanalytic theory.

Still under the impression of that clinical picture of my patient Jack, my random associations now glide to the figure of the Danish Prince with whom he shares the incapability of taking revenge. Like Jack, he has the "motive and the cue for passion" and he, too,

> must, like a trull, unpack my heart with words
> And fall a-cursing, like a very drab,
> A scullion!

Hamlet's aggressiveness exhausts itself in curses, abuses, and self-complaints. In the sense of Kretzschmer's theory he presents a mixed type of schizoid and cycloid temperament. His body build is described by the Queen: "He's fat and scant of breath." There are, however, many characterological features that point in the direction of a schizoid personality.

While my thoughts wander to other Shakespearean characters, to Othello, Iago, Richard, and Macbeth, a figure emerges in my associations, so voluminous and bulky that there is no place for others beside him: Sir John Falstaff. As in those sacred halls of the *Magic Flute,* vengeance is unknown in the Boar's Head Tavern of Eastcheap. Sir John is not revengeful and he does not understand how others could be. Poins warns the irritated Prince that Falstaff had spoken vilely of him before Doll: "My lord, he will drive you out of your revenge and turn all to merriment."

In omitting his figure, Kretzschmer has renounced the most representative example of the cycloid type as far as body build and temperament are concerned. Sir John is not just obese. He is obesity personified. He is sociable and jolly, full of zest of life and good humor. He has distinct features of oscillating between manic and depressive moods. There are sudden changes from an uninhibited *joie de vivre* to gloominess, from elation to a melancholic attitude. The greatest comical figure of world literature has conspicuous moments of sadness and expectancy of doom. He sighs, " 'Sblood, I am as melancholy as a gib cat or a lugged bear," and confesses that he is now "little better than one of the wicked." He is ready to repent and reform, but in the next moment he is very willing to rob some travelers. The Prince sees "a good amendment" in him "from praying to purse-taking." The knight himself brings his fatness in causal connection with his sadness: "A plague of sighing and grief. It blows a man up like a bladder." Is it not strange that Shakespeare, four hundred and fifty years before the analytic investigation of obesity, gives here an etiological explanation for the emotional genesis of overweight? Kretzschmer, who mentions the German expression *Kummer speck* (= grief-belly) in the context of his typology, has deprived himself of that classical explanation. There is even, comparable to the second clinical case described, a hypochondriacal fear in Falstaff that he might fall off in flesh, and, as in that case, the fear is clearly connected with guilt feelings and expectancy of impending personal calamity: "Bardolph, am I not fallen away vilely since this last action? do I not bate? do I not dwindle? Why, my skin hangs about me like an old lady's loose gown; I am withered like an old apple-john. Well, I'll repent, and that suddenly, while I am in some liking; I shall be out of heart shortly and then I shall have no strength to repent."

No doubt, that incomparable creation of a writer's imagination anticipated the scientific description of the cycloid character. More than this, we psychologists will have trouble catching up with it. Kretzschmer emphasizes, it is true, that the cycloid personality is generally earth-bound, realistic in contrast to the idealistic and sometimes fanatic and fantastic, eccentric, and lofty features of the schizoid type. Is there a better example of those traits than that pet mountain of a man? This full-grown and full-blown old man has kept the gaiety of a little boy, but also his sense of realism. He is not in awe of conventions, and the so-called sacred ideas do not impress him. He walks over them and laughs them off. He steals the show as he does any purse within his reach. He is amoral, a liar, a coward, a glutton, and a buffoon, a cheater, a reprobate, and invincible and irresistible in his charm and freedom, gained in humor. He sees through all make-believe and considers discretion the better part of valor. The self-protection and the absolutely realistic outlook, characteristic of the extreme cycloid temperaments, make him "a coward on instinct" while he is "as valiant as Hercules." His creed on honor will survive all the codes of nature. "Give me life!" cries Falstaff on the battlefield of Shrewsbury. The fear of death, so remote to the schizoid type, drives him to stuff himself with food.

He enjoys everything, but before all himself. This huge mass of flesh, this ton of a man will never "leave gormandizing," as the new King admonishes him. When we first meet Falstaff, he asks what time it is, and Prince Hal says: "Thou art so fat-witted, with drinking of old sack, and unbuttoning thee after supper, and sleeping upon benches after noon that thou hast forgotten to demand that truly which thou wouldst truly know. What a devil hast thou to do with the time of the day? unless hours were cups of sack, and minutes capons." Sir John is not only fun-loving, but funny, not only witty, but also the cause for other people's wit.

He does not think too much, he is fat and sleeps well, loves play and music. Caesar would not have considered him dangerous but would have wished to have him around.

The old rogue shouts a lot, but he barks rather than bites. He can abuse and curse as well as the next man. As well? No, much better. He is a genius at abusive comparisons and vile language, and has no par in the invention of invectives. But he is not sarcastic in his aggressiveness. He prefers biting into meat and fowl to making biting remarks on people. He lives on a minimum of activity if it is possible, and he is hurrying only to the set table, is not eager to arrive anywhere except to come and get it. He loves company and company loves him. He knows that he is loved and expresses the general liking people have for obese persons: "If to be fat be to be hated, then Pharaoh's lean kine are to be loved." He is the life of the party because he is the party of life.

We speak of fleeting thoughts, of the flash of an idea, but we have really no appropriate expression for the rapid speed with which thoughts cross time and space. In a split second I searched the little I know of world literature for obese and distinct cycloid personalities to be compared in some way or other to plump Jack, to the immortal figure of Sir John Falstaff. The express train of associations rushed from the stocky figure of the squire Sancho Panza, representing common sense, earthiness, and flexibility in contrast to the rigid insanity of his master, to the corpulent Nero Wolfe, the almost immobile gourmand and gourmet of Manhattan.

I heard my thoughts, so to speak, racing through the centuries of writing, but then I suddenly heard something very different. The *Rosenkavalier* waltz danced through my mind. The ¾ measures moved in casually and with sovereign indifference for the serious nature of the preceding associations, just as if they felt entirely at home in this intellectual environment. I had left the domain of purely theoretical reflections, it is true, but I was still searching for cycloid figures in world literature.

What business had that waltz in that sphere? To use a comparison, it was as if the secretary of a trust company were called to the conference of the board of directors, and in her place at the door of the conference room appeared a ballerina in short skirts.

I certainly had not called that abounding waltz. At this moment it was completely uncalled for, but I did not dismiss it immediately. It is psychologically interesting that sometimes we treat musical associations occurring to us in the middle of intellectual work differently than others. They are not violently ejected, but rather politely dismissed. We bow to them when we accompany them to the door of conscious thoughts, almost with regret that they appear at an inappropriate moment. And sometimes we welcome them although they come unannounced. Many men have stopped thinking of the brief they were working on and listened for a few moments to a barrel organ that played *Tea for Two* on the street. This by way of apology because I let the *Rosenkavalier* waltz dance through my serious thinking.

But then I began to ponder why it reappeared. What have those tuneful ¾ measures to do with Sir John of whom I had thought before? I had been in the England of virginal Elizabeth in my ideas and not in Vienna at the time of that other great queen, Maria Theresa. If the association had at least been the picture of the fat rogue as Edward Elgar painted it in the gargantuan boastfulness of his symphonic poem, the overture to the *Merry Wives of Windsor* by Nicolai, a composition I heard so many times, or the opera *Falstaff* by Verdi!

Only a few days ago, I had listened to the abundant flow of melody of that late work on the radio and had admired the vigor and the serenity of the old master. But the *Rosenkavalier* waltz? I thought of the first performance I heard of the opera in Vienna in 1911, and I saw in my mind's eye the corpulent figure of the bass singer, Richard Mayr, who always had the part of Ochs von Lerchenau in the Vienna Opera: the image of the aristocrat at the level of the marschallin, then making a pass at her maid who is young Octavian in disguise, the great scene of the tête-à-tête with the maid in that *chambre séparée*. Poor Ochs von Lerchenau becomes the victim of an intrigue, as does Sir John in the *Merry Wives of Windsor*. He is frustrated like the fat knight. The duel scene in which Ochs is afraid to die from a harmless wound and the battle scene from which Sir John escapes with the cry "Give me life!" And again that tender waltz, as background music to the images called up by the memory of that first performance.

Of course, that's it. I had thought of successors of Sir John in world literature, found none worthy of walking in his bulky shadow, and then in a long distance from that miraculous creation appeared Ochs von Lerchenau with his belly. There are so many differences between the two figures! Yet the coarse Lerchenau is a Viennese miniature edition of the knight with whom he shares the zest of life and an indomitable self-love. He is a weaker great-grandson of the British character, and in spite of all divergencies a certain family resemblance is unmistakable.

The emergence of the *Rosenkavalier* waltz made the impression of a hopscotch idea, but now it makes some sense. The line of thought, stimulated by Kretzschmer's characterological description of the cycloid type, went from that huge mass of flesh in the person of Sir John to the corpulent figure of the Austrian aristocrat, from the Boar's Head Tavern to a chamber in Vienna. Really there was a direct line from Falstaff in that Eastcheap tavern to Ochs von Lerchenau in a dubious restaurant in Vienna.

The surprising emergence of the waltz was only partly explained by the remote resemblance of the two corpulent men and of the situations in which they became the victims of an amorous intrigue. Force of psychological habit made me search for other connecting links between my associations. These links were few and far between: the characterological features of the obese cycloid type, the zest for life, the congenital optimism, the narcissistic self-love . . . Kretzschmer's careful description . . . my search for figures in world literature who resemble in body build and temperament that walking human barrel Sir John. . . .

But why the waltz? . . . Another waltz by another Strauss occurs to me . . . *Wine, Women and Song*. Perhaps that's it. . . . Sir John enjoys his liquor, of course . . . and so does Ochs von Lerchenau. (Here is again that waltz . . . the dinner-scene . . . Octavian Mariandl sings, "*Nein, nein, nein, nein, ich mag kan Wein.* . . .") But that other fat man, Nero Wolfe, drinks beer, many bottles daily. . . . It can't be the wine. . . . Besides that, overweight people become obese rather by excessive intake of food.

And women? . . . Yes, Falstaff is eager for amorous adventures with three women at Windsor, and Ochs wants to seduce the

chambermaid of the marschallin. . . . But again Nero Wolfe.
. . . He is not very fond of women. . . . Let me corroborate the
circumstantial evidence of that associative link. . . . Does not
the Prince express his astonishment that, in Falstaff's case, the desire survives the performance so long? . . . The fat knight pretends that he is a great ladies' man—he is not very discriminating
and they are rarely ladies—but is he really? He seems more attracted to the company of men. . . . There is Prince Hal, Pistol,
and Bardolph. . . . Sir John Falstaff has a distinct trend of latent
homosexuality that is unconsciously denied. . . . His love for the
young Prince has almost a maternal character, and its expression
is sometimes pathetic. . . . One of his sentences concerning his
young friend comes to mind: "If the rascal have not given me
medicine to make me love him, I'll be hanged." . . . And Ochs
von Lerchenau? It must have a secret meaning that the pretty girl
to whom he makes propositions is really a young man in disguise.
. . . He makes love to a male. . . . The third fat man, Nero
Wolfe, takes a vicarious pleasure in the seducing facilities of his
assistant, Archie Goodwin, and his relationship to him is characterized by a kind of contemptuous and protective affection. The
relationship of that fresh young man to his rotund boss is almost
the same, although mixed with much admiration for the old man.

Strange it is that I did not think along those lines, but it now
seems to me that these three obese men show a homosexual inclination for their young companions. . . . And those young
men, in turn, tease them, take them in, but admire them, nevertheless. . . . Should I have accidentally run into another characteristic trait of obese persons, not mentioned in Kretzschmer's
book or in other literature known to me? . . . Is there an unconscious, patronizing, almost maternal affection for younger
members of the same sex, a secret and denied homosexual trend
for son- or daughter-representatives?

Wine, Women and Song. . . . I don't remember anything
about Nero Wolfe's relationship to music, but Sir John is certainly fond of it. He declares to the Chief Justice that he lost his
voice in hallooing and singing anthems. (He does not mention
earthy and bawdy songs.) And Ochs von Lerchenau . . . but he
loves music, of course.

I just had an idea, but it faded away. It evaporated without any trace. We say that a man is lost in thoughts. Can thoughts be lost in a man? I have to find that idea that vanished. Where can I search for it? It must be hiding itself behind those other associations. I started from the question as to why the *Rosenkavalier* waltz occurred to me rather than any other tune; or, otherwise put, from the problem of selectivity of musical remembrances and associations. The figure of Falstaff should have suggested the emergence of Nicolai's overture to *The Merry Wives of Windsor* or some melody from Verdi's opera. But those compositions are centering on the figure of Falstaff, and I was roaming through world literature searching for comparable characters. Then the *Rosenkavalier* waltz emerged. Of course, it strikes nearer home than the music of Nicolai and Verdi. Home meaning Vienna. And Ochs von Lerchenau is really a distant relative of Falstaff.

But why should a musical association appear instead of a sober, rational thought, why a tune at all? . . . Wine, women, and song . . . Oh, song and the obese cycloid type and temperament. . . . By God, that is it! Did I not at the beginning think of Caesar's characterization of Cassius: "he hears no music"? This thought, the comparison of the lean, schizoid, unsmiling, and scheming type, in contrast to the other (Falstaff, Ochs von Lerchenau), must have lingered on without my being aware of it. Those obese, cycloid personalities hear music and love it. The memory of the *Rosenkavalier* waltz is also determined by that unrecognized, subterranean idea: by the contrast of the music-loving, sociable, jolly, and obese person with the other, represented by Cassius, the man who hath no music in himself and is, in Shakespeare's sense, so capable of treachery. Instead of the logical and reasoned thought that one of the features of the obese cycloid type is love of music—not mentioned by Kretzschmer—the *Rosenkavalier* waltz suddenly danced into my mind, so to speak, as a musical illustration of that idea. At the same time, the tune represented the appearance of that other rotund cycloid character, Ochs von Lerchenau, a Viennese chip of that old, big block, Sir Falstaff. As I later discovered, the characterological resemblance between Sir John Falstaff and the Baron von Lerchenau had been recognized by the composer and the librettist of the *Rosenkavalier*. In their

correspondence, published in 1926, Strauss reminds Hofmannsthal of the beautiful monologue of Falstaff in Verdi's opera and
adds: "I imagine the scene of the baron after Octavian's departure should be similar" [August 12, 1909]. Hofmannsthal claims
that a certain actor, considered for the part of Ochs von Lerchenau, does not have "just the most essential features" of the
character, namely, "the buffoonish, the Falstaffian, the easygoing,
the laughter-awakening" [January 2, 1911]. In the emergence of
that waltz, a condensation of thoughts had come to a musical
expression whose meaning I had not recognized.

While I am still wondering about the layer structure of those
thoughts, which unconsciously continued the Shakespearean contrast of the man who loves music and the other who does not hear
it, I am returning to the problem that had originally caught my
interest—namely, to the question of what happens to the cruel,
sadistic, and vicious drives of obese persons. I had found no
conclusive solution of the problem, only suggestions and conjectures, all concerning the primitive orality of this type. It seems
to me now that the love of music, which I now found as an overlooked characterological feature, also belongs to this instinctual
area. What is music other than sound, originally made by the
mouth, sound or scream that has become song? We speak of the
magic of music, of its soothing power. Perhaps musical expression
sublimates and masters our violent drives and has the magic
force to defend us against the evil dangers within ourselves, as
it originally banned the menace from without us. By that process
of transformation from a wild scream, which expressed primitive
aggression, to a melody, the violence was mitigated and another
oral gratification obtained. Did Bruno Walter, who wields the
pen as masterfully as the baton, intuitively reach this insight,
when in his book he asserted that music is unable to express the
evil, to communicate the vicious and cruel sadistic drives that
live in all of us?* In the analytic sense, the magic of music would
be mainly of the nature of an emotional defense against the
power of aggressive drives.

The emergence of the *Rosenkavalier* waltz indicated the sur-

* *Von den moralischen Kräften der Musik* (Vienna, 1935).

prising arrival of an unconscious thought that contributes another characterological feature to the analytic theory on obesity.
The love of music is another expression of oral activity and
gratification of the cycloid type. That neglected idea lingered
on and has exerted a remote control on the train of my thoughts.
They had consciously aimed at the solution of a problem, but
they arrived, invisibly directed to their goal when they were not
any longer endeavoring to reach it by way of rational conclusions.
The carefully aimed bullet went astray, and the shot in the dark
hit near the target. The facts, ascertained and verified by scientific research, and the fancy of the great writers in the form of
intuitive insights seemed to coincide with the views of the people
in a consensus about the love of music and the relative lack of
aggressiveness and viciousness in the character of obese persons.

While I am writing these final sentences, two lines, heard as a
child in grammar school, spring up as from a trap door. They
seem to confirm Shakespeare's views and the results of modern
psychological research:

> *Wo man singt, da lass dich ruhig nieder,*
> *Böse Menschen haben keine Lieder.*

> With people who sing you will get along,
> Evil men don't have any song.

5

There is an unknown melody that has been haunting me now
for several days. It appears sometimes very clearly, and sometimes
only the first bars are heard by the inner ear as a faint echo. It
came like an unannounced guest one has once known, but whose
name one has forgotten. Its repeated emergence irks me now, and
I try to turn it away as if the unrecognized guest had stayed too
long and has become wearisome. If I but knew what that tune is!
I am searching in vain in my memory. I must have heard it long,
long ago. Where was it?

Was it not in the Vienna Opera? It occurs to me that the melody I do not recognize must have something to do with my father. . . . My memory calls his image up . . . his face . . . his side whiskers . . . his beard was like Kaiser Franz Josef's . . . or rather like Jacques Offenbach's. . . . The image of the composer emerges quite distinctly as if it were a photograph. . . . The penetrating eyes and the pince-nez on a ribbon. . . . And then I know suddenly what the melody is: the aria of Antonia from *The Tales of Hoffmann*. As if a floodgate had been opened, an abundance of images emerges. When my sister and I went to the Vienna Opera for the first time in 1901, I was thirteen years old.

We had heard our father speak about *The Tales of Hoffmann* before. At the first performance of Offenbach's opera in 1881, a terrible fire had consumed the Vienna Ringtheater. Many hundreds of people had perished; my father had saved himself by jumping from a window. Many superstitious persons in our city, at that time, had tried to establish a connection between the catastrophe and the personality of the composer. They said Offenbach had an "evil eye" whose glances had magical power to harm people. They called him a "jettatore," meaning a wicked sorcerer. Poor Offenbach, whose picture we had seen and in whom we had discovered a likeness to our father, had in fact not lived to witness the opening performance of his opera.

The Tales of Hoffmann had not been performed in Vienna for a long time, in fact, not until 1901. My sister and I were agog with anticipation. In those days, the performances of the Opera were a frequent subject of discussion in the homes of the middle-class people of musical Vienna. We had often heard the orchestra praised and the individual singers evaluated. Then there was the new director whose artistic and creative zeal had revolutionized the old institution and who had become the subject of bitter contention and ardent enthusiasm. Every one of the performances which he conducted aroused a storm of controversy: his lack of respect for tradition which he had once characterized as "sloppiness," his startling innovations, his musicianship, and his inspired energy which demanded perfection from himself and those working with him. His name, which we heard spoken so often at home, was Gustav Mahler. We were told that he would conduct the orchestra.

Memories emerge of our first night at the Opera House; the crowded theater, the box reserved for the Court, the tuning of the instruments. The lights are out now; only stage and orchestra are illuminated. A man of small stature, with the ascetic features of a medieval monk, is seen hurrying toward the conductor's stand. His eyes are flashing behind his glasses. He glances, as if in fury, at the audience that applauds his appearance. He raises the baton and throws himself, with arms uplifted, ecstatically almost, into the flood of melody.

Slowly the curtain rises. There is a students' tavern, the young men drinking, boasting, and jesting. Hoffmann, the poet and musician, appears on the scene and is teased by his comrades because he has fallen in love once again. They ask him to recount the story of his foolish amours and he begins: "The name of my first beloved was Olympia. . . ."

The play takes us back, in the ensuing act, to what happened to young E. T. A. Hoffmann as he met Olympia in the home of the famous scientist Spalanzani, whose daughter she appears to be. It is love at first sight, with no realization that she is not a living woman but an automatic doll, fashioned with the utmost skill. The charming girl is seen at a party. When Spalanzani pushes a concealed button, she speaks, she walks, she sings and dances. Hoffmann confesses his love for her and is elated when he hears her "yes." She dances with him until exhausted, then her father or maker leads her to her chamber. Then, a malignant-looking man by the name of Coppelius enters in a rage and claims to have been swindled by Spalanzani. Vengefully, he manages to slip into Olympia's chamber and to smash the manificent doll Spalanzani's cleverness had wrought. E. T. A. Hoffmann is made the butt of the assembled guests' ridicule for having fallen in love with a lifeless automaton.

The second act takes place in Venice, at the home of beautiful Giulietta, who receives the young poet as graciously as she does all the other young men to whom she grants her favors. Dapertutto, a demoniac figure, bribes the siren to make a play for Hoffmann's love. She promises the ardent poet the key to her bedroom. He, however, gets into a fight with another of her lovers and kills him. She jilts Hoffmann, who finds her chamber deserted and espies her, in the embraces of another, entering a gondola which floats down the Canalo Grande.

The third act is laid in Munich, in the house of old Crespel, with whose fair daughter, Antonia, Hoffmann has fallen in love. The girl has inherited her mother's beautiful singing voice but also her fatal disease, consumption. Father and lover plead with her not to sing. But Dr. Mirakel, a physician and an evil sorcerer, makes her doubtful again when he reproaches her for giving up a promising career. In her presence he conjures up the spirit of her dead mother who joins with Dr. Mirakel in his exhortations to break her promise and to continue with her singing. Antonia yields and dies while singing her aria. Dr. Mirakel then disappears, emitting peals of triumphant, mocking laughter, leaving father and lover prey to their despair.

In the epilogue, we witness the same scene as in the beginning: the students singing and jesting, shouting "bravo" to Hoffmann's tale of his thwarted love. He, in turn, proceeds to drown his grief in drink.

When I went to the opera that evening, I had expected a light and amusing operetta in the manner of *La Belle Hélène* or *Orphée aux Enfers,* with sparkling melodies, debunking gods and heroes of Greek mythology. But this opera was so different, it made a deep impression on the thirteen-year-old boy. For many weeks afterward, some tune from *The Tales of Hoffmann,* such as the charming aria of Olympia, the chorus of the guests, the moving aria of Antonia, haunted me. Images from the performance recurred to the inner eye: there were the evil and demoniac figures of Coppelius, Dapertutto, and Dr. Mirakel, played by the same singer. They appeared as personifications of a mysterious power that destroys again and again the young poet's love and happiness. Also, the image of the pale face of Gustav Mahler himself reappeared, looking like a sorcerer, like a spiritualized Dr. Mirakel, performing wonders with the orchestra. And then the female figures, played, as they were, by the same singer: Olympia, Giulietta, and Antonia. They appeared to be three women in one, a triad which is always the same. There was, in the boy, a fore-knowledge or presentiment of a deeper meaning behind the succession of the three loves and their tragic endings, but this concealed meaning eluded him whenever he tried to penetrate the mystery.

When I heard the opera again, almost twenty years later, that which had been dark became transparent. It was like developing an old photographic plate. The chemical processes to which the plate had been subjected in the meantime had now made it pos-sible to obtain a positive print. The triad had revealed its secret in the light of what I had learned and experienced in psycho-analysis.

In every one of his attachments, young Hoffmann had met an antagonist called variously, Coppelius, Dapertutto, and Dr. Mirakel. This secret opponent was out to defeat the poet; he turned the beloved against Hoffmann or destroyed her. At the beginning we see Hoffmann infatuated or in love. We see him broken in spirit, in misery and despair, at the end. The easily inflamed passion of the young man meets an antagonistic power, self-deceiving and self-harming, which causes him to fail. That which makes him luckless and miserable is conceived as outside forces. But is it not rather some agent within himself emerging from dark subterranean depths? The sinister figures, who blind him about Olympia, who cause Giulietta to jilt him, and to bring death and destruction to Antonia, are personifications only of a foiling power which is an unconscious part of Hoffmann himself. This hidden factor, which frustrates him each time in the end, is already operative in his choice of his love objects. As if led by a malicious destiny, as if thwarted by a demon, he falls in love each time with a woman who is unsuitable: Olympia, a lifeless autom-aton; Giulietta, a vixen; and Antonia, doomed from the beginning.

The personalities of the three women themselves, as well as the sequence of their succession, seem to express a concealed significance, hint at a symbolic meaning behind the events. It is as if the author were presenting not only the particular case of this German poet and musician, Hoffmann, but beyond that a situation of universal significance. Does the play want to say that every young man follows such a pattern in his loves? Yet our feeling balks at such a meaning. We find ourselves at a kind of psychological impasse, both willing and recalcitrant to believe, feeling a fusion and confusion of emotions which oppose each other. We sense there is a hidden general meaning; yet what happens to E. T. A. Hoffmann, especially his loves for those strange female characters, is so specific and personal that it cannot relate to us.

The closest coincidence to the love life of the average young man may be seen in Hoffmann's infatuation for Giulietta the heartless Venetian courtesan, who wants to enslave him for reasons of her own. Her charm fills him with consuming fire, he puts himself in bondage to her, ready to sacrifice all to his passion. Need we search here for a deeper meaning? We have the lady of easy or absent virtue, who plays with all men and with whom all men play. Here we really have a type which is to be found in every man's life; the object of uninhibited sexual wishes, the mistress desirable in the flesh.

But what should we think of Olympia? We meet here with an odd love object, something almost incredible. The girl walks and laughs, speaks, dances, and sings. She is, as Hoffmann discovers later and too late, really only an automaton, and does not function unless her clever creator pushes certain buttons. Where is the place of such a strange creature in every man's life? Should we assume that the author wanted to give an exaggerated caricature of the baby-faced, doll-like darling who has no life of her own, the girl without brains and personality, the society glamor girl, the plaything and toy? Such an interpretation is tempting, it makes rational sense, but remains unconvincing. And Antonia? Should she be regarded as the woman who hesitates between choosing a man or a career? But her character does not tally with this concept. The outstanding feature, after all, is the menace of death connected with her singing.

If we tentatively accept these rational concepts, we arrive at the conclusion that the author wanted to portray three typical figures who play a role in a young man's life. They are the child-woman, the siren, and the artist, or a woman who oscillates between wanting to be a wife or to follow a career. Olympia, Giulietta, and Antonia would then represent three types whom every young man meets and finds attractive in different ways, appealing as they do to the playful, the sensual, and the affectionate part in him. Was this in the writer's mind when he created the three women representative of their sex? Have we now reached a better understanding?

If we have, we do not feel satisfied yet. Something warns us against contenting ourselves with such an interpretation. Should we give up our attempts at searching for a deeper meaning in the three female figures? Should we not rather take them at the value of their beautiful faces? We cannot do it. We cannot escape the haunting impression of a concealed significance. There is the repetitive character in spite of individual variations, the hidden logic which gives the play its tragic atmosphere. The sinister figures of the mysterious antagonist intensify the impression. They give to the events on the stage a sense of something pre-ordained and fateful which cannot be accidental. Other traits, too, make it evident that the author was well aware of the veiled significance, for instance, the remark of one of the students after Hoffmann has told the story of his loves: "I understand, three dramas in one drama."

Beside and beyond such small but telling items in the text, there is the force of this music in which the secret power of the inevitable, the shadow of near death, and the spell of destiny have been transformed into song. This power is felt in the playful and sparkling tunes of the students, in the Mozartian entrance of the guests, in the sweet aria of Olympia, and in the alluring Barcarolle of Giulietta. It laughs and mocks in Dr. Mirakel's tunes. It pleads in Hoffmann's confessions of love, in the exhortations of the dead mother, and in Antonia's swan song. There is something in the conjuring power of this music, in the depths of feeling it stirs, in the death fear and death desire it pours into unforgettable melodies, which does not allow you to escape from

this haunting sense of a concealed significance. Whether or not
the librettist meant to express a symbolic meaning, there can be
no doubt that the composer did. There is more in the events on
the stage and in this music than meets the eye and the ear.

Impossible that the interpretation of the three feminine figures
has reached the deepest level yet. They must be more than mere
types of women, even if they are also that. There is something
more meaningful in the three acts than the choice of three girls
and three disappointments in love. The rational concept of the
meaning of the three women all of a sudden strikes me as superficial, flat, and banal. It is very possible, even probable, that such
a commonplace was in the mind of the writer, but unconsciously
he said more than he consciously knew, expressed a meaning beyond his grasp. It should not be forgotten that the French
librettist took the material of the text for *The Tales of Hoffmann*
from various novels by the German writer Ernst Theodor
Amadeus Hoffmann (1776-1822), whom he then made the leading
figure of the opera. In these stories, Hoffmann showed a strange
mixture of the realistic and the fantastic, of the grotesque and the
tragic, creating a ghastly, haunting atmosphere even where he
depicts only everyday events. Offenbach's melodies communicate
to you the deeper insight; they speak immediately to your emotions, alerted as they are by the hidden element of the dramatic
action, although the plot itself presents only the surface aspect
of something elusive and mystifying.

In a situation like this, psychoanalytic interpretation comes
into its own, furnishing a key as it does to a locked room, allowing us to penetrate below the surface of conscious thinking. There
is not much of a mystery about Giulietta: she remains the "courtesan with brazen mien," as she is called in the play. What might
give us food for thought is rather her place in the sequence of the
female figures. She stands in the middle, following after Olympia,
the doll, and preceding Antonia over whom looms the shadow of
death. Since Giulietta represents the woman who arouses and
appeals to man's sensual desires, promising their fulfillment, her
middle position in the sequence suggests the interpretation that

in her is represented the figure which governs the mature years of a man's life.

More intriguing is the personality of Olympia. How does this doll, the child-woman, appear in the light of psychoanalytic interpretation? What can be the significance of her appearance in Hoffmann's life, with this mixture of features, both grotesque and pathetic? Freud has taught us that the hidden meaning of many dreams, neurotic symptoms, and other products of unconscious activity remains obscure as long as their manifest content alone is taken into consideration. In certain instances the concealed meaning of a dream, for example, can only be understood by reversing important parts of the dream plot. Then, and only then, and in no other way, may the meaning be unraveled from the distortions in such cases. Olympia is a doll who speaks and moves and sings only if and when appropriate buttons are pushed, when she is being led and manipulated. If we are to reverse the story, we get the picture of Hoffmann being led by hidden strings like a marionette. Or, if we go one step farther, he is made to walk and talk and sing and act like an infant. The reversal of this part of the plot seems thus to place the story of Hoffmann's first love in his infancy. The poet appears in the reversal as a little boy, and Olympia as representing his mother who plays with him. He cannot act independently of her, and follows her about. If we are willing to trust this psychoanalytic interpretation which, after all, does not sound any more fantastic than the story of Hoffmann's first love in the operatic plot, some meaning in the succession of the two figures dawns on us: Olympia and Giulietta. If Olympia represents the mother, the first love object of the small boy, then Giulietta is the woman loved and desired by the grown man, the object of his passionate wishes, the mistress who gratifies his sensual desires.

But what is hidden then behind the last figure? Who is concealed behind Antonia? When we trust to psychoanalytic interpretation, this riddle will not be hard to solve. Antonia vacillates between her love for Hoffmann and her love for music. She disobeys the warnings not to sing, and dies. When we reverse the contents again, as we did before, we arrive at the following meaning: Hoffmann, the poet, vacillates between his love and his art, and he dies. In the sequence of the plot, Antonia is the last image of woman as she appears to the old man. Antonia is the figure of death. The three female figures appear to us now in a new light: Olympia as the representative of the mother, object of the love of the helpless and dependent little boy; Giulietta as the desired mistress of the grown man, Antonia as the personification of death which the old man is approaching.

It is at this point in our attempts at unraveling the hidden pattern of meaning behind Offenbach's opera that the mental image of the composer himself emerges, shaded by the knowledge of his life story. Can it be incidental that he, already fatally ill, worked feverishly at this, his last opus which he hoped was going to be his best accomplishment? They called him then in Paris "Mozart of the Champs-Elysées." Mozart, his beloved and revered master, knew when he composed his *Requiem* that he would die soon. Offenbach, too, realized that his end was approaching. He put his full creative power into his work, and he died after it was completed like Antonia during her swan song. In the demoniac tunes of Dr. Mirakel are all the shudders of the approaching annihilation. All passionate longing for life and light is poured into the third act. Offenbach wrote to M. Carvallio, Director of the Paris Opera: "Hurry to produce my play. Not much time is left to me and I have only the one wish to see the opening performance." He knew he had to complete his work even if his efforts should accelerate his death. They did. He died a few months before the opening night. Like Antonia, he perished in his song.

It is not accidental that E. T. A. Hoffmann, the hero of the opera, was himself a musician as well as a poet. The identification of Offenbach with the figure of Antonia is also indicated in her passionate desire to become an artist like her mother, whose spirit exhorts her to sacrifice all to her singing. Offenbach's father was a singer in the synagogue and a composer of Jewish religious music.

The psychoanalytic interpretation here presented may seem forced to the reader unfamiliar with the methods of eliciting unconscious meanings. It will be helpful to point out that the symbolic significance here discovered is only a restatement in new form of an old motif well known from numerous ancient myths and tales. It can be called the motif of the man and the three women, one of whom he has to choose. Freud gave the first psychoanalytic interpretation of this recurrent plot in one of his less known papers.* He deciphered the concealed meaning in the material of *Lear,* which Shakespeare had taken from older sources. The old King stands between his three daughters, of whom the youngest, Cordelia, is the most deserving. Goneril and Regan vie with each other in protestations of their affection for the father, but Cordelia "loves and is silent." In the last scene of the drama, Lear carries Cordelia, who is dead, across the stage. Freud elucidated the hidden significance of this scene by the process of reversal. It means, of course, the figure of death who carries away the body of old Lear, as the Valkyries carry off the slain hero. Traces of this original meaning can already be seen in the scene of Cordelia bending over her "childchanged father." As is frequently the case in dreams about persons dear to the dreamer, Cordelia's silence in itself signifies unconsciously that she is dead, that she is death itself in a mythical form.

The same motif, displaced, distorted, and elaborated, appears in another one of Shakespeare's plays. The Portia scenes in *The Merchant of Venice* reveal to the interpretation of Freud an unexpected aspect. Portia will yield her hand to the man who, among three caskets, chooses the one which contains her picture. Here we encounter a hidden symbolism which we already know from Greek antiquity: boxes, chests, and other receptacles are symbolic substitutes for the female body. In the Bassanio scene of the play, the motif of the man who has to choose between three women is thus expressed in symbolic form. Bassanio prefers the casket which is leaden to the gold and silver ones:

> . . . but thou, thou meager lead,
> Which rather threatenest, than dost promise aught.
> Thy paleness moves me more than eloquence.

* "Das Motif der Kästchenwahl," *Gesammelte Schriften,* Vol. X.

The features of paleness, like silence in the case of Cordelia, appear frequently in dreams to signify that a figure is dead: persons who are deathly pale or who are voiceless represent dead persons or death itself. Antonia in *The Tales of Hoffmann* is a singer, it is true, but to sing is forbidden to her and it is her song which brings about her death, silences her forever. In unconscious productions, opposites may stand for each other, can replace each other. The secret similarities between the two Shakespearean plays become transparent: an old motif appears in the one in a tragic, in the other in a light version. What is in reality inevitable and preordained, namely, that in the end man has to yield to death, is here turned into a free choice. That which threatens is changed into wish fulfillment—a result itself of wishful thinking. There are hints which point to the orginal meaning, to the kind of a choice involved. ("Who chooses me must give and hazard all he hath," says the leaden casket, "which rather threatenest than dost promise aught," to Bassanio.)

Let me follow the old motif into the realm of the fairy tale where we meet with it frequently in its diverse forms, for instance, in the story of Cinderella who is the youngest of the sisters, and conceals herself. We can trace it farther back to the Erinyes, Parcae, and Moirai, the goddesses of fate who are standing guard over individual destiny. The third figure among them is Atropos, who cut the thread of life. Corresponding to the Parcae are the Norse in Germanic mythology, who, too, are conceived as watching over human fate. They rule over gods and men alike, and from what is decreed by them neither god nor man can escape. Man's fate is determined by them at the hour of the child's birth, by what they say to the newborn infant. The word fate (*fatum*) itself is derived from the same root as "word" or "that which is spoken." That what they say in magic words *is* a man's fate. Derived from the same Indo-German root, the word "fee" in modern German, the word "feie" in old French, and the Irish adjective "fay," which is contained in fairy, all originally denoted goddesses of fate. In many fairy tales the fairies are represented as bringing gifts to a newborn infant. In most instances they appear as beneficent, as kind, lovely, well-wishing figures. But in some of the stories their original fatal character re-emerges behind the benign aspect.

In conformity with the psychological law of the opposite which can replace one aspect by its protagonist in our unconscious thinking, the goddess of death sometimes appears under the aspect of the great goddess of love. In most ancient mythologies the same female figure has both functions like Kali in India, Ashtar with the Semitic tribes, and Aphrodite with the Greeks. Yes, indeed, it is wishful thinking which succeeded at last in transforming the most terrifying apparition into the desirable, the female figure of death into that of the beloved.

We look back at Offenbach's opera: Olympia, Giulietta, Antonia. Here are three women in one, or one woman in three shapes: the one who gives birth, the one who gives sexual gratification, the one who brings death. Here are the three aspects woman has in a man's life: the mother, the mistress, the annihilator. The first and the last character meet each other in the middle figure. In mythological and literary reactions, the representatives of love and of destruction can replace each other as in Shakespeare's plays, or they succeed each other as in Hoffmann's tales of thwarted love. In his three loves a reaction-formation unfolds itself: the woman chosen appears in each beginning as the loveliest, most desirable object, and always, in the end, represents doom and death. It is as if her true character reveals itself only in the final scene. For as long as the reaction formation is in power, the most terrible appears as the most desirable.

Behind all these figures is originally a single one, just as in the triads of goddesses whom modern comparative history of religion has succeeded in tracing back to their prototype of one goddess. For all of us the mother is the woman of destiny. She is the *femme fatale* in its most literal sense, because she brought us into the world, she taught us to love, and it is she upon whom we call in our last hour. The mother as a death-dealing figure became alien to our conscious thinking. But she may become comprehensible in this function when death appears as the only release from suffering, as the one aim desired, the final peace. It is in this sense that dying soldiers call for their mothers. I can never forget a little boy who, in the agonies of a painful illness, cried, "Mother, you have brought me into the world, why can't you make me dead now?"

It is noteworthy that the motif of one man between three women appears in an earlier opera of Offenbach, who took an active part in the choice and shape of the libretto. *La Belle Hélène* uses a plot from Greek mythology: Paris, son of Priamos, has to choose between Athene, Hera, and Aphrodite. The charming aria of the mythological playboy says: "On Mount Ida three goddesses quarrelled in the wood. 'Which,' said the princesses, 'of us three is the fairest?' " Here, again, we have the motif of choosing, this time in a frivolous version. To the young ladies' man, Hera promises power and fame, Athene wisdom, but

> . . . the third, ah, the third
> The third remained silent.
> She gained the prize all the same.

Is it not strange that Aphrodite, the goddess of love, remains silent? She does not speak, yet she is eloquent. In the end the young prince chooses her, only it is not choice, it is necessity. She is not only the goddess of love, but also of death. *The Tales of Hoffmann* tell and sing the role of women in a man's life; that is to say, in every man's life.

I now remember when the melody that haunted me for several days first emerged. It was a week ago, on my way back from the Public Library. I had looked up something there. Before leaving I had seen on a desk a book which was a biography of Jacques Offenbach. I took it, looked at the composer's picture, and ran over the pages, reading a paragraph here and there: the story of his childhood in Germany, his struggle and triumph in Paris, his way of composing, the feverish working on the score of *The Tales of Hoffmann*. He had a presentiment he would not live to see the opening night of the opera. He felt the end was near. He died a few months after he had reached sixty-one.

Walking home through the streets that evening, I thought of the book I am working on, and a sudden anxiety overcame me that I would die before finishing it. It occurred to me that I had passed sixty-one a few months ago. And then the aria from *The Tales of Hoffmann* emerged and the unrecognized melody began to haunt me as if it wanted to remind me of something one would like to forget.

6

After I recognized the melody that had haunted me as being Antonia's aria from *The Tales of Hoffmann,* I remembered with astonishment that this same tune had frequently occurred to me more than thirty years ago and that I had then written a paper on the unconscious content of Offenbach's opera. I found this piece in one of my folders and with it a letter which Freud had written to me after he had read the article. His letter was dated March 24, 1918, and reads in part as follows: "I liked your Offenbach article very much. I think it is correct. Only in one part of your presentation, in tracing back Olympia to the mother-image, you should have enlarged more freely and more fully and should have avoided giving the impression that you are fulfilling a prescribed task. You will perhaps rewrite that passage of your thoughtful contribution with your previous literary facility. With cordial thanks and regards, yours, Freud."

I rewrote that part and then put the manuscript away. It appears here in the main part of the preceding chapter. It was noteworthy that the same melody emerged thirty years later and led my thoughts back to a subject which had preoccupied me such a long time before. That early draft was not written for the day. It must have originated in some deep, unrecognized emotions. It survived the day together with the emotions which continued to live in the unknown underground. It may have hovered at the brink of conscious memory before, but only the re-emergence of that melody brought it back from its submersion after I had reached sixty-one years, the age at which Offenbach died. It cannot be accidental that its essential part was written and given to Freud when he had passed his sixty-first year.

The jinx was off: unlike Jacques Offenbach, I did not die upon reaching my sixty-first year. Recently I saw *The Tales of Hoffmann* once more, this time in the movies. It surprised me that during and after that performance my thoughts did not return to the hidden significance of the plot and its figures. It was as if writing that paper about the three women in a man's life had exhausted the emotional content of the subject for me. Or was it because there was so much to look at in the movie version that my attention was distracted?

At all events a conspicuous stage-set of the first act of the movie version turned my thought in a new direction. The scriptwriters went back to E. T. A. Hoffmann's novel *The Sandman,* from which the plot of the Olympia episode is taken, and gave much place and significance to the fabrication and acting of the marionettes. Not only was Olympia a puppet, but also the guest at her party. The figures of Professor Spalanzani and of the optician Coppelius are shown in this movie at their common work of manufacturing the puppets. Spalanzani's home is not a dolls' house, but a workshop full of dolls.

After that performance a memory came to mind which I had never recalled before. Psychology still cannot satisfactorily explain why memories of previously unrecollected childhood happenings emerge with full vivacity in one's old age. It seems to me that such occurrence of events and impressions belonging to the remote past of the individual are accompanied by a perceptible loss of emotional interest in the present. It is as if the diminution of the importance of actual situations facilitates a regression to earlier phases of one's life and gives them a heightened liveliness.

I had always believed the first theater performance I attended to have been *Orpheus in the Netherworld.* I clearly remembered that this had been a treat on my tenth birthday. The new memory, now emerging, revealed that I had been at a theater before that. I now recalled that a Moravian maid had taken me, then a small boy, to a puppet theater in the Prater and that I had enjoyed myself thoroughly. The marionette show was a fairy tale, and fairies and bad demons struggled with each other over the hero of the show, which ended, of course, with the victory of good over evil. The puppets appeared to me full of life and power. They acted under their own will and were led to heroic actions or bad deeds by their own good or evil intentions. It did not disturb me in the least that they were pulled by very conspicuous strings. I then believed in free will as do only our lawgivers and educators who conveniently overlook that we all are pulled hither and thither by invisible strings.

To playwrights and actors, as well as to women and children, the theater is so much nearer to material life than to us disenchanted realists. A patient remembered in his analysis that as a small boy he believed that going to the theater meant climbing up to the roofs of certain buildings on Broadway and standing up there during an evening. This strange idea had a simple origin in the thoughts of the child. When his parents took him on a walk, they sometimes talked of theaters and actors and referred to billboards on which new plays were announced high up on the houses of Broadway as they passed by. The boy also saw on these posters pictures of actors in wooden frames and the electrified letters of their names. What was more natural than to assume that his parents went up there when they announced to him that they were going to the theater?

It seems that these childhood convictions remain undisturbed and are as indifferent to the views of grownups as a Siamese cat is to the opinions of people around him. From that puppet show I must have conceived the idea that the theater was something like a palace of fairies, and the plot a fairy tale, not acted but brought alive. A remnant of this old concept of the stage as the meeting and matching place of superhuman forces has remained with me. The strings on which the puppets were pulled became invisible. They have been transformed into those threads by which the forces of destiny lead the figures to their destination.

In the tracks of this old concept, I was not astonished when I was told before my tenth birthday that I would see the gods and heroes of Greek antiquity at a performance of *Orpheus in the Netherworld*. The Greek and Roman gods had taken the place of sorcerers, fairies, and evil demons in my fantasies as they did in the real evolution of religious beliefs. My interest had shifted from the fairy tales of the Brothers Grimm and Andersen to the figures of the ancient mythology, to the sagas and myths whose figures were to be seen in the colored illustrations of a book, *The Most Beautiful Sagas of Ancient Mythology* by Gustav Schwab. I knew all the tales about Jupiter, Pluto, Mars, Venus, and Styx and, of course, Orpheus and Eurydice, whom I would now see on the stage, and I looked forward to meeting them in the flesh because the theater still appeared to me as illustrations come to life, as *tableaux vivants*. I have often asked myself since whether it is much more.

Thus, for me, the theater was a continuation of that puppet show seen as a small boy. There must have been, however, a psychological justification for my so long mistakenly believing that *Orpheus in the Netherworld* was the first show I had attended. It seems that the puppet show had been disavowed and forgotten because it was "kid stuff." But here was real theater, the place where adults go. The boy at the advanced age of ten years looked down contemptuously on the puppet show of his early childhood. It was strange that the memory of it emerged after that movie performance of *The Tales of Hoffmann* in which Olympia and her guests are marionettes. Perhaps an accidental impression facilitated the occurrence of this memory: leaving the theater and crossing Broadway, I saw high up on a building a poster on which another play was announced in electrified letters. Its title was *Guys and Dolls*.

Some months after this performance in the movies, I found in a folder two old yellowed sheets on which I had written some notes. Some of them were hardly legible. They were not dated, but their content, after having been deciphered, showed that they must have been jotted down when I was thinking of *The Tales of Hoffmann*, which means before 1918 when I gave Freud the manuscript of my paper. The notes of the first sheet already contained the outline of the concept I later worked out in my draft, but on the second were some words which to my great surprise pointed to an idea I had dropped or brushed aside when I wrote that manuscript early in 1918. The notes said: Olympia, Giulietta, Antonia, originally one woman-figure—the early pattern is Eurydice in *Orpheus in the Netherworld*—the revolution of the gods against Jupiter—death as punishment—Offenbach and Jehovah—Carl Blasel.

The last name brought back an abundance of memories of that performance on my tenth birthday. Carl Blasel was then a well-known Viennese comedian who sang and acted the part of Jove in that matinee. I still know that I connected the name of Blasel with his figure because the German word *aufblasen* means blow up, and the funny, obese old man was very fit to act as the helpless Jove in Offenbach's parodistic presentation.

Out of the submersion of almost fifty-four years, as from a trap door on a stage, his comical figure appeared in my mind, and I saw him as he emerged with all mythological attributes, including the lightning, as Jupiter amongst the gods who revolt against him. They are sick to death of sipping ambrosia and nectar and wish to drink champagne. I seem to hear that revolutionary song of the Olympians into which Offenbach skillfully inserted some bars of that other revolutionary tune, the *Marseillaise*. And by God!—or rather by Jove!—I remembered all of a sudden, after fifty-four years, the exact words of indignant Jupiter which did not appear, of course, in the libretto of the operetta, but were improvised and were pronounced in a broad Viennese dialect:

> *No wart's, ihr Mordsbagage,*
> *Ihr gebt's mir noch ka Ruah!*
> *Ich zahl euch keine Gage*
> *Und sperr den Himmel zua.*

> You bums, no peace by night and day!
> If you don't stop this uproar,
> I'll give you no more pay
> And close up Olympus' store.

Of course, I enjoyed the scintillating music, but I was much more fascinated by the debunking and parodying of the gods and half-gods of ancient Greece. Only later I learned to appreciate the "supreme form of wit" (Nietzsche's praising words) of the composer who expresses his travesty in music itself, as for instance in that solemn hymn in praise of Jupiter which suddenly jumps into that exuberant cancan, that *galop infernal* of all gods. Later I also began to understand that my extreme enjoyment of the mythological caricature introduced a phase of revolution against religion and tradition in my young life. The appearance of annoyed Jove in the middle of the outrage of gods represented a substitute memory of my father appearing in the nursery, extremely annoyed by the turmoil and noise we children made. That phase of rebellion against authority lasted to the end of puberty. I still remember that the mockery of the Greek and Roman gods and half-gods was followed by the debunking of the heroes of the German sagas in whom the boy had been interested for a short time. As the degradation and desecration of the figures of Greek mythology is connected in my mind with the performance of *Orpheus in the Netherworld,* the mockery and the debunking of the gods and heroes of Valhalla is tied to another operetta seen much later. It is *The Merry Nibelungs* by Oskar Straus, the composer who, later on, wrote *A Waltz Dream* and *The Chocolate Soldier.* In that early operetta, Straus parodies Wagner's operas, as Offenbach occasionally did Gluck's *Orpheus and Eurydice.* (Did not Wagner say about Offenbach as a composer, "Yes, he has warmth, the warmth of a manure heap"?) Oskar Straus, who follows, in *The Merry Nibelungs,* Offenbach's pattern of witty parody, must have recognized early the shame and nonsense of that racial glorification which was introduced by the Wagner cult and culminated in the Nazi terror.

While I am writing this, some of the enjoyment of that travesty comes back to mind with the memory of some lines which proclaim the Nibelungen treasure was not hidden at the bottom of the Rhine, but invested at the Rhine Bank at 6 per cent. The images of Siegfried, Gunther, and Hagen, of Kriemhild and her mother Utah, of all those Teutonic knights emerge together with some bars of Straus's witty music. I am humming the aria of Siegfried after he had killed the dragon and dipped into its blood:

I have taken a bath
Too soon after I did sup,
It didn't agree with me
I don't feel freshened up.

Or that other tune:

And how about Lady Utah?
She has not much to brag on,
Master Siegfried becomes her son-in-law
Who isn't afraid of any dragon.

The chorus sings:

So war's bei den Germanen
Seit alters Brauch,
So taten's unsre Ahnen
Und wir tun's auch.

That's a dear German custom
From early ages through,
Thus acted our ancestors
And thus we act too.

And this whole sordid mixture of *"Kraft durch Freude"* (in the tortures of Poles and Jews), of heroism and moronism, of bravery and depravity which that operetta shows as already present in the ancient Teutons appears now as a prophetic vision of the horrible things to come some thirty years later. The light and parodistically dancing tunes of the Straus operetta are relieved in my mind by the orgiastic cancan of Offenbach, by that irresistible galop which, according to a contemporary critic, could "awaken the dead."

Tearing the mask from the face of an age in which, as in our own, all vices hide behind the hypocrisy of decency and moralistic integrity, Offenbach's riotous and exuberant tunes bravely proclaimed enjoyment of life and made fun of all that official show of chastity, honesty and patriotism. They have a satanic spirit, those tunes, a *beauté de diable*. An American colloquialism says "ugly as sin." But sin is not only tempting, it is also very attractive. They should say "ugly as virtue."

The children of the Jewish ghetto have very few occasions to see pictures. In extension of the biblical commandment forbidding the making of images of God, the religious Jews do not permit illustrations of the figures of the Holy Scripture. There is really only one exception—the Haggadah, the book in which the tale of the exodus of the Jewish people from Egypt is told and which is recited at the festival of Passover. Here is the tale of the slavery of the Israelites in Egypt and of their miraculous salvation from Pharaoh's cruel oppression. There are also some very primitive pictures of these events in the old book.

There is an anecdote about how the first religious doubts awakened in a little boy who grew up in the pious atmosphere of a Russian ghetto. The child saw the picture of Moses in the desert in the Haggadah. The drawing showed the great lawgiver of Israel dressed as a Russian Jew, since the medieval artists gave the persons of the Bible the costumes of their times. After having looked long at the picture, the boy asked the Rabbi, "Why is Moses wearing a fur cap in the hot desert?" With this little problem began the child's doubt of the truth of the religious tradition.

As far as I can remember, my first doubt of the Jewish faith is also connected with the Haggadah, not with one of its pictures, but with one of the songs which is recited there. My father was an agnostic, but my grandfather was a fanatically religious man who demanded that we children attend the Jewish festivals. On the evening of the Passover meals that Haggadah was read aloud and also the traditional song was sung. It is called *Had Gadja* and is a kind of long nursery-rhyme tale. Its story is that a father purchased a little kid—two pieces were the prize—and that the cat came and ate the kid. Then came the dog who bit the cat, the stick came and hit the dog, the fire burned the stick, the water quenched the fire. Then came the ox and drank the water. The slaughterer killed the ox, but then came the angel of death and killed the slaughterer. The Most Holy (God) destroyed the angel of death who slew the slaughterer that killed the ox that drank the water that quenched the fire that burned the stick that beat the dog that bit the cat that ate the kidling, which "my father bought for two doggerel zuzim." As a child, I repeatedly heard that old Aramaic song, translated into German and chanted in the traditional style of synagogical cantillation. It illustrates the age-old law of retribution, the *ius talionis* as is appears in the laws of the ancient Orient. There are traditions that this *Had Gadja* is a symbolical presentation of the destiny awaiting the enemies of the chosen people.

My doubts started at the first verses, to which I returned in my childish thoughts after the recital of that stanza which was concerned with the first victim. If God was powerful enough to destroy the angel of death, why did he allow the cat to eat the poor kidling for which I felt sorry? Could he not have prevented that first murder? There I began to doubt the omnipotence of the Lord. My doubt continued until I realized that His omnipotence is infinite.

Not only the content, but also the tune of that song aroused my attention. At this time the little boy used to ask who had "manufactured" this or that melody he liked. He imagined, it seems, that tunes were made, manufactured like toys, in a mechanical, artificial way—an assumption which is correct only for the most modern compositions. He was interested in the name of the composer of melodies he had enjoyed, because names say much more about people to children than to adults. Children connect definite ideas with names which they do not yet separate from the person himself, but which they consider a significant and inherent quality of the individual. The name of the composer of the *Had Gadja,* thus my father told me, was Jacques Offenbach and he was a very famous man. For a long time I believed that the composer of *La Belle Hélène* and *Orphée aux Enfers* had also been the author of that song, *A Kidling*. I learned only much later that Jacques's father, Isaac Offenbach, who had been cantor of the synagogue of Köln, had composed the strange song that proclaimed the eternal law of retribution in a solemn tune which sometimes struck me as almost parodistic.

When Jacques Offenbach wittily mocked the Greek and Roman gods, he unconsciously made fun of his father as well, and of the moral and religious values of the tradition in which he had grown up. Yes, it is very likely that some of the satiric attitude he felt toward that traditional code of his Jewish environment was displaced to the Greek gods and heroes of antiquity, whom he made subjects of his superb mockery.

Yet he had never got rid of unconscious feelings of devotion and respect for those old values. In the celebrated composer, in the world-famous musician whose tunes reflect the spirit of Paris, of the mundane Second Empire and of the frivolity of the time of Napoleon III, a Jewish boy who had sung in the choir of his father's synagogue at Köln continued a subterranean life. Is it accident that in his arias there occur so many reminiscences of the synagogical tunes he had heard there in his childhood? In the great aria of Styx, in *Orpheus in the Netherworld, "Quand j' étais roi de Boétie,"* a typical bit of Jewish liturgic music appears as the end. The Barcarolle of *The Tales of Hoffmann* reminds the hearer in some of its bars of melodies of the synagogue. There is even a suggestion of that old song *A Kidling*, which his father, the cantor of Köln, had composed in a tune of *Une Nuit Blanche*.

The Jew-boy who went to Paris to study music when he was thirteen years old, and who later spoke French with a German accent and German with a French one, the destructive *moqueur* who had such an excellent sense for the incongruities of life and such sharp wit directed against tradition, remained ambivalent toward it. That revolutionary spirit was also conservative.

When the ten-year-old boy saw *Orpheus in the Netherworld,* he was mostly interested in the mythological figures whom the composer and the librettist had treated so disrespectfully. I am sure he did not understand many things, misunderstood others, and paid no attention to certain aspects of the plot. I heard the other day that a boy of this age came home from a movie whose title promised scenes from the wild West, and answered, when asked whether he enjoyed himself, "It was a waste of looking. It was full of love and such stuff." Like this boy, I was neither interested in nor amused by the love affairs of the gods.

The figure who interested me most was Orpheus, the only mortal amongst the Olympians. I had read about him in my book of mythology and I had often looked at his picture in it, which showed the master musician playing the lyre, surrounded by wild animals whom he had tamed by his sweet strains, and by rocks and trees he could move by the power of his tunes. I knew also that he had descended to the Netherworld to get his wife Eurydice, who had died, that he had returned without her and that the bacchantes had torn him to pieces during a Dionysiac orgy. His figure aroused admiration and pity in the boy.

I understood that in Offenbach's travesty no love is lost between Orpheus and Eurydice. I understood less well that public opinion compelled the great musician to follow his wife, whom he detested, into Hades. "I would not do that," I thought as a boy (and I think so now as an old man). "I would not die. To hell with public opinion!" Even before this I felt a kind of antipathy against Eurydice. She despises her husband as an artist and she dislikes hearing him play.

> The violinist
> Is very triste,

she says, and is terrified when he wants to play for her his recent concerto, which will last only one hour and a quarter. The humor of that scene was entirely lost on me. There was another feature that disturbed me: Eurydice changes at the finale into one of the bacchantes and sings a hymn in praise of Bacchus, that ecstatic and wild song:

> Evohé! Bacchus inspires me!

Was she one of the bacchantes who tore the marvelous musician limb from limb? Was she a member of that ferocious cult of Thracian women who killed the great singer? Did she kill him herself? There was, it seemed, a confusion in the writer's mind— or was it in my own?

Looking back at that performance, I wonder why the numerous anachronisms in the dialogue did not disturb me in the least. Jupiter, Styx, and other gods spoke genuine Viennese dialect, and made numerous jokes about Vienna local events or situations in their improvised lines. I took that in my stride and was not astonished that the Olympians spoke the language of my native town. There was, however, a tiny detail that annoyed me: Orpheus played the violin. I then played the violin myself—miserably enough—and I should have been attracted by the brother-musician, but I was disappointed. It was certainly not because of the anachronistic nature of this feature. I was annoyed because I expected to hear Orpheus play the cithara, that ancient instrument somewhat like a lyre. Before he appeared on the stage, I looked forward to seeing him with this instrument as he was pictured in my mythology book. I cannot be positive whether I was just curious to see what a cithara looked like or whether I expected that I would listen to some miraculous music. I had heard plenty of violin music in my young life, but never a cithara.

Looking back from a distance of fifty-four years at that stranger, that boy who was I, I know his main impressions at that performance were a very intense enjoyment of Offenbach's music and of his travesty of the gods, compassion for the figure of Orpheus, and a distinct antagonism against Eurydice whom—I don't know why —I held somehow responsible for the fact that the divine singer had to die.

How rich is life in childhood and how impoverished it becomes in old age! For the boy to whom the world unfolds, all is full of colors and sounds, life and movement, all new and interesting. How little of that remains when the shadows become larger, how cool and remote one's own life and that of others appear! You look at it as if from a far distance, as through the diminishing lens of binoculars.

A German writer, Jean Paul Richter, wrote more than one hundred and fifty years ago that memory is the only paradise from which we cannot be expelled. But it gets lost and is not often regained. We return to it in psychoanalysis when we remember early childhood impressions and events. But such memories surprisingly turn up outside the analytic treatment as well, when one gets old. Those memories of a very remote past occur then in a sudden flash, or they appear in a slow process of re-emergence that can even be observed on rare occasions, as in this instance. It is as if buckets are slowly raised from a deep well that has held them for a long time, and now they are sent up to the surface, filled with cool and refreshing water.

The preceding paragraphs form a too lengthy introduction to the main theme, a long runway, as it were, for a short flight. I rambled on about my childhood, the theater performance and that Passover song, *Had Gadja*. How will I find the way back to *The Tales of Hoffmann?* But I have never turned away from it in my thoughts, because numerous threads run from those memories to the opera in my mind. I need only pick them up and define them.

There is, of course, the personality of the composer. It is the same man who near the end of his life shaped the destiny of E. T. A. Hoffmann, who in his middle age wrote the travesty of the Orpheus myth and who, as I mistakenly believed when I was a boy, composed that Jewish song which in a nursery-rhyme manner presents the ancient law that the killer will be killed, the cat, the dog, the stick, the fire, the water, the ox, the slaughterer, the angel of death.

It is odd that the detail in the performance of *Orpheus in the Netherworld* that irked me as a boy of ten—namely, that the musician plays the violin instead of the lyre—now becomes a psychological clue. It is possible (more than this, it is likely) that the substitution of the violin for the lyre was necessitated for musical and theatrical reasons, that the fiddle replaced the ancient instrument because the tunes of the violin were more effective than those of the antique cithara. But beside and beyond these considerations, there is the fact that the violin (and later on the violoncello) was the instrument on which Offenbach excelled. As a young child, he played the violin well, and he went to Paris when he was thirteen to study violoncello. Yes, he played as soloist on this instrument in several concertos. Orpheus, playing the violin, represents the creator of that music, the composer himself. In a kind of self-persiflage, Offenbach demonstrates a potentiality of his own destiny in the figure of that mythological musician.

What destiny? Well, when you peel the comical and mythological covers from the plot and strip it to the essentials, there remains the story of an ambitious musician and composer who is thwarted in his profession and in his love life, dies, and goes to Hades. But is this not, raised from the level of fun-making to that of the tragic, the destiny of E. T. A. Hoffmann in Offenbach's last work? There the three demoniac figures of Spalanzani, Dapertutto, and Dr. Mirakel defeat the young musician and deprive him by a trick of his sweetheart as Jupiter does Orpheus. The Olympian god is here replaced by the three figures representing a mysterious and malicious antagonist with magical powers.

And Eurydice? Does she not appear at first as a spoiled child-woman like Olympia, then as a heartless bacchantic adventuress like the wanton Giulietta, and at the end like the ecstatically singing Antonia? Is she not a figure representing lust and death, as are those women in the opera? Here the three women are reduced to *one* fatal figure. Here is the primal image of death which later on reappeared in a veiled form in Antonia because Eurydice is dead and it is in search of her that Orpheus descends to the Netherworld, to Hades, which is easily to be understood as the symbolical expression of his own death. As in our interpretation of the Antonia-figure, we recognize in the mythological formation of Eurydice the threat of death for the man.

In the tale of Orpheus is the germ of what later on became the tale of Hoffmann. Here, as there, is the story of thwarted love, of frustrated ambition, of the expectancy of the end that is near. But in the early work all somber and fateful figures are dressed up in a gay mythological costume as at a fancy-dress ball, and they appear as butts of jokes and pranks. (By the way, Hoffmann is also the subject of mockery by the students in the tavern where he tells the story of his three frustrated amours.) The same fateful development that was first presented as funny will be seen as a tale of gloom and of defeat when the end draws near. Frustrated love, thwarted ambition—one's life as failure. Orpheus and Hoffmann, Eurydice and Antonia—they are the same figures seen in a comic light at first, and as tragic at the end. When the end is near, their composer gathers up all his energies, summons up all his musical power to achieve what had been his hidden aim, to express the best that's in him, all that is his inner self—before he goes down to Hades. He will show his adversaries what he can accomplish, if it is the last thing he does. It was.

The observer who follows with analytic attention the creative stream of Offenbach's imagination will find that the secret main theme remains the same in *Orphée aux Enfers,* in *La Belle Hélène,* and in *The Tales of Hoffmann.* When the trimmings are stripped away, the identical motif of love and death is discernible in these changing forms. There are rivers that disappear in the ground, flow on subterraneously for many miles, and re-emerge very far away from their previous place. Yet, it is the same river. Psychoanalysis enables us not only to interpret those different formations and to recognize their concealed meaning, but also to demonstrate the continuity of the emotional trends in so many varieties of shapes.

PART FIVE

Adventures in Psychoanalytic Discovery

Adventures in Psychoanalytic Discovery

I

1

WHILE FREUD was in the middle of his great discoveries he often found time and felt in the mood to study valuable works dealing with ancient history. In January, 1899, he wrote his friend Fliess that he was reading Burckhardt's *History of Greek Civilization* and that the book provided him with unexpected parallels to the psychology of pathological phenomena: "My predilection for the prehistoric in all its human forms remains the same." He kept this intense interest to the end of his life; in his last years it came even more strongly to the fore.

A few months after he wrote that letter (May 28, 1899) he reported to the same friend that he had bought Schliemann's book on ancient Ilios and had enjoyed the account of the archaeologist's childhood: "The man found happiness in finding Priam's treasure because happiness comes only from fulfillment of a childhood wish." In another letter he gave a definition of happiness which he considered "the deferred fulfillment of a prehistoric wish," and added: "That is why wealth brings so little happiness; money is not an infantile wish" (January 16, 1898).

What had happened to this Heinrich Schliemann as a little boy? In the cemetery of the little village in the state of Mecklenburg-Schwerin where he was born in 1822, there was the grave of a man Hennig who had once cruelly tortured and murdered a shepherd. People said that on a certain day of each year the left foot of the murderer stuck out from the grave. Little Heinrich patiently waited by the grave, and when the foot failed to appear asked his father to dig up the grave and find out why the foot of the monster did not emerge. The father, who was the pastor of the village, had told the boy many fairy tales and legends. He had also recounted the tales of Paris and Helena, Achilles and Priam, of Hector and of the heroes whose battles

473

around ancient Troy were sung by Homer. When the boy was seven years old, he was given as a Christmas present an *Illustrated History of the World* in which he saw a picture of Aeneas holding his little son by the hand and carrying his old father Anchises on his back as he fled the burning city of Troy. The boy Schliemann did not believe that the ancient citadel with its Cyclopean walls had been burned to the ground and that no one knew where it had stood. He announced that when he was grown up he would go to Greece and find ancient Troy and the king's treasure. In June, 1873, when Heinrich Schliemann was past sixty, he dug in the hills of Hissarlik in Asia Minor and discovered the golden treasure of a prehistoric king.

It seems to me that Freud could have reached still another conclusion if he had gone a few steps farther. (Perhaps he did by implication.) He points out that the fulfillment of a child's daydream meant happiness to the man. Although his father laughed at him, the boy Heinrich was convinced that the city of Troy was buried somewhere and, moreover, remained convinced although contemporary scientists considered Homer's description mythical. The same boy who decided he would some day dig out ancient Troy had clung a few years before to the belief that a dead murderer would stretch his leg out from his grave in the cemetery of Neu-Bukow. The belief that Troy and Priam's treasures were only covered up is the continuation of the earlier conviction that the dead, buried in the ground, are not entirely dead and still have a certain amount of will and power.

We do not doubt that the archaeological interests of the man Heinrich Schliemann had deep unconscious roots in the child's notion that the dead can express their wishes from the grave, can send messages to the living. This superstitious belief of the boy was perhaps the soil from which his passionate interest in archaeology grew. When the aging man discovered remnants of ancient Troy, he was overwhelmed because a childhood wish was fulfilled so late in life. Indeed, a great part of his satisfaction was the confirmation of that childhood belief that the dead are, in some form, still alive. Discarded when the boy became an adult and consciously dismissed long ago, that belief still continued its

existence in unconscious depths. On the surface, it had been replaced by a rational and scientific opinion about the state of men
who had perished a few thousand years before his time. The man
Heinrich Schliemann certainly smiled when he remembered that
he had once asked his father to dig out the leg of the murderer
who hesitated to stretch it out through his grave.

It may well be that we do not realize how persistent, tenacious,
and headstrong most of us were as children, or how we clung to
our preconceived ideas and early beliefs in spite of adults, yes,
even in spite of ourselves, and of our later, rational knowledge.
We analysts often are astonished when we realize with what
great energy those infantile opinions are unconsciously kept. For
example, we often wonder at the tenacity with which an infantile
theory explaining the nature of sexual intercourse is believed, although it has been consciously discarded long ago. In one of my
cases a little girl was convinced that her doll would speak to her
if she looked at her in a certain way. She once took the doll with
her on the subway, and from time to time glanced at the plaything in her arms because she expected that the doll would say
something about this new experience. As an adult woman she
was still sometimes inclined to believe that a bust of Shakespeare
in her husband's studio would suddenly begin to speak.

Another patient believed as a child that her uncle, a surgeon,
would one day perform an operation on her by which she would
be transformed into a boy and thus made equal to her envied
young brother. An alternative possibility to which she adhered in
her thoughts was that she would wake up some beautiful morning and discover that she had blond curls instead of her straight
black hair. Modern devices, by the way, make this miracle really
happen.

It is very likely that partial confirmations of childhood beliefs
often have a considerable place in the mental processes leading
to many new discoveries, that at their core they are returns to
early convictions that have remained unconsciously alive. Transformed and adjusted to a more appropriate concept, they recur
as new insights or as surprising hunches. Such returns to infantile beliefs, conceived as new, explain not only the genesis of

many discoveries, but also the nature of the emotions that accompany them.

For the child knowledge is power, and giving up his early notions means renouncing power. In his urge to understand the world, the child builds certain primitive theories which are destined to be deserted at a later time. The little boy slowly and reluctantly sacrifices his early notions and yields to the better knowledge and superior mentality of adults. In doing this the child sacrifices the uninhibited freedom of intellectual movement, the immediacy of experience, and the originality of his points of view. He will acquire certain thought-habits and self-discipline, but also mental clichés and rigid patterns of logical and rational thinking. In giving in to the adults in his thinking, he loses not only his immaturity and irrationality, but also the best part of his imaginative and creative faculties. Modern education to "emotional maturity" reaches its aim—if it reaches it—at the expense of the child's originality and intuition which continue to live only in the achievements of the best artists and scientists in combination with critical and rational intelligence. Full intellectual complaisance which deprives many children of their early independence of thought would make them merely conformers in later life.

Many discoveries are in this sense rediscoveries, returns to old views of childhood which have been dismissed, and are met again when the man is seeking new truths. Such an unconscious return is accompanied with the recovering of self-confidence. The boy in the man, who has been very sensitive to intellectual criticism and whose feelings have been hurt by the smiling superiority of the "grownup," has in his discovery asserted himself against the "better" judgment of the others and has, self-willed, followed his own way of thinking. (The "grownup" of his childhood had been replaced by the scientific tradition and by the conservatism of his colleagues.) But to assert oneself, to prove that one has been right in facing the intellectual resistance of the world means to experience a deep satisfaction. Here Freud's sentence that happiness lies only in the fulfillment of childhood wishes requires a continuation in the direction of intellectual achievement: the happiness of the explorer is often in the recovery of an old conviction.

The exciting and exhilarating character of a new finding, the felicity and the thrill of a new insight, the adventure and triumph of an analytic discovery are to a great extent founded on the unconscious gratification of such a return to early beliefs. They had been right after all! The feeling of victorious self-assertion in rediscovery is a good part of the satisfaction of search and research in the area of archaeological psychoanalysis. I am giving this name to the analytic study of prehistoric customs, beliefs, and religions by excavating and interpreting the remains of the emotional and mental life of the remote past. Those of us who are fortunate find out the truth about ourselves sooner or later, also the truth about the whole of mankind. And each finding, each dredging of a piece of prehistoric life also means a better understanding of our present, of the world around and within us.

Those who are doing creative work in a certain area rarely feel the incentive to reflect on the process of their mental productivity. This is valid not only for the writer and composer, but also for the explorer, the seeker of new truth, and it is also valid for the analyst who is eager to discover new laws in the dynamics of unconscious processes.

2

There was no necessity for me to probe into the course of psychoanalytic discovery in the area of the history of human civilization until I had to lead a seminar on research in the field of prehistoric religion and primitive customs. In the endeavor to give the students, psychiatrists and psychologists, a notion of the process which might bring new insight into still dark areas of many prehistoric phenomena, I was compelled to make clear to myself what the characteristics of this branch of analytic research were. I introduced my first lecture by pointing out that the premise for arriving at new insights in this field is still an original idea although the reading of many papers in the *Psycho-analytic Quarterly* seems to contradict this. If one can trust the statement of some analysts, an idea appears fully elaborated and ready, a finished product in their thoughts, as Pallas Athena sprang from the head of Zeus. The creative process is in reality much more complex, and comparable to that of impregnation and delivery. Some women assert that they can say with precision at what moment they were with child. But these are exceptional cases and most women realize that they are pregnant much later, yes, some only when they feel the first movement of the embryo. In a similar manner an analyst can but rarely say with certainty when the first still vague insight into a puzzling phenomenon occurred to him, the exact moment of the catch. In certain cases, however, it is possible to reconstruct the beginning phases of the creative process as examples in the following chapters will prove.

In three preceding books, *Listening with the Third Ear, The Secret Self,* and *The Haunting Melody,* I tried to present characteristics which distinguish the manner of psychoanalytic research from that of other sciences. The first feature concerns the nature of the instrument which is used nowhere else in reaching new and decisive insights, the second feature concerns the special inner experience in their emergence. That instrument, added to those of other explorers, is the unconscious of the analyst by which he receives and interprets the secret messages in the words of his patients. By this additional piece of instrumentation a new source of perception and understanding is made available to the analytic investigator. The nature of the inner experience in a new discovery is best described this way: The most important analytic insights, those that are crucial in the grasping of secret meanings, have the character of surprise for the psychoanalyst. From first indefinite impressions, which are almost intangible, vague hunches develop followed by a phase of haze or confusion and suspense. That chaotic pre-phase is ended with the emergence of a clear recognition of the unconscious meaning of the phenomenon that had been incomprehensible.

This development was described and illustrated by many instances taken from analytic practice in *Listening with the Third*

Ear. It was a surprise that new findings in the area of social and collective phenomena such as prehistoric rituals or primitive customs also follow the same course, that in the analytic understanding of a mysterious religious belief or of a puzzling social organization the unconscious of the analyst also functions as a receiver which is much more important and sensitive than his intellectual and rational thinking. But not only that, the phases of the discovery are also of the same or of a similar kind in the search and research of collective mental and emotional life. Here, too, the way goes from perceptions to haze and confusion, here, too, follows a phase of suspense out of which the new original concept emerges. We will discuss later on certain differences resulting from the fact that in clinical psychoanalysis individuals are treated, while in the case of analysis applied to the history of civilization we deal with groups and masses. Here, I like to emphasize that the manner of reaching new insights is essentially the same as far as the decisive operating of unconscious factors is concerned. I believe that this point of view secures a new approach to the exploration of social phenomena and represents a pioneer attempt on a new frontier of psychoanalytic thought.

The time when you become acquainted with material which becomes the object of analytic inquiry is not necessarily identical with the time when it makes an emotional and intellectual claim on you. For instance, such material as a strange ritual, a puzzling custom, a mysterious myth or legend makes, when first met, no special impression upon you. You take it for granted and treat it in your thoughts like another piece of tradition or social custom from ancient times or from foreign and remote lands. The moment of claim on you often comes later, sometimes many years later. I call this silent, but eloquent demand material makes on the analyst its "challenge." The challenge of the material compels him to turn his attention to its puzzling aspects. Here is the point of departure for a description and characterization of psychoanalytic discovery.

To my way of thinking, or rather observing, there are three phases which can be clearly distinguished in the process. In the beginning all seems clear and understandable. There may be some remarkable features in the material, but nothing to wonder about. Some things may strike the observer as curious, but they need not arouse his curiosity. The onset of a new approach is determined by the moment when you begin to wonder, to be astonished, when no easy and glib explanation of the observed seems to be satisfactory any longer. It is as if you had seen an object quite clearly on the table and had realized what it was, but in the next moment your sight became uncertain, the vision blurred, and you could not recognize it any longer. In moments like this, experienced by everybody, the temptation is strong to leave the matter as it is, or rather as it was before astonishment was experienced. In other words, to tell oneself there was a knife on this table just a second ago; it now seems as if something else is there. But it must be this knife. What else can it be? You dismiss the challenge of that moment. It can, however, happen that astonishment recurs and spreads out from a patch into a wider area, that the twilight can change into darkness. Some people then, and only then, bring their minds to bear on that strange business.

The transition from the conventional perception to this productive astonishment can easily be observed. It marks the initial phase of a new insight and often results in a kind of mental haziness or fog in which the old concept of things suddenly or slowly evaporates. In the endeavor to describe this initial chaotic phase, a sentence the composer Arnold Schönberg once said helped me: "When one observes well, things gradually become obscure." (I would like to replace the adverb "well" by "in a certain manner.") This statement sounds at first paradoxical, but it makes good sense in the area we are now discussing. A change in the quality of attention or observation makes you see things and people anew or makes you see new aspects of them. The light suddenly falls on them at an unusual angle and what has been transparent a minute before glides into twilight and even darkness from which later new profiles begin to appear. Before, you had taken things for granted, all was clear and obvious, and now they lose their distinctness and definitiveness. In other words, before a new discovery is made, substance has to become shadow again; the obvious, ambiguous or oblique, even enigmatic. Old views are not familiar any more, old figures seem to lose their contours before new patterns reveal themselves. This mental pre-phase precedes, consciously or unconsciously, the clarity of new findings. It is the dawn before the new day. Whoever has lost the faculty of wondering and of the dynamic change of view has become unable to do creative research work.

In that pre-phase you have to mistrust sweet reason and to abandon yourself to the promptings and suggestions emerging from the unconscious. You will even let the seemingly fanciful and irrational enter your thoughts and remain always ready to assume that there is something unknown even in the well known. The true enemy of original ideas is that kind of familiarity which breeds intellectual contempt for phenomena we thoroughly understand. Not only a little, but also much knowledge can be a dangerous thing, because it compels the "experts" to think in a certain groove and close their minds to an original view. Only when you leave your mind alone, will it throw up new patterns. We see things so often and so long that we scarcely see them any longer as they really are, and their presence has no meaning any more. They have to become strange again before we can see something new in them, before we rediscover them. The great divide is marked by the point where the obvious becomes obscure again, where order yields to chaos, where facts and figures do not matter so much and yield their place to novel factors and figurations. From here it is only one step to the moment when a new idea emerges with clarity and force and reveals a strange reality beyond the surface. When investigation and verification confirm what has been intuitively perceived, the circle is rounded.

It would be a mistake to assume that an original idea of this analytic type has to be born in an intellectual environment. It need not emerge—as a matter of fact, it rarely emerges—from profound thoughts and deep reflections. It is often stimulated by a chance observation, by some everyday impression, by a farrago of marginal thought-associations. The mental environment from which a far-reaching idea springs is of as little importance as the birthplace of a baby who will one day become a great man. Buddha was born as a prince in a royal place, but Jesus Christ saw the light of the world as a carpenter's son in a stable.

It need scarcely be said that the characterization of a certain group of analytic insights does not mean that results of research arrived at by different scientific exploration in this area are less valuable. The characterization concerns only the initial phases of the discovery process which continues along the way of other research methods. Finally, it is obvious that the area where the creative unconscious does its hidden work in finding new psychological truths becomes narrower, the more increased knowledge and conscious understanding conquer unknown areas. Also, in the intellectual domain of the analyst who investigates ancient customs and rites, the terrain that belonged to the It gradually becomes an area of the Ego. The task of the pioneers is different from that of the colonials who succeed them. There remain, however, many unknown areas in prehistory and in the early phases of civilization, and in these areas new far-reaching insights emerge only when the imaginative and intuitive faculties of the analyst are unleashed, when his unconscious leads him to the destination of unexpected meanings. The surprising is not reached on marked roads, and no guidepost points in its direction.

When is the right moment to get hold of such an idea? This is difficult to say. If I can trust self-observation, the best moment is not when the idea first occurs, but when it recurs, and then when it is, so to speak, at the zenith of conscious attention, on full swing. This last expression reminds me of a comparison I read the other day. A well-known musician discussing phases of musical performance speaks of the moment when the singer should start at the beginning of a song: "Have you seen a little girl anxiously watching a skip rope? . . . With one foot advanced ready to spring, her body sways forwards, backwards, forwards, backwards. . . . 'Now,' cry her companions. 'Now, now.' "* In the researcher there are unconscious mental

* Gerald Moore, *Singer and Accompanist* (New York, 1954).

movements, comparable to those of the little girl, in his approach to the secrets of his material. There are, alas, no companions helpful in timing. The explorer must trust a voice within himself that cries, "Now!"

3

The main material used in psychoanalysis is provided by a person's biography. We cannot understand the character, motives, and actions of an individual without insight into his development from early childhood. We cannot understand the general situation of human civilization without studying the history and prehistory of its evolution, without knowing the biography of mankind. In individual analysis we often have to reconstruct parts of early childhood which are no longer remembered by interpreting remnants in dreams, screen memories, and other productions of the unconscious. In the same manner we have to sketch the mental and emotional prehistory of our ancestors from myths, customs, legends, and rituals.

The difference between dealing with individual phenomena and with those of the psychology of masses and nations becomes immediately evident when you consider that the fact of the group itself creates divergencies in the emotional life, produces new emotions, and changes those within the individual to a considerable extent. But apart from these difficulties conditioned by the character of society, there is an added one which is connected with empathy. When you listen to a patient, you hear a person of your own time speak, a member of the same or of a similar civilization, of a common cultural atmosphere, however much his personality may differ from yours and however his disturbance may have changed his mental attitude. There is a common ground between you and him: you breathe the same air. But when you try to penetrate the secret meanings of the rites and customs of a past civilization, you live in a past remote from all human memory. When you set yourself the task of interpreting the legends of a primitive tribe in Central Australia, you have to learn to think entirely differently. You are living not only in a very distant country, but in the barbarous and remote atmosphere of the Stone Age. You are then a dweller in a period several thousand years before your time.

After emphasizing the differences in analytic research in these two areas, we still think that the methods of inquiry are basically the same, the ways of reaching the goals similar. The approach to the problems of mass-psychoanalysis shows the same phases in the experience of the explorer. Here also is the challenge of the emotional material; here also the haze or fog before the first insight into the hidden meaning emerges. Here also the surprise when the first hunch of the concealed significance occurs, and finally the extraordinary clarity which follows and illuminates not only the center of the special problem, but also its surrounding areas.

There are, however, specific characteristics of this kind of analytic research that have not yet been mentioned. It is not simply the night side of the human soul which demands our attention in analysis, but the side which is banned to darkness by powerful forces within us. The area of the repressed is thus defended against penetration by the inquiring mind. Other explorers are also prevented from reaching their aims by difficulties in the accessibility of their material as well as by deficiencies of their tools and instruments, by lack of knowledge, and by the limitations of their intelligence and imagination. The new factor added in the case of the analytic researcher is that active forces in himself resist the new finding. The haze or confusion preceding each fundamental and original insight is an expression of that resistance to the new idea which leads to the solution of the problem. That chaotic feeling indicates the mobilization of those undercurrents that defend the entrance into a forbidden territory full of intellectual dangers.

The feeling of helplessness caused by the repressing forces and the transition from haze into a surprising insight often acquires a quality which, as far as I know, is very rarely experienced in individual analysis. I shall facilitate the task of describing and defining the new feeling-tone by presenting three examples of analytic interpretation of similar problems in different areas. By contrasting the analysis of a neurotic symptom, of a poem, and of a prehistoric belief, I hope to show the quality of this new emotion accompanying many discoveries in the field of the analytic research of collective phenomena.

I take at random as an example from clinical experience the case of a patient, a woman in her early forties, whose history had quite a few obsessional features. She lived in a very modest furnished apartment in the suburbs of New York. One of her most frequent daydreams was that she would have a large apartment in the city, most elegantly furnished and with modern equipment in every room. Her husband, who had long been reluctant to spend the amount of money needed for a lavish apartment, learned by accident that an acquaintance had to leave town suddenly for South America with his family on business, and was eager to sell his large penthouse, which was modern and luxuriously furnished, for a moderate price. The husband of the patient bought the apartment with all the furniture, and the patient was suddenly the possessor of a most elegant residence. It was, she said, like a fairy tale. Overnight her most ardent wishes had become true. After she moved to her new home, the patient reacted in a strange manner. A short time of exultation and joyousness was followed by many weeks in which she felt very sad. In her depression she often complained that life no longer had any meaning for her. This paradoxical mood left her only for a few hours at a time. She often walked through the rooms of the new apartment as if in a wonderful dream and told herself it could not be true. The more she admired the luxury she now called her own, the more depressed she became. Strangely enough, she felt a little better and easier in her mind when she could find some small flaws in the furniture—for instance, a tiny spot on a carpet or a little scratch on a table. Such small imperfections seemed to diminish her melancholy for a few minutes. It was not difficult to guess that her depression emerged not in spite of the fact that her wish had been fulfilled, but because of it. It was the expression of an unconscious guilt feeling which reacted upon the unexpected stroke of luck. She expressed in her depressed mood her unconscious conviction that she did not deserve to be thus favored by destiny, that she felt unworthy of it.

The first insight into the character of the depression was gained when I realized that she felt better when she found some fault in the elegant apartment. Her intense guilt feeling was lifted for a moment when her good luck appeared less abundant and over-powering. The depression gradually decreased and finally evaporated after we worked its origin and unconscious motives through in analytic sessions. However, it was an unpleasant surprise when, after the disappearance of the depression, an unexpected new emotion appeared which was even more difficult to grapple with, which was more perilous and lasted several weeks. The patient now experienced a puzzling anxiety that filled her days. Of unknown origin, this new affect was without any recognizable content, an emotion without name. The anxiety seemed to increase the longer the patient was unable to say what caused it. What was the meaning of this aggravating new emotion and how could one explain that it replaced the depression which had yielded to analytic treatment? I understood neither the origin of this unexpected feeling nor its succession to the melancholic mood of the previous weeks.

The first ray of light fell into the dark situation when the patient once mentioned casually that yesterday she had had the anxious feeling that her little dog whom she loved might have been run over by a car. Soon other instances of thoughts occurring to her in the middle of her anxiety secured more insight: When she walked through her beautiful rooms she sometimes thought how terrible it would be if her husband who was on a business trip had a car accident and left her the apartment to herself. She was sometimes frightened that her sister who had flown to Europe would be killed in a plane crash. This first approach to determining some objects of her anxiety enabled us, of course, to guess its unconscious character as well as the reasons why it had replaced her depression. When she now looked at her luxurious apartment, she did not feel guilty or unworthy, but frightened. She had daydreamed of such elegance, but now it was as if her wish had brought about a reality which she could never hope for. But if her thoughts had such power to direct the course of events, was it not possible that other wishes, much less harmless than the desire for a luxurious penthouse, could be fulfilled? Old aggressive, hostile, and murderous impulses which had often led to fantasies in previous years re-emerged and were rejected. It was as if the realization of her wish for a penthouse had reawakened those other fantasies, had brought their realization within reach. Her anxiety was her unconscious reaction to the imagined possibility that those secret wishes could be fulfilled. The thought-danger to which she reacted with anxiety was the secret belief that persons she loved could be killed by the power of her thoughts. With the disappearance of the depression the door was opened to those exiled and forbidden wishes. The tiger had licked blood and this whetted his appetite.

In Schiller's ballad "The Ring of Polycrates," which is based on a tale of Herodotus, each wish of the tyrant of Samos is fulfilled and the monarch boasts of his extraordinary luck. Even a ring he throws into the sea is shortly afterward brought back by a fisherman who has found it in a fish. His friend, the King of Egypt, who becomes witness of Polycrates' good luck, is taken by a shudder:

> The guest in terror turned away.
> "I cannot here, then, longer stay.
> My friend you can no longer be!
> The gods have willed that you should die.
> Lest I, too, perish, I must fly."

The favorite of fortune is doomed; the gods want him to perish.

Let us add to this example the narrative of the Scripture which recounts the census of the Israelite tribes. In II Sam. 24, it is the Lord; in I Chron. 21, it is Satan who provokes King David to number Israel. Although warned by faithful Joab, who is ordered to undertake the census, the King insists that Joab go through all the tribes from Dan to Beersheba and number the thousands of men who could draw sword in Israel. But the Lord was displeased with this and smote Israel. The Destroying Angel with his sword stretched out over Jerusalem, and the people were stricken with the great pestilence. The King repented and offered sacrifice to reconcile angry Jahweh who finally said to the Destroying Angel, "It is enough; stay now thine hand!"

Comparing these three examples, we find that they present essentially the same emotional reactions in a neurotic, mythological, and theological garb. The fear which my patient experienced concerned persons whom she loved, while the friend of Polycrates feels the threat of impending calamity for himself. But the nameless terror in the face of extraordinary luck is the same. The mythological encasement of Schiller's ballad is absent in the biblical tale, but it is replaced by the theological garb of the historic report. The depression of my patient is the manifestation of an unconscious guilt feeling; Polycrates throws his precious ring into the sea to mitigate the envy of the gods, and King David atones for the mysterious offense against Jahweh. What is the nature of the crime common to the three cases? My patient was afraid that destiny would fulfill her secret wishes, of whose power she was unconsciously convinced. Polycrates boasts of his good luck and even tests it. The ancient Greeks would accuse him of *hubris,* of a form of conceit which makes men compare themselves with the gods and attribute to themselves the power of deities. The tyrant in Schiller's poem does not experience any presentiment of impending calamity, but his friend expresses his intense fear. In the biblical report David is warned by the voice of Joab, but insists and is severely punished. Instead of fear the consequences of his nefarious action are clearly demonstrated by the pestilence. The dark emotions of the patient found their interpretation in psychoanalysis, in which she recognized the depression as a symptom of her unconscious guilt feeling and her anxiety as reaction to her conviction of the power of her thoughts. But what is the crime of King David who ordered that his men should be numbered? J. G. Frazer attempted to explain the sin of the census with the superstitious fears many primitive and half-primitive people have about counting and being counted.* To quote only a few examples: among the Cherokee Indians of North America melons and squashes

* *Folklore In The Old Testament* (Abridged edition, New York, 1927).

must not be counted while still growing because otherwise they will cease to thrive. When a British officer in Columbia took a census of the Indians, many natives died of measles. The Indians attributed the calamity to their having been numbered. In Germany there was a belief that when you counted your money it would steadily decrease. Some people when asked how old they are answer, "As old as my little finger." Examples from the Lapps, the Scots, from the Greeks, Germans, and Armenians complete the list the well-known anthropological industry of Frazer has brought together. The scholar is of the opinion that the objection of the Jews to the taking of the census rests "on no firmer foundation than sheer superstition which may have been confirmed by an outbreak of plague immediately after the numbering of the people." He adds that the same repugnance lives to this day among the Arabs of Syria who are averse to counting the tents, the horsemen, or cattle of their tribes lest some misfortune befall them.

Frazer is certainly right in comparing the biblical story with the reports of anthropologists, missionaries, and travelers about the superstitions about counting of so many African, American, and European people. He need not have gone to Africa and America to find the same fears. When an Eastern orthodox Jew is asked today how old he is, he will answer, "Seventy to a hundred," which means: I am seventy years old and wish to reach a hundred. The superstitious addition means that he wishes to avert evil powers around him that might grudge his age. The same superstition appears when a woman is asked how many children she has. She will say, "Four—*unberufen!*" (Similar to "touch wood"). We regret that Frazer remained satisfied with the explanation that the Israelites at David's time had the same superstitions as other people and did not attempt to find the emotional motives of those beliefs.

In the biblical story the nature of David's sin becomes obvious in the fact that the punishment fits the crime. The King's army is decimated by the plague the offended Deity sends. In taking the census David put his trust in the number of his soldiers instead of in God. He was proud of his power and his ability to lead his people to victory, but should rather have believed in the power of Jahweh who taught him a theological lesson.

The psychoanalyst cannot acquiesce in the explanation that the case of David, like those of the primitive tribes, shows superstitious fears. He will search for the origin and motives of those beliefs. He will compare the superstitions of the people with those he has frequently met in analytic experience with neurotic individuals, and trace them back to their unconscious sources. The superstitious person unconsciously recognizes in himself the existence and activity of hostile and murderous wishes, and is compelled to project those unconscious tendencies into the external world since he cannot acknowledge them in himself. He constructs a supernatural reality, the existence of gods and demons who operate from the outside and direct his actions. It is the task of the psychoanalyst to retransform this construction into psychology of the unconscious, to resolve metaphysics into metapsychology. In the analysis of very intelligent obsessional patients we discover how often their superstitions originate in the repression of hostile and cruel tendencies. They are prevented from acknowledging that they often wish evil things to others; they have repressed those forbidden impulses, but unconsciously expect calamity as a punishment for their aggressive and cruel thoughts; death or serious damage as the penalty for the evils they wish to others. In that projection is also the fear of the power of evil wishes other persons have against them, of hostile and envious thoughts that could damage or kill themselves. They are thus afraid of the power of the same malicious or envious tendencies in others that they unconsciously experience in themselves. The antipathy against being counted, telling one's age, or saying how many children one has, has unconscious roots in the projection of the envious and hostile feelings we suspect in others because we have felt them in ourselves.

The fact that behind all those projections there are some psychological truths concealed is a leading principle in archaeological psychoanalysis, as developed in the following chapters. Scratch a superstition, a religious ritual, a myth or a legend, and you find unconscious facts. It is easy enough to dismiss all those strange beliefs and customs as superstitions. It is more difficult to discover that there is a psychological core of fact in old men's sayings and old wives' tales.

4

The purpose of the preceding comparison was not so much to give a minor example of analytic interpretation of different unconscious reactions to the same emotional problem, but to introduce some characteristics of psychoanalytic research into the nature of religious beliefs, customs, and rituals. The element of haze and suspense that can be observed before each decisive new insight often has an emotional quality of its own in the field of analytic research into ancient customs and beliefs. In the cases which were accessible to self-observation there was for a split second a definite feeling of the uncanny. I am prepared to meet the indignation of many readers at this point. Why should the first reaction of a scientific explorer to whom a new discovery dawns be an uncanny feeling? What has this emotion, rarely experienced by us, to do with the initial phase of new findings of social psychology? The expression "uncanny" is mostly current today in aesthetics; we speak of the uncanny impression made by a scene in a play or a movie.

That remote region of aesthetics was, however, considered worthy of Freud's attention when he wrote a paper on this neglected problem.* The emotion of the uncanny, akin to that of the terrifying, is there traced back to something that was once familiar which has been alienated to the ego by the process of repression. An experience appears uncanny when repressed infantile complexes are reactivated by an impression or when primitive convictions we have discarded seem once more confirmed. Freud differentiated two kinds of uncanny feelings, although he pointed out that sometimes no sharp demarcation can be made: the uncanny met in experience and the uncanny met

* "Das Unheimliche," *Gesammelte Schriften*, X, 369.

in fiction. Many things that strike us as spooky in fiction would not be reacted to in this way in real life.

I do not assert that the experience of the uncanny is felt in each case in which the analyst is on the track of a new discovery in the field of primitive religion and prehistoric customs, but it is often present in those exceptional cases when analytic research reaches an unconscious meaning that is at first entirely strange. In the following chapters I shall present examples of occasions on which the researcher felt that quality of the uncanny in the pre-phase of haze and confusion within the process of discovery.

We learned from Freud that the feeling of the uncanny often occurs when old, long-overcome infantile convictions seem to be confirmed by some impression. That is frequently the case when we hear or read reports of primitive customs, make the acquaintance of prehistoric rituals and magical performances. For a second those old, obsolete convictions and beliefs seem to have been right. We relapse for a moment into a phase in which we believed in the omnipotence of wishes and in magical powers around us, in which we did not consider death final, but thought the dead continued to live in some form, and so on. Such a momentary relapse into infantile, long-overcome ways of thinking not only produces a second of intellectual uncertainty, but also a kind of half-anxious feeling similar to that of a person who is under the impression that the ground beneath his feet threatens to slip away. This is also the case, because for that moment the reality function seems to fail and be replaced by magical thought-processes and animistic beliefs we have long discarded. The rational and logical structure of our *Weltanschauung*, founded on scientific results, gives way for a second to primitive superstitions.

The kind of material we study favors the emergence of this uncanny feeling and give special flavor to the haze and suspense that often characterize the pre-phase of a new analytic finding. Exotic and prehistoric rites, magical practices and other remnants from the infancy of mankind cannot shake our rational and mechanical view of the world, but they tempt us to return to the beliefs of our childhood that continue to live in our unconscious. We return for a second to the world of fairy tales and myths, of superstitions and magic. The feeling of uncanniness is an indication of the intrusion of those old beliefs demanding entrance into the region of our rational mind. But this second when we are in unconscious touch with convictions long relinquished is fruitful. It opens an avenue to the understanding of the hidden meaning of many puzzling phenomena of the remote past, to the discovery of the oldest in the most recent.

That phase of confusion or haze is almost identical with that of suspense before the new insight emerges. The twilight seems to be peopled with figures, shapes, and forms never seen before. Out of the silence of suspense strange messages reach the mind, vague noises like steps muffled in the fog. There a kind of mental mobilization takes place. In it the previously unidentified and unconstructed material obtains forms and patterns. Pieces fall into their proper place, and infinite affinities between areas far remote from each other become transparent. Theories which gave a slanted or unfaithful image recede and give way to suddenly revealed new meanings. Disengaged attention finds novel objects, and in this creative wondering and renewed imaginative act the solution of the problem is reached long before its validity can be proved. From the state of intellectual fermentation the explorer glides into a phase of reorganization of the material which slowly opens its possibilities like flowers their petals. What was once considered understood is reinterpreted, and new relationships of far-reaching significance are recognized. From preverbal perception the trend leads to thinking in formulated concepts. The circle which the new insight draws becomes wider. The magic lantern by which we see gives a stronger light. Also, the implications of a discovery have to be uncovered. The imaginative act separates the relevant from the immaterial. The mind marches ahead with lack of caution, with abandonment, leaving the necessary re-examination and verification to a later process. Now is the time to grasp the significance of clues; to snatch the wordless messages; to give rein to the functions of the unconscious; to become aware of the forces and counter-forces beneath the conscious surface.

This is the process leading from the moment of challenge to that of illumination. This is the analyst's response to the lure of the secrets of the human soul as they reveal themselves in ancient religion, prehistoric customs, and myths. This is the psychological stuff the analyst's daydreams are made of.

The old master Anatole France once said: "One gets tired of everything except of understanding" ("*On lasse de tout excepté de comprendre*"). The analyst who has once experienced the trial, the thrill, and the triumph of discovering the secret behind the prehistoric will always return to that ennobling adventure of the mind. He will always remain a searcher after the concealed truths of emotional life, and sometimes he will become a finder.

II

1

THE FOLLOWING chapter will present an example of one of the possibilities of future analytic research. An insignificant and everyday experience is reported, and it is shown at what new, unexpected, and unsuspected insights the analyst can arrive when he pursues the train of thoughts such a trifling incident provokes. None of the analytic results will be used in this new approach, none of the numerous results of analytic practice and theory will be applied, and none of the conclusions of our science will be quoted. They are not avoided. There was simply no place for them in the process here presented. Yet the way of thinking and of arriving at a new discovery is entirely analytic, is in the spirit of Sigmund Freud. I will endeavor to show that the insight was unconsciously already implied in the train of associations stimulated by that small slice of experience, and that it only had to be extracted from its context, extricated from the incidental entanglements of the original situation, and to be consciously conceived.

It seems to me that an analyst does not go out in search of a problem, but that the problem is rather within him and tries to be released, like a prisoner who makes all efforts to win his freedom. In his desperate efforts to be released the prisoner digs, unsuspected by his guardians, a subterranean corridor below the encircling walls. An unconscious idea thus works its way into the open in the darkness, works its way through and out. Much more search than research in its beginning, this new technique of analytic discovery is more akin to art than to science. But so was psychoanalysis in general at its departure, and it will always be at the crossroads of art and science when it starts a new expedition. It will first be led by hunches and guesses rather than by clear and objective directions. The conqueror wants to reach his destination and often recognizes much later which road led him there. The drawing of a precise map is not his task, but that of the geographers.

The thoughts provoked by this experience are in no way different from the jetsam and flotsam of everyday associations, they are fleeting impressions, carried away by the next wave. Also the thought-fragments which emerge later on are not recognized as significant. Only after they are spilled to the shore of conscious thinking is their meaning understood.

One evening a few years back I rested on the couch, tired after many analytic sessions, but not yet ready to go to bed. The visit I had paid to a hospitable family on the previous day came to mind. After dinner some new records had been played. I saw before me the cozy room, beautifully furnished and brilliantly lighted by a chandelier. I sat near the recording machine while listening to the gracious Symphony No. 83 by Haydn and reading the program notes on the jacket of the album. Some comments on the symphony were now recalled: that it is one of a set of six composed by Haydn for a Parisian organization and that the first audience called it *La Poule*. Its first movement came vividly to mind. I must have gotten up from the couch because I caught myself in the next minute walking the floor and singing the first strong, rhythmic theme which is replaced by the second subject with its beautiful oboe part sounding like the clucking noises of a hen. (I doubt if anyone listening to me would recognize the two themes.) While I thus walked across the room, reproducing the two themes half aloud, I moved my hands with great vivacity as if conducting an invisible orchestra. Marking the beat with the right hand and illustrating the phrase with the left, I became self-conscious or rather conscious of what I was doing. Before that I was naïvely enjoying the graces of the hen motif, heard with the inner ear, walking or rather dancing across the room.

Before I became fully aware that I was doing this, there was a split second in which I experienced a sensation the nature of which can be described only as uncanny. This distinct feeling was a mixture of strangeness and suspense, akin to anxiety, and bordered on the sense of dreamlike unreality. It became clear to me later on that this sensation set in as soon as I became aware of my odd activity and that it marked the moment of transition into a changed inner state. No uncanny feeling of this kind would emerge in a professional musician in the same situation. Such a person remembering the Haydn symphony and reacting to the recollection in tranquillity in the same manner would find nothing odd or uncanny in what is known as "mental conducting." I later recalled an anecdote, quoted by most biographers of Mozart.* It emphasized that emotional difference and made me more embarrassed. Mozart, who was eight years old and had made his first attempt at writing a symphony, was once left alone at home. When his parents returned after two hours, they became aware of an almost unnatural quietness. When they entered the apartment, they heard a series of light tappings and the sound of the boy's voice mumbling some indistinct phrases. But then he shouted, "You fool! Why don't you play your instrument as I conduct? Now we must begin over!" Wolfgang had the score of his first symphony on a chair before him, the orchestral parts were spread out on the bed. The boy had vividly imagined that he was conducting an orchestra playing his work.

* Adolf Schmid, *Language of The Baton* (New York, 1935), p. 10.

The fleeting uncanny sensation was followed by a moment of self-mockery. The slight feeling of anxiety was replaced by a humorous view, by making fun of myself and of my silly actions. Was I becoming senile? I had behaved like a little boy. I called myself an old fool. My conducting now appeared to me as an act and a miserable pantomime. That which strikes us as queer and uncanny in ourselves often changes easily into something that seems funny or ridiculous. I felt a little ashamed of myself and was ready to dismiss this incident as one of those *petits riens* of everyday life. (Did the thought of Mozart linger on?) Yet I did keep wondering about it. The sensation of the uncanny is very rarely experienced by me. What had happened in that moment? I have not the slightest knowledge of the art and technique of conducting. As far as I remember, I was never interested in it. That is, I never felt the wish to become a conductor. I don't even know the musical requirements of conducting, know nothing about baton technique, score studying, rehearsal and performance practice of a concert orchestra.

At this point I abandoned myself to "free" associations. Was I really never interested in conducting? . . . I was once, in my teens, it is true, enthusiastic about Mahler, but that was rather a fascination with his personality than with his function as conductor. . . . I suddenly see "in my mind's eye" Mahler rushing out from the Café Imperial on the Ringstrasse when the Burgmusik came marching on. (The Burgmusik was a military band with drums, wind instruments, and clarinets in Vienna during the old Austrian monarchy. At the stroke of twelve noon when the guards were changed, the Burgmusik marched to the Imperial Palace, and a crowd of grown-up Viennese and children marched over the Ringstrasse to the tunes of the band.) Richard Specht in his book on Mahler calls the march of the Third Symphony an *"ideale Burgmusik."* . . . Yes, I see Mahler standing on the sidewalk as if spellbound looking at the Burgmusik. . . . And then I seem to see him again at his desk in the Vienna Opera when he raised the baton for the overture. . . . The sergeant marching ahead of the Burgmusik, too, swings a big, ribboned baton. . . . The image of the bright uniform of the officer and then the black coattails of Mahler standing before the orchestra, illuminated by the light from the stage. . . . I now remember a series of silhouettes presenting the famous conductor and his various gestures. . . . The name of the artist who made those pictures, well known in Vienna, occurs to me: Otto Boehler. . . . Black pictures, silhouettes; only Mahler's eyes blazing. . . . Suddenly another band occurs to me . . . jazz players. . . . Negroes swinging it . . . the eyes wide open in the dark faces as if in trance . . . the violent movements of the jazz players. . . . Behind the picture of the jazz band appears now another one, different, yet alike in some ways: that of an early childhood memory. . . . I have not thought of that for ages. . . . The first time I saw Negroes. . . . When I was a boy, I was taken to the Prater by my parents: there were Negroes, a group of Ashantis, who had been brought to Vienna. . . . They lived in huts on a wide meadow, and the Viennese enjoyed the opportunity of looking at those exotic people and their primitive households. . . . The Ashantis were performing their dances. . . . I remember how they sat cross-legged on the ground, beating the drums. All of a sudden, a big fellow, perhaps their chieftain, jumped up and ran about dancing, howling, and wildly shaking his spear. Many other men followed him, danced after him, with unco-ordinated movements of their black bodies, raucously singing—if you could call it singing—and swinging their primitive weapons. . . . I stood there fascinated and did not want to leave when admonished by my parents. . . . And then, as if in contrast to the memory of the Ashantis of my childhood, the image of a parade I had seen in Manhattan emerges. . . . There is a band playing; at its head a majorette swirls her heavy baton. . . . The girl pirouettes, throws her baton into the air and catches it, trips and dances. . . . The half-naked Negroes in the Prater and the fantastic white uniform of the majorette . . . both appear in spectacles. (The contrast of appearance suggests the fact that in dreams and legends nudity is often presented by very rich dresses. . . . Damn those analytic associations which interfere with the freedom and spontaneity of thoughts. . . . But I am suspicious of my indignation. . . . In that contrast, especially in the picture of the pretty uniformed majorette, is perhaps more than meets the eye, namely, something the eye wants to meet. At this point I called myself some names and forced my thoughts back to the associations of the jazz band). Jazz players and Negroes in America, colored people in Vienna. . . . Then it occurred to me that the quarter where we now live in Manhattan is facetiously called Schwarzspanierstrasse by some Viennese people. Schwarzspanierstrasse (literally, Black Spaniard Street), because in that street and those surrounding it many Puerto Ricans live. . . . There is a Schwarzspanierstrasse in Vienna. It was thus called because the Benedictines, the "black monks" who came from France and Spain, had a church there. Beethoven died in the Schwarzspanierhaus. . . .

At this point I became painfully aware of how disjointed and disassociated my thoughts were, how they wandered all over in place and time. I said to myself that they had no rhyme nor reason. Yet they had one common feature, namely, rhythm. They circled around the central point of music. More than that, they described the cycle of musical development from Ashanti drums through military bands, Beethoven and Mahler, to jazz players, a condensed version, as it were, of the history of music from the primitive natives of Africa to modern composers. . . . There must be something meaningful in their sequence. They might contain the clues to the understanding of that uncanny moment that puzzled me, but I was unable to grasp them. When I finally dismissed that train of thought, I did not know that it really contained the solution of the problem. Everything was there, concealed but complete. Everything was already unconsciously perceived. At the moment I did not even recognize what was the real problem that unconsciously occupied my thoughts. I dwelt in an unknown building of ideas.

"Those free associations!" I thought. "Well, you have to let the chips of thought-processes fall where they may! You can always pick them up later on." I decided to jot down those associations and put the sheet into a folder. I felt discouraged because I had failed in a very modest intellectual task. "Some enchanting evening!" I thought ill-humoredly.

2

During the next weeks the memory of that evening emerged unexpectedly on several occasions. I added some notes on them to my previous memorandum, unfortunately without dating them. During a session a young psychiatrist who was in training analysis with me mentioned that he had compared two records playing the *Blue Danube* waltz by Johann Strauss. The one was by a well-known American orchestra, and the waltz was beautifully performed, with perfect phrasing and precision. He felt, said the physician, like singing with the instrumentalists. When he listened to the same waltz, played by the Vienna Philharmonic Orchestra, he did not feel like following the familiar melody, but was carried away by it. He wanted to dance and had to make an effort to keep his feet on the ground. I had in this moment a fleeting image of the Vienna Philharmonic Orchestra playing in the Konzerthaussaal where I had so often sat. But in that elusive mental picture the violinists on both sides of the conductor seem to sway with the tunes, to nod their heads and to tap their feet on the floor. . . . I realized, of course, that the grotesque image had been suggested by the words of the young psychiatrist, but why did the memory of my own conducting occur immediately after that image? There was, it seemed to me, no bridge except the general connection of music.

The succeeding occasions that brought the memory of that evening back were also accidental. It was, however, not accidental that they brought the memory back. We have to ascribe it to the selectivity of memory that the mental material which unconsciously preoccupied me was approached from different sides.

A few days later I listened to Dimitri Mitropoulos being interviewed by a lady on the radio. The artist said in the conversation that the conductor plays all the instruments of his orchestra and could be compared to an actor who plays not only Hamlet, but also the ghost of his father, Polonius and Ophelia, Claudius and the Queen. Here was at least a discernible thought-connection with the memory of my amateurish attempt at conducting, but why was the emphasis in my thoughts now on acting?

The third occasion had no manifest associative threads with conducting, except again the general one of music. It took my thoughts very far away from the Haydn symphony and Vienna, namely, to Africa. A friend kindly sent me a record of the various phases of the African initiation rites which take place throughout the equatorial forest once every five years. The expedition under the leadership of Armand Denis and Leila Roosevelt that visited the Belgian Congo in 1935 and 1936 prepared a sound recording of the primitive music that accompanies these religious ceremonies. The two records give an excellent idea of the circumcision ritual in the Northern Ituri Forest, where at a certain age the boys are segregated for many weeks and introduced to the beliefs and traditions of their tribes. You hear the ceremonial dances of the Negroes, their chanting and beating the drums. Then the "circumcision bird" appears. The part of this mythical animal is played by a Negro who hides in the bushes near the women's hut and utters the nasal cries of a huge bird. He is accompanied by another man who whirls a lath of wood on a short piece of vine. The whirring sound imitates the wings of the bird. You hear in the following flagellation of the boys the lashings of the whip and the cheering of the crowd. During the circumcision ceremony a stick orchestra is heard: rough sticks of wood, trimmed to different lengths, are struck by wooden mallets. After the initiation the boys shout obscene insults to the women of the tribe. Now they have left the women's care and are recognized as adult members of their people. Their triumphant shouting, accompanied by the cheering and laughter of the men to whom they now belong, presents the last phase of the ritual. The records transcribe the primitive music of a strange vanishing tribe. For the explorer of primitive culture they provide a valuable source which brings him as close as possible to prehistoric music and its performance in bygone ages.

Listening to the primitive rhythms of the Congo tribes took my thought, of course, back to the analytic study on puberty rituals of the savages which I had published more than forty years ago,* but it renewed also, strangely enough, the memory of the other evening. Clearly only a single feature connected the crude music of those Negroes with the Haydn symphony: the imitation of a bird. In the ceremony of the natives the nasal cries of the circumcision bird are produced. In the Haydn symphony an oboe peevishly repeats the same note while the first violin sings a piquant melody, adorned with many graces, imitating a clucking hen.

I remembered that on that evening the childhood memory of the Ashantis beating their drums, shouting and dancing had emerged. Here was the associative tie of primitive or prehistoric music. It did not matter that in one case Negro tribes of the Belgian Congo, in the other the Ashantis of British West Coast Africa produced the music. The essential factor was that the scene of the Ashantis dancing and making music must have impressed the boy I was then.

The last occasion renewing the memory of my acting the conductor came a few days later when I saw the film *Limelight*. Many people will remember Charlie Chaplin in the part of an old comedian who was once a success in the music halls and is now almost destitute. Chaplin's performance presents a strange mixture of genius and ham acting. When he talks about the dignity of the artist and about the ultimate goals of life, and so on, it is often not worth listening to. How much more eloquent was he when he was silent! There are, rare enough, a few moments when you feel that what he says is not contrived or merely high-sounding, but genuinely experienced. He is still far from being a philosopher, but when the old and dying clown says near the end, "Everyone is so kind to me. Makes me feel isolated," the voice of a long life's experience speaks.

One scene of the film made a strange impression upon me: the comedian is shown on the stage singing a song "Love, love, love" and accompanying it by his incomparable pantomime. The camera gently moves from the stage. It shows the upper part of the figure of the conductor who leads an invisible orchestra, with

* "The Puberty Ritual of the Primitives" in my book *The Ritual*, 1915 (English translation, New York, 1945).

his right hand beating the time, with his left expressing the phrases and the character of the tune. The scene of the comedian and of the conductor, so to speak, cut into half, below him, leading an unseen orchestra, made a bizarre, ghostlike impression. It was as if the two figures were a single one, and as if the pantomime of the actor and the gestures of the conductor comprised one movement. For a second there was just a trace of that uncanny feeling.

While I walked home from the movie theater, the memory of that experience many weeks ago came vividly back again. It was followed by vague thoughts and musings over the figure of the conductor in general. I wondered about his role and position in relation to the orchestra and within the orchestra, and about his function as a part of the musical performance. The figure of that man with the baton, so familiar to me, now appeared suddenly strange, problematical, even incomprehensible. It was, all of a sudden, a puzzling phenomenon which I did not understand any longer. As if pulled by a magnetic power, my thoughts were thrown back to that evening when I conducted the Haydn symphony alone in my room, as if in that scene were the clues to the solving of the mystery. But no helpful ideas occurred to me.

On reaching home, I looked at the manuscript on my desk—it was a book on Gustav Mahler on which I was then working—I remembered some sentences he had written in a letter to his friend Bruno Walter in 1909.* Mahler asked: "What is it, after all, that thinks within us? And what acts within us?" And then follows the sentence: "Strange! When I hear music—even while I conduct—I can hear definite answers to all my questions and feel entirely clear and sure or rather I feel quite clearly that there are no questions at all." Comparing my present situation with that of the composer, I realized that my study and experience could provide a general answer to Mahler's question—what it is that thinks within us?—but no more than that. Mahler felt that he no longer had any problems when he heard music or even when he conducted. Of course, music *was* for him the answer. Far from such a gratifying experience, my astonishment had just begun

* Quoted from Bruno Walter, *Gustav Mahler* (1941), p. 153.

when I caught myself mentally conducting a symphony in this very room. And that astonishment had been enlarged, had shifted from wondering at that feeling of the uncanny to the mysterious activity of conducting itself.

3

It is said that man is a creature of habit, and that certainly includes his personal habits of thoughts, his mental reactions to his experiences. It was thus unavoidable that analytic thoughts and reflections entered into my musing over the position and function of the conductor. Those analytic considerations emerged on two points, but I hasten to add that their result was, in both cases, negative. No light fell from my analytic knowledge and clinical experience on the puzzling phenomenon of conducting. Nothing I had learned in study and practice helped me to understand the significance of the part pertaining to the man with the baton. The purely mechanical application of analytic knowledge failed. What was explained when you thought of the conductor as a father-representative figure and of the instrumentalists and singers as son-figures who had an ambivalent attitude toward their leader? I imagined a young psychoanalyst who would point out to me that the baton of the conductor has a symbolic, phallic significance. I grinned at the thought: "Elementary, my dear Watson!" All such knowledge remains immaterial and irrelevant in this context, and we are none the wiser for such explanations.

There was nothing well considered or methodical about the fact that analytic thinking entered the area of my wondering at the function of the conductor, a domain where it had no place. It was rather by force of intellectual habit, almost automatically, that I began to see the problem of the conductor at an angle at which other difficult questions appeared in analytic practice. I had found that certain puzzling phenomena showed new aspects when I applied two mental techniques. Since both are almost unknown and have been acquired in personal experience, I shall demonstrate their character as simply as possible. We follow in psychoanalysis the principle of free-floating attention; in other words, we do not concentrate our observation on one or the other preferred part of the material because we do not want to cater to our pre-conceived psychological ideas. We turn our attention equally to all manifestations of the unconscious life as it unfolds in analytic sessions. Free-floating attention, comparable to a moving, equally distributed light, will sometimes be focused on certain points and can then be compared to a searchlight resting on one place. Such temporary concentration or overillumination will result in a kind of oversensitiveness, of hyperesthesia for the marginal, for phenomena or parts and aspects of them, which until then have been only casually observed, neglected or unappreciated in their significance. Thus, certain features appear isolated and overclear.

The natural consequences of viewing things this way were often artificially emphasized by me in the two directions, namely, of isolating and then of exaggerating these features in a kind of thought-experiment. Isolation in this connection means separating a symptom, for instance, from its environment, from the external and internal situation in which we are accustomed to see it. Thus detached, certain manifestations are sometimes seen anew or can reveal new aspects. Side by side with this mental device I recommend to my students another one, namely, that of exaggerating and magnifying selected features or trends so that they appear increased in size, look larger. Do we not use microscopes in science and industry to enable us to see objects better and more sharply? No one will deny that such an instrument—for instance, a thread-counter in weaving—is an artificial help for the eye, that it makes things appear much too large. Of course, this means that they are distorted; but no one will deny the great usefulness of the instrument. Why should we not also apply such expedient help in our thought-processes?

By this method of isolation and exaggeration, the full import of which as a means of finding psychological facts will be discussed elsewhere, certain features and trends appear conspicuous. After that mental experiment things are again reduced to their natural size and put back into their inner environment, into the context in which they belong. Only the results of this technique can decide if the experiment of isolation and enlargement was fruitful in the individual case and led to new insights and surprising views. The devices here recommended can have as their objects certain puzzling symptoms as well as character traits, features of behavior, habits of acting or speaking. In taking it from its frame and in exaggerating it in imagination, a special trait—for instance, a gesture—presents to the analytic observer a picture of sharp contours.

A patient had, for instance, a habit of looking around suspiciously in the consultation room before he lay down on the couch. This feature became transparent only after it was isolated in observation from such things as his walking into the room, his first words and gestures, the movements of his hands and legs. Loosening the trait from this particular situation and exaggerating it in thought, you tentatively imagine the patient looking around mistrustfully wherever he goes and you arrive at the assumption of suspiciousness and perhaps even of paranoid trends of which you were not aware before that time. Or here is another example from analytic practice: A patient generally began his analytic sessions speaking in his natural voice. After some time he spoke lower so that I had to make an effort to hear him. I had to ask him repeatedly to speak louder. He did so, but soon lowered his voice again. I recognized, of course, that this trait expressed his unconscious resistance. Since nothing in the material he reported seemed to justify the reaction at the time, the character of the resistance remained unclear until I applied those devices of isolating and magnifying this trait in my thoughts. I recognized then that his manner of speaking had the character of an aggression against me. I could tell my patient a little story I heard recently which illustrates beautifully this character of his behavior. The well-known actress Tallulah Bankhead, who usually speaks loudly and often shrilly, got into an argument with the comedian Jimmy Durante. At a certain point he said to her angrily, "Don't you dare to lower your voice at me!"

The drawbacks and uncertainties of such a mental experiment are not unknown to me, but its performance at appropriate occasions can open a new path to fresh insights and lead to original interpretations and bold and surprising concepts.

Is it venturesome to use those daring methods of tentative isolation and exaggeration in the approach to a problem so far remote from those of analytic practice? Let's try it. The task of isolating the appearance of the conductor from its frame is facilitated for us by a fact which otherwise has to be considered a decided disadvantage, namely, by our lack of knowledge and understanding of conducting. Since our notions of baton technique, of the signaling and expressive meaning of conducting gestures are very superficial and general, we have no difficulty in separating his appearance from the real, very complicated functions he has to fulfill. The mechanism of mental isolation is made even easier by the fact that there is a material technical device that supports our imagination. Did we not see the other day a television program presenting the performance of a symphony under the baton of Stokowski? While our ears followed the themes of the first movements, we saw the orchestra playing its instruments. The camera turned to the conductor, focused on him alone, and concentrated on him and his expressive gestures. Here is the figure of the leader isolated and in full limelight. (The memory of the conductor in Charlie Chaplin's film occurs here because the movie scene almost fulfilled the requirements of the experiment.)

How about the other part of our mental test, which should take place simultaneously, that of exaggerating or magnifying? No stretching of imagination was needed before since we had the reality of the television show, but to see the activity of the man on the platform in a magnifying distortion is obviously more difficult. Will we succeed when we try to imagine a very temperamental virtuoso-conductor who throws himself into the flood of melodies, and when we exaggerate the violence of his gestures and the spontaneity of his bodily movements? A felicitous accident comes to our aid: we remember at the right time reports of Beethoven's conducting methods, for instance, the one from an eyewitness that Ludwig Spohr presents. Let us imagine the great composer conducting his *Eroica* in the Palais of Prince Lobkowitz, a hundred and fifty years ago. He conducts holding a roll of sheet music in his hand. (The use of the baton was first introduced in Germany by Mosel in 1812.) Beethoven was accustomed, Spohr reports, "to insert all sorts of dynamic markings in the part and to remind his players of the marks by resorting to the most curious bodily contortions. At every *sforzato* he would thrust his arms away from his breast where he held them crossed. When he desired a *piano,* he would crouch and bend, when the music grew louder into a *forte,* he would literally leap into the air and at times grow so excited as to yell in the midst of a climax." This description does not provide the maximum of exaggeration we desired, yet it is the best at our disposal. And what better example than the conducting of the greatest of composers could we choose?

Now, ready for our thought-experiment, what do we see in this caricaturing picture, in this distorting mirror? We see a man alone, but aware that he has an audience, a showman who is violently gesticulating and moving his body about, who leaps and jumps, stamps around, and does astonishing things with his legs and hands. Here is, no doubt, an acrobat or a dancer performing in the rhythm he hears. Is he only a dancer? Is what he does only choreography? No, look at him, his face is as expressive as his body and his hands and feet. He is also a mimic, he is an actor and he acts the part the music dictates. You remember conductors, for instance, Felix Weingartner, who studied their parts before the mirror. The conductor is an actor devoted to his art, sometimes even in bondage to it. Toscanini puts all *passione* and *emotione* into his performance on the platform. Asking for a *pianissimo* from his orchestra he once fell on his knees, clasped his hands in prayer, and cried, "*Pianissimo,* please." A conductor certainly wears his heart on his sleeve or in his hands. In trying to transmit his interpretation of a composition to his players, he acts, he postures. Toscanini gesticulates "Like this the music should sound," or explains it should be like a mother rocking her baby to sleep while he actually rocks his hand in cradle fashion. The conductor is not only a dancer, he is also an actor. Is he a musician? That sounds paradoxical, but he does not play an instrument. Some people call him "a frustrated instrumentalist," but many excellent artists, like Ossip Gabrilowitsch, Casals, Koussevitzky, exchanged their instruments for the baton. The conductor plays all instruments. He is, so to speak, the all-round musician, the supermusician. But he is not heard, only seen. He is a silent musician. What a paradoxical figure! Not only improbable, but impossible. A musician who does not make music? Imagine a sculptor who makes other artists work on a monument or a painter who not only lets George do it, but also tells him how he should do it!

The audience at a concert will sometimes see only the conductor, will change into nothing but eye-listeners. The conductor is not only a musician, but also a magician who celebrates a composition with the solemnity of a priest who says Mass. When he conducts, he himself often feels inspired by a higher power. That violent Maestro Toscanini, who sometimes smashes his baton as Moses did the tablets, once said to a musician who had performed poorly, "You see, God tells me how the music should sound and you get in the way." We are momentarily under the impression that the conductor is the composer of the wonderful symphony played under his baton, as if he had not only reproduced but created it. And then we feel that we have been his dupe. He is not Beethoven or Mozart, only their interpreter, speaking for them as Moses spoke for God. Is he a prince of genius or only his butler, a creator or only the composer's hand and foot man? His signs and designs seem to have magical power and we are under his spell. Yet when we shake it off, he appears to us sometimes a comedian, a fraud and freak, a four-flusher and floor-flusher. No doubt, he occasionally attributes supernatural power to himself. Did Mahler not once say, "There are no bad orchestras, only bad conductors" as if he were almighty and the musicians of the orchestra only willing or reluctant instruments? Yet these musicians themselves adore some conductors as great artists and look down on others. We heard the other day the story of an orchestra player who was asked what a visiting guest conductor would perform and answered, "I don't know what he'll conduct, but we will play Brahms's First Symphony."

The image that emerges from our thought-experiment is, of course, only phenomenological. But in applying the devices of isolation and exaggeration, the phenomenon of the conductor appears even more mysterious than before; the signals he gives and which we know as rational and conventional seem even more fantastic. How can we reconcile so many contradictory features? What an enigmatic figure! A creative artist and the servant of the composer, a silent musician, a magician and a make-believe, a dancer, mimic, and actor, a man who is mute and who, as they facetiously say, "talks with his hands."

We tried to approach the problem from the analytic angle, once by direct approach and the other time by applying those artificial methods of isolating and magnifying the phenomenon. Both attempts were failures. The first supplied a clue which led into a blind alley, the second let us see the figure of the conductor with all its contradictions in an oversharp light, so glaring that it left us more confused than we had been before. It seems that the problem cannot be solved by analytic methods or by using or transferring analytic results to its area. Yet we know, somehow, that it cannot be solved without psychoanalysis.

Seeing that scene in *Limelight* had given me enough to think about, but thinking was not enough. Everybody can produce thoughts on a certain subject as a spider can weave a web on a corner. But such meditations have no more durability or substance than a spider's toils. In order to understand more about the function of the conductor, one has to know more about the history of that figure, to study why and how conducting entered the evolution of music, where it came from and what it came to.

4

A prominent historian of music* introduces his survey of conducting with the remark that the activity "is doubtless as old as music itself and was probably always employed whenever the

* Georg Schünemann, *Geschichte des Dirigierens* (Leipzig, 1913).

musical performance called for several or more participants."
That may or may not be correct, but we know very little about
the earliest times of conducting and cannot trace it back much
more than two thousand years. To make a short story shorter,
then, only a brief outline of the evolution of the art of the baton
is here presented. The ancient Greeks had two kinds of conducting. The leader of the chorus indicated the beat by stamping
his foot, which was iron-soled. Beside this way of marking the
beat, there was the chironomia, a system by which the progress of
a musical composition was indicated by arm, hand, and finger
motions corresponding to the rise and fall of the melody. In the
Vedic music the leader designated the sacred melodies with the
knuckles of the right hand, beating them with the forefinger of
the left hand.

Schünemann states that both kinds of directing "the noisy
beating of time as well as the chironomy form the point of
departure of a history of conducting." But the scholar, as all authorities in the field, emphasizes that music has no singular position within the ancient civilizations. It is not a separate and independent part of art, but part and parcel of the whole or united
art and intimately connected and interwoven with dance, drama,
and poetry. The factor of rhythm is the uniting principle of all
these arts. The choir leader led the dance and the music and
song with the choir. The great festivals and processions of ancient
cultures were not musical performances, but rhythmical presentations of cult, dance, and songs, accompanied by instrumental
music. The choragus leading his choir of twelve to fourteen men
originally marked the beat with his foot. His hand was also used
in the display, and ultimately replaced the foot. In the chironomic system, the measured movements of the hand signify the
beating of time. The Romans followed suit. With them the flutist
often seems to have marked the beat. The noises made by slapping the fingers won over those made by feet. In early ecclesiastical singing the beat was marked by backward and forward movements of the hands. The Gregorian chants which in some aspects
resembled our modern operative recitative were led by a pre-
ceptor who gave the pitch and the chironomic signs, sang himself,

helped with "voice and hand." Slowly the signs and designs became expressive and more differentiated.

With the entrance of the cembalo a new trend within the orchestra appeared. The conductor led the performance from the clavicembalo. Bach presided at the organ or cembalo while conducting; as did Handel and Gluck. Haydn appeared in London in 1791 and 1794 leading his symphonies sitting at the piano. The main part of the conducting was, however, done by his impresario, the violinist Salomon. The combined leadership, cembalo and first violinist, was, it seems, in general use during the eighteenth century. The first violinist led by beating with his bow. The keyboard player helped him by pulling things together. Two conductors shared the responsibilities of producing the music: one looked after the singers; the violinist was in charge of the instrumentalists.

Other methods of conducting emerged mostly from the Italian and French orchestra. Here the time-beater became, by and by, the *maestro di cappella, le chef d'orchestre*. The time-beater (*batteur de mesure* in France) kept strict discipline and marked the time beat very audibly. Rousseau told us in his *Dictionary of Music* (1769) of the noise of the conductor ("*le bruit insupportable de son baton qui couvre et amortit tout l'effet de la symphonie*"), and remarked that Paris is the only place in Europe "where they beat time without keeping it since in all other places they keep time without beating it." Because of the custom of conductors of striking their batons on the floor or on the desk, they were called "woodchoppers." Eighty years before Rousseau's complaint the famous French composer Jean Baptiste Lully had conducted a *Te Deum* for the recovery from illness of Louis XIV. In thumping the time on the floor with his long heavy baton, Lully struck his foot. He died from the consequences of the infection that resulted from his mistake.

The noisy knocking of the beat continued during the musical career of Bach. Leigh Hunt is still complaining in 1822 that the roll of paper which the conductor in the cathedral at Pisa wielded made a noise sounding "like cracking the whip." The period in which the conductor, *maestro di cappella,* and the time-beater stood side by side lasted a few centuries. They could not co-exist any longer. At the end of the eighteenth century Gluck was still leading from the piano, and the twelve-year-old Beethoven sat in the opera orchestra of Cologne and led the musicians from the harpsichord. The orchestra, until then conducted by a player at the harpsichord or the first violinists, did not react in a friendly fashion to a conductor who did not play his instrument. When Ludwig Spohr came to London to direct the Philharmonic Society in 1820, he was supposed to play his violin and conduct with its bow. It was no small sensation when he took a baton from his pocket and conducted from his desk.* The use of the baton spread rapidly. It was already being used by Carl Maria von Weber in Dresden in 1817, by Mendelssohn in 1835, and by Schumann, who tied a baton to his wrist with a special gadget. We stand here at the threshold of modern times, of the age of the great masters of the baton, of Bülow, Mahler, Nikisch, Toscanini. We followed the development from the time-beater, from the *Kapellmeister* to the conductor of the twentieth century who is no longer only a leader of the orchestra, but a master himself and the interpreter of the masters of great music.

It is only appropriate to add a brief history of the baton to the preceding sober and short survey of conducting. The baton is, of course, a late acquisition in music. The hands and legs were originally the best and only instruments to indicate time and rhythm. To focus the attention of early ecclesiastical singers, the leaders had devices ranging from abbot's and bishop's staffs to scrolls and kerchiefs, alone or tied to sticks. Some organists even tapped upon their instruments with their keys. Till the fifteenth century the leader directed choirs with a roll of paper. The conductor Anselm used a leather roll filled with calf hair, Carl Maria von Weber a paper roll, Gasparo Spontini an ebony stick. (Wagner describes that contrivance which had a billiard ball at either end, used by the Italian composer, "more to command than to conduct.")

The baton has undergone many alterations. It has decreased from a length of forty inches to about eighteen inches or less. There are no gold or ivory batons with ebony inlays any more.

* Schmid, *Language of the Baton*, p. 4.

The modern baton is a simple stick of light material such as vulcanite, celluloid, usually of light color. Also its significance has changed. It once had the same character as other musical instruments and was supposed to have magical power. Some superstitions still cling to it. When Richard Strauss was guest conductor at the Vienna Opera, he once forgot his baton but did not care and selected one of those on the stand. Just as he was ready to give the signal to begin, the principal viola player stepped forward and courteously handed him another baton, saying, "Please, master, take this one; the other has no rhythm." The baton was once akin to the scepter and later signified a staff of command. (A field marshal also has a baton.) In Lully's time it was a herald's staff. It has more than once been compared to a weapon. When Berlioz and Mendelssohn met at Leipzig in 1841, they exchanged batons, and Berlioz accompanied his with a letter in the vein of Fenimore Cooper, addressing the friend as "great chieftain." He reminds him of the promise to exchange their tomahawks. His own is simple; "only the squaws of the pale-face love ornate arms." He expressed the hope that when the Great Spirit sent them to the Land of Souls to hunt, their warriors would suspend their tomahawks at the door of their council hut. That little stick which was once the symbol of royal power and authority and seemed to emit sparks, became a signaling instrument, to prolong the arm and to amplify the movements of arm and wrists. Although some conductors like Stokowski, Mitropoulos, and Bernstein lead their orchestras batonless, the little stick remains not only the instrument, but also the badge and insignia of the master of the orchestra. We follow the designs it draws. We can read the "baton handwriting," and we unconsciously distinguish between the signaling and the expressive significance of the conductor's gesture.

5

An eminent historian of music tells us* that "not even the earliest civilizations that have left their traces in the depths of

* Curt Sachs, *Our Musical Heritage* (New York, 1948), p. 1.

the earth are old enough to betray the origins of music." The same historian informs us that the oldest civilization from which information about musical performance is accessible is that of Mesopotamia where excavations uncovered pictures of musical instruments. The music of ancient Egypt had already reached a relatively high standard. We cannot pursue the evolution of music more than a few thousand years. The attempt at investigation of primitive music of the savage and uncivilized tribes of today cannot hope to unearth the earliest phase of musical performance. Peoples on the lowest level of civilization, like the tribes of Southeast Australia, also have a long past behind them and have gone through many stages of evolution. Comparative musicology dealing with the music of those tribes is aware that it can reach only remnants of earliest art practice and can only observe and describe musical performance at a relatively progressed stage—so to speak, at a later phase of the childhood of mankind.

All observers agree that our division of the arts into music, dance, and acting is not valid for that period. They are inextricable in their beginnings. The whole or united art of which Richard Wagner daydreamed is not to be found in the future of human civilization, but in its remote past. Before speech, prehistoric man gave expression to his emotions in bodily movements and raucous screams. His shouts and the movements of his hands and legs gradually became song and dance. He danced and sang not for pleasure, but for magical purposes. "Dance," says that historian,[*] "is the mother of arts. . . . The creator and the things created, the artist and the work are still one and the same thing." Man creates the rhythmical patterns of movement, the vivid representation of the world "in his own body in the dance before he uses substance and stone or word to give expression to his inner experiences." The dancer did not possess his instrument. He inhabited it. His palms slapped together or against his thighs, his feet pounded on the earth. He had his own rhythmic and percussive accompaniment.

The only form of artistic manifestation that has been ob-

* Curt Sachs, *World History of The Dance* (New York, 1937), p. 3.

served among the lowest of all savages, the Wood Veddas of
Ceylon, consists of an exalted dance in which each dancer turns
around on one foot while performing some spasmodic movements
with the free leg.* The arms describe circles in the air and the
head is thrown backward and forward. The music is howled out
by the dancers, while the time is marked by strokes of the hand
on the nude belly. The dances of those savages like those of most
primitive tribes are mostly imitative. The "image dancer" is
possessed by his part. The animal or the spirit which he represents takes control of his body. The dancer becomes that animal
or spirit. Every imitative dance bears within it the germ of the
pantomime. Every dancer who feels himself into the living or
lifeless object recreates their appearance with his body. Imita-
tions in animal dances reproduce in a lifelike manner the characteristic bearing and movements of an animal and "are accompanied—almost as a matter of course—by sounds which are
appropriate to this animal. Every primitive hunter has the gift of
imitating convincingly the growling, grunting, howling, whis-
tling, yelling of the animals. . . ."** The dancer thus becomes an
actor, a mimic. We cannot imagine how those primitive howls
became simple melodies. From their character to that of an aria
is really a far cry, but there is no doubt that wordless singing, if
one can call it that, is the origin of music. The instruments enlarge and intensify the rhythm made by handclapping and
pounding of feet, later helped by wooden sticks, spears, and other
objects at hand. The example of our children who use pots and
pans or other available objects when they feel like making music
helps us to understand that development.

A prehistoric rock painting found in South Africa shows
women dancing.† A Bushman of today, a remote descendant of
those primitive cavemen, interpreted that early painting as follows: "They seem to be dancing for they are stamping with their
legs. This man who stands in front seems to be showing the
people how to dance, that is why he holds a stick. He feels that

---

* *Encyclopedia of Religion and Ethics,* I, 818.
** Curt Sachs, *World History of The Dance* (New York, 1937), p. 175.
† Quoted by Howard D. Kinny and W. R. Anderson in *Music In History*
(New York, 1940), p. 26.

he is a great man, so he holds a dancing stick because he is one who dances before the people that they may dance after him. The people know he is one who dances first because he is a great sorcerer." Here is, it seems to me, the prehistoric representative of the man with the baton who is still a great magician.

We have endeavored to detect the origin of conducting and the primeval functions of the conductor. The history of music and comparative ethnology have given us valuable information tracing musical performance back to very early practices. No record can take us back to those prehistoric times and to that no-man's land in which conducting originated. Neither the history of civilization nor comparative musicology reaches that far back. We cannot explore the character of prehistoric conducting and we know it as little as what song the sirens sang. We feel like throwing up our hands. But as if in contrast, the image of the conductor emerges, and his open hand urgently demands volume and "pulls out the sound," calling for a crescendo.

6

Our attempts to apply those mental devices of isolation and exaggeration to the material have perhaps not been entirely useless. Did we not see the figure of the conductor successively as dancer, actor, and musician? He was all these, but at one time, he was all these not in succession but simultaneously. When we condense and comprise all the traits which were artificially severed in that thought-experiment, it gives us heart to venture on a reconstruction of the prehistory of the conductor. The smattering of knowledge of the history of music-making will certainly lead us to the point where the work of the imaginative and combining function has to set in. In such an attempt at reconstruction we have, of course, to consider the mind of prehistoric man, which was so different from and yet so similar to our own.

Hans von Bülow's sentence "In the beginning was rhythm" shall introduce our venture. Tension and relaxation, breathing in and breathing out as upbeat and downbeat, are manifestations of the same rhythmic principle which governs music, dance, and poetry; the same principle, also, which shapes the expressions of our emotions. Rhythm, not melody, was the principle that gave prehistoric art its character.

Suddenly, driven and pushed by some intense emotion, one of the tribesmen of a prehistoric people jumped up and moved about in a primitive dance and act. He was inspired by the impression that he was a tree or a lion. His hands were flapping and flying together with the stamping of his feet. They slapped parts of his body which became musical instruments, the upper arms, the flanks, the abdomen, the buttocks. The stamping feet as well as the slapping hands were the original time-beaters. The other members of the tribe followed suit and danced after the initiator of the primitive song and dance. He was perhaps the chieftain of the tribe or he would become its head. We here introduced the first conductor, who is also the first dancer and musician. He is also the first composer because the raucous sounds he emits are created by himself. He is the first leader of the chorus and the first leader of a primitive orchestra without instruments. Much later, when primitive instruments magnified and complemented the subhuman voices of the group, that first dancer also became the first instrumentalist, because in dancing he struck something with a stick or a spear. There is not yet any division between composer and performer, nor any difference between dance-musicians and audience, because all the members of the group, inspired by their leader, perform. This division belongs to a much later phase of artistic production.

Until the beginning of the nineteenth century the leader will also be a player, will direct the others with his instrument, for instance, with the bow of his violin. The conductor is only *primus inter pares,* first among his peers. Priority and primacy of the feet as time-beaters will later yield to the hands which gesticulate and to the body which imitates and pantomimes. Prehistoric performance was a combination of dance, music, and acting or mimicry, and was an expression of emotions as well as magical ritual. But slowly there begins a differentiation of the arts. In the Stone Age they are still an inseparable unit, but they separate into individual and almost independent arts. The dance will become an important artistic branch and so will acting and music. There are still traces of their past unity: the dancer will make gestures like an actor and will be accompanied by music, and music will at first be an eminent factor of ancient poetry. But more and more the individual art will free itself from its former companions, go its own ways, and develop its own expressions. The ballet is now an independent art and so are poetry, acting, and music-making. That process of loosening of the primitive ties, of differentiation and isolation of one art from the others took place in different forms and in various tempi.

It seems that music first succeeded in getting loose from its connections with dancing and acting and detaching its production from its allied arts. This is perhaps due to the fact that, in contrast with choreography and pantomime, music had instruments which were not identical with the bodies of the performers and so was no longer restricted to voices, hands, and legs as its only organs of production. Yet we do not forget that the orchestra was originally that part of the Attic theatre on which the chorus danced.

It interests us more in which forms dancing and acting survived in the long evolution of instrumental music. The first conductor was a dancer and actor as well as a musician. With the suppression of dancing and acting and with the development of the orchestra, his fate seemed to be sealed. He was going to be absorbed into the instrumental body, submerged into the orchestra. There was the time when he was simultaneously the first violinist or the cembalo player or the choir leader singing with the others while he conducted. And now something strange happened: he became isolated and disassociated from the players. He relinquished the functions of an instrumentalist. He was pushed out from the middle of the orchestra and drawn up at the same time. He was removed by promotion. Just when it seemed that his function would be merged and submerged into the orchestra, an unknown emotional power lifted his figure and raised it to a position outside and above the orchestra.

We know what that hidden power was: the force of those drives that were there at the beginning of musical performance and which had been suppressed for so long. Those urges which had once expressed themselves in bodily movements, in gestures and dancing, in acting and pantomiming, had been more and more pushed back and suppressed in favor of the purely musical element, of the factor of sounds. They were suppressed, but they did not vanish. They demanded satisfaction and continued to call urgently for expression. In the emergency situation in which they were banned by the primacy of musical gratification and by the necessities of orchestral performance, they forced a side entrance. The underground activity developed by those forces led finally to a break-through, and to their at least partial victory.

When a conductor stood freely at his elevated desk and waved his baton or his hand at the orchestra, it was the success of a *coup d'état,* of a revolution of those powers which wanted bodily movement and acting within the musical performance. It marked the return of the repressed. The expressive gestures of the conductor are essentially dancing gestures, and the players dance with the maestro, dance to his tune. Those gestures are, it is true, only "hand dances," that is to say, they symbolize and express emotions only by means of arms and hands, but the whole body takes part in the movements. The gestures are also never entirely free, the impulses leading to them are controlled, canalized, and stylized. But, however conventional their designs become, there is enough spontaneity in them not only to express the emotions of the conductor, but also to stimulate the members of the orchestra. The facial expressions of the conductor and the movement of his body while leading his orchestra represent the element of pantomime and remind us of the part acting and imitation once had in primitive music performance. Degraded and almost disintegrated, debased, disassociated and disinherited, the primal impulses of prehistoric art production asserted themselves at last in the function of the conductor. He is still the leader he once was. He is again the dancer within the orchestra. He is the last musician as he was the first. As a remnant and revival of an art past beyond any human memory, he represents the earliest stage of music.

He is again the magician. His upbeat will open the door of a domain of miracle. He does not play any instrument, but his very gestures convey to us the significance of a symphony. His signal starts the performance, and his downbeat puts an end to it. The rest is silence.

7

When we now return to our point of departure, we recognize that the result of this expedition into prehistory was unconsciously anticipated in the intuitive understanding of the significance of my conducting the first movement of the Haydn symphony. There must have been, concealed to myself, a pre-recognition of the meaning of my activity, namely, that I had as in a flash experienced that conducting is a survival of the most primitive musical performance, in which singing, dancing, and acting were one thing. What else but a symptom of such unconscious understanding and its clash with a rational and conventional concept is the meaning of that momentary feeling of uncanniness? In that second, an old belief, a discarded concept was resuscitated, to yield immediately to an adult and "reasonable" view that rejected it as incongruous. For a second a recognition, swift as lightning, had penetrated the dull surface of conventional thinking. Instead of consciously grasping that hidden meaning, I took the part of intellectual and sober judgment which is superior only when it is put into the service of such intuitive insights. I made fun of such "fantastic" vision and pushed it contemptuously out of my thoughts. Many flashes of unconscious insight are lost in this manner to scientific research, destroyed by worship of common sense which, applied prematurely and inappropriately, is very insensible. The concept that conducting is the last remnant of dancing, once inextricably united with music-making, the revival of rhythmic performance, restricted to gestures, to finger dance, was submerged after it had occurred in that moment which was experienced as confusing and uncanny.

Following the train of my associations later on amounts to an attempt at recovering the lost insight. It was certainly not a methodical and well-considered psychological experiment, but an almost automatic way of proceeding, by now so familiar that it scarcely deserved the name of scientific exploration. It was close to a habit of thinking in this particular manner, my usual approach of exploration whenever I do not understand my own mental processes. This direction of thinking can be called psychology with as much or as little justification as adding your grocer's bill can be called mathematics.

A review of my train of thoughts reveals that the vanished insight was trying to re-emerge in personal reminiscences, to regain entrance into conscious thought by side doors. Those associations are signals which have to be deciphered, and their significance can be recognized only in their sequence and consequence. They illuminate the mental process in the same way as a blinker lights a dark street. It seemed that I was swimming in that stream of consciousness from the present to the prehistoric past, from the modern form of musical performance to that of forgotten ages. The train of association departed from the memory of Mahler whom I had seen conducting in the Vienna Opera when I was a boy. It flitted from there to the Burgmusik, to the jazz players, to the dancing and singing Ashantis, and to a drum majorette in a Broadway parade. The highly artistic gestures of one of the greatest of conductors are here not contrasted, but put side by side with those of the *Kapellmeister* of the Burgmusik and of the leader of a jazz band as if they were the same. In the swinging of the bodies of the jazz players and of their leader who trembles, wobbles, quivers whenever he conducts the original dance and mimicking of primitive music is still preserved. In the body movements of the majorette, who struts and tap-dances and twirls her baton, the primitive musician is resurrected. Here is an echo from the jungle of prehistoric performance. From here to the violent dance and music-making of the Ashantis is only one step.

In those associations visual perceptions appeared instead of formulated concepts. The occasions at which, in the following weeks, the memory of that evening occurred prove that the unconscious work of probing and searching continued. In the associations the basic idea announced itself, but remained invisible. The subterranean insight into the character of primitive music tried to break through to the conscious level in that bizarre visual image of the Viennese Philharmonic players swaying with the *Blue Danube* waltz, nodding their heads and tapping their feet on the ground. The remarks of Mitropoulos in the radio interview must have brought the idea of an original identity of conductor and actor closer to the threshold of conscious thoughts. The records of the African initiation rites led directly back to the concept of music-making of the primitive tribes, reminded me of mimetic dancing, imitating the birds (*la poule*, the circumcision bird), and reconnected the actual hearing with the memory of the Ashanti performance. The impression at seeing Charlie Chaplin's mimickings and the gestures of the conductor leading an unseen orchestra was that the actor, the dancer, and the musician appeared almost as one person. Those impressions are comparable to the thrusts of an unborn baby, are phases in the delivery of an idea. The attempt at applying the mechanisms of isolating and exaggerating helped to see the figure of the conductor in a sharper, almost caricatured manner and paved the way to the understanding of his function. The still vague perceptions, half formulated, then became fully clear in studying the historical material which preserves traces of the prehistoric music performance.

Reviewing the process by which the result was reached makes us wonder what kind of research technique is here applied. It seems that here is an innovation in the discovery process, since analysis is used only as a pervasive and general view of human emotional life and as a premise of thinking in a certain way. Neither the results nor the mechanism of analytic theory and practice were quoted. Yet it is due to the way of thinking which is characteristic of analysis that an insight was gained which none of the other sciences dealing with the same problem could obtain. The process itself will perhaps be called a psychological tour de force, but the decisive factor is whether such bold and daring enterprises reach their aim or not.

We cannot say if and to what degree the reconstruction of pre-historic music and of conducting within it comes close to reality. It does credit to its value or validity that the hypothesis here presented is in accordance with our knowledge of music in its earliest stages and with the information reaching back to the paleolithic culture in which human civilization started. More important than this result appears to me the new method by which it was reached. The still unknown and unacknowledged approach to analytic discovery in the area of prehistory is represented by this example in which the insight was unconsciously anticipated, and in which the problem was only to find a way leading to its conscious recognition. In other words, the inquirer had to explore what he had unconsciously thought. The study of the historical material is, in these cases, of course, taken for granted and has to be used to confirm or to invalidate, to modify or qualify the unconsciously anticipated insight.

In the beginning we had nothing but a trifling experience with its repercussions. We started on a mental shoestring, or on a thin string of associations, and arrived at a discovery which, however small, was not reached by the other sciences. The concept of pre-historic music and of the origin of conducting is perhaps not important, is only comparable to an instrument or ancient piece of pottery dug up in excavation. More important is the new technique of finding, since many rich treasures deep down in the earth await discovery. Future research workers in the field of archeological psychoanalysis, better equipped and more fortunate, will continue where we, their forerunners, left off. A past beyond all memory will become alive through their work.

It is good to feel the spade in one's hand and to break new ground. There is no reason to feel self-complacent when we consider how miserably we failed in the initial phase of our exploration. What a piece of work is man! How noble in reason, how infinite in faculty! Yet he is not even able to think all he knows, or to know all he thinks.

III

1

THE FOLLOWING PAGES seek to delineate a representative example of the process of psychoanalytic discovery together with its special result, the sources and the course of analytic findings. The findings present, in this case, the train of thoughts that led the analyst to the threshold of exploration. These thoughts are here reproduced, from the moment when his interest was awakened by a chance impression on Broadway to the point when the first vague notion occurred to him of the unconscious significance of a certain religious custom, and then to the stage where this concept became verifiable. In following the course of associations from the point of departure to that of arrival, I shall present a picture of analytic finding as it unfolds from personal impressions and fleeting images to the pursuit of objective truth.

Walking on Broadway one summer afternoon, I felt tired and depressed. The faces of the people I passed were tense, haggard, and harassed. Most of them appeared homely to me, men as well as women and children. The heat was oppressive. An old, bald man, badly shaved, with small and sad eyes, glared back at me in the mirror of a barbershop. On the next corner an old Jew, bent on a cane, walked slowly and heavily toward me. He was a small man with a long gray beard and glasses set slantingly on a long nose. He wore the caftan and black skullcap of East European Jews. Long gray sidelocks reached beyond the tips of his ears. He looked at me with a glance, timid and yet challenging at the same time, like a wild animal recently caught looking at its tamer. As if pushed by a sudden decision, he turned to me and asked me where West End Avenue was. He spoke Yiddish. His voice was as unattractive as his appearance. While I showed him that he had only a block to turn I looked at him and was intrigued by his long sidelocks standing out on both sides of his forehead.

Walking along I caught myself having an odd thought. The idea that crossed my mind like a bolt from the dark was: *God cannot be beautiful.* It was a sober statement and seemed to emerge from nowhere, spoken by an unknown self. In that moment nothing was farther from my mind than theological speculations. I understood only later that the irrelevant idea must have sprung from the impressions of the last minutes. I could easily trace it back to the impression people had made upon me, of looking at them, at myself, and at the old Jew. I corrected myself—at the other old Jew. The blasphemous sentence was, of course, a conclusion drawn from the premise: If we are created in His image, God cannot be beautiful. There is more than a superficial family resemblance between the creator and the creature. The book speaks of a distinct similarity. Do not people say of a child, "The very image of his father"?

From there I was gliding into musing about whether the quality of beauty is imminent to the concept of God in the monotheistic religions. I could not remember any biblical passage in which the Almighty is called beautiful. (The image of the Lord in Michelangelo's "Creation of Adam" flitted through my mind.) I doubt if the quality of beauty is to be found among the ninety-nine attributes the Mohammedans ascribe to Allah. I must look that up.

In that rambling manner of thinking I drifted from the idea that God cannot be beautiful to wondering whether an atheist can think blasphemous thoughts. At first that sounded funny—odd and ha-ha—but it made sense: you cannot abuse or revile a non-existent Deity. You cannot inflict indignity on a mere creature of your fancy or maliciously attack a non-entity. It would be as silly as hitting the air. Only persons who in some way believe in God, if only as a potentiality, can be blasphemous in word or thought.

I tested the argument on examples that occurred to me from literature. Lucifer's fierce defiance and his proud *"Non serviam"* is a defiance of the Lord rather than blasphemy. And so is Mephisto's accusation. The thought of the *Prelude in Heaven,* and of the fact that Goethe took its pattern from the book of Job, led me to the figure of this biblical patriarch. To my surprise a jingle formed itself in my thought:

> The sufferer Job made a fuss
> And did not cease to cuss.
> "I tell you to shut up,"
> Said God, "I know the rub
> Which I choose not to discuss."

Job denied neither the existence nor the power of the Lord who severely rebuked him. Crossing the bridge from ancient Hebrew to modern literature, that famous or infamous sentence of Renan's occurred: "To God all is possible even that He exists." In Huysmans' novel *Là-Bas,* a Catholic priest is introduced who has cut the name of Jesus Christ from his prayer book and has put it into his shoes so that he treads on it with every step. That priest who inflicts such unheard-of disgrace on the holy name cannot be called an atheist. Did not Huysmans himself land in a Trappist monastery after that period of morbid mysticism and satanism? Anatole France, who used to be one of his friends, was, it is true, convinced that the writer's conversion was due to a physical complaint and advised him to let his urine be examined. . . . Anatole France was himself a master of subtle blasphemy. Is the scene I now remember not from one of his novels? During the French Revolution a young aristocratic lady is taken to the guillotine. She turns to her lover and says, "Goodbye, sweetheart, in a few minutes I'll meet God. I am curious as to whether He is worth knowing."

Coarse or subtle, malicious or playful, flippant or taken seriously, blasphemy implies a latent belief. It is, I argued with myself, possible that someone may tentatively or vicariously assume the attitude of a believer in order to degrade or mock the reverence of religion. But such a temporary attitude, psychologically akin to irony, presupposes at least the mental potentiality of religious belief. Was it not in this vein that Freud once said to me, "The ways of the Lord are dark, but they are rarely pleasant"?

I wondered why some sophisticated theologian did not arrive at the idea that the very concept of blasphemy could be added to the proofs of God's existence. It could have its place beside the cosmological, theological, and ontological arguments. . . . There is perhaps something of this kind in the writings of medieval scholastics. Maybe there is more latent blasphemy to be found in the casuistic and scholastic literature than in the books of atheists. Someone better read in the field of theology and history of civilization than I would have no trouble in proving that there were many blasphemers among the great believers and many great believers among the blasphemers.

But how did I get into reflections of this kind? By what erratic thought-process did I arrive at such speculations which are otherwise alien to my way of thinking? Could it be true, as a friend half seriously asserted the other day, that the hound of heaven is after me? Considering my age, he has to race mightily to reach me.

When you come right down to it, it is strange that I am suddenly interested in the psychology of blasphemy. . . . It's funny on the face of it. . . . That is it, of course. . . . It started with the face of that old Jew seen on Broadway. . . . There was nothing funny about his face except the long sidelocks. . . . From them my thoughts drifted to God, to the God of his and my people. . . . Those ringlets standing forth under the skullcap—I remembered their Hebrew name: *payoth* or *payes*?—gave to his appearance not only a foreign and exotic character, but also something bizarre and unreal. . . . They are strange, yet they are familiar at the same time. . . . Familiar . . . of the family. . . . I recognized immediately of whom the old Jew had reminded me, of my own grandfather who still wore sidelocks. . . . When I first saw him, I was a little boy and very intrigued by the funny curls over his ears. I could scarcely turn my eyes away from them. The interest with which I looked at the *payoth* of the old man was a revival and renewal of my curiosity felt as a child.

Strangely enough, the memory of my grandfather, of whom I had not thought for many years, turned up again on the next evening when I jotted down a dream interpretation made a few hours before. A young psychiatrist, in training analysis with me, reported the following dream-fragment: *He saw me eating spaghetti.* There were no thought-associations concerning the content of the dream and helpful in its interpretation. . . . Only two day remnants, impressions from the day before the dream, occurred to the physician. He and his wife had been to dinner with a colleague who is like himself resident at a state institution. At the meal no spaghetti had been served, but a Jewish dish which the dreamer, who is Gentile, had relished. The other day residue was that during dinner my name had been mentioned.

When I asked the psychiatrist to divide the word spaghetti, he said "spa" and "ghetti." He remembered that yesterday evening his colleague had spoken of a trip to Europe made last summer during which he had visited various health resorts. Spa is, of course, the well-known Belgian resort, but the name is used for mineral springs in general. "Ghetti" is the plural of "ghetto." The interpretation of the dream was not difficult any more. The combination of "spa" and "ghetti" points to a mocking or ridiculing allusion to Jews who come from ghetti and visit fashionable mineral springs. A sarcastic thought of this kind must have occurred to the psychiatrist during dinner at which the Jewish dish was served and discussed as well as his Jewish colleague's visit to a health resort. The implied thought, transferred to the analyst, reveals an unconscious sneering impulse. The dreamer, who had several times before stated that he was free from racial and religious prejudices, expresses in his dream an idea which, translated into the language of conscious thinking, would be as follows: *Reik is also one of those ghetto Jews who visit French resorts.* The connection with eating is determined by the dish, which in the dream represents belonging to a national group. The element of spaghetti is overdetermined by the fact that the dreamer lived as a little boy near an Italian quarter and that his father often spoke of Italians and Jews with the same contempt.

When I jotted the dream down, it occurred to me that I had once really lived in a ghetto during two summer months. When my sister and I were children, Mother took us for a vacation to a little town on the Austrio-Hungarian border (Nagy-Marton, now Mattersdorf) where her father lived. There was still a kind of ghetto, a quarter in which the Jews lived separated from the other people. (I was told later on that one of them went to Vienna for a year to study the Gentiles and then wrote a book

entitled *The Goyim, Their Customs and Habits,* as if he had returned from an expedition to study a foreign people.) I still remember the narrow and noisy streets of the ghetto and its synagogue to which my grandfather took the little boy very much
against his will. He was a very religious, strange-looking man
whose long sidelocks ran into his white beard. I was afraid of
him. Do I only imagine that the old Jew I saw yesterday looked
like him?

At this point another, much more recent memory concerning
sidelocks occurred to me. In 1913 I moved from Vienna to Berlin
to finish my analytic training. Soon after my arrival a kind colleague took me sightseeing in the German metropolis. We
walked on the Kurfürstendamm, the broad avenue on which
elegant Berlin promenaded in the evenings. The colleague told
me that a certain part of the avenue was spoken of as *"vom
Kaufhaus des Westens zum Taufhaus des Westens"*—an untrans-
latable pun describing the section as being from the department
store of the West to the church of the West (*Gedächtniskirche*)
in which many wealthy Jews were baptized. He also turned my
attention to a new hair-do which had just become fashionable.
The sophisticated ladies of West Berlin then wore single locks
of hair reaching over their ears. "Look," said the psychiatrist,
"at the little curl on both sides of the forehead. . . . It is the
return of the repressed." In wittily using the psychoanalytic term,
he characterized the new hair fashion as a manifestation of the
prevailing style's Jewish descent. The long sidecurls their fathers
had worn before they were baptized had come back in the hair-do
of the Germanized daughters.

The subject of baptism of Jews or the more general one of
Israelites and other anti-Semites was picked up again in my
thought-associations later. The heat of the day had continued
into the night and I could not fall asleep. While lying awake in
bed I thought of the family S., acquaintances of mine. Mr. S.
is Jewish, his wife Irish-Catholic. He has broken off all ties with
his family, is proud of his purely Anglo-Saxon friendships and of
his exclusive club whose members favor the sport of fox-hunt-
ing. (Heinrich Heine once wrote that his ancestors belonged to
the hunted rather than to the hunters.) Mr. S. would, I am

sure, say that he has no prejudices and that some of his best friends are Jewish. His children have been christened and he wishes them to practice their Catholic religion. For some reason his youngest child was not christened until after his second year. During the Sacrament in the church the frightened little boy cried bloody murder when the priest sprinkled him with water and put some salt on his tongue. The child had been accustomed to eating almost everything, but after the ceremony he developed an intense reluctance to eating solid food. I ventured the guess that Christianity did not agree with him.

Following this train of thought, I remembered the last time I had been inside a church. That was long ago, in Austria during summer vacation. There were pictures on the many colored windows of the village church. One of them showed Jesus Christ surrounded by lambs . . . the Good Shepherd. . . . Surprisingly the question arose whether or not Jesus Christ had worn such sidecurls. . . . There was the doubt if those *payoth* were not rather introduced into Judaism by medieval rabbis. . . . Why, I mused, that hair style had perhaps already been started after the return of the Jews from Babylon and was perhaps in vogue at the time of the Saviour. . . . Did He not wear a prayer shawl, the tallith, and the fringes, the zizith on it, as other religious Jews according to the Gospel? . . . He wore perhaps sidelocks.

In this looser way of thinking, favored by sleepiness, the picture of the Good Shepherd brought up the association of the Lamb of God . . . the lamb that carries the sins of the world and is slaughtered as atonement. . . . There is perhaps more than a simile in it, the lamb was perhaps once a tribal totemistic animal. . . . "Mary had a little lamb" . . . I wonder whether He was not originally meant in that nursery rhyme. . . .

Still desperately trying to fall asleep, I, half amused, applied the old device of visualizing many lambs jumping over the fence. And then, already on the threshold of sleep, I had an odd experience. I was catching a hypnagogic picture, one of those puzzling visual images that sometimes mark the transition from the waking to the sleeping state.

A moment before I had imagined many lambs jumping over

the fence, then there was for a split second a blank or void in my thoughts, a chaotic mental sensation, *un moment d'absence*. I then saw distinctly "in my mind's eye" a big, powerful ram jumping over the fence, followed by a meek, little lamb, hesitantly doing the same.

For a moment I was flabbergasted and greatly puzzled by the surprising image. In the next second I experienced with full clarity the hunch which had been playing vaguely around the edges of my mind since yesterday when I had run into that old Jew on Broadway. The thought had come into the open in the shape of the hypnagogic image. I suddenly recognized the secret meaning of the sidecurls. I knew then that I would study the problem and not rest until I arrived at its core. Much reading and research work had to be done. The visual image had anticipated the solution of the problem, but what had to follow was the plowing of the long, hard furrow.

2

The name *payoth* is the plural form of *paya* which word means segment, border, or corner. There is no doubt that the custom of sidelocks in its present form is not very old. It cannot be traced back to the pre-exile era and it is not prescribed as a religious law. The custom developed as a result of the biblical law not to cut the hair around the head and emerged as a token of obedience shown by the Hebrews to this law of Jahweh. The main biblical passage in which this law is promulgated is Lev. 19:27. In this chapter the Lord repeats sundry laws concerning many things and speaks to the children of Israel: "Ye shall not round the corner of your heads, neither shalt thou mar the corners of thy beard . . . Ye shall not make any cuttings in your flesh for the dead nor print any marks upon you. I am the Lord." The Levitical law in its final form was promulgated in the year 444 B.C., and even when we assume that its draft brought laws and regulations, valid for centuries, into final form, we have to suppose that the prohibition concerning cutting hair is not old. The Lord speaks, in the words of Jer. 9:26: "Behold the days come . . . that I will punish all of them which are circumcised with the uncircumcised, Egypt, and Judah and Edom and the children of Amon and Moab, all that have the corners of their hair cut off." He predicts His judgment of the enemies: "And their camels shall be a booty and the multitude of their cattle a spoil and I will scatter into all winds those that cut off the corners of their hair" (Jer. 25:23; 49:32).

In obedience to this prohibition, the rabbis ordered the Jews to leave part of their hair over the temples and before the ears uncut. Ritual law has never given a final word as to a definite amount or length of hair. Length and form depended upon the customs of the Jews in individual countries, and differed at various times. Maimonides, the great scholar and religious philosopher (1135-1204), states that there is a norm for the sidelocks. Other early rabbis decided that four hairs in the proper place are sufficient to prove that their bearer is devoted to the law. The Shulchan Aruch, the codes which became the standard guide for the orthodox Jews, considers the proper length of the sidelocks to be from the temples to the point where the lower jaw begins. During the Middle Ages the Jews seem to have worn sidelocks of moderate length. The Sephardim, the descendants of Spanish and Portuguese communities, wear almost imperceptible sidelocks, while the Eastern Jews preferred them through many centuries in considerable length and conspicuous shapes.

Czar Nicolas I of Russia decreed in 1845 that his Jewish subjects should not wear either the Polish-Jewish costume or sidelocks. The Russian officers tried to enforce this ukase, but in vain. Many Jews used to shove the curls behind their ears to make them inconspicuous. The Jews of Eastern Europe and of the Orient still wear those ringlets extensively. The sidelocks are called *simanim* by the Jews of Yemen who let them grow long. The word means sign, because the sidelocks are considered to be a visible symbol of Judaism.

While the rabbinical literature offers very scanty information about the sidelocks, the Cabala, that mystical system of religious philosophy, frequently ascribes great importance to them. According to the Cabala, nothing exists but God and all things are emanations of the one Divine Being. Creation is a process of ten divine enumerations known as *sefiroth* (literally, "enumerations"). The Hebrew word for sidelock, *paya*, has the same numerical value as Elohim, the name of the Lord—namely, 86—which has, according to the developed Cabala, a great symbolic significance.* The sidelocks have, as have all parts of the human body, their specific symbolism: together with the beard they form an additional means of transmutation of God's attributes that stream from the ten *sefiroth* of the Divine Being into the so-called Lesser Face. Together with the beard, they are part of the reflection of God's appearance in the face of man. As a result of the Cabala, the Hasidim in Galicia, Hungary, Carpatho-Russia, and Palestine wear long sidelocks, often reaching down below the face and shining through the application of fat. Many Hasidim never cut their sidelocks out of regard for their sanctity and they even braid them.

Those are the essential facts about the sidelocks; not more than a handful. Their survey, far from satisfying our curiosity, rather whets it. The meager information available seems to raise several pertinent questions: how did that prohibition of the Lord lead to the custom of sidelocks? And what is their importance and significance? Above all, why should the Lord be so much concerned about the hair-do of His chosen people? We would think that their miserable political and economic situation would give Him cause for other and more urgent worries—not to mention their religious attitudes at the time. Had they not almost given up their monotheism and did they not pray to many other gods? In vain had the prophets tried to imitate their compatriots and announce the coming doom of the nation that had forsaken their God and His law. The times were ripe and rotten. And He should worry, He should care about the hair-do of this nation?

A more penetrating examination of the origin of the custom shows, however, that it is not the hair-do itself, but its symptomatic significance or religious meaning, which turns Jahweh's attention to this detail. However the authorities differ on various

* *The Universal Jewish Encyclopedia*, IX, 527. (Compare also *Jüdisches Lexikon* [Berlin, 1930], Vol. IV, article *Peot*.)

points, they all agree that the distaste of the Lord for the round-wise shaving of the hair had definite religious reasons. The main purpose of that prohibition in Leviticus was obviously to reject the idolatrous custom of the people who were neighbors of the Jews, a custom which many Jews had adopted.

The following paragraphs will review the main theories representative scholars have offered to explain the dislike the Lord shows for cropped hair. All of them quote the pertinent passages of the Scripture and discuss them. Immanuel Benzinger points out* that the peasant in the Near East, to this day, usually shaves his head and leaves only a tuft of hair on top. With ancient Egyptians the priests and perhaps also the higher priests shaved their heads. The statues from Telleh show that the Babylonians also wore closely shorn hair. It seems this was also the fashion among the Israelites in ancient times, and was observed as a token of mourning. Since the custom had a ritualistic significance as well, it was forbidden by the reformers. The Jewish commentaries** also state that the Law considers the shaving of the head in a circle so that only a strand remained in the center heathenish.† Some scholars point out that the hair of young people of the surrounding heathen nations was often shaved and consecrated at idolatrous shrines. Frequently this custom marked the initiatory rite into the service of a divinity (for Egypt, compare Herod. I. 65). It was therefore an abomination in the eyes of the Jews. One may compare the shaving of the hair of the Nazarite to these heathenish practices. The man who made a vow to God was responsible to Him with his whole body and being, and the conclusion of the Nazarite vow was marked by sacrifice and shaving of the head at the door of the sanctuary (Num. 6:11), indicating a new beginning of life. The long, untouched hair was therefore considered as the emblem of devotion to God. In New Testament times especially, the Jews frequently adopted the fashion of the Romans in cropping their hair closely (I Cor. 11:4). The fear of being tainted by the

* *Hebräische Archäologie* (edition Leipzig, 1927), III, 93.
** *Jewish Encyclopedia*, VI, 158.
† For instance, M. L. Lering in *The International Standard Bible Encyclopedia* (Chicago, 1915), I, 1320.

idolatrous practice of the heathen was so great that the sidelocks were untouched.

The commentaries of Jewish, Catholic, and Protestant theologians in general restrict their exegesis of the biblical passages to general remarks about the religious significance of the custom of shaving the hair as token of mourning. As far as I can see, this last view has been prevalent since Frazer's book *Folklore in the Old Testament* which was published in 1919.* There are only a few exceptions in books and papers dealing with more general subjects, but putting the biblical passage into a new context. As a representative example of such an original viewpoint, we choose George A. Barton's attempt to explain the mysterious prohibition of the Leviticus passage.** This scholar points to the special sacred significance supposed to pertain to corners of structures, fields, and other objects in the ancient Semitic nations. Numerous examples from the religious customs of Babylonians, Assyrians, Egyptians, Canaanites, and Hebrews prove this special belief. Do we not still speak of a cornerstone as a part of fundamental importance? Barton quotes among other passages the prohibition against rounding the corners of the hair, and thinks those corners belong to Jahweh and should therefore remain untouched. He believes that this regulation is responsible for the "curious custom of the curled sidelocks that present a peculiar appearance and distinguish the Jews of all other religionists in that land."

The other theory which is much more widely accepted is formulated by James George Frazer. The famous author of *The Golden Bough* dedicates a chapter of his book on comparative folklore in the Old Testament to the customs of mourning in ancient Israel. Those who lost their dear ones testified their sorrow at the death by cutting their own bodies and shaving part of their hair, making bald patches on their heads. He quotes many passages from the prophets, besides that of the codes, to prove these customs in mourning had been common to the Jews and their neighbors, the Philistines and Moabites. The reformers

* London, 1919. III, 270.
** *Encyclopedia of Religion and Ethics*, Edit. by James Hastings; IX, 20 f.

forbade those barbarous practices, putting the fear of God into the Jews.

Frazer shows that the custom of cropping the hair and mutilating the body has been widespread among many ancient peoples. An abundance of examples from the ancient Semitic people, but also from the Greeks, Assyrians, Romans, Huns, and Scythians is vividly presented. It is compared with similar customs from African, Australian, and American tribes who cut their bodies and shave their hair as token of mourning. With his usual lucidity and sense of discrimination, this writer presents an impressive collection of lore from the highly civilized nations of antiquity to the savage tribes still living in our time. Frazer shows the strength of his point by this abundance of instances in which the same mourning ritual appears in varied, but similar, forms. The affluence of this skillfully described material not only satisfies our scientific curiosity, but also our aesthetic sense. In the words of housewives testing the quality of meat, "Where there is no waste, there is no taste."

Another master of comparative history of religion, W. Robertson Smith, had another hypothesis about the custom of shaving the hair and the Lord's distaste for it. In his famous *Lectures on the Religion of The Semites** Smith explains the cuttings and shavings after death as an attempt to intensify the blood covenant with the dead. The Australians of Darling River have the custom, during the first two days of the ceremony of initiation into manhood, that the boys drink only blood from the veins of their friends who willingly supply the required food. In the same manner the mourners supply the souls of their deceased relatives with their blood. The hair is intended as a sacrifice to the dead to strengthen them, since it is a common notion that a person's strength is in his hair. The parallelism which runs through the mourning customs of cutting the body and polling the hair would be intelligible if both practices, so widespread throughout antiquity, served the worship of the dead. Frazer is of the opinion that this hypothesis of his revered friend W. Robertson Smith

* Third Edition. London, 1927, p. 325 f.

must be set aside because "it is not adequately supported by the evidence at our disposal."*

Smith's explanation of the cropping of the hair as part of the initiation ritual of youth is certainly valuable, especially if compared with the condition of the uncut hair of the Nazarites, and its solemn cutting at the sanctuary. There is a custom in Chasidic circles in Palestine to this day which seems to conform to Smith's view.** The hair of boys who have completed their fourth year is cut, and for the first time some tufts are left at the temples as *payoth,* sidelocks. It seems to me that Frazer dismissed Smith's hypotheses too early. But even if we attribute some merit to Smith's view, it is not specific enough. There must be a specific meaning to the ritual, a meaning which is not covered by the explanation that the hair is considered the seat of strength and is sacrificed to the dead.

Frazer's interpretation confuses two things because both concern the hair: the one is a certain hair-do displeasing to Jahweh and the other concerns certain mourning customs common to the Israelites and neighboring nations, who expressed their grief by tearing their hair out so that bald patches appeared on their heads. The temptation to connect these two things was great, since the prohibition of the roundwise haircutting appears side by side with those mourning customs which the Israelites shared with the Philistines and Moabites. What was more natural than to assume that the lawgiver also meant those mourning rituals when he forbade them to cut the corners of their hair?

Frazer was thus seduced to his hypothesis by the environment in which the prohibition appeared. George A. Barton is led to his explanation by the word "corner": the law forbids trimming the corners of the hair, and corners have a special sacred place in the thinking of the ancient Semitic nations. But the emphasis of the prohibition is not on the corners, but on the hair-do. Frazer's preconceived idea is that the law is directed against mourning customs; Barton's is that it is intended to prevent the Israelites from cutting corners.

We do not want to be hairsplitters—no pun was intended—but

* Frazer, *Folklore*, p. 300.
** *Jüdisches Lexikon* (Berlin, 1930), Vol. IV, article *Peot.*

the line has to be drawn as sharply as possible. It is disconcerting to see that most scholars have collected all the right facts from the four corners of the world that can be made to fit a wrong theory. Such a theory can be compared to pieces of a jigsaw puzzle that do not fit the place one tries to put them in, but its neighborhood. Let us assume that someone has to finish a jigsaw puzzle presenting Little Red Riding Hood in the forest. One of the missing pieces is the face of the little girl. Several bits are lying around. They are all fragments belonging to this puzzle, but they are part of the peripheral area, not of its center. Several pieces may form, for example, bits of the girl's hood, but they do not show her face, her hairline, or her curls.

3

Many of the commentaries and exegeses dealing with those passages in Leviticus and Deuteronomy casually refer to a remark of Herodotus, when they state that the prohibition of shaving the hair round is an attempt to set the Jews apart from neighboring pagan nations. In the third book of his work the Greek historian says of the Arabs that the only gods they believe in are Dionysus and Urania, and "they affirm that they poll their hair even as Dionysus himself is polled, for they poll it in a perfect circle and shave the temple and they call Dionysus 'Orotal.' " Herodotus, who traveled between 467 and 484 in Asia Minor, might well have seen Arabic tribes. He was, however, far from being a critical historian. Legends and traditional tales were interwoven in his record. "It is my business to relate what I am told, but I am under no obligation to believe it," he once remarked. However charming and artistic are his tales, the father of history, as he was called by Cicero, was simple and artless and tells his story, mixing facts and fancy, without wasting time on its critical discussion and inquiry.

How can we trust this historian telling us about the religion of the Arabs of his time? It is likely that his report is not only inaccurate, but also distorted by subjective concepts. His identification of the Arabic god Orotal with Dionysus is perhaps more or less arbitrarily founded on some impressions of superficial similar traits. His report can be helpful in defining the character of that god as well as misleading. But it needed more than a historian's imagination to invent the special feature that this god's worshipers polled their hair in imitation of him, that they shaved it in a perfect circle. When we consider the undoubtable testimony that the ancient Egyptian priests and higher officials shaved their heads, that the same custom prevailed in Babylon, and that the heathens are called round-cropped by Jeremiah (9:25; 25:23), we would be assuming too much coincidence if we rejected Herodotus' report to this effect. We believe that, whatever was the nature of Orotal in Herodotus' concept, his statement that the worshipers tried to imitate their god in their hair-do is correct. Such an attitude seems fantastic to us, but the deities of prehistoric times and of the primitive tribes of today are much more of this earth than the God of the monotheistic religions. An echo of that desire to imitate God is still perceptible in the admonition that the Israelities should be holy as Jahweh is holy (Lev. 19:2). Those worshipers needed little imagination to visualize what their god looked like, and it was not difficult to make oneself resemble him, to shape oneself in his image.

It seems that totemism, the primitive worship of animals, was once the universal concept mankind had of religion. Totemism marks the primal phase of ancient religions, and is thus a very important part of the *biography* of God. Only traces of that primal concept are to be discovered in the religion of the Israelites, but they are definite and distinct enough to make science assume that the worship of sacred animals was once the core of the Hebrew religion, as it was of that of the Egyptians, Babylonians, Assyrians, and Philistines. We are not concerned here with that prehistoric phase, but with a later period in which the gods had already regained a human or half-human form and in which only some of their properties, equipment, attributes, emblems, or companions reveal that they themselves had once been animals or animal-like. They were, for instance, depicted with human heads on animal bodies or animal heads on human bodies. Egyptian and Assyrian statues and pictures prove how long that half-totemistic, half-anthropomorphic phase of the concept of the gods lasted. We know that all those nations had certain festivals and ceremonies in which they, like the Arabs of whom Herodotus speaks, identified with their gods in one way or another. It must have been easy to do as the means to obtain a superficial resemblance were relatively simple: to put a hair ornament or a few bird feathers on one's head, or to cover oneself with the hide of the sacred animal, was enough.

But here is a new thought! Did we not get the impression from the theories of Frazer, Barton, Smith, and other scholars that here we have an entirely different set of circumstances? And did we not compare them to pieces belonging to a jigsaw puzzle in which the central bit is still missing? To continue our simile: What is needed is perhaps only to choose another fragment from the handful of pieces already at hand. It will perhaps fill the gap. The commentaries mentioning that passage from Herodotus' history show that at the time when the Pentateuch became a series of codes (that of Ezra about 445), many neighboring tribes polled their hair in a circle. The Arabs cited by Herodotus were such a nation. The other fact that the Arabs shaved themselves as they did in order to resemble their god Orotal was, of course, mentioned, but none of the scholars I know made use of this fact, drew conclusions from it, or considered it worthwhile availing himself of it to explain that puzzling prohibition of the Lord.

The Arabic god Orotal, whom Herodotus compares with Dionysus, had, no doubt, certain features in common with the Thracian god of vegetation. It is very likely that he was originally a totemistic god like Dionysus who was believed to assume the form of a goat. We know that an animal sacrificed to the god was first regarded as a divine incarnation. Just the Dionysiac cult provides an excellent example of the belief that a god may incarnate himself temporarily in animal form. In the frenzied observance of the cult, an ox or a goat, representing the god, was rent by the maddened worshipers and the raw flesh was devoured. In such a sacramental feast the Dionysus-worshipers clothed themselves in goatskins. Whatever may have been the similarities of the Arabic Orotal with Dionysus, one of them was most likely that he had still a half-totemistic character, and was believed to resemble a goat or a bull. When now Herodotus reports that the Arabs tried to be like him by polling their hair in a circle, is it not plausible that they imitated him in his animal form? It seems that this hypothesis presents a new approach to the understanding of the Lord's mysterious prohibition against shaving the hair. There is a line in the prologue of Shakespeare's *Henry V* which explains what I mean:

> . . . a crooked figure may
> Attest in little place a million.

A mere naught put in the right place—for instance, after a row of figures on a check—can push the number up into the millions. A fact put into the right place, that is, alongside other particular facts, can give an enormous significance to a certain situation and elucidate a question which has been a mystery. It seems to me that there is such "a little place" where "a crooked figure may attest" an unimagined lot. The unnoticed second part of Herodotus' statement, about the Arabs who polled their hair roundwise to resemble their god, points the way to the solution of the problem of why Jahweh felt an intense antipathy against a certain hair-do of His chosen people. He wished to set them apart and to prevent them from relapsing into an animal cult, a totemistic worship in which they would identify with a barbarous god in imitating him with hide and hair as the Arabs, the Philistines, the Egyptians, and Assyrians did. If, as I believe, this interpretation which makes use of a neglected trifle of information is correct, it again conforms to that sentence of the Psalms: "The stone which the builders refused is become the headstone of the corner."

4

The endeavor to make oneself resemble a sacred animal or a totemistic god or spirit is ubiquitous on certain levels of the evolution of human civilization. The reports of anthropologists, historians, and travelers, of missionaries and explorers are filled with descriptions of the manner in which the ancient nations and the savage tribes of today try to identify with their individual totem gods. In the following small selection of examples I shall restrict myself to the area in which we are here interested, namely, in the hair-do. A particular way of arranging the hair was the mark of the tribe of the ancient Indo-German Europeans.* The Acheans wore their hair in curls, the ancient Britains and Ligurians let their hair grow.** The ancient Thracians combed their hair backward and tied it together, braiding it on top of the head. Cutting of the hair is a celebration with the young Hindus; some families allow only one curl, others three curls to grow; some men wear the curl in front, some behind. In commentaries the religious significance of the different hair-dos is discussed. Different families in ancient India wear their hair in different manners. According to Xenophon the ancient Medes combed their hair to one side to differentiate themselves from other tribes. The Longobards cut their hair at the neck, but let it hang down loose in front. The Alans and the Scythians had similar language, weapons, and dress, but the Alans, according to Lucian, wore their hair short, the Scythians long. H. Hirt, from whose book I took these instances, states that style of hairdressing is a definite tribal mark. The Jowa clans in America have each a distinguishing mode of dressing their hair. The Buffalo clan, for instance, wear their hair in such a way that it imitates horns.† Among the Omahas the smaller boys of the Black Shoulder (Buffalo) clan wear two locks of hair in imitation of horns. The Hanga clan wear a crest of hair two bunches long, standing erect and extending from ear to ear in imitation of the buffalo. The Small Bird clan of the Omahas have a little hair in front over the forehead and some at the back of the head to resemble a tail with much hair over each ear for the wings.

Different tribes have their individual ways of cutting a child's hair. Thus the Pawnee Indians "cut the hair close to the head, except a ridge from the forehead to the crown where the scalp-lock was parted off in a circle, stiffened with fat and plaited, made to stand erect and curved like a horn, hence the name Pawnee, derived from pariki-horn."‡ The Dakota parted the hair in the

* Herman Hirt, *Die Indogermanen* (Strassburg, 1907), Vol. II.
** Plinius III. 27.
† *Third Report of Bureau of Ethnology* (Washington, 1884), p. 238.
‡ *Encyclopedia of Religion and Ethics*, IX, 467.

middle from the forehead to the nape of the neck; the scalplock was always finely plaited. The long hair on each side was braided and wrapped in strips of beaver or otter-skin hanging down in front of the chest." The Bechuana warriors in Africa wear the hair of an ox in their own hair and the skin of a frog on their coat, in the belief this will make them as hard to hold as those animals. We remember R. Smith's theory of the sacrifice of the hair as part of the initiation ritual, when we learn that a subclan of the Omahas cut off all the hair from their boys except six locks on each side, on the forehead, and one hanging down the back in imitation of the legs, head, and tails of a turtle. Livingstone reports that the boys of the Menuganga tribes in East Africa "train their locks till they take the admired form of the buffalo's horns; others prefer to let their hair hang in a thick coil down their back like that animal's tail." In Frazer's book there is an abundance of instances of this kind showing the variety of forms in which the worshipers of ancient nations and of present savage tribes affect a resemblance as close as possible to the totem god. The impersonator of the sacred animal, of course, preferably uses the skin or other part of the beast, but the arranging of the hair is not the smallest part of the attempt to identify in appearance with the totem ancestor and totem god. Dr. Marcel Baudouin considers the role of the hair in this function a *"totem partial."** Another French writer, Maurice Bensson, calls it *"la carte d'identité"* of the worshipers.

We venture the thesis that the prohibition of Leviticus is directed against the temptation of the Israelites to imitate totemistic gods whom they had once worshiped as did all their neighbors. Herodotus' report states that the Arabs polled their hair in imitation of their god. But this god, whom he compares with Dionysus, still had a half-animal form, was perhaps half a bull or a goat. Was not Dionysus himself once identified with a goat or a ram? Do not his companions, the satyrs, still wear the horns and hoofs of the goat? All the neighbors of the Israelites worshiped gods who still had totemistic features, and the Israelites themselves had adored images of a bull at Dan and Beth (I Kings 12:28). The Bible itself still compares the power of Jahweh with

* *Le Courrier Medical* (October 23, 1938).

that of the horned beast Reem. That prohibition is part of the great wall erected against identification with the barbarous totem gods whose appearance his worshipers tried to imitate in their dressing and their hair-do.

The correct interpretation of the Lord's forbidding his worshipers to trim their hair roundwise contains a premise without which it is impossible to understand why and how the Jews arrived at the custom of sidelocks. They let a few hairs on each side grow as token of their obedience to the Law given by the Lord. This became a visible sign, an emblem or badge showing that the wearer was devoted to God and belonged to the chosen people. From the few hairs indicating obedience to the Law evolved, later on, the custom of wearing locks or curls. But are those sidelocks as they appeared much later only a token of the devotion to Jahweh's prohibition, a badge of a religious and national community?

At this point the reader as well as the writer visualizes the variety of forms that the *payoth* of the Eastern Jews show. There are nearly as many kinds of those curls as there are mustaches, thin and broad ones. Some are short and some small, some straight and some curled, some neglected and others carefully oiled and fatted. The common feature in all this variety is that the curls stand out from the surface of the beard and the other hair, and have a definite, recognizable form.

In visualizing the many sidelocks we have seen, we get a distinct impression of those curls standing out from the skull-caps of orthodox Eastern Jews. Are we victims of delusion, do we play a mental trick on ourselves? There is no doubt that the conspicuous examples of those sidelocks reaching over the ears, sticking up from the head, look like the horns of a bull or, if curled, of a ram. That is certainly a surprising impression, but we have to trust our eyes. We are confused and do not understand how such a hair-do can develop from a few hairs left uncut to show that religious Jews did not shave their head roundwise like the pagans of the nations surrounding them. How did that new hair style evolve?

An attempt to explain this development will have to start from the phase in which the Israelitic tribes worshiped totemistic and half-totemistic gods besides Jahweh. At this time they certainly tried to imitate those gods, including their appearance, especially in ceremonies initiating the young men into the tribe. In hair style, headdresses, in badges and dress, they tried to impersonate those gods who had only partly gained human form. There are still distinct traces of that phase in later times. The religious reformers and the prophets made desperate efforts to bring the people so far that Jahweh alone would be their God, but the Israelites, who are a stiff-necked people, did not easily or rapidly give up customs they had followed for centuries. We have also to assume that the custom of cropping and shaving the hair in imitation of some totemistic deity was still followed in spite of the prohibition of the Law and of the attacks of the prophets against that heathenish hair-do. In the Diaspora the Jews cropped their hair like people among whom they lived and left only a small amount of hair untouched, thus indicating that they were faithful to Jahweh's law.

The following development can easily be guessed. The stronger the temptation grew to conform with the customs of the other people, the more intense the pressure became of the rabbis upon the community to observe the Law. Instead of a few hairs as a token of religious observance, a kind of bunch was developed to testify that its bearer was loyal to Jahweh and belonged to His chosen people. It became a sign of one's difference not only from the heathen, but also from those Jews who had joined the new covenant. Sidelocks were small and inconspicuous during the early Middle Ages. Under the influence of the Cabala, that half-mystical, half-religious system of Judaism, the *payoth* became longer and were carefully displayed; they became, so to speak, a national or religious badge.

Such elongation and emphasis was a reaction against the negligence increasingly shown to the biblical law. Out of fear of sinning by default, the sidelocks were now displayed and were no longer a token of religiousness, but almost of saintliness. Driven into defensiveness by the untiring pressure of their rabbis, who insisted on strict observance of the Law, the Jews overshot the mark of the Law. But in reaching as they did they lessened their vigilance against the hidden antagonist, paganism, which had now the disguise of the most intense religious zeal. It is as if the devil should slip into church in a monk's habit, wearing a hood through which only slight elevations reveal the horns. The side-locks that had become longer and more conspicuous were not only symbols of Jewish loyalty to the Law as it is prescribed in the Bible, but also renewals of an ancient idolatrous cult which imitated the totem god in the hair-do of the tribe. Under cover of religious zeal the prehistoric totemistic custom entered, unrecognized, Jewish orthodoxy. The sidelocks were unconsciously shaped and curled in a manner resembling a bull's or ram's horn and thus renewed the most archaic and primitive form of idolatry, the same barbarous totem worship which Jahweh had forbidden. Out of the bottom of the pit into which the idea of an animal-like god was banished the old totemistic concept had victoriously returned. Masked as an expression of high devotion to Jahweh, a visual badge of a despised, primitive idolatrous concept had re-emerged. In their anxiety to avoid a sin by neglecting the observance of a biblical prohibition, the Jews committed a much more serious sin in their unconscious relapse into heathenism. In the display of their sidelocks an expression of sacredness reveals itself as a sacrilege. In the strict observance of religious Law a blasphemy is acted out. Angelo, in Shakespeare's *Measure for Measure,* says:

> Let's write good angel on the devil's horn
> 'Tis not the devil's crest.

This is the outline of a development sketched with the help of all available data from history and archeology. The result of this reconstruction, namely, that the sacrilege not only slips into a highly progressed religious institution, but is conceived as an expression of special religious zeal, is so bizarre and odd that it appears scarcely imaginable. It is not only that at the height of devotion an act of religious rebellion emerges, but also that this sacrilegious act pretends to be a manifestation of unusual zeal and thus mocks all traditional belief. The process is so extraordinary that it seems unlikely to find analogies.

5

Yet there are similar processes in an area very distant from that of religious cult and custom: in the sphere of neurotic symptoms, especially in the typical manifestations of compulsive and obsessional neuroses. This form of mental disturbance sets in with measures of defense against the intrusion of forbidden hostile and sexual impulses which have remained unconscious. Strange thoughts and actions emerge in the patient who tries to protect himself against the assault of trends which are repressed and now attempt to break through to the surface. The ego of the patient who is frightened by puzzling sexual and aggressive tendencies within himself sharpens his vigilance. In order to keep those unwelcome and alien impulses away, he erects measures of defense which become the more severe the more urgently those forbidden impulses demand satisfaction. The longer the neurotic disturbance lasts, the more desperate and irrational those defenses built against the danger from within become. The obsessional and compulsive symptoms, which were at first formed of the rejection of unwanted trends, become more and more manifestations of a compromise between the controlling forces and the repressed tendencies. Finally, those repressed impulses force their entrance into the carefully reserved area of the ego, and the exiled emotional trends infiltrate the personality. They either overrun its bastions of protection by a sudden and surprising attack at an unexpected place or infest them in the form of slow penetration. There is a phase in which the situation of the symptoms resembles the picture of an undecided battle in which the antagonists are entangled in an inextricable melee and in which the outcome is dubious. Finally, the rejected and repressed ideas get the upper hand and the symptomatical picture is governed by their superior power.

Here is a representative case in which an obsessional idea emerged in a surprising manner. The patient, a young girl, lived a double life. At home she behaved as a "nice girl" whose dates with young men had a harmless social character. In reality she was promiscuous and even liked to take the initiative with men. She had discovered that a man could easily be seduced when, in the phase of petting, she put her tongue into his mouth, which she considered an invitation to sexual intercourse. One evening when she left home to go to a man she was tortured by the feeling that she had by mistake put her tongue into her father's mouth when she kissed him good night.

The emergence of such repressed tendencies is not restricted to the area of obsessional thinking: occasionally they flow also in distorted forms in our dreams or sometimes appear in wit and in break-throughs, even in the disguise of naïveté. Such an anecdote is told about the great composer, Anton Bruckner. The celebrated symphonist who had led a chaste life was in the company of women often shy and gauche. A young lady who was his neighbor at a banquet tried desperately to begin a conversation with the old man. Finally she said, "I dressed especially beautifully for you, professor. Did you not notice it?" The simple-minded composer answered, "Oh, for me you need not have dressed at all."

An example from obsessional symptoms will well illustrate the dynamics of such a break-through at the peak of the defense and bring us at the same time closer to the area of religious phenomena. The patient, a woman in her early forties and a pious Catholic, had a little plaster bust of St. Anthony on her mantelpiece. Once when she dusted the room, she thought she had pushed the figure of the saint whom she considered her personal patron rather irreverently aside. She made amends by caressing the bust and putting it at a favorite position in the middle of the mantel. Still not satisfied, she carefully changed the place of the figure once more. It now seemed to her that it was not standing straight. In an effort to give it the right angle she set it down too energetically and, to her great consternation, broke it.

The counterpart to this symptomatic action is found in an anecdote Anatole France once told his secretary. The writer spoke of the great familiarity Italian peasants show in social intercourse with their Catholic priests. A Roman woman who had her baby in her arms got into conversation with her priest as he was coming from Mass carrying the holy host. The bambino, attracted by the sacred wafer which he perhaps confused with a butterfly, wanted to grasp it. The priest tried in vain to keep the little hands away and protect the Sacrament from their touch. But the child wished to get hold of this consecrated bread. In his desperate effort to protect it from the sacrilegious contact, the priest finally could not help warning the child and saying, "Kaka!" In his most zealous defense he was led to uttering an atrocious blasphemy.

6

We have stated that the sidelocks of the Eastern Jews represent, unknown to them, a totemistic symbol and are to be compared to the hair-dos, headdresses, animal skins by which totem tribesmen indicate that they are descended from this or that sacred animal, to whom they affect a resemblance. To take the bull or the ram by the horns, we need only remember that the Scripture itself admits that images of bulls were worshiped at Dan and Beth, that the ram was sacrificed to Jahweh, and that His power is compared to that of the horned beast Reem. All these features are remnants of a prehistoric totemistic phase in which the Israelites also tried to resemble their animal gods in appearance, covering themselves with their skins or polling their hair to be like them. Is it necessary to remind the reader that all the nations who were neighbors to the Israelites had gods with much more distinct animal characters?

The Hittite deities wore caps with several pairs of horns, Melkarth of Tyre was represented as an almost bestial god with two short horns on his head; so was the Syrian Hadad. The Phoenician goddesses usually have the horns of a cow, and with Hathor, whom Isis was identified, is depicted with a cow's head and horns. Cows were sacred to Isis who sometimes wore a ram's horn. Ra sometimes wears a disk with a ram's horn and Kneph wears a ram's head with horns, curving, long, or project-ing. In Greece, Dionysus also appeared in the form of a bull and is often called "horned" or "bull-horned." The Canaanites wor-shiped Baal as a bull. At Mendes at the Delta in Egypt as well as

at Heraclopolis, Osiris was worshiped as a ram, and at Mendes
and Elephantine burial places and sarcophagi of sacred rams
have been found. The long twisted horns of a ram are often
attached to the headdresses of the Pharaohs who became Osiris.
Attis was honored by the sacrifice of rams. The shophar or keren
of the Israelites which is blown on Jewish New Year's Day was
made of a ram's horn. But why add examples to examples when
any textbook of comparative history of ancient religions shows
an abundance of the worship of bull- and ram-headed gods of
antiquity and of the custom of the Mediterranean nations to
affect a resemblance to their animal-shaped deities?

It is better to look back at the road by which we came to this
point where saintliness and sacrilege seem to meet and merge in
the custom of curled sidelocks. Having finished the circle, we
have to return from a long detour to the point of departure and
to trace our steps back to the result that emerged from the fusion
and confusion of notions.

Was not the sight of that old Jew with his conspicuous sidelocks followed by the blasphemous idea that God cannot be
beautiful? In falling asleep the next evening, that hypnagogic
picture appeared in which a big ram jumped a fence, followed
by a little lamb. In retrospect that visual image appears as the
most important lead in the research that followed, as preconscious
anticipation of its result. Jesus Christ, adored in the figure of
the lamb, became the *Agnus Dei*. Is it not logical that the lamb
follows his father who is a ram? Godfather and Godson emerge
here in their original animal forms; their concept is, in that
image, so to speak, re-translated into the language of prehistoric
totemism. The impression the two sidelocks had made upon me
had sunk into the unconscious, had there been elaborated, and
had led to a conclusion. The sidelocks looked like a ram's or
bull's horns. From some unconscious depth the idea was dredged
up of the prehistoric appearance of the god the Israelites once
worshiped. Was there perhaps an unconscious memory operating
that brought up the biblical scene of Abraham sacrificing a ram
instead of his son Isaac? I knew, of course, that in prehistory, the
sacrificed animal originally replaced the animal god himself.

However this may be, at the sight of those sidelocks the concept of the resemblance of the children of Israel to their creator occurred. Instead of the impression which had remained unconscious, the thought occurred that God cannot be beautiful. The blasphemous thought was stimulated not only by seeing the old Jew, but also seeing the faces of tired people around me and my own melancholy visage: all of us His creatures. The old Jew must have reminded me of the god of our forefathers and of the low and humble beginning of his concept, of that phase when he was worshiped not in the image of a ram, but simply as a ram. In prehistoric times, the figure of deity was really crude and barbarous, ugly and terrifying. God needed thousands of years to emerge from this beastly shape and to become superhuman. St. Anthony saw, in that grandiose vision which Flaubert presented, the succession of gods following each other in the evolution of civilization, but he did not visualize the earliest beastlike appearances of God on earth.

We return here to the thought that God cannot be beautiful when we are made in His image. Did we not learn that the Cabala taught that the face of God is reflected in that of a man, even in the beard and sidelocks of His worshipers? I must have seen His face in the old Jew on Broadway who made such an uncanny impression upon me.

It is not so long ago that blasphemy was considered a crime and was severely punished by common law. Was not C. B. Reynolds, whom Robert G. Ingersoll defended in that famous *Argument,* condemned for blasphemy under the laws of New Jersey in a trial at Morristown in 1887?

Some train of thought connecting the ugliness of the people with their creator had led to that blasphemous idea that God cannot be beautiful. If this be crime, it has a new form. It is guilt by association.

In his lectures on the gods Robert Ingersoll once said, "An honest God is the noblest work of Man." He pointed out that the concept of the Deity is a projection of our own ideas into a metaphysical world. Voltaire had expressed the same idea long before the forceful American advocate of enlightenment. He said:

"If God has made us in His image, we have certainly got even with Him."*

Was the result reached here worthy of so much search and research? It is not for us to decide. The little curl on both sides of the forehead certainly casts a long shadow of meaning. It is satisfactory that the psychoanalytic approach could elucidate the secret significance of the sidelocks, could solve a problem that the history of religions and archaeology were unable to clear up.**

A tiny stick put into the earth can indicate the position of the sun as well as the obelisk of Luxor. Small bricks also make a house. We are content with the discovery of why all God's chillun got not only wings, but also sidelocks.

IV

1

A DISCUSSION which recently† took place in the columns of the New Statesman, a serious British magazine, made me take out and open old folders in which many notes on the psychological question of prayer were preserved. The controversy concerned the value of prayer, and took as its point of departure a service at which the congregation prayed for rain. A critic, who was a priest, called such an incantation a "blasphemy in prayer." Many correspondents of the New Statesman derided belief in the prayers of rainmakers, while others defended their psychological value. A correspondent wrote that the expression of even a foolish petition that elicits no direct response makes us more aware of ourselves and of the nature of the Deity, and added that "perseverance in prayer has a psychoanalytical effect"—whatever that

* Les Sottisier, XXXII.
** It is very likely that the custom of the tonsure which is a symbol of Jesus' crown of thorns can be traced back to the same origin.
† October, 1954.

might mean. Another correspondent is reminded by the debate of some verses of unknown authorship called "Prayer for Rain":

> In vast and unimaginable space
> Where countless Suns send forth their fecund rays,
> Each to its group of whirling satellites,
> There rolled a little miserable ball,
> And on this ball a minute microbe knelt
> And prayed the Great Controlling Force of all
> To wreck the order of the universe,
> Unchain the Suns and bid ungovernable chaos come again.
> For what? To damp the dot whereon the microbe knelt.

Reading the notes I had accumulated over many years, I became aware that only a little work was needed to shape their essential content into a paper which would fit admirably into the frame here presented. The continuation and elaboration of that first draft led to a not unimportant new insight in the field of prehistoric and primitive civilization. The result of that analytic exploration is significant not only for the remote past, but is, as the controversy in the *New Statesman* shows, of some importance for the present situation of our civilization. The course of the investigation illustrates the process of analytic discovery, but with a difference that is interesting because it promises new developments of future research in which the function of the unconscious as a receptive and interpretative organ will be more appreciated than at present.

The instances of psychoanalytic discovery presented in the preceding chapters showed how impressions of everyday life led to a problem which had resisted the efforts of other sciences, but could be solved by the method of analytic penetration. In the following instance the problem was there in the beginning. It had been clearly stated and frequently discussed by anthropologists, students of the evolution of religion, and historians of civilization, but it could not be solved. It remained obstinate and unsolvable. It did not yield to analytic exploration either until some apparently accidental impressions led to certain decisive insights whose analytic interpretation opened the way to its solution. It is the same distance covered in the opposite direction;

going from the maze with its mysterious network of paths to the street and everyday life.

When—more than forty years ago—my first psychoanalytic papers on the psychology of religion were published, several problems that had occupied my thoughts were skirted because I had nothing to contribute to their solution. The answers that anthropologists and historians of civilization had given to certain fundamental questions did not satisfy me. One of those problems concerned the relation between magic and religion, one of the most obscure and controversial of subjects. The aspect most interesting to me within that problem was the transition from magic to religion. None of the attempts made to clarify this question was satisfactory. When you tried to make a sharp distinction between the two areas, the facts of ancient and primitive civilization made the separation appear questionable. When, on the other hand, you assumed a complete continuity between magic and religion, it was very difficult to subsume the two under a common heading.

J. G. Frazer lays stress on the "fundamental distinction and even opposition of principle between magic and religion," and is of the opinion that, in the evolution of thought, magic "has probably everywhere preceded religion."* The human race which passed through that age of magic tried first to exert mechanical control and attempted "to force the great powers of nature to do their pleasure." The phase of magic gave place to an "age of religion," in which men courted the favors of those powers by offering sacrifices and prayers. The last motive for this replacement was disappointment in magic. Man understood that his efforts to work by means of imaginary causes had been vain or, to use Frazer's words, that "he had been pulling at strings to which nothing was attached." When he gave up magic in despair, man found religion as a truer theory of nature.

Frazer's theory was subjected to sharp criticism by R. R. Marett,** R. S. Hartland, A. Lehman, H. Hubert, M. Mauss, and other prominent anthropologists, who called his distinction too

---

* *The Golden Bough,* 2nd ed.; I, 16.
** *The Threshold of Religion* (2nd ed.; London, 1914), pp. 47 ff., 147 ff.

intellectualistic and unjustifiably sharp. In spite of those arguments, it is now assumed that the concept of magic preceding religion in the evolution of civilization is generally correct. It is obvious that the transition phase from magic to religion lasted a long time, perhaps a few thousand years. There is a strong conservative trend in human nature which resists sudden change. The old does not disappear when the new emerges, but survives a long time and co-exists with the new before it gives place to it— if it ever yields to it entirely. Magical rites existed side by side with religious ones; belief in spells and sorcery at the same time as worship of the gods. The texts of the oldest Babylonian, Egyptian, and Greek hymns and prayers prove that there were mixed forms of both systems of thought, magico-religious concepts.* The fact that there is a tendency to retain the previous form or to revert to it does not deny that there are fundamental differences of attitude in magic and religion. Magic involves an attitude of compulsion and coercion; religion an attitude of dependence and humility. In magic the medicine man or the average tribesman performs an act by which he, in his imagination, controls or sets in motion the events he wills. In religion the worshiper has renounced this sovereign attitude and submits to the supremacy of God or of several divine beings. Although the existence of magico-religious rites cannot be disavowed, "the apprehension of a qualitative difference must be taken as primary and fundamental."**

The qualitative difference between magic and religion is best

---

* M. Jastrow (*Die Religion Babyloniens und Assyriens*. Giessen, 1905-1912) shows in his collection of hymns how prayer grew out of spells. H. Oldenberg (Religion der Veda. Berlin 1917) presents an analysis of the relation of prayer and spells in India. J. Goldzieher (Zauberelemente im islamitischen Gebet. Orientalische Studien Theodor Nöldeke zum 70. Geburtstag gewidmet. Giessen 1906 I. 303 ff.) discovers in the formulas and ritualistic gestures of Mohamedan prayer remnants of magical rituals. A. I. Wensinck (Animismus und Dämonenglauben im Untergrund des jüdischen und islamitischen Gebets. Der Islam 1913. 219 ff.) does the same with late Jewish prayers. R. R. Marett (From Spell to Prayer in The Threshold of Religion. London 1914, p. 29 ff.) shows how prayer originates in magic; similarly L. R. Farnell (*The Evolution of Religion*, London, 1907, p. 16 ff.) F. B. Jevons (The Idea of God in Early Religion. Cambridge 1911. 108 f.) maintains that prayer and spell were originally one thing and became differentiated later on.

** Stanley A. Cook in *Encyclopedia of Religion and Ethica*. X, 615.

characterized by contrasting the attitude of the magician who performs a spell with that of a religious man who prays for rain. The
first attitude is expressed in the words: "My will be done"; the
second by the sentence: "Thy will be done." Magic endeavors to
influence the course of events by means of rites without inter-
vention of divine beings. It is coercive. In religion man tries to
cultivate the good will of gods by means of hymns and sacrifice,
and so to induce them to bestow the benefits which man desires.
Prayer is pleading and persuasive. In magic man is master of his
destiny; in religion he has submitted to God and entrusts his fate
to Him. No transition phase seemed possible between the two
attitudes. No bridge could, it seemed, lead from "My will be
done" to "Thy will be done." The second concept was apparently
a reversal of the first. Even if you assumed that there must have
been an intermediary phase, what could have been its character?
It was obvious that many magical features survived in religion. It
is a long way from the Malay charm in which the tribesman treats
the soil, saying:*

> It is not earth that I switch
> But the heart of So and So.

to the man who desires to bring sickness or death upon an enemy,
and says:

> Lo, I am burying the corpse of So and So.
> If you do not make him sick, if you do not kill him,
> You shall be a rebel against Muhamed.

Here magic has already passed into the category of prayer.

It was, of course, easy to assume that in his urge to control
nature and the course of events himself, man learned to influence
the Deity in his prayer to the extent that his wishes were fulfilled.
The transition from magic to religion would thus be made by a
phase which could be expressed by the formula: "My will be
done with Your help." But the key problem is not solved by such
a concept. The gap between spell and prayer was still too wide.
None of the theories presented could fill it. The question seemed
unanswerable.

* W. W. Skeat, *Malay Magic* (London, 1900), pp. 569-71.

2

After I had decided to leave the problem alone because it was too difficult for me, I turned my curiosity to other questions. But the problem did not release me. It crept up on me or set traps for me along my way. It emerged surprisingly at other points of my research work. It did not appear in its previous form of a general question contrasting the principles of religion and magic, but in a more specialized shape. It came up unexpectedly, and not, as before, as a theoretical problem, and not from the point of view of the study of religion, but directly out of various experiences. Such re-emergence can be compared with a common experience: You have been introduced to a man at a cocktail party, and a few days later you run into him on your way to the office. You see him again when you go to lunch, and catch sight of him again when you leave your office in the late afternoon. It seems that this must be more than coincidence.

The impressions leading back to the problem came from two areas which were as remote from each other and had as little communication with each other as two planets. The first kind of impression, received on various occasions in the course of the following years, originated in psychoanalytic practice.

The instances of prayer remembered by neurotic persons in analytic sessions are not very different from those of other persons. The differences we observe are such as develop from neuro ic symptoms, or from the interference of aggressive, hostile, or sexual impulses. A patient remembers, for instance, that when he prayed as a boy that a member of his family should have a long, healthy life, he had to add "here on earth," because he was suddenly attacked by the thought that God might misunderstand and give eternal life to that person. In the case of a patient who grew up as a practicing Catholic, sexual thoughts often disturbed the smooth flow of his prayers. He had, for instance, to think that the word "ejaculation," used for short, spontaneous prayer exclamations, referred also to sexual discharge. When he once prayed before the statue of the Holy Virgin, the thought occurred to him that her legs had not always been together, thus expressing the blasphemous idea that she had sexual intercourse. Some patients remembered that they had sometimes experienced an inability to pray, that emotional dryness (*"sécheresse du coeur"*) about which St. Teresa di Jesus complained.

The symptomatology of neuroses, especially of the obsessional neuroses, is full of magical thinking, but here I am choosing examples not of irrational thoughts, but of magical rites performed by persons consciously opposed to any superstition. A young girl who is a college student has many difficulties in keeping the content of textbooks in her memory. When she gets tired of reading and studying, she puts the book under her pillow. Although her intelligence contradicts this superstition, she still believes that she remembers the material she has to study by sleeping with the book. This belief in mental osmosis leads to the performance of the magical ritual, to the practice of "contagious magic," as Frazer would call it, by a modern, free-thinking girl.

Here is another case of magical acts, this time in a negative form. A young man who has many difficulties in social intercourse with women and shows distinct paranoid characteristics told me that he had received a package of cookies from a girl and explained why he had immediately sent it back to her. He had made the acquaintance of this girl in L. where he had worked as an engineer for several months. He had sexual intercourse with her and suspected that she had plans to marry him. After he had left L. because of work that had to be done in another town, the girl had written him several times and had sent him cookies she had prepared for him. He had liked them in L. and relished them again now, but eating them had a disastrous effect. As soon as he had digested them, he felt, as he reported in his analytic sessions, an intolerable desire for the girl and in the following days was tormented by sexual fantasies in which he vividly recalled intimate scenes with her. At the same time he was afraid to see her again since he was well aware that she had matrimonial designs he was unwilling to fulfill. The well-educated man first playfully, but later seriously, assumed that the girl had "bewitched" him with the cookies, that she had put some mysterious ingredients into them which aroused that extraordinary desire in him which he had never felt before. He pointed out to me that certain aphrodisiacal drugs and hormones could well be mixed with the other food and began to study the properties of those materials in scientific books. His conviction that the girl had used love magic to arouse his desire for her was essentially the same as that of ancient and half-civilized people who believe in love charms. Here, thus, was a modern variation of the theme of the potion which made Tristan and Isolde bound to each other by an imperishable love. Putting a book under a pillow and returning a parcel of cookies are magical performances which prove that these persons believe in a mystical power emanating from themselves and others. That conviction is, in both cases, connected with material objects. But this is not important because in other cases magical words or even gestures without words are supposed to direct the course of events.

These cases are now to be contrasted with others in which neurotic symptoms appear garbed in a form between magic and prayer. Here are two representative examples: A patient who suffered from a serious obsessional neurosis recounted an experience in which he mastered a severe attack of his compulsive inhibitions. One evening he found himself unable to pass a lamppost in a lonely street, because to go on the right side meant in his obsessional thinking that his father would soon die, while to pass on the left meant that he himself would die. Shocked by the assault of those sinister thought-conceptions he stayed at the lamppost for a long time unable to move one way or the other. Leaning on the post, he sighed and moaned, "O God! O God!" Only when he finally said, "Why have You forsaken me?" did he become aware that he, transfixed on the lamppost, had stretched out his arms as if he were being crucified like Christ on the cross. One moment later he felt he was released from his obsessional detention and could walk on.

A patient, educated in an orthodox Jewish milieu, reported the following memory from his childhood: According to tradition the destiny of men in the following year is determined in heaven on New Year's Day (Rosh Hashana). Once the two older brothers of the patient, who was then not yet six years old, play-acted the scene which in their imagination took place in heaven on this holiday. They predicted which relatives and acquaintances of the family would die in the year just beginning, and in so doing they carefully considered the age and state of health of the people in question. The youngest brother, listening to their decisions, suddenly interrupted them with the words, "Why don't you make Aunt Fanny die?" The two brothers broke into laughter when the little boy expressed his dissatisfaction at their having excluded the aunt he did not like. Here is certainly a magical performance within the framework of religious tradition. As in the previous instance, the identification with the Deity—there in the Crucifixion, here in usurpation of the function of Supreme Judge —is the determining factor in those performances which belongs to a transition phase from magic to religion. God is absent in the examples mentioned before.

These clinical experiences were complemented by another set of impressions which also led me back to that problem of the relation of religion to magic. Those impressions came from old experiences to which I sometimes returned in my thoughts. On a walk in Vienna I once entered a Catholic church at the beginning of a Mass. I had been in churches before, but this was the first time I had attended a High Mass. From my studies of ritual I had no more than a superficial knowledge of the significance of the service and of the prayers of the Eucharist. I had missed the Introit, but I followed attentively all the parts of the holy action until the end, very much aware of all the postures and gestures of the priest and of the congregation. While I thus observed the course of the Mass, I suddenly had a most extraordinary sensation. I would unhesitatingly call it uncanny if there were not certain nuances and shades which qualify that feeling. In one sense the uncanny has the character of something mysterious or fateful, bordering that of the unearthly or weird; in another that of odd, fantastic, or queer, the tone of the timid or even of the anxious. In this particular case neither anxiety nor awe was felt, but the sensation was close to that feeling experienced when something long-forgotten, a buried memory, reawakens. I tried to define the character of this sensation or to recognize its content as precisely as I could after leaving the church. It was for a second as if I had attended the ritual of a very ancient people,

for instance, of the Sumerians or Egyptians more than four thousand years before Christ, the bloody ritual of the Aztecs or of a
cannibalistic tribe of Southeast Australia. The uncanny feeling
had lasted only a moment, and was acutely experienced at the
Consecration when the substance of the bread is changed into
the body of Jesus Christ and the substance of the wine becomes
His blood.

When much later Freud's paper on the uncanny appeared—the
author mentioned in a footnote the insignificant assistance I
could render—I understood that the sensation of uncanniness indicated a relapse into mental habits I had consciously outgrown,
a reaction to the emergence of old, repressed beliefs. Later on I
had learned by self-observation that, in my case, an uncanny feeling sometimes heralded the emergence of a new psychoanalytic
insight in the field of prehistoric civilization, but nothing of this
kind followed that moment of uncanniness on this occasion.

When on several occasions I attended services of the Catholics,
Protestants, and Jews, in the following years, I tried in vain to
re-experience that puzzling feeling. (Once I had been present at a
Mohammedan service in the Balkans during the war.) I did not
succeed in reliving that sensation until I accidentally visited a
Jewish service on the Day of Atonement (Yom Kippur). Passing a
synagogue, curiosity propelled me to enter. I had not been in a
synagogue on that highest holiday since my early teens, and the
interval of more than fifty years had almost erased all memories
of the service, so that what I saw appeared new. A touch of that
uncanny feeling emerged when I looked at the many men in
their white prayer shawls who swayed as they said their prayers,
but the sensation became intensified and very distinct toward the
end which marked the most significant celebration of Jewish
liturgy. Near its end the service reaches the highest degree of
solemnity, similar to that of the High Mass. It is the moment
when the rabbi pronounces his blessing on the community. He
stands opposite the congregation and has drawn his prayer shawl
over his head. Thus veiled and almost fully covered, wrapped up
and cloaked, he spreads his hands in a strange gesture. The fourth
and fifth fingers are spread away from the others and remain in
this artificial position during the ceremony. You can see a repre-

sentation of those two hands spread in that characteristic gesture on tombstones of the Aaronites. Strange notions about the magical effects of the priest's blessing are widely spread among the Jews. The people are supposed to turn their eyes away from the rabbi while he recites it and while he makes the symbolic gesture. It is believed that he who looks at the priest who, spreading his hands, pronounces "The Lord bless thee. . . ." will become blind or even die.

After forty years I had again experienced that uncanny feeling during a religious ceremony, the same sensation of which I had been aware during the consecration of the Holy Mass. What did it mean? What traits do the two ceremonies have in common? It was not difficult to find an answer.

3

It was easiest to determine where the uncanny quality of the impressions I had received on those two occasions originated, since Freud had explained to us in general to what kind of impressions we attribute such a character: to those that seek to confirm the animistic mode of thinking after we have reached a stage in which we have intellectually abandoned such beliefs. Such impressions were there at the High Mass as well as at the Atonement Day service. The general impression was that I was present at the ritual of a lost or long-forgotten people of antiquity, that I became witness to an archaic and barbaric ceremony of some savage tribe. The Consecration of the Mass as well as the priest's blessing mark the climax of the service and its holy actions. They have another feature in common: in both, the Divine Presence is supposed to be most acutely felt. When the priest comes to the Consecration, which is the heart, the core, and the soul of the Mass, he changes bread and wine into the body and blood of the Lord. The priest assumes the person of Christ and uses the same ceremonies that Christ used at His last supper. "This is My Body. . . . This is My Blood. . . . Drink. . . . Do this in commemoration of Me. . . ." No one who knows the evolution of religion and studies the totemistic rites will deny that that ceremony is a substitution for the ancient totem meal, in which the clansmen who eat the sacred animal together identify themselves with their ancestor-god in incorporating him. The object sacrificed is now worshiped as God. The ancient totem meal was revived in the form of Communion, and the congregation consumes the flesh and blood of the Lord. The French use the expression *manger du Bon Dieu* for Communion. In the ceremony the priest is identified with Him.

The Christian Communion has absorbed the primitive sacrament, the old feast of kinsmen who took the manna, the power of an admired and envied person, in themselves in eating the substance of his body. The celebration of the totem meal, in which the tribesmen acquire sanctity by taking into themselves the sacred life, is really a commemoration of the original killing of the god. Christ is present not only in the person of the priest who speaks His words, but in all the members of the congregation who take part in the holy action. Eating His body and drinking His blood makes them Christ-like; in the same sense, originally, that Australian savages believe that they absorb the power and magic ability of the missionary whom they have killed and eaten. The unconscious memory of those cannibalistic features that continue to live in the concealed core of the Eucharist explains the emergence of the uncanny feeling. It was only later that the researches of Robertson, Smith, Frazer, and Freud who traced the Christian Communion back to the primitive totem meal came to mind. What was decisive for the uncanny impression was the suggestion contained in the Consecration that God is really present in the sacrifice. The most conspicuous feature of this most solemn part of the Mass is that the priest acts the part of Christ, who sacrifices Himself.* It was mainly this suggestion of

* Nobody who has attentively followed the Mass will deny this character of the holy action. I am quoting from the passages in which the Consecration is described by a Catholic priest (Ronald Knox, *The Mass in Slow Motion*, New York, 1948, p. 110 f.): "The priest finds himself . . . acting the part of Jesus Christ. . . . But he is not content merely to tell the story; he acts it; he suits the action to the word. When he says the words 'He took bread' or 'He took the cup,' the priest suits the action to the word." The writer explains further the difference of the activity of the priest and of the acting in a play: when you act you pretend that somebody—for instance, Hamlet or Macbeth—who

the Real Presence of God, whose body is eaten and whose blood is drunk before our eyes, which is responsible for the impression that I was attending the ritual of a prehistoric people or of primitive Australian tribes.

This quickly passing impression was not revived until many years later when I saw part of the Jewish Atonement Day service. Why did the same impression arrive at that time? Why did the uncanny feeling emerge at the priest's blessing? Is the archaic character of the ceremony enough to explain that strange sensation? Certainly not; there must have been some specific features reviving the childhood belief that God was present in the synagogue. And there are such features; they are not as outspoken, but they are as eloquent as those at the Mass. Only during the liturgy the tabooed name of Jahweh was once pronounced. The rabbi, covered with the prayer shawl, acts the part of the deity. Is not the prohibition to look at him while he speaks the priest's blessing another form of the biblical prohibition to look at Jahweh? And which God is it who is present at that solemn moment? The rabbi garbed in the cloth made of the hide of the totem animal makes that strange gesture of both his hands. The position of his spread fingers imitates the cloven-footed animal that was once worshiped by the Israelite tribes. The prayer shawl is a substitute for the ram's hide, the artificial gesture of the hands is an imitation of the ram's hoofs—no doubt, God is present in the ceremony: the prehistoric god in its original, totemistic shape. The magic and mimic performance of the rabbi proves that the priest took the part of this primitive god.**

Those most solemn portions of the Catholic and Jewish liturgy contributed the main impressions of a prehistoric ritual, but there were others, so to speak, at the fringes of my observation, although scarcely perceived at the moment, which introduced and intensified that odd sensation. Gestures, movements, and positions

isn't there is really present. "But the priest, in this interval of drama, doesn't pretend that somebody is there who isn't there. Jesus Christ is really there. . . . He is really there, not merely in the sacred Host, but also in the person of the priest. . . . The priest has become a kind of dummy through which, here and now, Jesus Christ is consecrating the Sacrament, just as He did, but in His own person, nineteen hundred years ago."

** Compare Karl Abraham, *Der Versöhnungstag, Imago* (June, 1920).

suddenly appeared strange, although I had seen them often before and had taken them for granted.

Two of them were focused as distinctly auxiliary factors in the genesis of the uncanny feeling: the one was the sign of the cross, so often made during the Mass, and the other was the swaying of the praying people during the Jewish service. Crossing oneself is obviously the expression of the Christian's identification with the Lord and later became the symbol of the Divine Victim. The cross is only the visible sign of this closest association, according to the words of Paul: "I am crucified with Christ; nevertheless I live; yet not I, but Christ liveth in me" (Gal. 2:20). The swaying of the body during prayer has been explained as the expression of religious trance or ecstasy. Shortly after leaving the synagogue, it occurred to me that the swaying is the last remnant of the original ritual dancing in which primitive nations imitate the movements of their totem animals. My thoughts went from there to the dancing of David before the Ark, to the jumping of the Jews during the Esre prayer, and to the religious dancing of the Hasidim, to the pantomimic dances of the natives of Northwest America and of the Arunta and other tribes of Australia. These thoughts were the only theoretical result of my attending the service in the synagogue. That result was poor enough, but it became the point of departure for far-reaching considerations about gestures in magic and religion much later.

In some cases presented in preceding chapters the emergence of uncanny feelings heralded the occurrence of new analytic insights and even of discoveries. This was not the case in these instances. The impressions received at the Catholic and Jewish services had made me wonder, but they did not lead to any new insights.

4

My daughter Theodora, recently graduated from Bennington College, once asserted that I am "intelligent in a dull way." From the preceding conversation, it could not be clearly concluded whether she meant that I lack the spark that gives light or whether I am slow on the uptake. In the case here sketched, she would have been right in both directions. Not the slightest notion occurred to me that the impressions received on both occasions could cast some light on the problem that had preoccupied my thoughts in my younger years. I did not connect those impressions in any way with that unanswered question of a transition phase from magic to religion. Yet there was some circumstantial evidence pointing in this direction, there was a path leading back to that problem, too early relinquished. The idea that there are certain similarities between the most important parts of the Eucharist and the Atonement Day service remained isolated and disconnected. I remained content with the recognition that in both liturgies God is supposed to be present at the altar and that the priest acts the part of the Deity, that he (and with him, of course, the religious community) is identified with Him. Similarly, the significance of the gestures and postures of prayer, which I had unconsciously recognized, was not followed up in my thoughts. The situation can well be compared with that of a paleontologist who has been very interested in a certain dinosaur and who, when much later he finds footprints of an extinct gigantic reptile in a part of Central Australia, is too indolent to pursue those traces further until he discovers bones of the prehistoric beast. Some new impressions had to be received to revive the old ones, and it took a coincidence of certain circumstances to lead me back to the unsolved problem.

On one occasion I visited a family I had known for some years, and had a chance to observe the couple's three-year-old child. The boy played by himself and obviously did not pay much attention to the grownups in the room. He was pretending that he was an engine, and with his arms and legs made the appropriate movements and imitated the different noises an engine makes in running and in arriving at a station. He then changed the object of his imitation and moved slowly around, opening his eyes wide and then closing them for some time. When he had revolved in this strange manner for a while, his mother asked him who he was, and he answered, "A lighthouse." Later on he acted out the part of a tiger with suitable jumps and spitting. I was told that he also acted the part of a policeman when he got a whistle, walked seriously and gravely around on his beat and pursued imaginary criminals. I looked smilingly at the little boy, engrossed in his play which was for him not acting, but real life. While he identified with a steam-roller or an animal, he was a steam-roller or that animal. He did not act them. Only at a later period the boy, after being transformed into a terrifying animal or an admired person in his play, sometimes said, "But I am really Peter Smith." Thus distancing himself from the object of his metamorphosis, he began to "act" a part instead of "being" that object. In a few years he will, we can be sure, have forgotten that he "was" an old watertank or an elephant, and will, if reminded of those games, either be ashamed of them or disavow that they ever existed. But what will happen to those wishes—they were obviously wishes— which were fulfilled in his vivid imagination when he was transformed into various beings whose power he coveted or of whom he was afraid? They will be replaced by others—for instance, by the desire to become an engine driver or a prize fighter when he is grown up. By this time perhaps he has already reached the age when he has been told about God and been taught to pray. Maybe he now asks God to make him an excellent boxer.

Such thoughts, stimulated by looking at the boy playing, led to all kinds of scientific daydreams out of which emerged the picture of a theory, a shadowy picture sharply focused only at its edges. The games of the child were magical in their character. They were the individual counterpart of the magic performances which ancient peoples and savage tribes produced in their rituals. The boy was transformed into a steam-roller or a tiger by an act of his will, by the omnipotence of his thought. The magical ceremony performed by self-produced noises and gestures is not only the means by which the metamorphosis is achieved, but also its result. It already follows the fulfillment of the wish to change into that object, a wish that was first realized in simple fantasy by way of "delusion," if you can use a psychiatric term in this case. If there was an age of magic in the prehistoric development of mankind, the imagined realization of the wish must also have preceded the magical rite.

In his play the boy does not differentiate between the kingdom of plants, of animals, and of men. He can as easily change into a lighthouse as into a policeman. This is quite as true of the primitive mind which ignores the boundaries between different areas of beings, all animated and tied together by the "solidarity of life," as Ernst Cassirer called it.* The objects the little boy imitates— better, which he becomes—in his games are obviously such as he desires to be. In this direction his games reminded me of the concept of totemism, a mode of thought that governs the whole religious and social life of the most primitive tribes we know, and which left deep traces in the religion of advanced culture. In the totemistic system, the aboriginal Australian tribes derive their origin from a certain animal, plant, or stone and identify themselves with this worshiped object. Their identity with it is not conceived as symbolic, but as real: the ethnologist Karl von Steinen reports that a certain Indian totemistic clan stated that they are aquatic animals or red parrots.** The Dieri tribe in Australia have a totem consisting of a certain sort of seed: the head man of the tribe is spoken of as being the plant itself.† Totemism is not only a social system in which the tribe traces its descent back to a certain animal to which it is tied by an indestructible bond, but also the oldest and most primitive form of religion. The clansmen worship the particular species of animal whom they consider their ancestors, and renew their unity with them in totemistic rites in which they imitate the animals by dressing in their hides and by moving in the same way. The little boy who pretended he was a tiger behaved exactly like an African tribesman whose totem is the tiger. God acquired, in later religious development, a human, mostly terrifying shape, he became anthropomorphic. There is even a duplicate of this stage in the pretending of the little boy when he identified with a policeman, a feared and admired human being who is as close to the concept of a godlike power as a little boy—and not only a little boy—can reach. When, much later, he learns from his mother, his teacher in school, and finally in church of the existence of God, he will already have advanced to a phase of evolution in which he will expect the fulfillment of his wishes by Christ. He has in his individual life traveled the way from magic to religion, from

---

* *An Essay on Man* (New York, 1944), p. 109.
** *Unter den Naturvölkern Zentral-Brasiliens* (Berlin, 1897), p. 307.
† Frazer, *Lectures on the Early History of Kinship* (London, 1905), p. 109.

spell to prayer, the same distance which mankind has gone in many thousand years.

A few days after I had visited that family and had been witness of the boy's pretendings, I was reminded of his imitating different objects when I read the *Essay on Man* in which the noted German philosopher Ernst Cassirer, who taught at Yale and Columbia until his death in 1945, presented an introduction to a philosophy of human culture. One of the chapters of the book on "Myth and Religion" brought my thoughts back to the relation between magic and religion which is in Cassirer's words "one of the most obscure and most controversial subjects." It annoyed me that the philosopher in this chapter somewhat haughtily dismisses the principle of the "omnipotence of thought" by which Freud explains the psychic dynamics of magic. Absorbed in his highly abstract speculations, some of which are undoubtedly very profound, the philosopher, who has no clinical experience of psychoanalysis, can afford to ignore the method by which depth-psychology reached its results. I then thought of the games of little Peter. If Cassirer could have observed that performance, which was magical in its character, he would have better understood why Freud spoke of the "omnipotence of thought" as the principle of magic.

At the same time I remembered another book in German by the same author, which I had read many years before and which dealt with the philosophy of symbolic forms.* Cassirer calls gestures reproductions of the inward in the outward, and presents a theory of the sign language whose forms he recognizes as imitative. The memory of that earlier book paved the way back to earlier thoughts about the concealed significance of gestures, thoughts that had occurred to me after that visit to the synagogue and after observing the strange position of the rabbi's hands at the blessing. I had thus returned to the old problem of the relation of religion and magic, and again turned my full attention to its possible solution.

It is easily recognized that the way to the solution of the prob-

* In three volumes (Berlin, 1923-1929). The translation of the first volume of the *Philosophy of Symbolic Forms* was published in 1954 by the Yale University Press.

lem was not smooth. All the various impressions I had received on different occasions, separated by long intervals, all the fragmentary and disconnected thoughts stimulated by them, were, so to speak, tossed into a mental pot. When I later saw what it boiled down to, I was astonished to find that it was a full theory of the transition phase from magic to religion. This theory surprisingly emerged as the result of the process of unconscious elaboration, as a concept that owed its existence to the confluence of several rivers of thought. It was astonishing to realize that certain thoughts, as it were, attracted others and merged with them, that there was an affinity between them and that an unconscious order controlled their movements. The space of our thought-processes seems to be infinite and chaotic. In reality it is finite and is controlled by invisible forces. The old cliché can also be used for the cosmos of ideas: It's a small world.

5

When we imagine Truth as one of the symbolic figures which, as Justice and Virtue, appear in pictures or sculpture a theory would correspond to her dress, and a person who formulates a theory could be compared to a dress designer. He designs a dress which will be exactly right for this particular lady, will be ideally suited to her figure and personality. The dress designer creates the best style, but he works in his imagination drawing the pattern. The dressmaker follows the designer's plan working directly with the material, and fits it to the lady herself. During the fitting it will be necessary to make allowances for the real figure of the lady, to make slight alterations, for instance, with regards to measurements. The dressmaker will perhaps lower the bodice or let out the waistline, and so on. In other words, he will have to take into account more precisely the realities of the figure which the dress designer considered in a more general way. There is no such thing as an ideal dress, because there is no ideal dress designer or dressmaker, nor are there measurements exact enough for perfect fit. The dress designer can be compared to the theorist, the dressmaker to the research worker who takes the pattern and fits it to the real facts. It is unavoidable that during the fitting some changes will have to be made before the dress fits the figure of Truth. There are, to continue the metaphor, bad and good dress designers and dressmakers. There are trends in research just as there are fashions in dress designing. The work of the dress designer is creative and imaginative, that of the dressmaker requires skill and labor, has to be precise and conscientious. In scientific research both processes are performed by the same person. The explorer conceives the theory and tries to verify it; he tests its value by investigating the facts.

The theory of a transition phase from magic to religion had to be verified on the basis of facts which the comparative history of religions and anthropology had collected and described. The study of the following months, taken up at the point where I had interrupted it more than three decades before, concerned, of course, the literature on the subject, especially an abundance of new books and articles, but it could follow a certain line through the manifold and many-sided material. All the experiences that had made their contribution to the formation of my theory had one factor in common: the central point of observation was the gestures and postures in magical rite and prayer.

When we think of spell and prayer as representative manifestations of magic and religion, we obviously think of a word or words as vehicles of their power. But words, and especially sentences or formulas as they appear in rites, are late developments of expression and communication. The more you study the ritual of the most primitive tribes and the culture of antiquity, the stronger will be your impression that the word served as the elucidation of the action, gesture, and posture. The language of the body is older than the spoken word; it is the primal and most primitive language. The visible expression of men was only much later replaced by the audible.* Scholars agree that voice language is already a substitute for body language. Missionaries and anthropologists who have lived many years among savage tribes state that the aborigines of Australia and Africa express much more by gestures than by words. For the nations of antiquity the exter-

* E. Saglio, *Adoratio* (Paris, 1877), p. 90.

nal actions of the ritual were of greatest importance. A scholar says that "they were religion itself." R. R. Marett asserts* that religion "according to the savage is essentially something you do," and lays special stress on the importance dance and rhythm had for the savage. "Religion pipes to him and he dances." The people of the Mediterranean, among whom civilization made the transition from magic to religion, would, as M. Jousse says,** "be without gestures like birds without wings." It is very well known that there are wordless magical rites, but it is less well known that there are prayers that are pure gestures, for instance in Japan and New Guinea,† godless prayers (*sine Deum*).

What is the concept of the scholars as to the origin and the meaning of the different gestures and postures in prayer, of those genuflections and prostrations, processions and circumambiences, of bendings and bowings, kissings, fondlings, and other caresses, turning and knocking, of clasped and raised hands, and so on? Just because those gestures and postures are traditional and come to us from prehistoric times, their interpretation is very difficult. While the older school of historians of religion did not hesitate to see in them a symbolization of the attitude of the worshiper to God, expressions of submission and surrender, of petition and reverence, the new school of comparative history considers these gestures remnants of magical practices aiming to secure the help of the gods or to protect an individual against their dangerous power. To convey an idea of this contrast, we need only compare the views of two representative scholars of two schools of thought on the same gesture—for instance, about the raising of hands in prayer. The German historian G. Meiners‡ is of the opinion that, in spreading out his arms, man tried to pull down the gifts that were slow in coming, and in great emergencies to force down quick help from the gods. Gold-

* *Faith, Hope and Charity in Primitive Religion* (New York, 1932), p. 11.
** *Methodologie de la psychologie du geste;* quoted by Thomas Ohm, *Die Gebetsgebärden der Völker und das Christentum* (Leiden, 1948), p. 90.
† Compare books on the gestures in prayer, quoted by Thomas Ohm and Friedrich Heiler, *Das Gebet* (München, 1923), p. 98-109.
‡ G. Meiners, *Allgemeine kritische Geschichte der Religionen* (Hannover, 1806/07), II, 272.

zieher* considers the raising of the hands in Islamic prayer a residue of old magic gestures. It was originally a gesture of cursing, and served as defense against evil demons.

The newest trend in the science of comparative religion does not deny that the magical interpretation of various prayer gestures contains correct elements, but is inclined to accept the older symbolic interpretation as the simpler and more obvious explanation. According to Friedrich Heiler, whose book on prayer is considered a classic in this field,** both interpretations neglect to refer to the customs of greeting. Heiler considers the gestures of profane salutation the key to understanding of prayer gestures and postures. Most of them were, he considers, and he tries to prove his point by abundant examples, originally gestures of salutation and respect, later on transformed into forms of petition. In the salutatory gestures, submission, reverence, and adoration, many kinds of *Socialgefühlen* find expression.

Heiler's reconstruction of the primal prayer gestures as residue of profane forms of social intercourse, especially of greetings, is nowadays accepted by many theologians and historians. The little that is justified in it, is, of course, adaptation of misunderstood or not understood, much older meanings to social customs of a newer phase of civilization. The concept represents one of the many superficialities in which science is so rich, and is hopelessly flat and rationalistic.

It is obvious that the gestures and postures of prayer date from different times, and that even the oldest of them have undergone some changes and were adjusted to different environments. Very few have kept their original meaning or, better, have returned to it in new, transformed shapes. Most of them are remnants of magic gestures by which man conjures something up by reproducing it or protects himself against something he is afraid of— for instance, evil coming from sorcerers or demons. We are certainly not able to penetrate the significance of all these magical gestures, but we can venture to express some informed guesses about the meaning of quite a few of them.

* J. Goldzieher, *Zauberelemente im islamischen Gebet* (Giessen, 1906), I, 303 ff.
** *Das Gebet* (5th edit.; Munich, 1923).

6

Returning to the various occasions on which the first decisive impressions about the meaning of such gestures were perceived in my experience, a survey reveals the character of those which mark the transition from magical to religious performance. You remember the instance of the young girl who put the book she studied under her pillow in order to remember its contents on the next day. Here we are still on the ground of pure magic. Compare the instance of the obsessional patient who was transfixed on the lamppost and was surprised to find himself with arms outstretched as Christ on His cross. The gesture and the words that occurred to him leave no doubt that the patient unconsciously identified with Christ. As a matter of fact, he felt released by that union with the Saviour. Progressing to the chronologically next impression in the same sphere, we remember the High Mass at which I experienced a decidedly uncanny feeling while looking at the Consecration. The actions and gestures of the priest, as representative of the community, prove that he is identified with Christ in the Sacrament. He not only speaks the words of the Lord, but renews in the "breaking of bread" the "tablefellowship" which the apostles shared with Him in His ministry. But the identification with God goes here far beyond the symbolic and reaches the oldest and most primitive manner of becoming one with the Deity: God is eaten by the community. In emptying the chalice and in eating the Host, the blood and flesh of the Saviour are incorporated in the most literal sense. Behind the Eucharist appears the image of the primitive totem meal in which the tribe periodically ate the worshiped totem animal with whom they renewed the bond of consanguinity. The position of the fingers when the priest raises his hands to his head and pronounces the blessing indicates that he has taken the part of the ram, of the primitive totem animal of the prehistoric Israelite tribes. In the person of the priest mimicking and disguising the sacred animal that was God, Jahweh appears before the descendant of the ancient Hebrews during the most solemn service, renewing the old covenant.

The congregations in the church and synagogue are identified in those rituals with their gods in the person of the priest who represents them, but also by means of their own gestures. Did we not see how frequently the faithful crossed themselves in church? And did we not see them covered by their shawls, swaying in prayer at the synagogue? Clearly, making the sign of the cross has the significance of sharing the fate of the Divine Victim. In the swaying in prayer we recognized a remnant of original danc- ing movements, a last trace of those mimetic dances in which ancient people and the savage tribes of the present imitate the totem animals whose descendants they consider themselves.

When we now return to the last occasion, the observation of the boy who in his playing changed into an engine, a steam- roller, a tiger, or a policeman, the circle we here draw is closed. The child does not pretend to be those objects, he does not act; he is, in his imagination, transformed into them. In observing the boy's behavior the magical character of his postures and gestures was conspicuous. He sometimes made noises imitating, for in- stance, a train leaving the station, but he did not speak except when asked by his mother "who" he "is." The metamorphosis was mainly performed by the omnipotence of movements or ges- tures. He became a lighthouse revolving and opening and closing his eyes. Here, certainly, is a magic performance expressed by gestures alone. An instance quoted by Fennichel* shows that the belief of children in the omnipotence of such gestures is not restricted to their own person: one child had the idea that when the conductor closes his eyes, the train passes through a tunnel.

Surveying the development from magical gesture to the ges- tures in prayer and liturgy in general, we dare to formulate a theory bridging the gap from magical to religious ritual and show the gradual change in the emotional attitude expressed in this evolution. In magic the person controls the course of events by gestures and spells. George Thompson has concisely written that "primitive magic rests on the principle that by creating the illusion that you control reality, you can actually control it." When religion entered the world of thought, primitive man did

* Otto Fennichel, *The Psychoanalytic Theory of Neurosis* (New York, 1945), p. 48.

not give up his belief in the omnipotence of his thoughts and wishes. He was afraid of the gods or demons, originally in the form of admired animals whose power he wanted to possess. In identifying with this totem animal (and later with the god in his anthropomorphic form), he had part in its strength and other coveted qualities. He became this admired god originally by taking him into his body, by eating the totem animal, later on by imitating its appearance and movements, by disguise and in mimetic dances. Thus transformed into God, he could still direct nature and fulfill his wishes because he became God. Only much later did he hesitantly make God his helper, and try to bend the will of the Deity in his favor by sacrifice and prayer. Even in this phase man had not entirely renounced his belief in his own power. He himself is not omnipotent any more, but powerful enough to influence the god to whom he has ceded most of his power. He now participates in the god's strength. The god who was once only feared gradually becomes a kind and benevolent being and an ally. He was threatening the person; now he is put into the service of his wishes, at his disposal whenever prayed to. "Whatsoever ye shall ask in my name, that I will do," says Christ. Magical incantation becomes prayer. For a long time God still retains the shape of an animal, of a tiger, an eagle, or a ram, but slowly becomes human and superhuman. He had already been asked to help and to assist with his superior strength as long as he was an admired totem animal. The tribesman who was afraid of him did not hesitate to assume that he would come to the rescue of his descendants.

An anecdote Otto Fennichel reports* presents the analogy of this attitude in the mental life of children. A mother asked her child not to open the door in her absence. She remembered after leaving the house that she had forgotten her keys, and rang the bell. The child did not answer for a long time, but finally he said, "Go away, you dirty thief, there is a huge lion here." From petition, from asking God for His assistance, from a childlike trust in Him and His power is a long way to resignation and subjecting oneself to His decision, to understanding of one's own weakness

* *The Psychoanalytic Theory of Neurosis*, p. 481.

and His might, to the heights of Christ's prayer: "Father, into Thy hands I commend my spirit." With such sublime surrender to the will of God, religion has reached the peak of its evolution, a peak neighbor to that other summit on which an agnostic bends to unchangeable laws of nature.

If we remain aware that subsequent phases are prepared by certain features of previous development and that no sharp demarcation lines can be drawn in primitive civilization, we can sketch the evolution from magic to religion in the following manner: In magic the person feels: "My will be done." In the phase of transition, we discovered, man has identified with the god whose superior power he has usurped and whose strength he has arrogated as his own. Full of self-confidence he now claims: "My will be done because I am God." In the following phase man acknowledged his weakness and helplessness and tried to secure the support of the Deity whom he influenced by prayer and sacrifice. The formula for this period can be stated: "My will be done with God's help." The principle of the last development is immortalized by the final words of the Lord's Prayer: "Thy will be done."

This characterization of the change from magic to prayer and its intermediary stages shows how difficult it was for man to renounce the belief in the omnipotence of his thoughts. The analytic method enabled us to bridge the gap which the science of history of civilization could not fill. Our finding of the missing link between primitive magic and earliest religious beliefs is certainly open to all kinds of argument, but, as far as my knowledge goes, no such theory has been published.

7

It is not up to me to decide whether the thesis here presented is valid, but to the scientists who have dedicated their lives to the study of prehistoric civilization and the history of religion. They would certainly not object if I myself express a little doubt before presenting my theory to their judgment, as follows: Is analysis of the gestures in magic and prayer not too slender and fragile a bridge to span the distance between the two areas? Is the carrying power of the bridge sufficient? The newer research of anthropologists and historians, like R. R. Marett, Th. Ohm, E. Saglio, and others will convince any unbiased reader that the role of words in primitive religion is of subordinate importance compared with its gesticulatory part. The omnipotence of movements, observed by psychoanalysts in early childhood, has here its collective counterpart. In the sense of my thesis this importance of the gesture can be followed up from the most primitive state of religion to its most elevated phase. The Bantu of Ruanda in Africa worship an animal god Mandwa Rumana.* At the initiation ritual of this bull-god the novices run around on all fours. In the Indian temple dances the postures of the images of the gods are imitated in such a way that each pose of the fingers and legs has a different significance of devotion.** The Mongolian Lamas in Tibet retire with the imago of the deity whom they have selected as their patron, in order to shape the body of this god by concentration in thought.† When at a late date magic was absorbed by religion, gestures originated in the older phase were taken over by the newer ritual, often acquired another significance, but sometimes remained almost unchanged.

Certain gestures of the fingers are still used for magical purposes, good or bad. Such a use is reflected in the story in Exodus that reports that Israel prevailed in battle when Moses held up his hand while Amalek prevailed when he let his hands down (Exod. 17:10 ff.). I cannot now pursue this thread through all forms and ages of religion and will restrict myself to a single representative instance which proves that the magical gesture has kept its meaningful significance in the religious concepts of today. The well-known minister of a Presbyterian church on Fifth Avenue in New York, John S. Bonnell, reports‡ in his recent book

---

* E. Johannsen, *Mysterien eines Bantuvolkes* (Leipzig, 1925), p. 38.
** Cf. Coomaraswamy, *The Mirror of Gesture*, quoted by Th. Ohm, *Die Gebetsgebärden*, p. 108.
† Cf. K. Bleichsteiner, *Die gelbe Kirche*, quoted by Ohm, p. 109.
‡ John Sutherland Bonnell, *The Practice and Power of Prayer* (New York, 1954), p. 12.

that he found himself overpowered by the subway crowd when he had to make a daily trip to the Presbyterian Medical Center at 168th Street. He had to share the subway with the swarm of jostling, perspiring, weary people and became uncomfortable and confused. "Then one day I happened to notice that my hand holding the strap in the center of swaying was lifted up in the attitude of prayer." It occurred to the pastor that all these men and women were also God's children on whom life was pressing hard, and that he should pray for them and himself. From then on the dread of the subway journey disappeared; praying for those around, he found peace of heart. Here is an excellent example of an individual case in which a certain attitude of the hand secured the symbolic-religious meaning of charity.

Such a sublimated meaning was given to most gestures which originally served magical purposes. The individual case just reported can well be compared with similar phenomena of congressional worship. I am choosing the habit of the swaying of Jews during their prayer, those movements of their bodies that made such a strange impression upon me when I attended the service. The explanations of that prayer habit that have become known to me are much too rationalistic. The *Encyclopedia Judaica* expresses the conjecture that the habit originated in circles of mystics and had the purpose of making the blood boil to transport the worshipers into an ecstatic state.* L. Dembitz presents, as the most rational explanation,** that the Jew has a nervous temperament and that he likes to speak with his whole body, not only to God, but also to his fellow-men. H. Fischer, who discusses the same habit of the Mohammedans in their devotions,† is of the opinion that prayer is spoken in a certain rhythm and "one is compelled by the movements of the body, to feel this rhythm, to experience the prayer." As will be remembered, the sight of the men swaying backward and forward in their prayers stimulated the idea that the movements are remnants of a ritual dance as it was performed by the Greeks in their crane dance, and by almost

* Vol. VII, p. 130.
** Lewis N. Dembitz, *Jewish Service in Synagogue and Homes* (Philadelphia, 1898), p. 301.
† "Ist der Islam modern?" *Moslem Review* 10, 1934, p. 63.

all primitive tribes of Australia and Africa at religious ceremonies in which they imitate their totem animals (compare the fox trot). This kind of worship, especially with masked dancers, can be called a prayer. The Tarahumare Indians of Mexico, for instance, think* that "the favor of the gods may be won by what, in want of a better term may be called dancing, but that in reality is a series of monotonous movements, a kind of rhythmical exercise, kept up sometimes for two nights. By dint of such hard work they think to prevail upon the gods to grant their prayers. . . . The Tarahumares assert that the dances have been taught them by the animals. . . ." (As an aside might here be inserted that a very intelligent priest, Monsignor Robert Hugh Bension has, compared the Catholic High Mass** with a religious symbolic dance, in which the gestures and movements of the priest are described as "figures.")

The meaning of the imitative and magical dance of primitive Bedouins who identified themselves with an animal god has been forgotten and lost to conscious thinking for many centuries. In its place a second, spiritualized—psychoanalysis calls it anagogic—interpretation for the habit of swaying had to be given by the theologians. They found it in the verse of Psalm 35:10: "All my bones shall say, Lord. . . ." Such reinterpretation of the significance of magical gestures is entirely in the spirit of the religious tradition that disavows the past when a certain state of progress is once reached.

The great Rabbi Israel Baal Schem Tov, the founder of the sect of Hasidim (1699), who considered prayer as the great way to union with God, was aglow with unsuppressed emotions when he prayed. His opponents laughed at his swaying and grimacing in prayer, but Rabbi Israel told his disciples the following story: There was once a wedding feast. The musicians sat in a corner and played upon their instruments, and the guests danced to the tunes and made merry. They swayed this way and that way, and the house was filled with noise and joy. A deaf man passed the house and looked in through the window and saw the people

* *Encyclopedia of Religion and Ethics*, IX, 361.
** *Papers of a Paria* (New York, 1913). Compare the remarks of Ronald Knox in *The Mass in Slow Motion* (New York, 1948).

whirling about the room, leaping and throwing about their arms. "How they fling themselves about," he cried out. "This is a house filled with madmen." For he could not hear the music to which they danced.* It is very likely that we, too, have become deaf to the music that propels the praying people and cannot see any sense in their gestures. The essential result of this analytic exploration is the reconstruction of an until now undiscovered transition phase from magical ritual to prayer. We did not forget that after an interval of forty years my interest in the problem was reawakened by the editorials in the *New Statesman*. The president of the National Farmer's Union has asked the Archbishop of York to call for prayers for fine weather. A debate started on the question of whether the Deity can be cajoled by the rainmakers. Even in this collective petition, the belief in magic continues to live and operate.

In the first World War a poem described a worried God listening to all the prayers for victory from the Germans, the French, the Britons, and the Russians. God sighs, "My God, I've got my work cut out." It is prescribed to Him by His believers. Prayer is only the last link of a chain which began with the belief in the magical power of man's own thoughts and desires. In this phase we discovered man still believes in his own magic in identifying with the god or totem animal. Secretly, he will always believe in it and listen to that tempting, false promise he had already heard in paradise: "You shall be as God knowing the good and evil. . . ."

V

1

THERE are coincidences which seem to have significance even for those of us who are not superstitious. It certainly was coincidental that I read on two successive days some magazine

* Jacob S. Minkin, *The Romance of Hasidim* (New York, 1935), p. 90.

articles in which the malignant spirit of the Pharaoh was discussed. It was not accidental that this casual reading reawakened interest in a subject that had preoccupied my thoughts when I was eighteen years old. An American magazine reported that the two little daughters of an Egyptologist who had assisted in the discovery of the two solar ships of Cheops beside the Great Pyramid of Gizeh had suddenly died. The journalist linked these deaths in mysterious connection with the spirit of the Pharaoh whose solar ships were unearthed. On the next day an issue of the Paris *Match** fell into my hands: in it two special correspondents sent to Cairo presented in an article, illustrated by wonderful colored photographs, the story of the discovery of the tomb of Tutankhamen by Carter and Lord Carnarvon. The article, written in sensational terms, tried to revive the romance of that nineteen-year-old Pharaoh whose wife put flowers on his golden coffin at his funeral thirty-three hundred years ago. A tiny wreath of flowers was found around the symbols on the forehead of her husband. The vivid description of the life and of the treasures of Tutankhamen is followed by the story of the Pharaoh's curse.

The article revives the memory of the story of a mummy's vengeance, a story we all heard back in 1923, when that perhaps most important of all archeological discoveries was made in the Valley of the Kings. From 1923 to the beginning of the thirties we heard story after story of "the curse of the Pharaohs." The legend started when Lord Carnarvon, the Maecenas and friend of Howard Carter, died on April 6, 1923, from the effects of a mosquito bite. People began to talk about a punishment the spirit had visited on the disturber of his resting place. The world press of the following years had headlines like "New Victim of the Curse of Tutankhamen." The nineteenth victim, the seventy-eight-year-old Lord Westbury, committed suicide. He was the father of the former secretary of Howard Carter: his son had been found dead in his apartment the year before. Archibald Douglas Reid, who was going to X-ray the mummy, suddenly died. Also the Egyptologist Arthur Weigall, who had discussed that super-

* No. 287 (Sept. 25-Oct. 2, 1954).

stition of the curse of the Pharaoh, died of an "unknown fever." He was considered the twenty-first victim of the Pharaoh's vengeance. Howard Carter's partner, A. C. Mace, who had assisted his friend in his work on the tomb, died; he had been ailing for a long time, it is true; Lord Carnarvon's half-brother, Aubrey Herbert, committed suicide, and Lady Elizabeth Carnarvon died in February, 1929. A man named Carter died under mysterious circumstances in the United States. He appeared as the latest victim of the Pharaoh.

Howard Carter, who had discovered the tomb, continued to live. He died many years later (in February, 1939). He himself condemned the "ridiculous" stories of Tutankhamen as a form of "literary amusement," adding that "in some respects our moral progress is less obvious than kindly people generally believe." The German Egyptologist George Steindorff emphatically stated that there is no such thing as the curse of the Pharaoh. Also Carter himself wrote: "So far as the living are concerned, curses of this nature have no place in the Egyptian ritual." The protective formulas found inscribed on the magical mannikins left in the burial chamber like "Death will come on swift pinions to those who disturb the rest of the Pharaoh," were designed to frighten away the enemies of Osiris, the deceased king. Yet, the legend of the Pharaoh's vengeance continued to live. More than twenty years after the discovery of Tutankhamen's cadaver, a report from the atom city Oak Ridge expressed the guess that the ancient Egyptians had known the secret of the atom and had put radioactive stones into their tomb whose rays were fatal after many thousand years. Arthur Weigall, who functioned as general inspector of antiquities for the Egyptian government, expressed another view which seemed to be more appropriate. In his book dealing with the discovery of Tutankhamen, the scholar quotes several examples of curses found in Egyptian sepulchers, for instance, the inscription written upon a mortuary statue of a certain Ursu.* Ursu, who was a mining engineer and lived less than a hundred years before the times of the young Pharaoh, composed the following curse: "He who trespasses upon my

* *Tutankhamen and Other Essays* (London, 1923), p. 111.

property or who shall injure my tomb or drag out my mummy, the Sun-God shall punish him. He shall not bequeath his goods to his children; his heart shall have no pleasure in life; he shall not receive water [for his spirit to drink] in the tomb and his soul shall be destroyed for ever." On the wall of the tomb of Harkhut, at Aswân, dating from the Sixth Dynasty, these words are written: "As for any man who shall enter into this tomb . . . I shall pounce upon him as on a bird, he shall be judged for it by the great God." Such curses, Weigall says, should have frightened the tomb robbers who already systematically plundered the sarcophagus of the dead Pharaoh and whose activity reached a peak during the Twentieth Dynasty.

We know that thieves broke into the tomb of Tutankhamen within ten years after his death. In Weigall's opinion, only the robbers would come under the curse. The mummy and the tomb were the earthly home of the disembodied spirit, and the fear of the Pharaohs was that robbers might desecrate their graves and endanger their permanent security by destruction of the mummy. By the beginning of the Eighteenth Dynasty hardly a mummy remained undamaged in the vicinity of Thebes, and almost all royal tombs had been robbed. The consuming fear of a Pharaoh thus concerned the integrity of his mummy around which the soul of the king hovered. Weigall emphasizes the factor of this fear that the tomb and the body might be broken up and argues that the "scientific excavators whose object is to rescue the dead from oblivion which the years have produced might be expected to be blessed rather than cursed for what they do." Weigall himself reports some uncanny experiences from his Egyptian excavations, but doubts that "the possibilities of that much underrated factor in life's events, coincidence, have been exhausted" in the search of an explanation of many tragic events of that kind. While he considers the rumor of the malevolence of the ancient mummies nonsense, he tries "to keep an open mind on the subject." A German writer, Otto Neubert, who visited the tomb of Tutankhamen at the time when Carter discovered it, adds some new data in a book published in 1952.* He tells us

* *Tut-ench-Amun, Götterfluch und Abendland* (Hamburg, 1952).

that Lord Carnarvon died from the bite of a scorpion, not of a mosquito, and the scorpion was a sacred animal in ancient Egypt. He quotes a fellah who said about the daring excavators; "Those people will find gold and death," and reports that the nurse who took care of Lord Carnarvon in his illness soon died.

He tells a story he had heard during his visit in the Valley of Kings from Howard Carter, who also told it to Arthur Weigall. During the excavations that led to the discovery of the tomb, Carter had in his house a canary bird who sang happily. On the day on which the entrance to the tomb was laid bare, a cobra entered the house and swallowed the bird. People imagined that the cobra was the spirit of the newly found Pharaoh, especially since the Pharaoh wore the form of the royal cobra on his forehead, symbolizing his power to strike and sting his enemies. It was at the end of this season's work that Lord Carnarvon was mysteriously stung upon the face. Mr. Neubert seems to believe in the vengeance of the dead Pharaoh. The sovereignty of his logic allows him to overlook the fact that the discoverer of the tomb, Carter, continued to live to an old age, that most Egyptologists, working with Carter, as well as hundreds of workers remained unharmed, and that he himself, Mr. Otto Neubert, is, as he assures us, hale and hearty twenty-five years after his visit to the fatal sepulchral chamber.

When, at the end of 1922, the mummy of Tutankhamen was found, I followed the news of the excavations with great attention and interest in that summit of archaeological success. The description of the fabulous treasures found and of all the commodities for the dead king fascinated me. Such accumulation of riches energetically contradicted the contemporary opinion that "you can't take it with you." The succession of tragic deaths and illnesses marking the path of many Egyptologists who collaborated with Carter intrigued me, as it did most people, but, strangely enough, I never felt the intense feeling of uncanniness they experienced at the mystery. The spooky events made, of course, an impression upon me, but there was none of that emotional reaction observed in many educated people around me. It could not have been that I was specially insensitive to uncanny sensations, because I had sometimes experienced the uncanny in life and fiction with considerable intensity. Only much later it occurred to me why I was relatively unaffected by the reports of the malignant spirit of the Pharaoh. I had been intensively preoccupied with that same problem sixteen years before the discovery in the Valley of the Kings, and had then been stirred up by an experience which had made a strong uncanny impression upon me. People say that lightning does not strike the same spot twice.

2

My father died in the summer of 1906 when I had just reached my eighteenth year. I have described and analyzed the emotional upheaval following that event elsewhere.* Guilt feelings and remorse tortured me, an upsurge of sexual impulses frightened me, and I was the helpless victim of an inner conflict that lasted almost a year. A few days after my father's funeral I picked up a book entitled *Der König von Sidon* by Paul Lindau in a lending library. The name of the writer was then unknown to me,** and the title promised a historical novel. The book made a mysterious and lasting impression upon me; its plot entered my dreams of that time and I identified myself with the leading figure. After reading it, I misplaced it and found it again several years later. It is the only book from my young years I still possess, and whenever I now see it I still remember that I had to pay the lending library for it—I was very poor—and I think of the unconscious motivation of that symptomatic misplacement which resulted in my keeping it.

Not only the style of printing, but the red box framing each page and the decorations at the head of the chapters are old-fashioned. Its style and diction, typical of German writing at the turn of the century, is also hopelessly out of date. Here is the outline of the plot: A young archaeologist, Andreas Moeller, who is devoted to his science, gets a long-expected telegram from Constantinople calling him to Saida, the modern site of ancient

* *Fragment of a Great Confession* (New York: Farrar, Straus and Co., 1949).
** *The King of Sidon* was published in 1898. Paul Lindau was a well-known Berlin writer of novels, plays, and travel books.

Sidon, to co-operate on excavations with Hamdy Bey, nominated as conservator of antiquities by the Turkish government. Moeller, now lecturer on archaeology at Berlin University, is still young, but already well known because he had deciphered a mysterious Phoenician inscription and thus earned the respect of the famous French scholar, Ernest Renan. Moeller lives in a boarding house; he is a tall, narrow-chested man of an almost pastoral appearance, a bookworm, and rather lonely. A few weeks before, his landlady, who respects him highly, had asked him to give a young girl who lives in the same house and takes stenographic dictation some information about the spelling of an ancient Phoenician name. The girl Sabine appears; she is employed by Dr. Scholl, a younger colleague and student of Moeller. The name she cannot spell for her stenographic record is that of Eschmunazar, the King of Sidon, son of Tabnit. Andreas Moeller tells her how to spell the name and mentions the anthropoid sarcophagus in which Eschmunazar was buried and which was discovered in 1855. He also explains the meaning of the word anthropoid as manlike, resembling the face and body of the dead who rests in the shrine of the mummy.

During the following weeks Andreas Moeller falls in love with the pretty, simple girl, asks her to help him as a stenographer, and is confused by the contradictory emotions his romantic feeling awakens in him. Being with his attractive neighbor, who now transcribes what he dictates, he feels elated and his work makes excellent progress. The relationship between the young professor and the secretary becomes more and more friendly, yet Moeller is still too shy to declare his love for Sabine. He feels slightly jealous of Dr. Scholl for whom Sabine still works. The telegram from Constantinople calling him to the excavations near Beirut throws him into a conflict. Here is a long-desired opportunity to make what may be important archaeological discoveries, but he must separate from Sabine whom he now loves. There were perhaps archaeological findings of greatest scientific value to be made down there between the Lebanon and the sea.

Sabine encourages his wish to leave as soon as possible, and when he tries to speak of his feelings for her advises him to write to her on his journey. He lands in Syria, always thinking of the beloved girl, and finally writes her asking her to marry him after his return. Arrived at Beirut, he can scarcely control his impatience to hurry to the place where Hamdy Bey, in the meantime, has discovered wonderful Greek sarcophagi. The German consul and his gracious young wife treat him with great hospitality, but he is driven to reach Sidon as soon as possible. His guide, an old Arab, Hassan, brings him in a few hours to the place where Hamdy Bey meets him, welcomes him with all signs of friendship, and leads him to the shaft in the rock. Deeply stirred up, he admires the wonderful coffins and cannot fall asleep for a long time.

The following weeks are filled with work and with dreams and daydreams in which the young archaeologist imagines new findings. His health suffers as a result of his morbid zeal which does not allow him any rest and because of the Mediterranean climate to which he is not accustomed. He is enthusiastic about the marvelous Greek sarcophagi whose walls are covered with colored figures in perfect relief, and he is filled with a passionate desire to be the first to discover a beautiful prehistoric sarcophagus. When the newly found treasures are finally brought on board the ship which brings them safely to Stambul, Andreas refuses to leave. In spite of all the pleading of his friend, who is afraid that Andreas is ill, he declares he wants to stay. Left alone he writes Sabine who has not answered his proposal, and tells her of the strong impressions he has received and of his desire to awaken one of the proud sleepers of the prehistoric past to new life. He cannot leave; it would be like a cowardly flight, like stealing away deceitfully without paying his debt to destiny.

In feverish unrest he descends into the shaft and finally finds an unsuspected opening in a corner of the ceiling of the sepulchral chamber. The hole is enlarged, the walls of the rock removed, and behind them an empty room is found. It is a rock grave, and remnants of human bones are on the ground. A terrible smell of decay in the small, sticky room makes him feel exhausted. On the next morning he starts again to search for a still undiscovered second shaft. Tortured by impatience, he has to stay in bed for several days. Scarcely convalescing he discovers a gigantic block of stone and, after it is removed by long, hard work, a cranny. When the light of his lamp falls into the depths, he trembles as he sees an immense sarcophagus of black stone. Who is the proud, lonely sleeper hiding in this recess? Andreas feels blood rushing to his head; his pulse hammers. Drops of perspiration are on his forehead and an anxiety, never before experienced, makes him choke. . . . Alone he stands before the anthropoid sarcophagus from which a face with wide-open eyes seems to smile at him, and discovers a hieroglyphic inscription which he deciphers. The dead one is Tabnit, King of Sidon, father of Eschmunazar. Shaken by fever, he looks at the signs which seem to revolve like a terrible merry-go-round. The last words he can speak are a command to Hassan to wash and brush the walls of the sarcophagus: he is seized by a fainting fit and breaks down beside the sarcophagus. On waking he looks at the mortal remnants of the man who had once been a great and mighty king here on earth. Andreas, looking long at the cadaver, feels that a terrifying, threatening glance from the empty sockets of the eyes is directed at him and steps back. He kneels down beside the stone and, fingering the letter groups with the left hand, jots with his trembling right the translation of the engraved hieroglyphs. They say: "I, Tabnit, priest of Astarte, King of Sidon, am resting alone in this chest. Whoever thou art who discovers it, man, do not open my death closet. Do not disturb my rest. Neither silver nor gold nor other precious things are to be found with me. I am alone in my closet. Do not open it because doing it is an abomination before Astarte. If thou open my death closet and disturb my rest, thou shalt have no rest on earth. The blood shall boil in thy veins. The woman whom thou lovest shall forsake thee. Thy mind shall become confused. Thy limbs shall grow stiff. Thou shalt be a living corpse and when thou die, thou shall continue to live without rest. Thus is the will of Astarte. And thus it is pronounced to thee by her priest, Tabnit, King of Sidon."

When Andreas has finished the record after several hours, he timidly steals away, putting his left hand like a blinker at his temple so as not to see the priest of cruel Astarte whose curse echoes in him. He runs as if haunted to his home, pursued by the furious glance of the king who has cursed him. He closes his eyes so as not to see the irate look and wants to cover his ears so as not to hear the words "Thou shalt have no rest on earth." He wants to barricade himself in his room and close windows and doors against intrusion. When he arrives at his room, he finds a letter from Sabine, forwarded by the German consul in Beirut. The girl writes that she feels honored by his proposal and that she admires him, but has become engaged to Dr. Scholl. He seems to hear that voice: "The woman whom thou lovest shall forsake thee. . . ." When old Hassan enters, he shouts at him, "Don't you know before whom you stand? I am the King of Sidon. Get out." His mind becomes confused and his limbs grow stiff. He takes a carton on which Hamdy Bey had sketched a blueprint of the shaft and slowly writes angular lines and round marks. Then he extinguishes the lamp and walks slowly to his bed. Hassan finds his body the next day. Round his head a towel is tied covering the forehead and the hair, the arms are pressed on the body. A sheet covers the body closely so that the form is delineated only at a few places. At the foot of the bed is a white carton covered with Semitic characters. Many months later a young archaeologist is told about the carton considered to be an inscription play of the dying scholar. The young archaeologist states that the three lines are beautiful and correct Semitic hieroglyphs and, fingering the groups of characters and reading from right to left, he deciphers them: "Let no one dare to disturb my rest! I am the King of Sidon."

3

My experience in life and in reading fiction has been such that strong impressions I receive are not lasting. Their power exhausts itself, so to speak, in the emotional explosion of the moment. There are other impressions which have no immediate intense effect but whose emotional power increases with time. The novel *The King of Sidon* belongs to the second group. While reading it, I felt, of course, that special emotion of uncanniness, but the feeling was not strong and was soon mastered. But images awakened by the novel occurred to me repeatedly during the next months. The impression grew with distance from the time when I had put the book aside, which meant in this instance so carefully away that it could not be found again. What had happened to the archaeologist Andreas Moeller had got under my mental skin. It crept into my dreams and often intruded on trains of thoughts which were very remote from the characters and the plot of the story many weeks after I had read it.

Much later I understood that the uncanny impression during the reading of the novel was in more than one way intimately connected with the emotions stirred up by the death of my father. My rational thinking fought vainly in those weeks against superstitious beliefs that he continued to live in some form of existence and knew what I did and thought. I tried to shake off remorse because I had often caused him grief and had fallen short of his expectations. A furious ambition that had been alien to me until then had taken hold of me, and I daydreamed I would accomplish something remarkable to honor the name of my father. I did not know yet what I would study, but I was determined that I would discover something of importance in that field. Here already was a trace of my unconscious identification with the archaeologist Andreas Moeller. Another symptom of mental preoccupation with that story was that I felt a strange interest in the history of the Phoenicians. During high-school years I had not learned much about that ancient people and biblical lessons provided no more than a smattering on the subject of their relations with the Hebrews. Strangely enough, I had not fully realized that they were, so to speak, cousins of my ancestors, that their language differed only as a dialect from the Moabite and Hebrew, and that they also wrote those square letters found in Hebrew inscriptions.

Some passages of Paul Lindau's story had the character of a straight report of facts, as if the discovery of that mummy of Tabnit and the death of the archaeologist had really taken place. It was mentioned, for instance, that Andreas Moeller's archaeological work had awakened the interest of Ernest Renan, who recommended the young scholar to the department of antiquities of the Turkish government. The name of Ernest Renan was known to me as that of a historian of religion, especially of early

Christianity (*La Vie de Jésus*), but I soon learned that the French orientalist had been on an archaeological mission in Phoenicia from which he had brought back valuable inscriptions to Paris.* I wrote Paul Lindau asking him whether the plot of his story was founded on real events, but received no answer. I no longer remember how and where I found out that the tomb of Tabnit was really dug up near the site of ancient Sidon. O. Hamdy Bey, director of the Musée Impériale de Constantinople, and his collaborators discovered that well-preserved anthropoid sarcophagus of black stone covered with Phoenician hieroglyphs. Hamdy Bey is introduced into Lindau's story, and also the terrible heat in the sepulchral chamber as well as the fever and fatigue of which Hamdy Bey speaks reappear. The writer had followed the report presented by Hamdy Bey and created only the figure of the German scholar, Andreas Moeller. Hamdy Bey even mentions that he was a bit scared of becoming the victim of the curse of the priest-king whose tomb he had opened and whose mummy he transported in an ordinary box of zinc. ("*Je m'attendais un peu d'être l'objet d'une malédiction . . . de la part du vieux roi prêtre, dont j'avais ouvert sans scrupule la chambre sépulcrale et dont j'emportais le corps dans une vulgaire boîte de zinc. . . .*") Théodore Reinach has presented a scientific report on the discovery of Tabnit's mummy and the translation and historic evaluation of the inscriptions found in the tomb in the second volume of a scholarly work published in 1892.** I still remember with what interest I read the explanations of the French archaeologist, and that I, a boy of eighteen, identified with the prominent French archaeologist who had the same first name as I. It seems to me that he and Andreas Moeller of Lindau's story became merged into a single figure in my ambitious and ambiguous daydreams during those months.

I understood only later the personal note in the impression which that second-rate novel had made upon me: it hit home, the home which had just been struck by the death of my father. All the ambivalent feelings toward the deceased were brought close

* Published in his *Mission en Phoenicie* (Paris, 1864).
** Théodore Reinach and O. Hamdy Bey, *La Nécropole Royale à Sidon* (Paris, 1892-96).

to the threshold of pre-conscious thoughts by the novel. Here were love and hate, honor and disgrace; here were furious hunger for achievement, burning ambition and its punishment. Here the goal and the price you had to pay for reaching it. Here were the mystery and majesty of death.

In the forty-eight years since that summer I have sometimes been reminded of Paul Lindau's story, but it was never in connection with any personal experience. Certain clinical cases of obsessional neurosis, especially those whose compulsive thoughts circled around the problem of death and of life after death, reawakened the memory of the fate of that archaeologist in the story. I recall a case in which a younger man complained about strange pains in his breast. The medical examination showed there was no organic cause for those painful sensations. I did not understand the unconscious motivation of the mysterious symptom for several weeks. One day the patient again complained about the pain and described it with the words, "It is as if a heavy stone had been put on my breast." A few minutes before he had spoken of the unveiling of a tombstone for his father at which he had been present. It dawned on me only then that he had unconsciously identified with his dead father in his grave. I am omitting other cases which brought that story back to my mind because their presentation would lead us too far astray.

The reading of the article in the Paris *Match* as well as the paragraphs in the American magazine about the calamity in the family of an Egyptologist who had co-operated in the unearthing of Cheops' solar ship had reawakened my interest in the superstitious fear connected with the excavation of ancient sarcophagi. In pursuing certain thoughts about the psychology of those fears, I again recalled the plot of Lindau's story. When I read it again, the uncanny feeling had almost disappeared or was only present like the faint echo of a forgotten tune, but I realized why the report about the twenty-one victims of Tutankhamen's curse had made a much weaker impression than the novel about the vicissitudes of a German archaeologist. The uncanny feeling I experienced reading the novel had been more intense than that occasioned by the contemporary news account of the havoc caused by the malignant spirit of the Pharaoh. Fiction was stranger than life in this case, because the interest awakened in the story concerned the fateful events in the life of an individual, while in the news report, the very accumulation of victims of Tutankhamen proved injurious to the psychological effect. It moves me more when I hear that an old man who lived in the next house, and whom I have seen once or twice on the street, died from hunger than does a report in the newspaper that a thousand people perished in a famine-stricken part of China. The news in one case concerns a human destiny, the other is almost a matter of statistics—such is life. Furthermore, it cannot be denied that the vividly presented details in the novel contributed to its interest, while the enumeration of Tutankhamen's victims made an impression almost like that of a list of also-rans, or rather of also-rans to the grave. Adding to these factors the personal significance the book had for me at the time will make it understandable why the rumor of Tutankhamen's curse affected me less than the tale of the malediction of Tabnit, King of Sidon, priest of Astarte. Our age and personal circumstances at the time we read a book often give it an experiential meaning which is not commmensurate with its artistic value.

My reawakened interest in those superstitious beliefs was not concerned with the facts reported—if facts they were—but with the psychological factors, with the origin and motives of the fear aroused by excavation of the mummy. Those superstitions were obviously not of recent date; they could be traced back to the dawn of history. What were the roots of those magical beliefs? To understand them one has to study the development of the concept of death to be found in the traditions of ancient peoples, has to understand how they felt and thought about the relationship between the living and the dead, the prehistoric and later ways of burial and disposal of bodies, how ancestor worship developed, and so on. From all we know of the complicated burial customs, the artificial preservation of the body and the elaborate care provided for it belong to a relatively late phase of Egyptian history. The paleolithic natives of Egypt buried their dead in rock shelters. In the earlier stages of the evolution of humanity little attention was paid to the disposal of the dead. How did this desire to preserve the dead as long as possible to "those on earth who love life and hate death," as an Egyptian funeral prayer says, develop? What were the Pharaohs afraid of when, still young and healthy, they made careful provision for the preservation and protection of their mummies? What were the living afraid of when they entered the tomb chambers, of what the excavators who transported the coffins to the light of day? What was the nature of the desecration inflicted on the mummy, and why those terrible curses threatening anybody who disturbs the rest of the dead? It is easy to understand that the mummy was considered the habitat of the Pharaohs for whose life after death so many objects were prepared when they were buried, but that does not explain the deep-rooted fear, the superstition that whoever digs the body up will die.

That fear of the vengeance of the dead cannot be traced back to the belief of taboo, of the dead killing anyone who touches the body or any object belonging to the dead king. That power works like electricity, which must be insulated lest it blast the unwary. Its effect is automatic and indiscriminate. It destroys at touch. The concept of primitive taboo cannot be separated from contagion. "Everything," says Jevons, "which comes in contact with a tabooed person or thing becomes itself as dangerous as the original object, becomes a fresh centre of infection. . . ."* Nothing of this kind has been observed in the case of Tutankhamen's mummy. There is not a trace of infectious unluckiness for the hundreds of fellahs who touched the coffin, nor for the many who carried and transported it until it landed in the glass cases of the museum of Cairo. This immunity would be impossible if the magical nature of the mummy were that of a tabooed object. The mummy would not have spared the lives of many hundred visitors, workers, and newspapermen who touched it. And did not Howard Carter who discovered Tutankhamen in his hiding place live many years after having examined the body and the four shrines? The mummy of Tutankhamen was, it seems, highly discriminating and made a careful selection among those who approached it. The taboo belongs without any doubt to a rudimentary phase of social and religious development, but the

* F. B. Jevons, *An Introduction to the History of Religion* (London, 1896), p. 61 f.

fear-inspiring character of the curse of the Pharaohs is of a much more primitive, one would almost say, primeval kind. There is a secret that cannot be reached by rational thinking and rationalistic arguments. Was there a desire or an urge in the primitive mind that has been lost with growing civilization, a barbaric concept we can no longer fathom? What is the nature of that nameless and impending dread?

We know that the mummy was the earthly home of the disembodied spirit, and the identity of the living corpse depended on its remaining inviolate and intact, but we can guess that such a belief is already a late and secondary concept. What is concealed behind the fear that the mummy might be injured? Those terrible curses from the tomb, the threats of death and perdition to anybody who meddles with the dead king or his property, are difficult to understand, if we exclude taboo as the principle of explanation. Yet that belief is older than the taboo fear, is, so to speak, an ancestor from which the taboo superstitions descended. All elaborate protective measures concern the body and its sacredness; yet it is not the body as such, but some spiritual factor represented in the body. Here is, it seems, an idea that is so archaïc it is utterly alien to us. We too preserve the bodies of our dead and take care of their tombs, but we cannot imagine inscriptions in our cemeteries threatening any intruder with annihilation and death. But is the spirit of those curses really so utterly alien to us? Is it not rather alienated? Is the way of thinking expressed in those threats really so remote from our own? If it belonged to a circle of prehistoric superstitions entirely inaccessible to our ideas, we would be unable to feel what prompted Shakespeare to write those lines for his epitaph:

> Good friend, for Jesu's sake forbear
> To dig the dust enclosed here.
> Blest be the man that spares the stones,
> And curst be he that moves my bones.

Here is a curse quite similar to that of the Egyptian Pharaohs and of the Phoenician kings almost four thousand years later. And do we not detect an echo of the same feeling when we in the funeral Mass wish an undisturbed rest for the dead (*Requiescat in pace*)?

In studying the rich material which the history of burial customs of ancient peoples provides and in searching for a clue to the secret of those curses, I had arrived at certain provisional hypotheses comparing the Egyptian provisions and protections for the mummy with obsessional thoughts of neurotics about life in the beyond. I assumed that at the concealed core of the fears that led to the development of such elaborate measures for the body was a special, single fear of damage to some of its parts, and that this particular fear had been displaced and generalized to the mummy and its property. Such assumptions are harmless as long as you remain aware of their character as preliminary attempts at the elucidation of puzzling things, and as long as you do not confuse them with a valid explanation. They have a suspicious resemblance to the daydreams of an explorer, having in common the fact that they produce a temporary feeling of gratification.

In my case, such transient satisfaction was disturbed by two facts. Some of the features found in the material of my study did not tally with that assumption. One need not give up a hypothesis because of such minor contradictions, but they serve as warnings to be especially cautious, because they sometimes lead to the discovery of irreconcilable and fundamental inconsistencies. The second factor was equally discontenting and came as a surprise: at a certain moment of my research—I do not know where and when—the odd idea occurred to me that I had read or heard some French sentence which contained the clue I searched for.

What were the words of the sentence? I tortured my memory in vain for many weeks. Among the many French words or phrases occurring to me, there were a few which seemed to refer to the subject under discussion in my thoughts in one way or another, but none that opened an avenue to the solution of the problem of the Pharaoh's curse. There was, for instance, that old exclamation "*Le roi est mort, vive le roi!*" but how did it relate to the Pharaoh except by the title of royalty? I remembered that sentence saying that the dead have to be killed ("*Ce sont les morts qu'il faut qu'on tue*"), but in it is only reflected the thought that the living had better lay their ghosts. One is scarcely allowed to stretch the meaning of that sentence so far that the excavation of a mummy could be brought under that heading. For some time the French phrase I had forgotten played hide-and-seek with me, but it did not let itself be found. (I read somewhere the definition of a little girl: "Memory is what I forget things with.") I sought for it at all possible and quite a few impossible places. Had I read it in the issue of the Paris *Match?* It was not there nor in Théodore Reinach's report giving full details of the objects in Tabnit's tomb. It was not in the few French books and articles by Egyptologists I had read in the last months. Had I perhaps heard it in Paris or read it in a French novel? Such questions remained, of course, unanswered, since I had not the slightest notion of what the forgotten phrase had said or meant; only the fact (or was it a delusion?) that it provided the solution of that problem.

Don't get me wrong! The idea that a lost sentence contained the answer to the question was not welcome to me. It did not come as a guest, but as an intruder into the home of my thoughts. It did not appeal to me because I had marched along on a certain path and I did not like to learn that I had taken the wrong turn, that the right path was somewhere else, and that I was not told where. It is a most uncomfortable situation to know that something exists somewhere and not be able to catch it, to possess something that is not available. At that time I had not the slightest inkling that the phrase I sought was being shut away by myself, that it was a repressed idea which eluded me because I did not want to catch and face it. Only after I found it in a strange way did I realize that the phrase had been kept prisoner in the underground vault by myself, that I had been its unconscious jailer.

The point of departure for my hypothesis had been that the careful preservation of a mummy was a custom founded on emotional reactions to intense aggressive and hostile feelings toward the deceased Pharaoh, a reaction-formation of a structure similar to those to be found in the symptoms of obsessional neuroses. My recent notion that a forgotten French sentence pointed in another direction shook the beautiful trust I had in my thesis. It was the first indication of a surprise awaiting me: what I was driving at was very different from what I was driven by.

<h1 style="text-align:center">4</h1>

It was a strange situation: there were some French words or sentences, the key to the problem, but the key was lost and the door could not be opened. Actually, the key was not lost, it was only misplaced, or rather had been put unconsciously into an excellent hiding place. I found it just as I was ready to give up the project of exploring the subject. I wanted to turn my attention to other themes, but all of them mysteriously led my thoughts back to the problem I wished to put away.

The great German dramatist Christian Friedrich Hebbel, whose works are almost unknown in this country, wrote, looking back to his youth, in his diary: "First the cup is lacking, then the wine." Youth has an overflow of ideas and does not know how to put them into shape. Old age has learned the method, but there is a scarcity of new ideas. Thus I returned in my thoughts to the projects that had preoccupied me in younger years, and all ways of thinking led, often on strange detours, to that problem of the relationship of the living and the dead, and indirectly to the curse of Tutankhamen and Tabnit.

When I had finally decided to drop the research plan on this subject, that inaccessible French sentence suddenly sprang up in a dream. The dream is unique in my personal experience because it is the only one in which the solution of a problem presented itself to me. I know that I do not belong, alas, to the chosen ones to whom the Lord unveils His secrets in their sleep.

Before going to bed I had cleared the deck, that is to say, I had tried to bring about an appearance of orderliness to the helter-skelter of books, magazines, and manuscripts that littered my desk. Among the scattered things were the many sheets on which notes on Tutankhamen, burial customs, Egyptian prehistory, and primitive ancestor worship were jotted down. I looked at them before I put them together and into a folder, to be sunk in the depths of one of the drawers. So much work and no result! When

I put the Paris *Match* away, the magazine opened to the pages which showed the beautiful pictures of Tutankhamen's mummy and its shrines and of the objects found in the tomb. It was very stupid of me not to have taken the train from Alexandria to Cairo when I was in Egypt on my way to Palestine in 1937. I was then too eager to see my son in Jerusalem; I should have allowed myself a week's sojourn in Cairo. I could have seen the golden coffin of the Pharaoh and the other treasures of the museum. What a pity! I should have at least gone on a tour with other tourists to the Pyramids. The memory of a movie recently seen, *Valley of Kings*, emerged. In the movie people ride to that famous necropolis on camels. The plot of the picture was worse than melodramatic, it was almost moronic, but the photography showing the desert landscape, the colossal statues of the kings, and the tombs of the Pharaohs was exciting. I should have gone there. I have never ridden on a camel.

This was my last thought before falling asleep. I woke up in the middle of the night and felt that well-known pressure from my gallstones. I took decholine from the medicine chest and tried in vain to fall asleep again. Lying there in the dark, I was prey to all kinds of depressing thoughts. There was no pain, but an intense discomfort. If painful attacks should occur, an operation will be unavoidable. I put on the light and smoked a cigarette, but it did not taste good. It occurred to me that a few years ago I had severe pains in the throat which were not alleviated by gargling or drugs. I had been worried and had consulted Dr. Vogl. The excellent physician carefully examined me and smilingly said, "Not every prominent psychoanalyst has to die of cancer of the throat." He wrote a prescription and the complaint soon disappeared.

The visual picture of Freud as I saw him last emerges: a very old man, his beard white, his hands covered with wrinkles. . . . I really should give up the study on Tutankhamen's vengeance and spend my time, rather, on the translation of the letters Freud wrote me. Did I not promise John Farrar to deliver the manuscript before New Years? . . . I now have permission from the Freud Foundation in London to publish the letters. What is it that makes me postpone the work? . . . I was always a good procrastinator and there was never a lack of self-excuse. . . . What would Freud himself have said to the publication of his letters? . . . He would not have objected to it. . . . He allowed me to publish his letter on Dostoyevsky and wished only a few sentences concerning personal things to be excluded. . . . But he once declared that he was quite indifferent to what was published about him after his death. He did not believe in an existence in the beyond. I remember the remarks he made about it in a conversation with George Sylvester Viereck in London. . . . Yet I have some scruples about publishing certain passages in his letters to me. He would perhaps have frowned on it, although they, too, show that he was one of the noblest of men.

The pressure in the gall-bladder region was still acutely felt. . . . I must have made a mistake in my diet, perhaps eaten some fat. . . . What did I eat at dinner? I cannot remember. No use trying to sleep. I took a new book which I had begun reading earlier in the week. . . . It is the report a French missionary, André Dupeyrat, wrote about the twenty-one years he spent among the barbaric Papuans in New Guinea.* It is a realistic portrayal of the life and customs of a truly barbaric race of humans who still live as their remote ancestors did in the Stone Age. Father Dupeyrat penetrated a region of Papua never visited by a white man, where cannibalism still flourishes. He describes, for instance, how one of his native friends called Golopoui once took him to his hut. When he crawled through the narrow doorway into the oppressive atmosphere of the dark hut, he saw two skulls and some human bones on the floor. They were shiny and polished like ivory. The priest asked the Negro where his parents were. "They're here," said the man, and pointed to one of the skulls with his big toe. "That is my father and that one is my mother." Without the least embarrassment he told the priest that his parents became old and feeble, and that he realized that their time had come. He asked friends in another village to take care of them. They invited the old couple to a banquet at their village, where they brained them with clubs, cut the bodies up, cooked them in a stone oven, and ate them. "Afterward they

* *Savage Papua: A Missionary among Cannibals* (New York, 1954).

washed and cleaned the bones and I brought them back here. You can see what good care I take of them. . . . But then, I am a dutiful son." Father Dupeyrat gives other descriptions of such horrifying repasts at which the Papuans drink bowlfuls of liquid from the body with avid movements of their tongues. Once the priest was told that the natives ate the flesh of their dead chief to absorb his strength and other virtues.

I put the book aside before I had read its last pages, and fell asleep. The dream that followed was like a novel. Some psychoanalysts assert that we all become poets when we dream, and many of those productions of our fantasy resemble novels. It is rare that my dreams have this character, but I remember that some of them have made the same impression as a long story. They were dreamed when I was young. The dream of this night was not simply a succession of isolated pictures, but was really like a novel or a movie. Such an exception does not contradict the assumption of my lack of imagination. This dream used, in the main, material from the novel, *The King of Sidon*, as well as from the report of the discovery of Tutankhamen's mummy, a real event whose fantastic character surpasses the imagination of most science-fiction writers.

Here is the dream: *I am in an airplane that flies over Alexandria and slowly descends. I am looking at the Pyramids and the wide planes of yellow sand surrounding them. I am riding at a gallop on a camel, and I am wearing high cavalry boots. I am giving the spurs to the camel. Our cavalcade arrives at the foot of colossal figures of Pharaohs. I dismount easily and throw the reins to a fellah who is waiting. I am entering the sepulchral chamber of an Egyptian or Phoenician king, but it is, at the same time, the hut of a savage tribesman. There are human bones on the ground covered by leaves. It is very hot and there is a stench. It is windy. It is very dark, but I have an electric torch which I turn around. The chamber is crammed with precious things piled up. The flashlight falls on an anthropoid sarcophagus. The first thing I see is a gigantic canary bird with widely spread wings, sitting on the breast of the mummy. There is a snake about to jump at the canary which will devour it. I know it is the death bird. It opens its beak and sings in a very low, ghostlike voice. The mummy is an old man with a white beard. He looks at me with wide-open unblinking eyes. The canary has stopped singing. There is a silence without end. On the sarcophagus is an inscription in hieroglyphs like Hebrew letters. I am reading the lines from right to left. It is not difficult. I stand near the sarcophagus, but I cannot move. I am scared stiff. In the midst of the long silence a voice says in slow singsong: "Qui mange du Pharaoh en meurt." I have always known it. A feeling of relief. I feel great.*

I am not sure whether the last sentences still belong to the dream, they may be a part of the beginning of conscious thinking. It is doubtful whether the words "I have always known it" mean that I have always known that whoever eats of the Pharaoh dies or that I have always known that sentence. The latter is more likely, because, immediately when I awoke, I recognized that this was the elusive phrase for which I had searched so long in my memory. Not trusting the forces of repression that had so often pulled a dream clearly remembered at awakening back into the unconscious, I jotted down its text and began, comfortably leaning on a pillow, its analysis.

I am in an airplane that flies over Alexandria and slowly descends. I am looking at the Pyramids and the wide planes of yellow sand surrounding them. These first sentences revive the memory of my trip to Palestine in 1937 when I really landed in Alexandria. Why is the dream renewing those impressions? In making order on my desk and putting the notes on Tutankhamen away, I had thought of the journey and had regretted missing the opportunity to see the Valley of the Kings. The dream gives me a second chance in starting again at this point. *I am riding at a gallop on a camel and I am wearing high cavalry boots. I am giving the spurs to the camel.* The grotesque picture of wearing cavalry boots and giving the camel the spurs has the following origin: In the film *Valley of Kings,* seen a few days before the dream, a group of people are riding camels in an easy trot to the tombs. In a later sequence, a sandstorm surprises them and they ride at a furious gallop to escape it. Looking at the scene, I had wondered what it would be like to ride on a camel in such a situation. It seemed difficult. The dream disposes of this doubt, reminding me that I had been a good rider when in the Austrian army in World War I. I treat the camel as if it were a horse, giving it the spurs. It is quite easy to ride on a galloping camel. Transferring the scene from the picture to the dream, this scene expresses my impatience to see as soon as possible the ancient monuments, the grandeur that was Egypt. *Our cavalcade arrives at the foot of colossal figures of Pharaohs.* This also is taken from the movie. In the picture a man walks on the arm of a statue. The colossal sizes of the kings' statues, so often seen in photographs but vividly presented in the film, had impressed me. *I dismount easily and throw the reins to a fellah who is waiting.* Memories of such situations in which I, as an officer, returning from riding, threw the reins to the soldier who took care of the stable. The easy dismounting from the camel removes the doubt that it would not be as easy to jump off a camel as a horse.

So far, so to speak, we have the prologue to the play. What follows is the central scene of the dream, in which I discover the subterranean tomb of a prehistoric Pharaoh. *I am entering the sepulchral chamber of an Egyptian or Phoenician king, but it is, at the same time, the hut of a savage tribesman.* This scene fulfills the ambitious wish to make discoveries as sensational as those of Howard Carter and Andreas Moeller in *The King of Sidon*, at the same time to find something remarkable in the field of psychoanalysis. We are accustomed in thought and speech to conceiving of the unconscious as a subterranean region of the mind, and to comparing our work with that of archaeologists. In this particular case the secret meaning of the curse of the Pharaoh, and specifically that French phrase, the keywords in the literary and metaphorical sense, are to be dug up. The dream exaggerates the importance of this possibility, comparing such a finding with the great discoveries of archaeology. *There are human bones on the ground covered by leaves.* Again impressions from the book *Savage Papua*, read before falling asleep, where Father Dupeyrat sees human bones covered with leaves in the hut of a native. *It is very hot and there is a stench.* Again taken from the description of the French priest. The bad odor appears in his tale, but I am suspicious that in this dream element at the same time there is perception of a bad smell, of the flatulence of my own digestive process. *It is windy.* The feature of strong wind was perhaps stimulated by the perception of the weather and of the fluttering curtains at the half-open windows. I surmise that it concerns also gas in the bowels. *It is very dark, but I have an electric torch which I turn around.* Taken from the movie in which an old tomb in the Valley of the Kings is found. Carter also used electric light. *The chamber is crammed with precious things piled up. The flashlight falls on an anthropoid sarcophagus.* The chamber piled with precious things is, of course, the tomb of Tutankhamen of which I have seen so many pictures, the last ones in the Paris *Match.* At the same time the room is that of Freud, in which there were many Egyptian and Etruscan antiquities. As during the whole dream, the sepulchral chamber also represents the intestines. The crammed feeling concerns the bowels. In sleep the need to empty them is perceived. The contents of the chamber thus also symbolize feces (contrast: gold, ebony, precious things). The word "anthropoid" is taken from *The King of Sidon* in which the archaeologist Moeller explains the meaning of the word (as equaling "manlike") to Sabine with whom he fell in love. The dream makes a compound of the two discoveries of the sarcophagi of Tutankhamen and Tabnit. I am identified with the discoverers of both mummies.

A scene repeats the experience of Howard Carter who describes the appearance of the sarcophagus: *The first thing I see is a gigantic canary bird with widely spread wings, sitting on the breast of the mummy. There is a snake about to jump at the canary which will devour it.* The canary bird appeared in the story Carter told Weigall and Neubert. The small singer was devoured by a cobra. Some people saw in that incident a bad omen, especially since the newly found Pharaoh had worn the symbol of a cobra on his forehead. On the breast of Tutankhamen's mummy the soul bird, protecting the Pharaoh with widespread wings, was modeled. *I know it is the death bird. It opens its beak and sings in a very low, ghostlike voice.* The expectation of impending doom for myself in the role of the sacrilegious disturber of the Pharaoh's hiding place. There is an allusion also to a sexual theme in which the canary represents a penis symbol. The allusion uses not only the general sexual symbol of the bird, but also associations of Vienna slang. The vulgar expression corresponding to the English word "fuck" is in Vienna *vögeln,* alluding to the erection of the penis. The death bird has nothing to do with the findings in the tomb. The element is taken from associations arising while reading books on ancient Egyptian theories about life in the beyond. The memory of the last movement of Mahler's Second Symphony had occurred to me during the reading. In this movement the composer presents a sound picture of the day of last judgment, when the dead rise from the grave and the Great Summons sounds in the Valley of Jehoshaphat. The dead march to their court. They tremble and quiver with fear because none is just before God. In the words of Mahler himself: "Finally, after all had cried out in the worst turmoil, only the long-lasting voice of the death bird from the last grave remained." Here, thus, is the low, ghostlike song of the canary: an omen of the terrible fate awaiting me.

As readers of my last book *The Haunting Melody* know, the tunes of the last movement of the Second Symphony of Mahler pursued me in a meaningful way after the death of my friend Karl Abraham.* The resurrection chorus unconsciously became the musical leitmotif of my ambition, of a silly wish to become immortal by my accomplishments. I do not know why at this point *The Magic Flute* by Mozart occurred to me, but then I remembered that the voice of the death bird in Mahler's symphony is imitated by a flute. This cannot be the only associative connection. Other, more important ones emerged later on. *The mummy is an old man with a white beard.* The old man with the white beard is, of course, Freud, but also my father. *He looks at me with wide-open, unblinking eyes.* The wide-open eyes appear in the etching of Freud at his desk by the Viennese artist Max Pollak. The picture hangs in my room. The unblinking eyes were a peculiarity of a patient I had seen a few days before. It made an odd impression that the man blinked his eyes so rarely.

* *The Haunting Melody* (New York: Farrar, Straus and Young, 1953).

The canary has stopped singing. As in Mahler's symphony the death bird before a long pause. Again a sexual allusion: The bird that becomes silent equals being unable to reach an erection. Threat of impotence. *There is a silence without end.* Again from Mahler's symphony. The silence without end is, of course, that of death.

On the sarcophagus is an inscription in hieroglyphs like Hebrew letters. I am reading the lines from right to left. It is not difficult. A conglomerate made up of various materials. The hieroglyphs are taken from descriptions of Tutankhamen's grave, but the Hebrew letters are a slight distortion of the inscription on the Phoenician sarcophagus. I had read that Phoenician letters in their early forms are practically identical with those of Hebrew. Also the Phoenician language belonged to that North Semitic Canaanite which includes Hebrew. The inscription also represent, of course, letters of Freud which I will translate and publish. I am excavating Freud in publishing memories and letters of his. Hebrew and Phoenician are read from right to left. When I was a boy, I was taught to read Hebrew by my grandfather and did it quite well. I can scarcely read it any more and regret that. The dream also fulfills the wish to understand Hebrew. Andreas Moeller in Lindau's story, with whom I identify in the dream, is an authority on Semitic languages and reads and translates the Phoenician inscription on Tabnit's sarcophagus quite easily. *I stand near the sarcophagus, but I cannot move.* Taken from *The King of Sidon* where Andreas Moeller stands near and kneels down on the sarcophagus. I cannot move, like Moeller who felt his limbs grow stiff in accordance with the curse of Tabnit, priest of Astarte. I am as terrified as he who stepped back in awe of the lonely sleeper who had provided a concealed recess for his body. The inability to move is, as so often in dreams, an indication of a powerful inhibition. It concerns my hesitancy to penetrate further the realm of the secret of Pharaoh's curse. Deeper than this: I cannot bring myself to publish the Freud letters, to excavate the body of the beloved man.

I am scared stiff. The word "stiff" has in this context several meanings: scared stiff is a well-known colloquialism, but the word "stiff" has also the sexual connotation of the erected penis. I had recently read the slang expression "a stiff," denoting a corpse in a mystery story. A high degree of condensation is reached in this dream element which includes not only paralysis by fear, but also the contradictory meanings of intense sexual desire, indicated by a strong erection, and of the state of death. As other elements in this dream this one is very overdetermined. *In the midst of the long silence a voice says in slow singsong . . .* The voice is my own; at the same time that of Tutankhamen and other Pharaohs or of the god Osiris into whom the Pharaoh is transformed after death. Where does the feature of singsong come from? In *The King of Sidon* as the young archaeologist dictates his scientific paper on Phoenician prehistory to the girl, he sometimes falls into Semitic singsong when he recites inscriptions. Here also is an echo of the monotonous up-and-down rhythm in which the Code of the Old Testament is recited in the Jewish service. The voice does not emphasize the words it speaks. It does not sound solemn, but sober as a judge, as the Supreme Judge on judgment day. Thus the singsong has a parodistic touch as if to make fun of the expected or feared verdict.

The whole sequence of events also points to the last movement of Mahler's Second Symphony: after the death bird has sung, there is a long silence as in the dream. Then the chorale sets in, at first mysteriously and darkly, until it leads to the powerful unison of voices. Their message says or rather sings that resurrection is a certainty and that there is no punishment in the beyond, that suffering has not been in vain and that wishes and ambitions will be fulfilled: "I shall die to live. . . ." It seems here that I treat the resurrection chorale, which appeared to me in my young days as a prediction of power and glory, very irreverently, calling it singsong. I make fun of its message of resurrection and of a life in the beyond. (While I write this, a sentence Anatole France once wrote in a review of a novel by Paul Bourget occurs to me: "If we may believe Mr. Bourget, none of us can help arriving in paradise—unless there is no paradise, which is very likely.") At the same time I express my disbelief:

I do not believe in nor care for becoming immortal by achieving something remarkable. Again the ambivalent attitude to my youthful striving for accomplishment and fame. *"Qui mange du Pharaoh en meurt."* At first sight or sound, this is the verdict on the criminal who has done an unspeakable thing. But the second consideration says that the voice is not laying down the law, but quoting it. What happens here is not that sentence is pronounced, but that a sentence is recited. What sentence? Of course, the phrase for which I searched so long, that French sentence with the keywords, unraveling the mystery of Tutankhamen's and Tabnit's curses.

The sentence proclaiming that who eats of the Pharaoh dies as a result is, of course, the center and climax of the dream. The manifest content of it seems to make sense. It is coherent and consistent and forms a whole. On the surface there is a story; a beginning, middle, and end: I go to Egypt and discover a mummy, like Carter; decipher a hieroglyphic inscription, like Andreas Moeller in the novel. The dream obviously fulfills an ambitious wish of this kind. In the dream I experience the panic I imagined is connected with disturbing the peace of the dead Pharaoh and I hear the sentence pronounced: I have to die. So far so good. There are at least two factors disturbing the appearance of unity and continuity of the dream tale. Let me introduce their psychological evaluation by pointing out that the sentence "Who eats of the Pharaoh dies" does not correspond to the exposition or the premises of the plot. Howard Carter, Andreas Moeller, and Theodor Reik—who is identified with the two archaeologists in his dream—have not eaten the body of the Pharaoh, but have discovered it. Now it is conceivable that the crime we committed in digging up the mummy could be called cannibalism by the stretch of a Shakespearean fantasy. And, as a matter of fact, Shakespeare makes Queen Margaret call her son's murderers "bloody cannibals" (*King Henry VI*, Part III, V, v, 61). They at least were killers, but we, on the contrary, have given new life to the hidden bodies of the kings. Not to mention that such a use of the term "cannibal" is even, in abuse, alien to us who are not contemporaries of the virginal Elizabeth. The phrase stating that the eater of the Pharaoh dies must have a meaning within the dream, because each part of the dream content is psychologically determined, but the eating of the Pharaoh does not tally with the plot.

We remember at the right moment that it corresponds rather to something else, to one of the important day remnants of which the dream is made. Before that sentence there is a dream part saying that human bones are on the ground covered by leaves. But this feature, like several others, is taken from the description of life with the cannibalistic Papuans. In his report the French missionary describes in a matter-of-fact way the Papuans' bloody meals. No human bones were, of course, found in the tombs of Tutankhamen or Tabnit. And now it occurs to me that the dream itself points to the book *Savage Papua* as one of its sources: in it I am entering the sepulchral chamber of an Egyptian or Phoenician king, but it is at the same time the hut of a savage tribesman. How does this sound? If it is not sheer nonsense—and we do not believe that dreams are nonsensical—it can only mean that there is in my thought some connection—perhaps a comparison?—between the prehistoric Egyptians and the Papuans in faraway New Guinea. Be that as it may, there is no doubt that *"Qui mange du Pharaoh"* corresponds to the tales the French missionary tells about the man-eating Papuans.

The best is yet to come. For a moment I had the impression that Father Dupeyrat's being French had something to do with the emergence of that French sentence in my dream, but then I remembered that I had searched for a lost French phrase which would unveil the mystery of the Pharaoh's curse many months before reading the book *Savage Papua*. The only connection could be that the author's French nationality had reawakened the idea of that forgotten sentence, had revived the wish to call it to mind. In the middle of such reflections it struck me suddenly that that French sentence I heard in my dream is not correct. In reality, the proverb says: *"Qui mange du Pape en meurt"* ("Who eats of the Pope, dies of it"). The saying, I was told later, originated at the time when the exiled popes resided in Avignon, and it means, of course, that whoever attacks the Pope has to fear the worst. But the dream changed this meaning in two directions: it took the word *mange,* "eats," literally, as the presence of human bones and the allusion to the cannibalistic Papuans show. It thus returned from the metaphorical to the crude, realistic meaning of the word. Furthermore, the dream replaced the Pope with the Pharaoh, so that the person who eats of the Pharaoh has forfeited his life.

The first change is easily understandable; it fits the story which deals with the discovery of a prehistoric Pharaoh. In ancient Egyptian religion the place of the Pharaoh not only equals but transcends the status of the Pope in the Catholic Church. The Pharaoh not only represented the highest mundane and religious authority, he was the god Osiris himself, on earth and in the beyond. One can say that the dream transferred the French saying into the Valley of the Kings, and thus had to replace the Pope by the Pharaoh in the interests of coherence and local color. It is as if an American play were produced in London, and the director replaced American names and places by familiar English proper names, so that the English audience could understand the meaning of allusions, and so on. Yet even such a transformation must have its secret significance in the dream, and has a certain bearing on its unconscious meaning. The change must also serve another purpose. Here, clearly, is a gap in the dream content, a gap similar to that we found before between the excavating and eating of the Pharaoh—perhaps it is the same, seen from a different point of view. "Once more unto the breach, dear friends, once more!" One would like to shout with Henry V.

The unconscious memory of the lost French sentence was awakened by reading the book about the Papuans. Of course, that's it! The title! From *Savage Papua* to *Pape,* the French word for Pope (compare papacy) was not far. The fact that the book was written by a French Catholic priest helped, of course, to push the forgotten sentence still nearer to the threshold of pre-conscious thinking. These two factors joined an ardent wish to remember those keywords, and their combined efforts succeeded in calling them up from unconscious depths. But why didn't the saying appear in its original form? Why not *"Qui mange du Pape en meurt"?*

We have already said the saying had to be changed in the interests of uniformity and coherency with the manifest dream text. But there is another, more important, reason. In its original form the word *Pape* is easily recalled by its sound connection with Papua. (The word Papua is derived from a Maluccan word which means "frizzy" or "curly," used to designate people with curly or frizzy hair.*) It is not only adaptation to the new environment, the Egyptian milieu, which is responsible for the replacement, but also the avoidance of the word *Pape*, which equals "father." The expression *Pape* had to be avoided because it was too close for comfort, namely, to the idea of eating one's father. Consider that the dream also returns in its language to a kind of children's talk. We called our father Papa. The dream takes the word *Pape* as if it were Papa. Here is an instance of such literal-mindedness in children: The German word for parrot is *Papagei*. When my son Arthur was a small boy, a parrot was shown to him and its name was mentioned. Arthur asked, "Where is the Mamagei?"

It is the experience of almost all analysts who have interpreted many dreams—and I am an old hand at it—that the emotions felt in dreams can be considered a more reliable clue than the logical sequence, which is often deceptive. After hearing that sentence which sounds like a verdict, I do not feel like a person about to die, but, instead, *a feeling of relief*. That surely does not correspond to the character of impending capital punishment.

The logic of the manifest dream content seems to be stringent and conclusive: after I have committed the abominable crime of entering the sepulchral chamber, I hear that sentence pronounced. But all surface logic in the dream is only apparent and specious. Those treacherous cracks in the dream structure indicate that there is a secret compartment behind the open sections of the dream. The appearance of unity and continuity is already a result of the secondary elaboration operating in the dream production to give it the appearance of a logical or reasonable tale. The result is make-believe, or rather make-me-believe, which means pretense before the dreamer who remembers his vision after he awakens. The wish forming the dream was not a desire

* *Encyclopedia of Religion and Ethics,* IX, 628.

to discover the sarcophagus of a Pharaoh or of a Phoenician king, but to find out the secret of the curses threatening the discoverer. In order to find that out, I had in my dream to take the place of an archaeologist discovering a mummy and to have the same emotional experience.

The basic wish of the dream does not aim at archaeological findings, but at a psychological discovery in the field of archaeology, at the solution of a problem that prehistorical and archaeological research had not been able to master. The unraveling of that puzzle was, in my unconscious thoughts, connected with a forgotten French sentence. And what is the central scene of the dream? That French sentence is found, is spoken. After I have experienced awe and fear, after recognizing the approach of doom, a voice—a voice within me—unveils the secret: Who eats of the Pharaoh, dies of it. In other words, the curse of the Pharaohs originally had as its purpose frightening away those who approached the body of the Pharaoh in order to eat a part of it. That seems to be an atrocious statement, but this is not the appropriate moment to discuss its validity, but merely its presence in the dream. There can be no doubt that is what the French phrase says and what I recognize as the keywords, as the clue to the mystery of the Pharaoh's curse. The following sentence of the dream text confirms it: *I have always known it.* This concerns both: I always knew somewhere—namely, unconsciously—the French sentence, and I have always known that intimidation of cannibalism was the primeval purpose of those mysterious curses. *A feeling of relief* is connected with the finding of that phrase at last, but also with the cheerful certainty of having arrived at the solution. The last sentence of the dream text, *I feel great,* is the natural continuation of that exalted feeling in the sense of American colloquialism: I feel very good or fine. At the same time, it is a last echo of that megalomaniac idea that I achieved something remarkable in solving that problem of prehistory.

I do not know whether or not the last three sentences were thought in the minutes of awakening. They denote the emotional state or mood in which I found myself when I emerged from the dream. Also the ambiguity of the expression "I feel great" shows that this sentence belongs to the transition phase of the dream. While I sometimes felt "great" in the sense of that colloquialism, I never—except in dreams—considered myself a "great man." Dreaming can be compared to a ride in one of those tunnels of love in our amusement parks. You enter a tunnel in which you see wonderful and terrifying pictures, heroes and monsters, beauties and witches, fantastic landscapes and palaces. You start the ride in full daylight, and then gradually it gets darker and darker until suddenly those pictures appear. Entering and leaving the tunnel your eyes adjust themselves to the darkness and to daylight. There are similar threshold sensations in gliding from conscious thinking into the region of dreams and in the transition phase from the dreamland to the realm of material reality. The last sentences of the dream belong, it seems to me, to that no-man's land, to the in-between region.

5

While I immediately recognized the French sentence as the one I had so long been seeking, I, too, was at first taken in by the pretense of logic and consistency in the dream. I considered the French phrase the death sentence for myself, the criminal who had committed an outrageous sacrilege. It is the purpose of elaboration to make the secret meaning of the dream unrecognizable to the dreamer. It succeeded for just a minute, but then those minor inconsistencies paved the way to a better psychological understanding. The appearance of consistency and continuity is not only the work of the primary dream process, but also of the censorship operating while the dream is produced and interfering with too frank an expression of the impulses that are satisfied in it. I am choosing a single part of the dream to prove my point, the bird that reminded me of Mr. Carter's canary and with it of the superstitious belief that the spirit of the Pharaoh in the shape of a cobra devoured the cheerful singer. In the dream, too, this is a warning in symbolic form. When the bird ceases to sing there is silence without end, the silence of death. But does it not rather express a fear of death? Identified

with Carter and Andreas Moeller, I feel that intense anxiety before opening the lid of the sarcophagus and facing the body of
the Pharaoh. (The reader has certainly not forgotten that behind
this fear is hidden the hesitancy to publish the letters of Freud,
as if this would be a sacrilege against the dead man.)

The canary is the death bird whose song is heard in Mahler's
Resurrection Symphony. In the dream as in the symphony, the
last sounds of the bird are followed by long silence. But while
this silence is ended by the voice pronouncing the sentence in
the dream, in Mahler's symphony it is followed by the relieving
and releasing hymn which proclaims that there is no punishment,
there is only reward for the striving of men, the message of immortality.

Here then, is a full reversal of the panic on judgment day. All
inner circumstantial evidence, contradicting the manifest dream
content with its deceptive appearance of homogeneousness,
points in the same direction. Also found in the dream is a release from anxiety; a sentence is not pronounced, but a lost sentence is found. My goal is reached.

It will be remembered that in my thought-associations to the
death bird *The Magic Flute* surprisingly emerged. The connecting link was the fact that the sounds of the death bird in Mahler's symphony (as those of the bird in *The Drunkard in Spring*
of *The Song of the Earth*) are produced by a flute or a piccolo.
But this thought-association led far beyond this point. In the
simple fairy tale-like plot of Mozart's last opera a serpent appears
pursuing Tamino into a cave. But not only that, there is Papa-
geno who sings *"Der Vogelfänger bin ich ja"* ("A fowler merry
and gay am I") and appears with a large birdcage and various
birds (the canary and the cobra!). Not only that, there is the subterranean temple of the second act. No doubt, the cult of that
secret society is Egyptian. The priest Sarastro sings that beautiful aria:

> O Isis and Osiris, grant
> The spirit of wisdom

The goddess has imposed a holy silence on Tamino who, under
the spell of Sarastro, has to undergo various ordeals so that he

may become a member of that secret circle. Here, too, as in Mahler's symphony are increasing fear, rising to panic, and then sudden release from fear. Here, too, is the wonderful message that there is no punishment, or vengeance, a message sung in an Egyptian temple! And the words?

In diesen heil'gen Hallen
Kennt man die Rache nicht.

Within these sacred halls
Dire vengeance is unknown.

It is certainly accidental that the resurrection chorale and this aria of Sarastro's proclaim essentially the same message. It is not accidental that both musical works emerged in my thought-associations into which they were introduced by the death bird. In both works the dread of death is suddenly removed and replaced by the certainty of immortality. In both works the trembling creature is reassured that there is neither punishment nor vengeance. In both Mozart's opera and Mahler's symphony the struggle ends with the triumph of the hero. In those two works as in my dream the long silence is relieved by a momentous message. The last shred of doubt is removed: the French sentence of my dream does not proclaim death, but conquest of the fear of death. Only much later another concealed connection between Mozart's opera and thoughts on Freud emerged: *The Magic Flute* symbolizes the rise and ideals of Freemasonry in which Mozart was very much interested. Freud was a brother of the Jewish Freemason organization B'nai B'rith in Vienna, and so was I. Here is an allusion to certain ideas on Judaism common to both of us, and to the ideals of that brotherhood. On Freud's seventieth birthday I wrote a salutation in the magazine of the B'nai B'rith. Freud liked the phrasing of the article and thanked me in a letter praising a passage.

From here a train of thoughts leads again to his letters, their personal character, and the problem of their publication. Although there is not the slightest reason against publication—there are many for it—I unconsciously considered it a kind of profanation of Freud. Why? Every letter of his does credit to his memory which I hold sacred. Yet the inner dispute about publi-

cation of the Freud letters is one of the important day remnants
for the dream, in which translating and commenting on these
letters was the same as the excavation of the mummy of an
Egyptian Pharaoh. All this sounds absurd, but we remember at
the right moment that the discovery of Tutankhamen's body was
an immortalization of the dead king in the eyes of science, while
superstition considered it a desecration of the Pharaoh. It is also
meaningful that the publication of the Freud letters took in my
thoughts the place vacated by giving up research on the Egyptian
problem. We have to wait for an explanation of what this replacement means.

While the conflict about the Freud letters was the secret psychological source of some significant dream thoughts, the perception of pressure from the gallstones was the somatic stimulus
determining their formation. This physical complaint, felt just
before the dream, led to thoughts about a possible mistake in my
diet and to doubts about what I had eaten at dinner. The dream
picks up this thread and draws it to the point where it joins that
other thread of Pharaoh's curse. If I am the sacrilegious criminal
who has eaten from Pharaoh's body, this would be a mistake in
my diet indeed, and we are not in the least surprised that the
meal did not agree with me. But that sounds fantastic and ludicrous and leaves us with a feeling of suspense because we cannot
imagine its meaning.

With those uncertainties and unanswered problems, we have
already entered the central theme of the dream and of the discovery supposedly conveyed by that French sentence. The French
phrase was supposed to be the key to the problem of the superstition concerning the excavation of Egyptian mummies. At the
same time, it should explain the reason for those terrible curses
dreadening the intruders. If we tentatively assume that the
French proverb really presents in a few words the quintessence of
the answer to this question, a radical change in my first hypothesis becomes necessary. Two assumptions of that original approach
to the problem can, however, remain intact, when we believe
that the original purpose of Pharaoh's curses was the intimidation
of cannibalistic desecrators of their bodies. The first is that the
superstitious fear was of a much older date than the highly de-

veloped religious system of dynastic Egypt. It must have had its roots in a past in which cannibalistic impulses were still very much alive and intensively felt, so that a strong and efficient warning was necessary. That fear certainly antedated the development of the highly complicated pantheon of Egyptian gods, but also the careful preparation for the burial and preservation of the body. The custom of hiding and protecting the cadaver was already a manifestation of a new morality that fought against the old barbaric impulses, long before the Egyptian gods had established their regimen. The battle against cannibalistic appetites of the original natives of Egypt lasted perhaps many hundred, if not a few thousand, years, and accompanied the most significant phase of development from savagery to primitive culture. That means it reached from early prehistory to the dawn of the first Egyptian dynasties and beyond that phase. Religion then became the strongest weapon and the firmest stronghold in the defense against cannibalistic impulses, and the gods were the most energetic protectors of the dead. We know that cannibalism has been practically uprooted among the North African tribes who were man-eaters, through the increasing influence of Mohammedanism.*

Father Dupeyrat's report shows that Christianity in New Guinea is slowly and gradually gaining ground in its endeavor to make the Papuans renounce their cannibalistic practices. In a similar way, the fear of punishment by the cruel gods of Egypt and Syria was once used to deter the barbaric natives of those countries. The names of gods later appear in inscriptions and curses in the sepulchral chambers, those narrow cells which the Egyptians called "houses of eternity." The primal purpose of the protection of bodies became repressed in a later phase and was replaced by more developed religious and magical concepts in the preservation of the dead and of their possessions. The late belief in an existence in the beyond as the most important idea of Egyptian religion covers and conceals earlier measures of defense to prevent the survivors from eating parts of the body. The second assumption is that the superstition, expressed most vividly

* *Encyclopedia of Religion and Ethics,* Vol. III.

in the fear of the Pharaoh's curse, does not belong to the category of the taboo, but to a much older and more primitive stage of cultural development, even when it continued to live far into the time of blossoming Egyptian civilization. Those superstitions do not show the characteristics of the taboo that operates automatically. The fear of tabooed objects and persons makes curses and warnings superfluous. If the superstition partook of the nature of taboo, the inscriptions on sarcophagi and tombs would not necessarily put the fear of God, in this case of Osiris and Astarte, into the clansmen.

The next and most urgent question at this point is, of course, the validity of the view that the origin of that superstitious fear is the belief that eating parts of Pharaoh's body will be punished by death. Instead of discussing the merits and demerits of this hypothesis, which can only be examined by historians of ancient civilization and Egyptologists, I shall try to find how that view unconsciously emerged in my thoughts. While I studied the historical works of Egyptologists like Petrie, Breasted, John A. Wilson, and others, I received certain impressions about the power and glory of the Pharaohs. The Pharaoh represented the sun-god Ra or Osiris, or his son Horus. But increasing knowledge provides us with clues pointing to the fact that, at the dawn of Egyptian history, the divine kings of the tribes on the Upper Nile were slain before old age: "Behind the impressive figure of the omnipotent and deified Pharaoh looms the shadow of a divine king as Frazer depicted him, who holds his sovereignty by virtue of his magic power and as its prize must lay down his life ere that power grow enfeebled with the decay of his body."* The ritual of the identification of the dead king with Osiris, who was himself killed and resurrected, is very impressive. Osiris was held to have weaned the Egyptians who ate human flesh in neolithic times from their earlier cannibalism. From here was only a step to the idea that Osiris was not only killed and torn to pieces, as the traditional tale reports, but also eaten. This idea must have remained unconsciously, but was in its subter-

* W. Gordon Childe, *New Light on the Most Ancient East* (New York, 1953), p. 6.

ranean existence fed by new impressions. There is no doubt
that in prehistoric Egypt, as in North Africa, Europe, and Asia,
cannibalism was general in paleolithic times. This cannibalism
was not due to hunger but was of a magical nature, as it still is
today with some African and Australian tribes. To eat a man has,
in the mind of primitive tribes, the result that one obtains his
strength and magical power, all those qualities one had admired
in him. The corpse-eater acquires in the animistic concept the
soul of the deceased, his "mana," the spiritual essence which is
contained in his body.

The identification of the dead Pharaoh with Osiris who, according to the legend, had made the oldest Egyptian tribes renounce their cannibalism thus formed one of the unconscious
thought-bridges from the area of the dead king to the subject
of cannibalism. The blueprint of another thought-bridge must
have emerged at another point of my study. In the Pyramid
Texts of the Old Kingdom I came across a "cannibal hymn,"
which Breasted quotes*: King Unis is there portrayed as he
eats various gods in order to possess himself of their powers. King
Unis, the text says:

> is one who eats man and lives on gods, . . .
> It is "He= who= is= upon the Willows
> Who lassoes them for him.
> It is "Punisher-of-all-Evil-doers"
> Who stabs them for King Unis.
> He takes out for him their entrails.
> He is the messenger who King Unis sends out to punish.
> Shesmu cuts them up for King Unis
> And cooks for him a portion of them
> In his evening meals.
> King Unis is he who eats their charms
> And devours their souls
>
> . . . .
> Their charms are in his belly
>
> . . . .
> He has swallowed the knowledge of every god
>
> . . . .
> Lo, their soul is in the belly of King Unis.

* Breasted, *Development of Religion and Thought in Ancient Egypt,*

This deceased Pharaoh devours gods and men to incorporate into himself. The Pyramid Texts say in a new translation* of the gods whom King Unis gobbles up:

> The biggest of them are for his breakfast,
> Their middle sized are for his lunch
> And the littlest of them are for his supper.
> Their old males and females
> Are for his kindling.

The Pharaoh himself eats gods and men.

The impressions received during reading such passages and others I have forgotten** must have led to the unconscious idea that the primary and primeval purpose of the Pharaoh's curses was to terrify cannibalistic intruders. At a certain point of my unconscious thought-activity, I must have arrived at the conclusion that the original purpose of the burial customs of the ancient Egyptians was the protection of the body against the cannibalism of the natives. All those germinal thoughts were only potentially present, and remained unconscious. In their place emerged a kind of *idée fixe* to the effect that there was a French sentence containing a key to the mystery. But I had forgotten not only that phrase, but also its meaning! That mysterious idea was in certain directions comparable to the belief in God: it was present without any objective reasons, remained unknown in its nature, and did not tolerate another idea beside it. It could not be defined and was as vague and forceful in its effect as the Deity which conceals itself.

That insight into the prehistoric motivation of the Pharaoh's curse had remained unknown to me, or was known only in the vague form that a forgotten French proverb pointed in this direction. In place of that repressed insight, I formed a thesis to the effect that the artificial preservation of the body, the elaborate care with which it was provided with covering and ornament, was a late reaction to impulses of an aggressive and hostile nature.

---

* John A. Wilson, *The Burden of Egypt* (Chicago, 1951), p. 146.
** In the meantime, I remembered that I must have read somewhere in Flinders Petrie's writings that the disturbed condition of the bones in most of the neolithic graves in Egypt is due to ceremonial cannibalism.

What happened then was described: when I was ready to give up the search for the forgotten sentence and the whole research plan, the repressed idea returned in that dream.

How did that phrase succeed in breaking through the defensive walls just at the moment I was willing to forget my thought-preoccupation with that puzzling subject? It is, of course, undeniable that there was a second of regret when I put my notes away. It amounted to an admission of failure. My thoughts then turned to the other work I had to do: the translation and publication of the Freud letters. Some unknown powers in me had prevented me from penetrating the mystery of the Pharaoh's curse. They were withholding the solution and blocked my way. It seems the same inhibiting forces would not allow me to work on the preparation of the Freud letters. There seems to be not the slightest connection between the two subjects. Yet if there is no visible connecting link (Freud's great interest in ancient Egypt and the excavations in the Nile Valley were later remembered), there is a subterranean thread leading from the second task to the first. There had been that inhibition against beginning the translation of the Freud letters, as if their publication were a sacrilege. Is that the only reason for my procrastination in preparing the letters? I recognized that publication of the great man's letters was unconsciously considered by me as self-aggrandizement. (I thought of those letters, for example, in which Freud in quite a few passages acknowledges my psychoanalytic talent and expresses appreciation of various books or papers.) The dream presents this reflection in the form that I am feeding on Freud, that I am eating a part of him. From here thoughts easily to be guessed led to the comparison with those prehistoric cannibals who ate of the Pharaoh for magical reasons, namely, to acquire the power and the strength of the dead king. Reading the French missionary's book on the cannibalistic Papuans and the description of their meals propelled those thoughts more into the pre-conscious, because those savage Australian tribes were in the dream compared with the prehistoric desecrators of Pharaoh's tomb. They both still live in the Stone Age. The gall-bladder complaint was a significant somatic dream stimulus and lent itself easily to the dream-presentation because the mistake in my diet could well take the place of having eaten human flesh.

In the dream in which I act the part of an archaeologist, I commit the crime of excavating the mummy of an ancient Pharaoh (= publishing the letters of Freud). I am terrified and I expect to be punished. I hear the sentence of death. But this same sentence provides the solution to the problem that had occupied my thoughts. The dream does not compare the publication of the Freud letters with cannibalism, but presents it as such in the characteristic magnifying way of dreams. In it I have done the horrible deed of eating of the Pharaoh (= Freud), but that outrage marks at the same time my triumph: I found the solution of the problem that eluded all my conscious efforts.

In the magical and animistic concept of ancient peoples and of savage tribes of our time, eating parts of a dead person means not only acquiring his qualities, but incorporating him, becoming him. Whoever eats of the Pharaoh becomes himself the King. I have eaten of Freud, I have picked his brain, I have incorporated him. The deepest level of the latent meaning of the dream reveals itself: in publishing those letters, I wish to become Freud. Did not Andreas Moeller, who excavated the mummy of Tabnit, become himself, in his delusion, the King of Sidon, the priest of Astarte? But with such wish-fulfillment the Pharaoh's curse is also realized, because after reaching his aim the researcher has to die.

The discovery I was making in the dream is really a rediscovery, because I must have unconsciously arrived at the insight into the meaning of Pharaoh's curse long before. The emergence of the French sentence whose text had so long remained inaccessible proves that such an unconscious understanding had been reached. The idea percolated, but did not boil over into conscious thinking.

The horror of excavating the mummy of Tutankhamen and of exposing it in the glass case of the Cairo Museum is a sacrilege only in the eyes of the superstitious. Its discovery is one of the proudest achievements of archaeology. The same action that had been condemned was praised as honoring the memory of the dead king.

We are not unmindful that in my dream, too, the analytic interpretation of the Pharaoh's curse is looked upon both as blasphemy and as achievement ("I feel great"), as an insult and as an expression of respect and awe. The same deed from which I am shrinking as sacrilegious, the publication of Freud's letters, immortalizes his memory for "those on earth who love life and hate death," as the ancient Egyptian formula says. The minor discovery in the dream has been made possible by the supreme penetration of the meaningfulness of dreams which we owe to the genius of Freud. When I think of the creation of psychoanalysis, lines of the writer Friedrich Hebbel, mentioned before, occur to me:

> From His unfathomable depths
> The Lord comes to the fore
> To gather the torn threads
> And intertwine them once more.

6

A few minutes before seven o'clock the morning after the dream—no one is yet awake—I am as usual at Horn & Hardart for breakfast. It is cool and there is a strong wind. I am hungry as a wolf. The dream with the leitmotif of cannibalism does not interfere with my appetite. The pressure from the gallstones has disappeared. I am thinking of the diet I have to observe, but I feel like the patient in the cartoon who says to his nurse, "But I don't want nourishment. I want something to eat."

During breakfast I am skimming through the newspaper. Since my sixty-sixth birthday I have acquired the ridiculous habit of looking at the obituaries. It is too silly! When I read that So and So has died at sixty-one or sixty-three, I feel a little contemptuous of the man besides a ludicrous feeling of satisfaction as if I have accomplished something in having passed sixty-six. Before leaving Horn & Hardart, I notice a sign saying "No smoking please!" The writing on the wall! I light a cigarette.

I just read in the New York *Times* that they have placed a bust of Friedrich Schiller somewhere in New York, and two lines of the poet occur to me:

> *Das Leben ist der Güter höchstes nicht,*
> *Der Uebel grösstes aber ist die Schuld.*

> Life is not the highest good,
> But guilt is of the evils the worst.

Hm . . . I am not so sure. . . . The scrambled eggs and the coffee tasted fine. . . . The fresh morning air is delightful. . . . I enjoy the sight of a pretty girl holding her skirts down with both hands against the impudent pass of the wind. . . . Nonsense, my dear Mr. von Schiller! Guilt is by no means the worst of evils, and life is decidedly of all goods the highest. . . . Besides that, is it the only one of which we are sure. . . . I would not want to change places with the Pharaoh Tutankhamen with all the pomp and circumstance of dynastic Egypt. . . . The Viennese used to sing "You live only once. . . ." And a grim counterpoint (with the voice of the Austrian writer Karl Kraus) sounds, "You don't live even once!"

PART SIX

Letters of Freud

Letters of Freud

THE FOLLOWING pages present all Freud letters still in my possession (except, of course, the letters published in other parts of this volume). Many of his letters to me were lost, some on my flight from the Nazis, some on account of other circumstances. Among them, alas, was the longest and perhaps most personal one he wrote me. That letter discussed the study on Goethe and Friederike which I had published in the psychoanalytic magazine *Imago,* edited by Freud, in 1929. Freud called this monograph (later published as a book and now part of my *Fragment of a Great Confession**) very courageous and correct in its analytic penetration and conclusions. He added some critical remarks to the effect that I had neglected the analytic elucidation of Goethe's unconscious motives from the ego-side. There followed a discussion of some still unobserved character traits of Goethe's personality. I only remember that Freud contrasted the unique sincerity and straightforwardness of the great writer with his reserve and discretion in other directions. While Goethe did not hesitate to shape his novels, plays, and poems into "fragments of a great confession," he showed a strange secretiveness about certain domains of his personal life about which he kept all people, even his most intimate friends, in the dark. In the last lines of the letter Freud praised my book and expressed the hope that I would continue with my creative research work. When the Nazis confiscated the files of the Internationaler Psychoanalytischer Verlag in Vienna, they also seized this letter which I had lent to the press for copying. It seems to be irretrievably lost.

In the letters the translations of which follow I have, of course, omitted all remarks about other psychoanalysts and about patients. A few sentences referring to persons still alive are also left out. I considered it inappropriate to omit Freud's critical comments on my own shortcomings and weaknesses. Whenever he

* New York: Farrar, Straus and Co., 1949.

had to make critical remarks, he did it with such obvious benevolence and in such a form that he almost never hurt my feelings. I remember that he sometimes said, "It makes me sad that you did this or wrote that," almost always emphasizing that he had great expectations for me and wished I would show more moderation and self-control. On the few occasions on which it became necessary to censure me, he spoke and wrote plainly and without mincing words.

It is unforgettable that he always expressed his belief that I would do valuable psychoanalytic research work and was convinced (in contrast to the opinion of many members of the New York Psychoanalytic Association) that I had a special talent for psychoanalytic work. In praise and in disapproval, in encouraging as well as in warning me, he was the great educator whose words left indelible traces in my memory. I shall not speak here of the personal character of the style of his letters because every line of them shows the kind of man who wrote them.

The first lines in my possession are written on a piece of paper without date (probably 1911), and refer to an article on psychoanalysis which appeared in the German magazine *März:*

Excellently written and very well organized, like most of your work that I have read. However, they will say that you are a "passionate'" follower, and that will settle it.

With hearty greetings,
Freud

The beginning of the letter of December 13, 1913, is quoted in the introduction to my notes on a lecture of Freud's that remained unpublished. The continuation of that letter refers to a draft of a review I had written about a paper on Hamlet published by the German psychiatrist E. W., in which I had accused the author of plagiarizing articles by Otto Rank and Ernest Jones on the problem of Hamlet. Freud's critical remarks about my review follow:

I cannot, however, praise your essay. It is too rude, biting, and contains a superfluous suspicion. I suggest to you the following disposition: W.'s paper awakened much interest; he is considered as representing psychoanalysis. Some remarks on that. W. reports that he has not read the papers of R. and J. [Full quotation.] Criticism: you can neglect reading the literature before finishing your paper, but not at its publication. After your work is done you have to read and get informed. Otherwise, it would be a too comfortable way of disregarding predecessors. Now the question: Did that precaution help W.? It is very likely that he has read my remarks. [Quotation.] Very likely a case of cryptomnesia. If not, it is in no way permissible to repeat discoveries made thirteen years ago. Humor—as much as you wish like that at the end of your review, but no insults! More cheerful and superior.

Cordial greetings,
Freud

November 1, 1913

Dear Herr Doktor:

May I ask you to do something for me, a little task which I hope will not cost you more than an hour? I have let myself be persuaded to pledge some material for a biography and portrait for a French literary project, *Nos Contemporains*. The article they wrote turned out so stupidly that I objected to it, whereupon the editor urged me to write the text myself. The idea is odious to me. I think, however, that by using the present copy with my criticisms you will easily be able to whip a decent article into shape which will bring out what is essential for the reader without sounding like publicity, and will at the same time be accurate and in good taste.* . . . By the way, I would like to speak with you on the next possible occasion about your difficult position at Heller's.

Cordially,
Freud

The critical remarks and corrections on the French article are of biographical interest:

* A few lines of a personal nature are here omitted.

1) Too subjective, without interest for the public. I did not say anything about sleep.

2) As far as I know, I have done just that, namely, presented a complete theory of the dream. Whether it is "definitive," only the future can decide.

3) However flattering this may be, I have to repeat that I consider discussion of personal relations in such an article inappropriate.

4) Why only *"quelques années"*? It was the regular study of medicine.

5) There is no such examination. It should run: took up his residence as lecturer on *maladies nerveuses*.

6) Incorrect. I became a practicing physician in 1886, and still am today.

7) I got the title of professor in 1902.

8) Entirely misunderstood. After I had given a lecture at the celebration of the foundation of Clark University at Worcester, Massachusetts, I received the honorary title of LL.D.

9) Please will you put the German names beside the French ones:

    a) *Zur Auffassung der Aphasieen*
    b) *Die zerebralen Kinderlähmungen*

10) To parenthesize as addendum to the previous:

11) *Studien über Hysterie mit J. Breuer:*

    c) *Die Traumdeutung—L'analyse des rêves*
    d) *Zur Psychopathologie des Alltagslebens*

12) e) *Der Witz und seine Beziehung zum Unbewussten (l'inconscient)*

13) *Drei Abhandlungen zur Sexualtheorie:*

14) g) *Kleine Schriften zur Neurosenlehre* (3 Volumes, 1906-1913)

    h) *Der Wahn und die Träume . . .* etc.

15) *Totem und Tabu. Uebereinstummungen im Seelenleben der Wilden und der Neurotiker (Le Totem et le Tabou. Quelques concordances entre la vie psychique des peuples savages et les neuroses).*

16) *Le* "Intern. Zeitschrift für ärztliche Psychoanalyse" *et le*

journal Imago *destiné à l'application de la psychoanalyse aux sciences non-medicales et la collection des* Schriften zur angewandten Seelenkunde.

17) The special science of psychoanalysis created by me is cultivated by numerous societies in Germany, England, and America and stands in the center of discussion in the medical world. The method of treatment of nervous patients founded on that science is already practiced by many physicians. The application of psychoanalysis to mythology, pedagogics, science of religion and history of civilization makes rapid progress.

Obviously not satisfied with the translation of misunderstood titles of his books, Freud himself suggested some changes. I wrote the article and gave it to Freud.

September 17, 1913

Dear Herr Doctor:

I am sending you the pages for correction and delivery to Mr. Clement Deltour, Wien I, Hotel Bristol.

Cordially,
Freud

Should you not mention the *Jahrbuch* which I have taken over entirely myself so that Breuer and Young need not be named?

I do not know whether the work *Nos contemporains* was published.

January 1, 1914

Dear Herr Doctor:

All my work of the last weeks and my departure immediately afterward have made me put off answering your letter and expressing my thanks for the dedication of your fine book.

Let me now tell you the following: don't believe that I told Heller anything negative about you. He has communicated his objections to you from his own experience, and I had to confirm them after I had defended you for a long time. I would have liked to contradict him if I could have. Heller is a violent man, and has obviously acted according to the principle: "Throw him out, he breaks my heart!" He is certainly not a mean person.

I would be pleased if you would learn from these experiences, instead of suffering and being grieved by them. Your talent which is manifest will survive these years. If I can do anything to speed you on your way, it will be out of inner necessity that I do it.

Perhaps you have to conquer in yourself a streak of masochistic guilt feeling which sometimes compels you to spoil favorable opportunities.

Courage and good luck in 1914!

Cordially yours,
Freud

The book dedicated to Freud was *Arthur Schnitzler als Psychologe* which was published in 1913. To explain certain paragraphs in the preceding letter: I had been very poor and Freud had secured a job for me with the Viennese bookseller and publisher, Wilhelm Heller, who had just published *Totem und Tabu*. At this time Freud visited Heller's bookstore almost daily. At Heller's office I read and reviewed the new books, edited monthly brochures, and so on. I must have made myself quite objectionable to my boss, who was a quick-tempered man of whose explosions of anger I was afraid. During the conflict Freud had taken my side. He defended Heller here against accusations I had expressed and explained the man's behavior by alluding to a well-known Jewish anecdote: A *schnorrer* (beggar) most vividly describes his poverty and the misery in which he and his family live to Rothschild. The millionaire is deeply touched and, crying from pity, he calls his butler and pointing to the *schnorrer* shouts, "Throw him out, he breaks my heart!" A short time after that I left Vienna and moved to Berlin where I finished my analytic training.

April 20, 1914

Dear Herr Doctor:

I heartily approve your writing the report on the congress on sexuality for us, and I also would like the idea of your taking over the reviews on psychoanalysis for the new magazine on sexual research. You have, however, to restrain yourself in writing them.

With cordial wishes for your success in Berlin,

Yours,
Freud

The magazine here mentioned is the *Zeitschrift für Sexualforschung,* which was published in Berlin.

June 14, 1914

Dear Herr Doctor:

I acknowledge with great pleasure that you are now our most industrious contributor. I don't like to learn that otherwise you have no cause for satisfaction. I know that you are again successfully engaged in spoiling for yourself as many opportunities as possible. All this because of a few people whom you would like to kill! Too much repentance!

Your couvade paper seems to me really a hit. For practical reasons, I restrict myself to a few adverse criticisms. You must take the praise for granted. a) The psychoanalytic explanations, which can be easily altered, are in my opinion not formulated clearly enough for lay readers. b) I would not in your place easily renounce the main argument for your thesis. Women themselves lay the blame on the father when a child dies. That speaks a clear language. c) With the Busch quotation you've dug one layer too deep. You might rather have said: With primitive man it is just the contrary of what is described in this passage from Busch. Becoming a father is often difficult; being a father, however, is mostly easy.

Which of the two papers you should favor? Hard to advise. I should say: both. But do not produce too fast. As for the Heine project, you should probably wait for the other volumes of the letters. It is an utterly attractive subject.

You know that I have made arrangements with Abraham so that you may turn directly to him in situations of emergency.

I wish you a sclerotic conscience and swift success for your immediate plans.

Cordially yours,
Freud

I had sent drafts of two papers, one of which was on couvade, to Freud. His criticisms were, of course, highly appreciated by me and carefully considered in the final presentation. The paper was read before the Berlin Psychoanalytic Society in April, 1914, and published in *Imago* of the same year.*

The emergencies of which Freud speaks are such as originated from my precarious financial situation. For many months Freud generously furnished me with a certain amount of money. The last sentence refers to my moral scruples of that period, particularly to guilt feelings because of thought-crimes.

Karlsbad, July 15, 1914

Dear Herr Doctor:

I have just received news about your interesting person from Abraham and from you at the same time, and I am, of course, annoyed that you have wasted your time recently with so much neurotic nonsense. First of all, therefore, I have had the Wiener Bank send you 200 marks for the last four months. I had no intention of stopping the promised subsidy, but I assumed that you had fled to Berlin to avoid such pensioning, and I hoped by the arrangement with Abraham to put an end to your jokes of starvation.

Thus everything remains as it was, and nothing must interfere with your taking all other steps to provide promptly a decent measure of comfort for yourself and your wife. We really liked your essay on couvade very much. I have great hopes for you and I am glad to criticize you mercilessly, although I consider it inadvisable to exercise a similar control in our magazine over authors who do not demand such criticism with as much urgency, for that would end in intolerable monotony and in the flight of many contributors to rival publications, at a time when our magazine is hardly on its feet.

Your remarks on the attitude of different neurotic types to psychoanalysis are interesting, and we must give the idea more discussion.

* For English translation, see my book *Ritual* (New York: Farrar, Straus & Co., 1946).

We shall never forget that Abraham took you under analysis. He is really a wonderful person. Stick to him if you must stay in Berlin, which might not be unfortunate for your future. Those who belong together need not always be thick as thieves.

With cordial wishes for you and your fiancée—or wife?

Yours sincerely,
Freud

Dr. Karl Abraham had suggested that he would take me under analysis, of course, without payment. Freud had without my knowledge arranged with Abraham that he should give me money whenever I needed it. I had tried to save money by cutting down on meals, and often felt hungry. The other allusion in Freud's letter refers to my request that he should criticize my papers mercilessly because I wished to accomplish the best I was capable of—an expression of my perfectionism at that time. I married in August, 1914.

July 17, 1914

Dear Herr Doctor:

You know I would never have written the article, but I do not feel justified in changing anything in it. Your planned contributions will be very welcome. Please send all to Rank who will give them to me to read. With urgent wishes for your welfare in Berlin (where you do not seem to be lonely).

Yours very cordially,
Freud

Otto Rank was editor of *Imago*. The teasing allusion in parenthesis refers to the presence of my bride in Berlin.

Karlsbad, July 24, 1914

Dear Herr Doctor:

I have satisfied your need for merciless criticism in speaking with Ferenczi and accusing you of various naughtinesses in your reviews. The "*à qui le dites-vous*" is a Jewish joke, too good for those goyim, and makes a bad impression. I am, of course, in agreement with the content of your criticism.

I asked L. about his article in the *Theologische Literatur-zeitung* and I then got the article and the enclosed letter. Please return it. You will perhaps be persuaded by it to show more understanding in your criticism of the poor pastor's soul vacillating between the upperworld and the netherworld.

Cordial regards,
Yours,
Freud

Freud's critical remark concerns a review I wrote on an article by one of our Swiss contributors who was a pastor for the *Zentralblatt für Psychoanalyse*. I had made fun of the author who endeavored to explain to his readers that psychoanalysis not only deals with repressed sexual and aggressive tendencies, but also with unconscious moral trends. The French phrase *"à qui le dites-vous"* ("you are telling me?") is here, of course, sarcastic. Dr. S. Ferenczi was editor of the *Zeitschrift für Psychoanalyse*.

September 27, 1914

Dear Herr Doctor:

a) p. 9 Kleinpaul, *Das Fremdwort im Deutschen* (Göschen, 1905): Heiopopeia is an old Greek lullaby which a princess from the Greek court in Constantinople brought to South Germany, namely, the refrain *Haide, mo paide,* thus: Sleep, my child, sleep.

b) *Mit Rosen bedacht*
   Mit Näglein bedeckt
Are *Näglein* not, rather, carnations?

I want to put these two remarks at your disposal for your essay on lullabies.

Cordial regards,
Yours,
Freud

Freud's remarks refer to an essay on lullabies which I did not publish. Heiapopeia is an expression Viennese mothers often use rocking their babies to sleep. In the Brahms lullaby I had mistaken *Näglein* for little nails.

November 15, 1916

Dear Herr Doctor:

I congratulate you on your promotion and gratefully acknowledge the receipt of the manuscript, which has already found
its way into our staff file. From there it will be sent to the printing
press as soon as our snail's pace permits.

The contribution is original, contains much worth reading,
and pleased me very much. I am glad to see that your writing
is developing well in spite of the war.

With hearty greetings,
Freud

I was serving at the front of the Austrian army and was pro-
moted to lieutenant.

November 7, 1918

Dear Herr Doctor:

Once more your work seems to me penetrating and thoroughly
correct in interpretation. I am happy that you are treading such
rewarding paths. But the article is poorly organized, in a way
making for obscurity, and you have given insufficient consideration to the fact that the essay is written for nonanalysts.

Please telephone me as soon as you receive this so that we can
arrange a meeting.

Cordially yours,
Freud

I cannot remember to which paper Freud refers here.

July 11, 1919

Dear Herr Doctor:

The Moses paper which I have now read is very ingenious and
convincing. It can, however, lead to one misunderstanding. One
could be led to believe that there was once a revolution of the
son in which the father-god was replaced by the son-god. This
seems to be impossible because totemism is entirely a father-
religion, and the son-religions only begin later after the anthropomorphic deity had long been established and only traces of

totemism remained. Therefore, it follows that a much later revolt of the son was, so to speak, regressively displaced forward and told in totemistic language. All other things are valid.

I would also not conclude that the change from bull to ram represented a change of totems. Such things are quite unwarranted. It is probable that there was a condensation of the myths of two tribes with different totems. Hoping that you will have a good summer,

Cordially yours,
Freud

The essay on Moses is contained in my book *Das Ritual* which was published with a preface by Freud in 1919.

Seefeld, August 26, 1921

Dear Herr Doctor:

I am acknowledging that your demands are justified. The first one for an appropriate chest of drawers is the easiest to fulfill. Please secure one and I shall give you the amount after my return. The typewriter is also only a question of money. If you find one which is not too expensive, there is no reason why you should not buy it. I expect your suggestions about both expenses.

It is more difficult to deal with the third point. I believe that the magazines can best be edited in Berlin. There will be a meeting in which our moneygiver Dr. Eitingon, Abraham, and Jones will take part. At that time I will present your complaints and we will discuss what can be done.

With cordial regards to you and
your family,
Yours,
Freud

At this time I was busy introducing a Zentralstelle für psychoanalytische Literatur, a scientific center of information on analytic literature which would help young analysts in their research work, provide scholars with psychoanalytic bibliographies, and so on. The requests mentioned here concern office material.

March 10, 1921

Dear Herr Doctor:

I send you the enclosed for authoritative answer. By the way, can you tell me where the following lines (which I need for the book on psychology of the masses) are to be found?

Christophorus trug den Christus
Christus trug die ganze Welt.
Sagt, wohin hat Christophorus
Eigentlich den Fuss gestellt?

I have searched in vain in Goethe's works.

Cordially,
Freud

Freud who overestimated the scope of my reading often asked me for the source of a passage from literature. In this case I could find it.

The following two communications were written on visiting cards and were brought to me by patients whom Freud referred to me.

August 20, 1922

Lady from Australia, 26 years old, suspicious of psychosomatic attacks. Psychoanalytic examination of 2 to 3 weeks to decide. Eventually full treatment. Patient speaks a little German. Don't neglect to get lungs examined.

Freud

June 9, 1922

British, special circumstances, please occasional analytic sessions on his visits to Vienna.

The trial analysis (in Vienna analytic sessions were daily) of the first case confirmed Freud's diagnosis. The second patient who was in diplomatic service could only come to Vienna occasionally.

Badgastein, July 8, 1922

Dear Herr Doctor:

Thanks for your prompt settlement. My expectation of getting rid of some members has not been realized. Not paying the contribution has, of course, no consequence for those members.

Cordially,
Freud

Refers to some function I had to fulfill as secretary of the Vienna Psychoanalytic Society.

Lavarone, August 17, 1922

Dear Herr Doctor:

When the countess writes to me, I shall support you very energetically. But you have to be prepared for the fact that the rupture will then take place. Has the father no influence whatsoever? The contribution of your little son is very beautiful, deserves a commentary. I am preserving it.

With cordial regards to you and your wife,

Yours,
Freud

The countess was the mother of a young man whom Freud had referred to me for psychoanalytic treatment. By her interference, she made continuation of analysis impossible. The contribution of my son Arthur is contained in my book *Geständniszwang und Strafbedürfnis* ("Compulsion of Confession and Need for Punishment") which was published in 1925 and is not yet translated into English.

Salzburg, August 10, 1922

Dear Herr Doctor:

"By general request," which is to say with great reluctance on my part, I have consented to give an address at the Congress. May I be granted the privilege of not revealing the subject until I make the address?

I have read with disappointment your private memorandum on the state of the reviews. It shows how the analysts themselves are still slaves to the pleasure principle. I know no remedy, but your proposals will be awarded the most serious consideration at or by the Congress.

> Cordially yours,
> Freud

The memorandum I gave Freud concerns the reviews for the analytic magazines. I had been dissatisfied because many contributors did not keep their promise to deliver reviews on time. The next letter refers to the book *Geständniszwang und Strafbedürfnis,* mentioned before.

> January 13, 1925

Dear Herr Doctor:

I have read your thoughtful and extremely important book with great interest. At first it seemed to me that you come all too easily to the conclusion that the examples of self-betrayal through slips of the tongue are really meant for the confessions that they are in effect, and you could have emphasized that initial ambiguity. But the following presentation makes your thesis increasingly plausible as you expand upon it. Your attempt to demonstrate the role of the superego in all neuroses seems as legitimate as it is fruitful. The whole is on rather broad scale, but is clear and demands attention. There are many ingenious thoughts strewn throughout. On reading a few passages I have felt inclined to remind you with red pencil to look over a sentence again. Although, true to my custom, I am avoiding pronouncing final judgment on a work I have just read, still I hazard the impression that here you have produced something especially valuable. Now dispose of the manuscript.

> Cordially yours,
> Freud

> February 28, 1926

Dear Herr Doctor:

I really should react to your "Pro Memoria" of February 2 with an invitation to take a beautiful walk with you. I should like to do that if I, as you know, were not inhibited by all my minor and major complaints and symptoms. At all events, I was very amused in reading it even where I was not entirely in agreement with you. And, of course, you will not have expected complete agreement in matters so personal. A single correction of your presentation you will have to accept without contradicting. It is the following: you accuse me of having addressed Romain Rolland as "incomparable," which appears inappropriate to you. But when you read the *Liber Amicorum* or the excerpts in the *Neue Freie Presse,* you will find that my word was "unforgettable" which adjective you will certainly not censure. This is not important, but is perhaps interesting.

In spite of your own confession that you are vindictive, I consider you a rather kind and benevolent man and can thus trust that you will treat my shortcomings and weaknesses with leniency.

Cordial regards,
Yours, Freud

I had written Freud that he overappreciated Romain Rolland whom I did not like very much. Freud had contributed a salutation to the *Liber Amicorum* published on the occasion of the writer's birthday.

January 23, 1928

Dear Herr Doctor:

If I failed to answer your letter, it was certainly not with the purpose of keeping you away. Rather because I in my laziness thought you would at the meeting of the society have occasion to make an appointment with me. We had such informal social intercourse during the summer that you need not ask for an appointment like a strange interviewer.

Eitingon will be here by Friday; thus a conversation among the three of us would be most appropriate. But if you will be in Paris by the 27th of the month, please phone me before about the time of your visit and I shall plead your part with Eitingon.

I know that you are not satisfied here. I regret very much that your mood and your attitude to life have become so dissatisfied just when your intellectual achievement is developing so splendidly, and I admit that I cannot contribute much to the solution of your problem on account of my isolated position due to my illness.

Cordially yours,
Freud

During the previous summer Freud and his family lived at the Semmering, a resort near Vienna, and I and my family spent the summer months in the Südbahnhotel nearby. I then saw Freud almost every day. The remarks on my situation again concern my financial worries.

February 26, 1928

Dear Herr Doctor:

Of your three contributions I appreciate the first as a well-justified, ingenious continuation of an analytic theory and the third one as a beautiful contribution to the interpretation of dreams and to self-analysis. It is difficult for me to relate to the third one. The darkness which still covers the unconscious guilt feeling does not seem to be lightened by one of the discussions about it. The complication only increases. This contribution will, of course, also be published, if you wish it.

Cordially yours,
Freud

The three papers together with others are contained in a book *Der Schrecken* ("Fright") which was published in 1929, and has been translated into English. The following letter also refers to this book.

Tegel, October 23, 1928

Dear Herr Doctor:

I have read all the essays. They are all significant and finely written. Their merits in respect to psychological depth are, of course, uneven. I am most impressed by the first on traumatic neuroses. I cared least for the one which presented the idea of masochism turned outward.

The dedication and the introduction are, of course, impossible.

Also the scattered remarks on colleagues, some witty and some merely spiteful, should be expurgated. They betray that the writer is still too close to the subjective material of his investigation, and in this way puts convenient weapons right into the critics' hands.

Cordially yours,
Freud

Berlin Tegel [without date]

Dear Herr Doctor:

I have by no means forgotten about inviting you to visit me, but I am merely waiting for a favorable stage in the course of my treatment. Today I write simply to ask you for a bit of information out of your superior literary knowledge. The question: Where in Schiller or Goethe is the well-known maxim: "He who has art and science has also religion," etc.? My notion that it was in the *Xenien* has not proved correct. Goethe's maxims in verse perhaps?

With cordial greetings,
Yours,
Freud

P.S. Of course, also the full text.

April 10, 1928

Dear Herr Doctor:

I cordially congratulate you on the second edition of your *Ritual.* A beautiful success in the midst of a hostile environment! Your later contributions have kept the promise that was given in those first ones, and one may expect even more from your future work.

With many others I only regret that you give so much expression to your personal moods in your objective studies. I regret still more that my circumstances have made it impossible to change something in the factors that awaken those moods, excuse them, but do not justify them in a higher sense.

Cordial greetings,
Yours,
Freud

October 28, 1928

Dear Herr Doctor:

In memory of one of your former duties, may I ask you to look after the enclosed manuscript? Heard with pleasure that your brilliant lecture was a success.

Cordially yours,
Freud

Tegel, September 13, 1928

Dear Herr Doctor:

I cannot explain your attitude except in the following way. You send me those remarks, submit yourself to my decision as to whether they should be printed, and anticipate that I shall condemn them as unworthy of you in form and content. In doing that you give expression to your feelings and discharge them without any risk.

The calculation is correct, but it grieves me much that you even need such therapy. Your hostility transgresses all justified measure, blasts the frontiers of what is permissible, spoils your presentation, and must sadden anyone who, as I, has the interest of a friend in you and highly appreciates your achievements. It cannot possibly go on like that.

I would have asked you long ago to see me, but I am at present in a bad state of transition, still unable to do anything and compelled to hide like a crab that changes its shell.

Cordially yours,
Freud

I had written a letter full of bitterness against some colleagues who had hurt my pride, and I had given uninhibited expression to my indignation. Freud's letter was, of course, well justified in its criticism of my attitude.

Tegel, October 20, 1929

Dear Herr Doctor:

The famous story of the mandarin (*tuer son mandarin*) comes from Rousseau, after all. Could you tell me without going to too much trouble where it is to be found?

Cordially yours,
Freud

November 18, 1929

Dear Herr Doctor:

Please don't bother yourself any longer about the "inch of nature" and forgive me for having bothered you with it. I've done without the quotation. No one was able to locate it. Where I could have picked it up remains a mystery, for it is hardly likely to be of my own coining. Since, besides Shakespeare, I used to read only Milton and Byron, there is still the possibility that it might be found in Byron. But please do not look for it, and accept my best thanks for your trouble.

With cordial greetings,
Freud

Berchtesgaden, August 21, 1929

Dear Herr Doctor:

In my judgment, you do my little essay too much honor by commenting and elucidating upon it, but I do not wish to quarrel with your intentions. Certainly you have added those very things which the analyst must add to supplement the presentation. But the psychologists of religion have got along without it, and after your elucidation they will not understand it any better nor accept it less grudgingly. Naturally, I was not writing for those readers.

You have my permission to publish whatever appears appropriate to you from my letter. I am sure that you, too, wanted to exclude the passages I marked with red pencil, alluding to our personal relationships.

My prothesis compels me to consult Professor Schröder again. I am planning to arrive at Berlin on September 15. And this time you have to come to dinner with us.

Cordially yours,
Freud

The letter refers to my note on Freud's paper on a "religious experience," contained in this book. The other passage concerns Freud's letter on Dostoyevsky, published in this volume. Freud periodically came to Berlin for readjustment of his mouth prothesis. He lived on these occasions at Tegel near Berlin, where I visited him. I had moved from Vienna to Berlin.

Berlin Tegel [no date]

Dear Herr Doctor:

I certainly want to see you and talk to you. My stay here will still take some weeks. At present I am in my most helpless state, comparable to a change of shell, and have to hide.

Cordially yours,
Freud

March 23, 1930

Dear Herr Doctor:

You know that I try to forbear from criticisms of recent works of our school. When I make an exception in your case, you must take that as proof of my special appreciation of your work.

I read your last contribution to the *Psychoanalytische Bewegung* with some uneasiness. I have been troubled by a change in me which was brought about under the influence of Looney's book, *Shakespeare Identified.* I no longer believe in the man from Stratford.

Cordially yours,
Freud

Freud's remarks refer to an article *The Way of All Flesh* I had published. The paper deals mostly with the problem of death in Shakespeare's *Hamlet.**

April 6, 1930

Dear Herr Doctor:

Thanks for sending your article on my "Civilization and Its Discontents." It is the best and most dignified of all I have read

* Translated in my book, *From Thirty Years with Freud* (New York, 1940), p. 197.

about it until now. I hope to be in Tegel at the beginning of May.

Cordially yours,
Freud

My paper had been published in *Imago*. It is contained in this volume.

Tegel, July 10, 1930

Dear Herr Doctor:

Just received your book and letter. Cordial thanks. I am wishing a beautiful time to you and your wife.

Freud

May 30, 1931

Dear Herr Doctor:

Thanks for your birthday salutation which gives me special pleasure. I considered the doubt of your little son if one is justified in congratulating someone very reasonable.

Cordially,
Freud

I had published an article on Freud's birthday in the magazine of the Jewish organization B'nai B'rith. My son Arthur, then six years old, was quoted in it: the boy could not understand why you congratulate a person on his birthday rather than his parents. My article, beginning with a discussion on the fact that we all still believe in the omnipotence of thoughts when we convey our good wishes to someone, ended with the sentence: "We congratulate ourselves on Freud's birthday."

May 8, 1932

Dear Herr Doctor:

To the enjoyable thoughts on your literary gift the satisfaction was added of getting some information about you, for instance that you now live in Berlin. People said that you had moved and had accepted a commercial job in Czechoslovakia.

One feels even more helpless in these miserable times, but one does not renounce one's interest.

Cordially yours,
Freud

I had sent Freud my newly published book, *Nachdenkliche Heiterkeit* (not translated into English) on his birthday. The depression in Austria made me decide to move once more to Berlin.

September 9, 1932

Dear Herr Doctor:

I was very happy to see that, after emerging from your retirement, you have lost nothing of your critical or literary abilities. Your book is very interesting. I share your doubts concerning certain planned applications of psychoanalysis, and I appreciate the skill with which you discover the decisive ancient and primal behind the modern. The objection to the book will, of course, be that it is essentially negative—which does it no harm.

My daughter whom I expect this evening will certainly bring me some latest dispatches about your personal life.

I do not indulge in any complaints about failing bodily functions, since at my age I obviously have no right to expect much. Still I was able to complete seven new lectures to supplement those that were published in 1917. And a few other bagatelles.

With cordial wishes for you and yours,

Your Freud

The book is *Der unbekannte Mörder* ("The Unknown Murderer"), 1932 (English translation by the Hogarth Press, 1936).

[without date]

Dear Herr Doctor:

I would be very glad if I knew that you had found a permanent home in the charming Hague. You must again strike root somewhere. I have decided not to leave Vienna, no matter what happens here.

Fine that you are working, which means creating. I can do so no longer, which clears me of much responsibility, but also leaves me so impoverished.

With cordial wishes,
Yours,
Freud

I had moved to the Hague where I lived until 1938 when I came to the United States. Austria was already endangered by the Nazis.

January 4, 1935

Dear Herr Doctor:

Thanks for your New Year's letter which at last brought the news so long expected by me that you have settled down in a foreign country, are entering into good social connections, and earning what you need. Some stability and security seem to be a requirement for our difficult work. I count upon it that you will still present us with valuable achievements of the same caliber as your first studies.

I analyzed Mahler for an afternoon in the year 1912 (or 1913?) in Leiden. If I may believe reports, I achieved much with him at that time. His consultation appeared necessary to him, because his wife at the time rebelled against the fact that he withdrew his libido from her. In highly interesting expeditions through his life history, we discovered his personal conditions for love, especially his Holy Mary complex (mother fixation). I had plenty of opportunity to admire the capability for pschological understanding of this man of genius. No light fell at the time on the symptomatic façade of his obsessional neurosis. It was as if you would dig a single shaft through a mysterious building.

Hoping to hear good news from you, with cordial wishes for 1935,

Yours,
Freud

This letter is the answer to one of mine in which I asked Freud for information about his meeting with Gustav Mahler (in 1910). A discussion of the significance of this letter is to be found in my book *The Haunting Melody.*

January 9, 1936

Dear Herr Doctor:

You did not predict correctly that I will not read your new book. I consider it clever and stimulating as everything you write, but I would have preferred your concentration on a single problem. The danger threatening you is to get scattered.

Hoping that you will be victorious in the fight with your difficulties,

Cordially yours,
Freud

The book here referred to is *Der überraschte Psychologe,* published at Leiden in 1936.

April 29, 1936

Dear Herr Doctor:

Thanks for your thoughtful gratulation. Au revoir in August.

Cordially yours,
Freud

Before moving to Holland, where I had a psychoanalytic practice and worked as training psychoanalyst in the Hague, I asked Freud for a letter of recommendation:

Certificate

No one who knows psychoanalytic literature can be ignorant of the fact that the numerous contributions on applied psychoanalysis by Dr. Theodor Reik, especially those concerning religion and ritual, belong to the best and most successful in this field. They are unique of their kind. Whoever has the opportunity should feel obliged to support Dr. Reik in his career and to promote him so as to make the continuation of his work possible.

Prof. Dr. Sigm. Freud

The following letter is Freud's answer to two questions I had asked him. A few remarks about the occasions on which the two questions emerged will be necessary for the understanding of Freud's opinions. The situation to which the first part of Freud's letter refers was the following: Toward the end of her analytic treatment, which had been successful, a wealthy patient of mine, Miss S. in The Hague, wanted to express her gratitude to psychoanalysis by establishing a foundation. She discussed with me her plans which were greatly influenced by her interest in child psychology and education. At the time there were no competent child psychoanalysts in Holland, and Miss S. wished her foundation to give grants to gifted Dutch psychiatrists and psychologists who would study and be trained in child psychology and psychoanalysis in Vienna. The foundation would support those students during their years of study and training and help them to establish themselves after their return to Holland. The patient, who had undergone analytic therapy, had no theoretical knowledge of psychoanalysis and wished, in mistaken tolerance, that the students be trained in psychoanalysis as well as in Jung's therapeutic methods. The Dutch psychiatrist Dr. K., whom she knew and who had just returned from a long psychoanalytic training in Vienna, and I tried to convince her that such a combination was inappropriate and was not available at the Vienna Psychoanalytic Institute.

The second question concerns the case of a psychiatrist who had applied for membership in the Amsterdam Psychoanalytic Association, of which I was a member and in which I took an active interest. The candidate was a practicing Catholic, and some officials of our association expressed their doubts as to whether such an attitude could be reconciled with the therapeutic tasks of psychoanalysis. I was asked to find out what Freud thought about this problem. His answers to the two questions, which are still applicable in the area of psychoanalysis, are of considerable historical and theoretical interest.

November 21, 1937

Dear Herr Doctor:

I entirely agree with your and K's opinion that a practical co-operation of psychoanalysis with other psychotherapeutic directions in pedagogics and mental hygiene is hopeless at this time and that such an attempt is not desirable. Psychoanalysis would come off badly in the venture. It is permitted to assume that the analysts would consider valuable suggestions from the other methods, but it is certain that the others would not appreciate analytic points of view. They understand too little of them. Perhaps it will be different later. Today I would have to advise you to refuse participation in the work of such a foundation. It is easier for me to advise you than the noble-minded donor. I would like to see the lady, but only *after* she has made her decision. If her inclinations and her opinion vacillate between both schools of thought, the best way out would be for her to create not one, but two foundations remaining independent from each other. I cannot be put in authority and bring about a decision where I am undoubtedly partial.

In the case of Dr. St., on the other hand, the decision seems to be easy. Psychoanalysis is not much more contradictory to the Catholic faith than to any other religion, and not more decidedly than any other science. To act consistently, one would have to exclude all other believers from visiting a university when they do not want to study theology. It is certainly more justified not to be concerned about the faith of a candidate and to leave it to him which attitude he can take in the undeniable conflict between religion and science.

Cordially yours,
Freud

January 21, 1938

Dear Herr Doctor:

I have no objection to your remark on the influence of analysis on S's perversion. I did not remember that the passage V 356 you refer to concerned S.

Cordially yours,
Freud

I asked Freud for permission to quote certain passages from his paper on masochism contained in Vol. V of his *Gesammelte Schriften*. The passage concerns the case of a masochist who had been under Freud's psychoanalysis for a long time, and whom Freud had referred to me for continuation of the treatment.

The last three letters I received from Freud, who was in London, are from the year 1938 and addressed to New York.

After I realized that I could no longer stay in Holland without the risk of becoming a prisoner of the Nazis who were threatening to invade that country, I immigrated to the United States in June, 1938. Most members of the New York Psychoanalytic Society treated me condescendingly, and I was strongly admonished against practicing, or rather forbidden to practice, psychoanalysis. I complained about this when I wrote to Freud. I asked him if he could suggest some way in which I might continue my work. The first letter, dated July 3, 1938, was his answer to this request. It was accompanied by the second letter which was a recommendation written in English. The last letter is clearly a reaction to another letter of mine in which I again complained about the hostility and indifference of my New York colleagues.

> 39 Elsworthy Road
> London, N.W. 3
> July 3, 1938

Dear Herr Doctor:

What ill wind has blown you, just you, to America? You must have known how amiably lay analysts would be received there by our colleagues for whom psychoanalysis is nothing more than one of the handmaidens of psychiatry. Could you not have stayed in Holland longer?

I am, of course, glad to write any certificate that would be useful to you, but I doubt that it will help you. Where over there is an institution which would be interested in supporting the continuation of your research? Have you attempted to get in touch with the German Academy in America [Thomas Mann, Prince Lowenstein, and others]?

When I think of you, sympathy and annoyance fight within me.

I could feel well in England if I were not incessantly subjected to all possible demands, and if I were not reminded of my powerlessness to help others.

With my best wishes, which you will well need at this time.

Yours,
Freud

I am surprised to learn that Dr. Th. Reik has gone to America where the fact that he is not a medical man is likely to interfere with his activity as an analyst. He is one of the few masters of applied analysis, as is shown especially in his earlier contributions, while his later work is more concerned with matters of general psychological interest. In both ways he has given proof of a high amount of intelligence, criticism and independent thought. Any man who is interested in the progress of the Science of Psychoanalysis should try to lend his assistance in the continuation of his work.

Prof. Sigm. Freud

I am ready to help you as soon as I get the news that I am equipped with the omnipotence of God, if only for a short time. Until then, you must continue to toil alone.

Most cordially yours,
Freud

I did.

July 3d 1938

39 ELSWORTHY ROAD
LONDON, N.W. 3

I am surprised to learn, that dr Th. Reik has gone to America where the fact that he is not a medical man is not likely to interfere with his activity as an analyst. He is one of the few masters of applied ana-lyses as is shown especially in his earlier contributions while his later work is more concerned with matters of general psychological interest In both ways he has given proof of a high amount of intelligence, criticism and independent thought. Any man who is interested in the progress of the science of Psychoanalysis should try to lend him assistance in the continua-tion of his work.

Prof. Sigm. Freud